Diagnostic Methods in the Cardiac Catheterization Laboratory

Diagnostic Methods in the Cardiac Catheterization Laboratory

Edited by

Pedro A. Lemos
Heart Institute (InCor)
University of São Paulo Medical School
and
Sirio-Libanes Hospital
São Paulo, Brazil

Paul Schoenhagen
Cleveland Clinic Foundation
Cleveland, Ohio, USA

Alexandra J. Lansky
Cardiovascular Research Foundation
New York, New York, USA

CRC Press
Taylor & Francis Group
Boca Raton London New York

CRC Press is an imprint of the
Taylor & Francis Group, an **informa** business

CRC Press
Taylor & Francis Group
6000 Broken Sound Parkway NW, Suite 300
Boca Raton, FL 33487-2742

First issued in paperback 2017

ISBN-13: 978-1-84184-658-3 (hbk)
ISBN-13: 978-1-138-11411-1 (pbk)

Library of Congress Cataloging-in-Publication Data

Diagnostic methods in the cardiac catheterization laboratory / edited by Pedro A. Lemos,
Paul Schoenhagen, Alexandra J. Lansky.
p. ; cm.
Includes bibliographical references and index.
ISBN-13: 978-1-84184-658-3 (hardcover : alk. paper)
ISBN-10: 1-84184-658-9 (hardcover : alk. paper) 1. Cardiac catheterization. I. Lemos,
Pedro A. II. Schoenhagen, Paul. III. Lansky, Alexandra.
[DNLM: 1. Coronary Angiography–methods. 2. Heart Catheterization–methods.
3. Coronary Artery Disease–diagnosis. 4. Diagnostic Imaging–methods.
5. Radiography, Interventional–methods. WG 141.5.C2 D5365 2009]
RC683.5.C25D535 2009
616.1′20754–dc22

2009035198

Visit the Taylor & Francis Web site at
http://www.taylorandfrancis.com

and the CRC Press Web site at
http://www.crcpress.com

Foreword

It is remarkable that it has now been 80 years since the German surgical resident Werner Forssmann inserted a small catheter into his antecubital vein, walked to the radiology suite, and took an X-ray of the catheter's position in his right atrium (1). Now a designated landmark in medical history, this revolutionary event demonstrated that the heart could be safely accessed from the forearm, but resulted in the immediate termination of Dr. Forssman from his training program. Unfortunately for Dr. Forssman, who ended his career as a rural practitioner, it was not until 25 years later in 1956 that Forssman's discovery was appropriately recognized when he shared the Nobel Prize with pioneers Andre Cournand, MD, and Dickinson Richards, MD, for their combined work in developing cardiac catheterization (2,3).

Over the next 30 years, the methodology for diagnostic cardiac catheterization advanced markedly, but was primary focused on ventricular hemodynamics, shunts, and cardiac physiology. I recently pulled out the dusty hemodynamic textbooks that I used during my Cardiology Fellowship Training program at the University of Texas Southwestern Medical Center in Dallas under the mentorship of Dr. L. David Hillis (4,5). Paging through them now, these textbooks were quiet dense, even for an energetic cardiology fellow, with plenty of mathematic derivations for cardiac output, intracardiac shunts, and indices of ventricular performance and coronary physiology. In the clinical laboratory during my fellowship training, we used oximetry, thermodilution and green dye curves to detect cardiac output and shunts, Douglas bags to determine true oxygen consumption, and Millar catheters and contrast ventriculography to assess left ventricular performance and pressure volume relationships. Because these calculations were manually derived, a right and left heart catheterization took several hours and a full morning to complete. As fellows, we were masters of ventricular performance and coronary physiology. Little did we know that our world as interventionalists had already changed, as a result of the events that occurred in September 1977 by a humble interventionalist in Zurich, Switzerland (6).

The use of balloon angioplasty dramatically expanded over the 1980s, even after the tragic death of Andreas Gruentzig in 1985. The focus of the catheterization laboratory then changed substantially – detailed hemodynamic evaluations were replaced by therapeutic interventions coupled with diagnostic imaging. As we began to understand the limitations of balloon angioplasty, including abrupt closure and restenosis in the early 1990s, the diagnostic components of the catheterization laboratory evolved to advanced imaging and plaque characterization, most often using intravascular ultrasound(IVUS). We developed a parade of new devices to address the specific morphologic components of the plaque (e.g, rotational atherectomy for calcified lesions; directional coronary atherectomy for bulky lesions, excimer laser ablation for in-stent restenosis). Seminal work using IVUS also identified that restenosis after balloon angioplasty and directional atherectomy was primarily due to arterial remodeling rather than intimal hyperplasia, a transformation finding at that time (7,8). We also learned that atherosclerosis was ubiquitous in the "normal" appearing coronary vessels in patients undergoing coronary intervention (9), and that we needed to treat the patient, and not simply the lesion. These findings obtained from diagnostic imaging completely changed our understanding of coronary atherosclerosis and restenosis. At the same time, we learned the importance of providing more quantitative methods of coronary stenosis severity, and this expansion to vascular intervention has allowed the extension of these techniques to the peripheral vascular bed.

Diagnostic Methods in the Cardiac Catheterization Laboratory, edited by Pedro A. Lemos, MD, Paul Schoenhagen, MD, and Alexandra J. Lansky, MD, is a contemporary textbook that reviews the more timely topics in diagnostic imaging required for the evaluation and treatment of patients with complex coronary artery and myocardial disease. Both students of cardiac catheterization and seasoned interventional cardiologists will benefit from a thorough read of this insightful textbook.

Diagnostic Methods hits the mark on so many different levels. I still find occasional coronary anatomy that I have not seen, or if I have, it was so long that my memory is a little fuzzy. These rare anatomic conditions are concisely reviewed in *Diagnostic Methods* in "Coronary Anomalies and Fistulae. An Overview of Important Entities". Furthermore, having spent my academic career studying quantitative angiography, I keenly appreciate both the value and the limitations of these methods. *Diagnostic Methods* focuses on a number of outstanding challenges of quantitative angiography, including the "Practical uses of online QCA", "Pre-intervention evaluation of CTO, "Myocardial perfusion blush evaluation", "Challenges in the assessment of bifurcation lesions" and "The Vulnerable Plaque and Angiography " Each of these chapters provide keen insights into the state-of-the-art of quantitative angiography in several practical and clinically relevant sections. *Diagnostic Methods* also provides superb reviews of the expansion of quantitative angiography to the peripheral vasculature. These include, "Peripheral Qualitative and quantitative angiography of the great vessels and peripheral vessels", "Tips and tricks of the angiographic anatomy of the carotid arteries and vertebrobasilar system", "Invasive Evaluation of Renal Artery Stenosis", and "Angiographic Assessment of Lower Extremity Arterial Insufficiency".

Intravascular ultrasound (IVUS) holds a special place in my heart, having worked side by side with Gary Mintz, MD, at the Washington Hospital Center for 7 years. I must admit that after comparative studies in thousands of patients during the 1990s, Gary finally convinced me that IVUS provides much more extensive and accurate diagnostic information than angiographic alone. *Diagnostic Methods* provides a contemporary overview of IVUS in several chapters, including "Merits and limitations of IVUS for the evaluation of the ambiguous lesion", "An in-depth insight of intravascular ultrasound for coronary stenting", "Intravascular ultrasound to guide stent deployment," "A practical approach for IVUS in stent restenosis and thrombosis", "Pharmacological intervention trials, and "IVUS and IVUS-derived methods for vulnerable plaque assessment". These chapters are essential for the complete understanding of IVUS in contemporary practice. A final chapter "Optical coherence tomography" addresses very important clinical role of high-end imaging for assessment of lesion composition and healing response to stenting.

I remember first hearing Nico Pijls talk about Fractional Flow Reserves while I was an interventional cardiology fellow at the University of Michigan over 15 years ago. At that time, we were testing angiographic measures of coronary flow reserve using digital subtraction methods, but the techniques were cumbersome and poorly reproducible. Doppler flow catheters were just being developed, but, as I sat in the audience listening to Dr. Pijls, I was struck with the simplicity and relevance of measuring fractional flow reserve. Although we were primarily focused on intermediate lesions, coupling both FFR and Doppler flow may provide a more complete assessment of coronary flow and microvascular disease. The FAME study has substantially altered our approach in patients with multivessel coronary artery disease, and a precise understanding of both fractional flow reserve and intracoronary Doppler measurements is critical (10). *Diagnostic Methods* includes important updates on the state of the art for physiologic assessment of lesion severity in several chapters, including "Evaluation of acute and chronic microvascular coronary disease", "Collateral function assessment," and "Merits and limitations of FFR for the evaluation of ambiguous lesions". I would highly recommend that all interventionalists are fully familiar with the physiologic assessment of coronary lesion severity.

Our world is changing rapidly, and I am certain that the interventionalist for the next decade will also have a keen understanding of non invasive cardiac imaging. This is not only due to the rapid transition toward structural heart disease, for which a multimaging assessment is essential, but also for assessing coronary anatomy using less invasive methods. *Diagnostic Methods* also provides an extensive review of noninvasive imaging, including "Cardiac magnetic resonance imaging: viability assessment and cardiac function", "Cardiovascular interventional MR Imaging", "Role of MDCT for the diagnosis of coronary anomalies and fistulae", "A practical overview of coronary CT angiography", and "Multidetector computed tomography imaging for myocardial perfusion, viability and cardiac function". This comprehensive overview will provide the interventionalist with an integrated knowledge of noninvasive and invasive images. *Diagnostic Methods* also provides a very focused review of several challenging clinical conditions. These include, "Evaluation of LV function in cases of global and segmental disease", "Obstructive hypertrophic cardiomyopathy", "The role of the cath lab in patients with advanced heart failure and cardiac transplantation", and "Evaluation of common congenital heart defects in the adult".

Diagnostic Methods is highly recommended for all clinicians who wish to provide "State of the Art" care to their highly complex patients in the catheterization laboratory. With our rapidly evolving knowledge base and continued quest for evidence based practices, *Diagnostic Methods* will be an important addition to the interventionalist's core library.

Jeffrey J. Popma, MD
Director, Innovations in Interventional Cardiology
Beth Israel Deaconess Medical Center
Associate Professor of Medicine
Harvard Medical School
Boston, Massachusetts, U.S.A.

REFERENCES

1. Forssman W. Die sondierung des rechten Herzens. Klin Wochenschr 1929; 8:2085.
2. Cournand AF and Ranges HS. Catheterization of the right auricle in man. Proc Soc Exp Biol Med 1941; 46:462.
3. Richards DWJ. Cardiac output by catheterization technique, in various clinical conditions. Fed Proc 1945; 4:215.
4. Grossman W. Cardiac Catheterization and Angiography. First ed. 1974, Philadelphia: Lippincott Williams and Wilkins.
5. Yang S, Bentivoglio L, Maranhao V, et al. From Cardiac Catheterization Data to Hemodynamic Parameters. Third ed. 1988, Philadelphia: Davis, F.A.
6. Gruntzig A. Transluminal dilation of coronary artery stenosis. Lancet 1978; 1:263.
7. Kimura T, Nobuyoshi M. Remodelling and restenosis: intravascular ultrasound studies. Semin Interv Cardiol 1997; 2(3):159–166.
8. Hoffmann R, Mintz GS, Popma JJ, et al. Chronic arterial responses to stent implantation: a serial intravascular ultrasound analysis of Palmaz-Schatz stents in native coronary arteries. J Am Coll Cardiol 1996; 28(5):1134–1139.
9. Mintz GS, Painter JA, Pichard AD, et al. Atherosclerosis in angiographically "normal" coronary artery reference segments: an intravascular ultrasound study with clinical correlations. J Am Coll Cardiol 1995; 25(7):1479–1485.
10. Tonino PA, De Bruyne B, Pijls NH, et al. Fractional flow reserve versus angiography for guiding percutaneous coronary intervention. N Engl J Med 2009; 360(3):213–224.

Preface

Coronary angiography has revolutionized the diagnostic approach to patients with coronary artery disease and plays a central role in modern, pharmacological, transcatheter, and surgical treatment approaches. It has transformed the field of cardiology and defined the subspecialty of interventional cardiology.

However, despite the increasing understanding of the atherosclerotic disease process and advanced diagnostic and therapeutic options, coronary artery disease remains a major cause of morbidity and mortality worldwide. These facts demonstrate the need for additional anatomic and physiologic assessment of coronary disease beyond angiographic luminal stenosis, which has led to the development of several secondary transcatheter diagnostic modalities.

In modern catheterization laboratories worldwide, diagnostic evaluation of coronary artery disease has evolved far beyond angiography alone, allowing not only anatomic assessment of the artery lumen/stenosis but also of the wall/plaque, and physiologic assessment of hemodynamic lesion significance. In addition, more recent developments of noninvasive modalities, and in particular cardiac computed tomography and magnetic resonance imaging, allow complementary assessment with the future prospect of hybrid laboratories. Such comprehensive diagnostic evaluation of coronary lesions is the basis for advances in transcatheter interventions.

This expanding focus of coronary multimodality imaging in modern catheterization laboratories requires knowledge of several diagnostic modalities. In this title an international group of authors and editors including cardiologists and radiologists have collected comprehensive state-of-the-art information about the evolving diagnostic approach in the catheterization laboratory. The use of qualitative and quantitative angiography of the coronary arteries, great vessels, and peripheral arteries is discussed in the context of routine and challenging clinical scenarios (chronic total occlusion, bifurcation lesions, plaque vulnerability). Additional chapters discuss further catheter-based anatomic evaluation with intravascular ultrasound and optical coherence tomography, and assessment of lesions significance with fractional flow reserve and intracoronary Doppler. The emerging role of complementary noninvasive imaging with cardiac computed tomography and magnetic resonance imaging is the topic of dedicated chapters. The chapters describe diagnostic assessment and therapeutic consequences.

This title provides a comprehensive guide to the diagnostic approach in modern catheterization laboratories and its impact on interventional transcatheter treatment strategies. Directed toward cardiologists and radiologists performing diagnostic and interventional procedures in the catheterization laboratory, this title gives an up-to-date perspective but also a look into the future.

Pedro A. Lemos
Paul Schoenhagen
Alexandra J. Lansky

Contents

Contributors

Alexandre Abizaid Instituto Dante Pazzanese de Cardiologia, São Paulo, Brazil

Stephan Achenbach University of Erlangen, Erlangen, Germany

John A. Ambrose University of California, San Francisco-Fresno, Fresno, California, U.S.A.

Chourmouzios A. Arampatzis Interbalkan Medical Center, Thessaloniki, Greece

Pareena Bilkoo Gill Heart Institute, University of Kentucky, Lexington, Kentucky, U.S.A.

Michael Bock Deutsches Krebsforschungszentrum (dkfz), Heidelberg, Germany

Daniel Chamié Instituto Dante Pazzanese de Cardiologia, São Paulo, Brazil

Kamaldeep Chawla ICPS, Institut Hospitalier Jacques Cartier, Massy, France

Clarissa Cola Sant Pau University Hospital, Barcelona, Spain

John Coletta Harrington-McLaughlin Heart and Vascular Institute, and Cardialysis-Cleveland Case Laboratories, University Hospitals Case Medical Center, Case Western Reserve University School of Medicine, Cleveland, Ohio, U.S.A.

J. Ribamar Costa, Jr. Instituto Dante Pazzanese de Cardiologia, São Paulo, Brazil

Marco A. Costa Harrington-McLaughlin Heart and Vascular Institute, and Cardialysis-Cleveland Case Laboratories, University Hospitals Case Medical Center, Case Western Reserve University School of Medicine, Cleveland, Ohio, U.S.A.

Ricardo A. Costa Instituto Dante Pazzanese de Cardiologia, São Paulo, Brazil

Milind Y. Desai Cleveland Clinic Foundation, Cleveland, Ohio, U.S.A.

Richard T. George The Johns Hopkins University, Baltimore, Maryland, U.S.A.

C. Michael Gibson Beth Israel Deaconess Medical Center, Boston, Massachusetts, U.S.A.

Steffen Gloekler University Hospital Bern, Bern, Switzerland

Giulio Guagliumi Azienda Ospedaliera Ospedali Riuniti di Bergamo, Bergamo, Italy

Anuj Gupta Columbia University Medical Center, New York Presbyterian, New York, New York, U.S.A.

Ziyad M. Hijazi Rush Center for Congenital and Structural Heart Disease, Chicago, Illinois, U.S.A.

Claudia P. Hochberg Boston Medical Center, Boston, Massachusetts, U.S.A.

Angela Hoye Castle Hill Hospital, Kingston-upon-Hull, U.K.

Hussein M. Ismail Castle Hill Hospital, Kingston-upon-Hull, U.K.

Usman Javed University of California, San Francisco-Fresno, Fresno, California, U.S.A.

Samir Kapadia Cleveland Clinic Foundation, Cleveland, Ohio, U.S.A.

Ryan K. Kaple Massachusetts General Hospital, Boston, Massachusetts, U.S.A.

Kakuya Kitagawa The Johns Hopkins University, Baltimore, Maryland, U.S.A.

Zsolt Kulcsár University Hospital, Geneva, Switzerland

Philippe L.-L'Allier Montreal Heart Institute, University of Montreal, Montreal, Quebec, Canada

Albert C. Lardo The Johns Hopkins University, Baltimore, Maryland, U.S.A.

Thierry Lefèvre ICPS, Institut Hospitalier Jacques Cartier, Massy, France

Pedro A. Lemos Heart Institute (InCor), University of São Paulo Medical School, and Sirio-Libanes Hospital, São Paulo, Brazil

Yves Louvard ICPS, Institut Hospitalier Jacques Cartier, Massy, France

Akiko Maehara Cardiovascular Research Foundation, New York, New York, U.S.A.

Eulógio Martinez Heart Institute (InCor), University of São Paulo Medical School, São Paulo, Brazil

Bernhard Meier University Hospital Bern, Bern, Switzerland

Gary S. Mintz Cardiovascular Research Foundation, Washington D.C., U.S.A.

Marie-Claude Morice ICPS, Institut Hospitalier Jacques Cartier, Massy, France

Debabrata Mukherjee Gill Heart Institute, University of Kentucky, Lexington, Kentucky, U.S.A.

Koen Nieman Erasmus MC, Rotterdam, The Netherlands

Guillermo E. Pineda Gill Heart Institute, University of Kentucky, Lexington, Kentucky, U.S.A.

LeRoy E. Rabbani Columbia University Medical Center, New York Presbyterian, New York, New York, U.S.A.

Henrique Barbosa Ribeiro Heart Institute (InCor), University of São Paulo Medical School, São Paulo, Brazil

Expedito E. Ribeiro Heart Institute (InCor), University of São Paulo Medical School, São Paulo, Brazil

Carlos Eduardo Rochitte Heart Institute (InCor), University of São Paulo Medical School, São Paulo, Brazil

Marco Roffi University Hospital, Geneva, Switzerland

Dieter Ropers University of Erlangen, Erlangen, Germany

Manel Sabaté Sant Pau University Hospital, Barcelona, Spain

Paul Schoenhagen Imaging Institute and Heart and Vascular Institute, Cleveland Clinic Foundation, Cleveland, Ohio, U.S.A.

Karl H. Schuleri The Johns Hopkins University, Baltimore, Maryland, U.S.A.

Tiago Senra Heart Institute (InCor), University of São Paulo Medical School, São Paulo, Brazil

Ilke Sipahi Harrington-McLaughlin Heart and Vascular Institute, Case Western Reserve University, University Hospitals Case Medical Center, Cleveland, Ohio, U.S.A.

Dimytri A. Siqueira Instituto Dante Pazzanese de Cardiologia, São Paulo, Brazil

Christian Spies The Queen's Medical Center, Honolulu, Hawaii, U.S.A.

Daniel H. Steinberg Medical University of South Carolina, Charleston, South Carolina, U.S.A.

Nobuaki Suzuki Harrington-McLaughlin Heart and Vascular Institute, and Cardialysis-Cleveland Case Laboratories, University Hospitals Case Medical Center, Case Western Reserve University School of Medicine, Cleveland, Ohio, U.S.A.

Kengo Tanabe Division of Cardiology, Mitsui Memorial Hospital, Tokyo, Japan

Jean-Claude Tardif Montreal Heart Institute, University of Montreal, Montreal, Quebec, Canada

Stanley N. Thornton Ochsner Heart and Vascular Institute, New Orleans, Louisiana, U.S.A.

Vasilis Voudris Onassis Cardiac Center, Athens, Greece

Frank Wacker Charité, Universitätsmedizin Berlin, Berlin, Germany, and Johns Hopkins School of Medicine, Baltimore, Maryland, U.S.A.

Christopher J. White Ochsner Heart and Vascular Institute, New Orleans, Louisiana, U.S.A.

Khaled M. Ziada Gill Heart Institute, University of Kentucky, Lexington, Kentucky, U.S.A.

1 Coronary anomalies and fistulae: An overview of important entities

Chourmouzios A. Arampatzis and Vasilis Voudris

INTRODUCTION

Coronary artery anomalies (CAAs) are an infrequent incident in the general population. Although they are far less common than acquired heart disease, their implication is important since they are related with sudden death, especially in young individuals.[1] By definition, CAAs are an anatomic variant with a rare occurrence (0.3–1.3%) in the general population,[2–5] even though in a well-documented angiographic study 5.64% of the total population had CAAs.[2] Indeed the exact proportion of the general population with this abnormality might be underestimated for the following reasons: (a) the majority of the anomalies have a benign course since they are discovered as incidental findings during diagnostic catheterization and moreover their course may be totally silent without any signs, symptoms, or complications; (b) data derived from necropsy studies are hampered by lack of diagnostic criteria, entry bias, and limited sample[2] size.

DEFINITIONS AND PATHOPHYSIOLOGY

Several investigators have published classifications using the correlation of the anatomic variant with the clinical manifestation.[3,6,7] Conversely, our knowledge is limited regarding the pathophysiology and the natural history of the anomalies. In addition, the anatomic variations seem to be endless since a vast number of case reports illustrate and underline extraordinary cases. Therefore, we adopt the definitions and classifications proposed by Angelini et al.[8] as depicted in Table 1.1. Any morphological feature observed in >1% of an unselected population is defined as *normal*. *Normal variant*, an alternative, relatively unusual morphological feature seen in >1% of the same population; and *anomaly*, a morphological feature seen in <1% of that population. In addition, and according to Greenberg et al.,[9] coronary anomalies can be categorized into three groups as delineated in Table 1.2.

Coronary anomalies may be associated with chest pain, dyspnea, syncope, cardiomyopathy, ventricular fibrillation, myocardial infarction, and sudden death.[2] In a large prospective cohort study, young athletes carried a twofold risk compared to nonathletes for sudden death.[10] The most common cause of sudden death in the aforementioned cohort was congenital CAA. The exact mechanisms involved in the spectrum of manifestations are sometimes unclear and insufficient. There is a definite and clear relation between preset ischemia and anomalous origin of left coronary artery from the pulmonary artery (ALCAPA), ostial stenosis, and ostial atresia. Possible reasons for secondary myocardial ischemia are tangential origin of coronary artery, anomalous origin of a coronary artery from the opposite sinus of Valsalva (ACAOS), myocardial bridge, coronary ectasia, fistula, and adult ALCAPA. Recently obtained solid data from an intravascular ultrasound study proposed that the clinical manifestations of the ACAOS are associated with the specific pathway the artery follows.[11] Indeed in this study, intussusception related with coronary hypoplasia and lateral luminal compression is the only documented mechanism found to cause ischemia in the case of ACAOS. It is interesting to note that diagnostic exercise stress tests and myocardial perfusion scans often provide confusing or even false-negative results.[2,12] Individuals with coronary fistula, coronary ectasia, ectopic origin, and proximal muscular bridge may possibly have an increased risk for atherosclerotic disease. Large coronary aneurysms, fistula, and ALCAPA may be associated with aortic-root distortion and aortic valve disease. Fistulae are possible, though not definite, related with bacterial endocarditis, volume overload, and ischemic cardiomyopathy. Lastly, there are certain variants that have direct relation with technical difficulties during coronary angioplasty (ectopic ostia) and complications during surgery (ectopic ostia, muscular bridge). Despite the fact that we do not

Table 1.1 Normal features of the coronary anatomy in humans

Feature	Range
No. of ostia	2–4
Location	Right and left anterior sinuses
Proximal orientation	45° to 90° off the aortic wall
Proximal common stem	Only left (LAD and LCx)
Proximal course	Direct: from ostium to destination
Mid-course	Extramural (subepicardial)
Branches	Adequate for the dependent myocardium
Essential territories	RCA (RV free wall), LAD (anteroseptal), OM (LV free wall)
Termination	Capillary bed

Abbreviations: LAD, left anterior descending artery; LCx, left circumflex artery; RCA, right coronary artery; RV, right ventricular; OM, obtuse marginal artery; LV, left ventricular.

have clear evidence about the occurrence of the variants, coronary anomalies may account for 19% of sudden death in young athletes.[13]

CONSIDERATIONS AND TREATMENT APPROACHES

Anomalies of origin

High takeoff of the coronary arteries has no major clinical impact, but selective engagement of the vessel during coronary angiography may be sometimes extremely difficult. In multiple ostia, either the right coronary artery (RCA) and the conus branch arise separately or there is virtually no left main stem and the left anterior descending and circumflex artery come up separately (double barrel). Although there is no clinical risk in both entities, there is a moderate risk of injuring the conus branch during heart surgery manipulation. Single coronary artery (Fig. 1.1) is an extremely rare anomaly reported in only 0.0024 to 0.044 of the population.[14] Patients with this anomaly may have no clinical manifestations. However, in case a major branch follows an interarterial path, in between the aorta and the pulmonary artery, there is an increased risk for sudden death. In addition if a proximal blockage occurs, the result would probably be fatal. The ALCAPA entity is one of the most serious congenital anomalies of origin. The incident is very rare[15] and 90% of untreated infants die before the first year of their life.[16] In the majority of the cases, left coronary artery (LCA) arises from the pulmonary artery and RCA arises from the aorta (Bland–White–Garland syndrome). Treatment of ALCAPA consists of re-creation of dual coronary artery perfusion. Direct re-implantation of the LCA into

Table 1.2 Coronary artery anomalies

Anomalies of origin
High takeoff
Multiple ostia
Single coronary artery
Anomalous origin of coronary artery from pulmonary artery
Origin of coronary artery or branch from opposite or noncoronary sinus and an anomalous course
Retroaortic
Interarterial
Prepulmonic
Septal (subpulmonic)
Anomalies of course
Myocardial bridging
Duplication of arteries
Anomalies of termination
Coronary artery fistula
Coronary arcade
Extracardiac termination

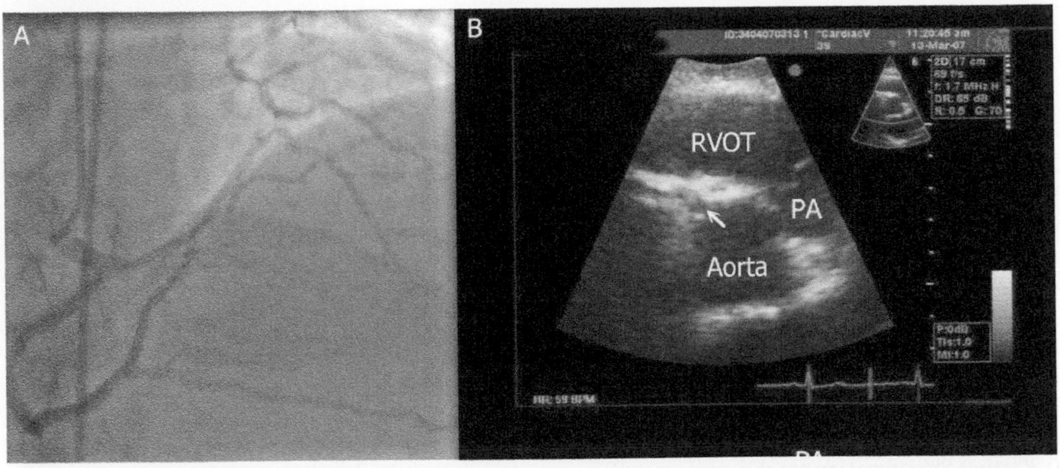

Figure 1.1 (**A**) Coronary angiographic image of a single coronary artery (LCA) originating from the right sinus of valsalva. (**B**) Transthoracic echocardiographic image, short axis view. Arrow indicates the origin of the LCA from the right cusp. *Abbreviation*: PA, pulmonary artery; RVOT, right ventricular outflow track.

the aorta or creation of an intrapulmonary conduit from the left coronary ostia to the aorta (Takeuchi procedure) comprises the treatment approaches in the infants and ligation of the LCA combined with bypass operation in the adults.[15]

Anomalous origin of a coronary artery from the ACAOS is also a rare incident, which follows five alternative pathways[17] as depicted in Table 1.2. Of those, the interarterial course (between the aorta and the pulmonary artery) is associated with a severe prognosis.[8,18] On the other hand, the most common LCX anomaly in this category, which is an LCX origin of the right coronary cusp with a course behind the aortic root[2] (Fig. 1.2), is associated with benign prognosis.

The following points are noteworthy: a large number of patients with ACAOS have prodromal symptoms such as chest pain, syncope, or dyspnea, and exercise during such symptoms plays a pivotal triggering role in patients' death.[18] The RCA arises from the left sinus of Valsalva (right ACAOS) in 0.17 to 0.96 of patients who undergo angiography[2,5] and when it has an interarterial course, it has a 30% rate of sudden death.[19] The LCA (left ACAOS) arises from the opposite sinus in 0.09 to 0.15 of patients who undergo angiography.[2,20] Importantly, in up to 75% of the patients, the course is interarterial[20] and suspected to fatal events. ACAOS presents an excellent paradigm in which recent studies have demonstrated new mechanisms involved in the pathophysiology of the disease.[21] Symptomatic patients may be treated with β-blockers[22] and provided to avoid heavy exertion, stent implantation when justified (symptoms, stenosis more than 50% evaluated with intravascular ultrasound, large dependent myocardial territory, and detected reversible ischemia) in case of right ACAOS.[23] The use of stent in the case of left

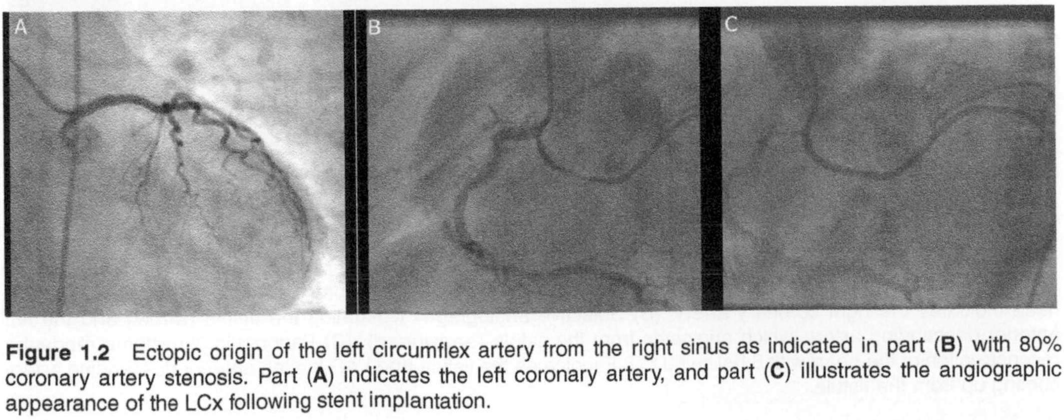

Figure 1.2 Ectopic origin of the left circumflex artery from the right sinus as indicated in part (**B**) with 80% coronary artery stenosis. Part (**A**) indicates the left coronary artery, and part (**C**) illustrates the angiographic appearance of the LCx following stent implantation.

ACAOS[24] carries a greater risk for the patient than the risk of stenting right ACAOS. Indeed, surgical intervention is the preferred treatment option in the case of left ACAOS.[11]

Anomalies of course

Myocardial bridging should probably be considered as a normal variant, as it is present in >1% of the general population.[2] The classic "milking effect" during coronary angiography induced by systolic compression of the tunneled segment offers a clear and firm diagnosis. Although their course is relatively silent, sometimes they may be associated with angina pectoris, myocardial infarction, life-threatening arrhythmias or even death.[25]

Anomalies of termination

Vascular connections between arteries and extracardiac structures are commonly called fistulae,[2] but few of them have any effect upon coronary functioning. A true fistula of the circulatory system is characterized by a clearly ectatic vascular segment that displays fistulous flow and connects two vascular territories ruled by large pressure differences. This condition is seen in 0.3% to 0.8% of patients who undergo diagnostic angiography.[3,12] Communications, especially to the left ventricle, can also be secondary after myocardial infarction, biopsy, or heart surgery (septal myomectomy). Fistulae are usually detected by coincidence on coronary angiography. However, diagnosis of coronary artery fistula can be made by detecting a continuous heart murmur in the upper precordial area. The implicated coronary artery is dilated and tortuous, and the drainage site may have single or multiple communications forming sometimes a diffuse plexus-like network. The clinical presentation of the fistula is related with the drainage site. The right cardiac chambers are the most frequent sites of drainage [right ventricle 45% of cases, right atrium 25% (Figs. 1.3 and 1.4)] followed by the pulmonary artery (15%).[26] The fistula drains into the left cardiac chambers in less than 10% of cases.[27] When the shunt leads into a right-sided cardiac chamber, the hemodynamics resemble those of an extracardiac left-to-right shunt; when the connection is to a left-sided cardiac chamber, the hemodynamics mimic those of aortic insufficiency. The clinical presentation of coronary fistulae includes dyspnea, congestive heart failure, angina, endocarditis, or even myocardial infarction. However, most of the fistulae are silent. Symptomatic patients must have true fistulous flow accompanied by sizable shunting of coronary flow and volume overload. It has been advocated that coronary steal phenomenon in the majority of the patients is the principal cause of secondary ischemia, but it seems unlikely to be such a mechanism to promote critical reductions in myocardial perfusion.[28]

The treatment options are surgical closure or endovascular exclusion/occlusion. Surgical closure is safe but recurrence ranges from 16% to 18% and mortality rates increase with age. Several studies have shown that surgical closure is safe and effective.[29–31] A safe and effective

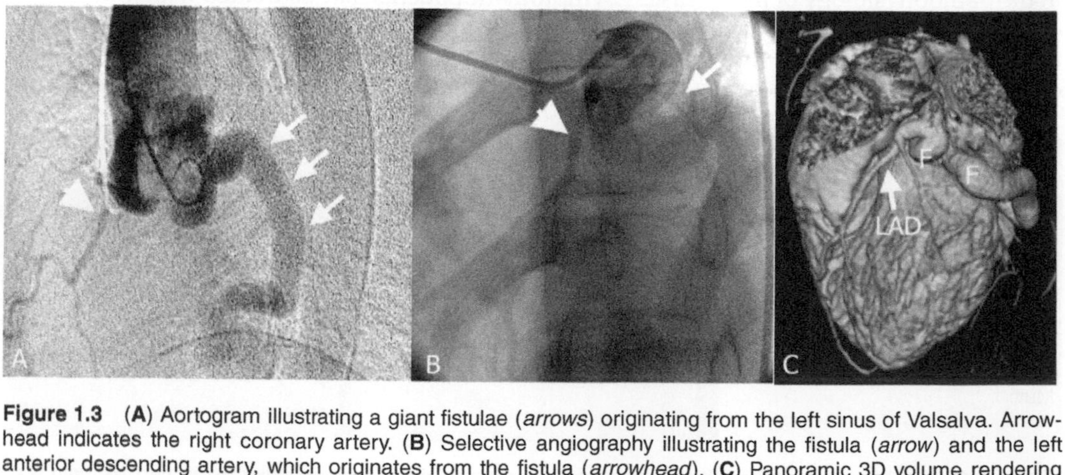

Figure 1.3 (**A**) Aortogram illustrating a giant fistulae (*arrows*) originating from the left sinus of Valsalva. Arrowhead indicates the right coronary artery. (**B**) Selective angiography illustrating the fistula (*arrow*) and the left anterior descending artery, which originates from the fistula (*arrowhead*). (**C**) Panoramic 3D volume rendering reconstruction of the heart with 64-slice MDCT. F indicates the fistula and LAD the left anterior descending artery coming up from the fistula.

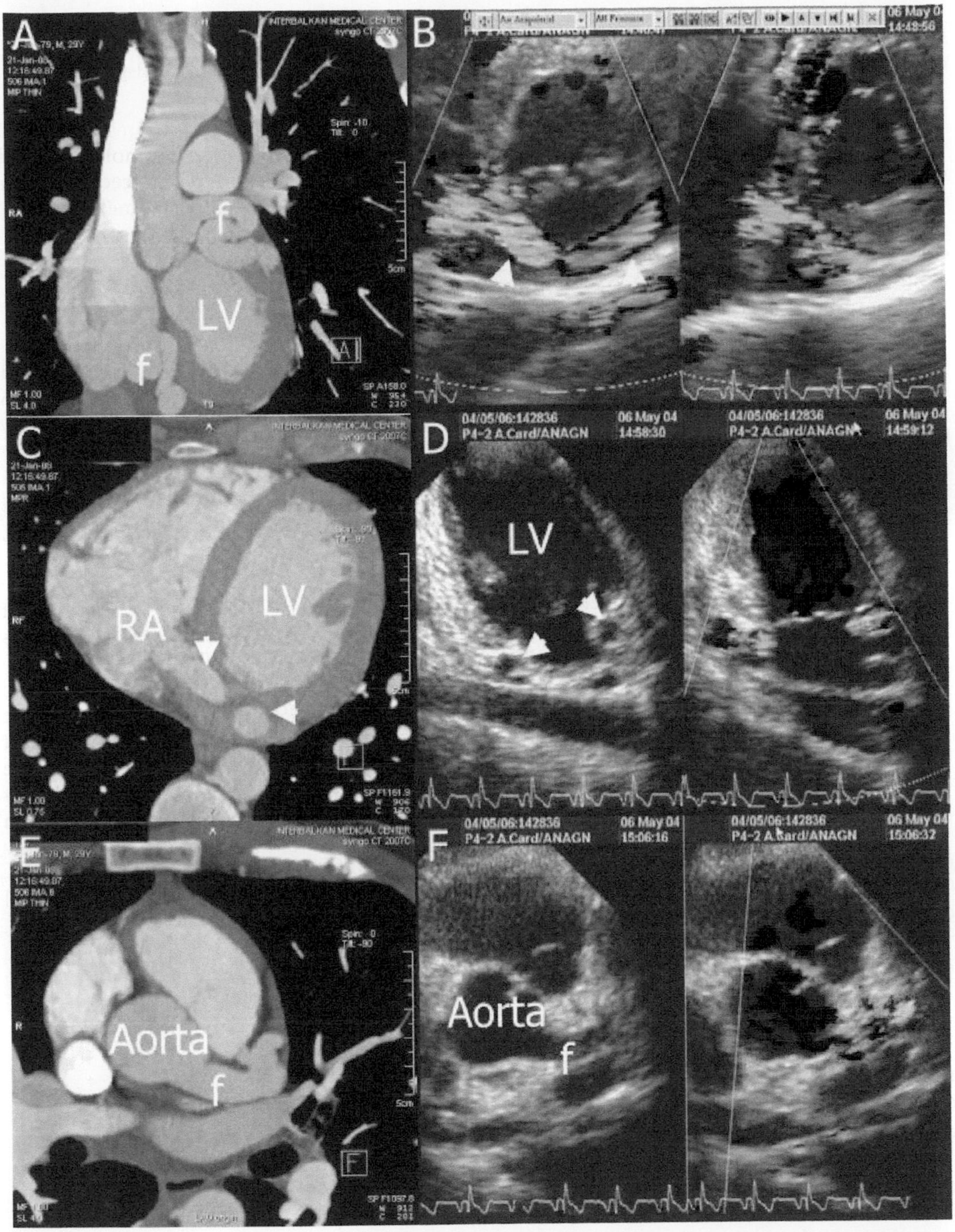

Figure 1.4 (**A**) Multiplanar reconstruction of the heart and the great vessels. f indicates the giant fistula originating from the left sinus and drain into the right atrium (RA). (**B**) Transthoracic echocardiographic image. Arrowheads illustrate with color the fistulous flow. (**C**) Multiplanar reconstruction of the heart. Arrowheads indicate the fistula corresponding with the arrowheads of the TTE image in (**D**) that shows a two-chamber view of the heart. (**E**) Multiplanar reconstruction of the great vessels indicates the origin of the fistula (f) as a virtually giant left main stem in total association with panel (**F**) which shows a TTE image of the aorta and the fistula (f).

therapeutic approach is endovascular exclusion/occlusion. The majority of the reported cases have been treated with stainless steel coils with a success rate of 50% to 92%.[32] In addition, embolic occlusions with alcohol, double-umbrella devices, and stent grafts have also been used.

NONINVASIVE IMAGING AND SCREENING METHODS

Conventional coronary angiography has long been the gold standard for the diagnosis of coronary anomalies. However, this method is hampered by the invasiveness of the procedure itself, the inability to visualize the arteries three dimensionally, and since some of the anomalies have a rare ectopic origin, they are prone to injuries, dissections, and complications. On the other hand, correct angiographic correlation is difficult[2] and importantly less accurate than electron-beam computed tomography (EBCT), magnetic resonance imaging (MRI), or multislice computed tomography (MSCT).

Transthoracic echocardiography is simple, noninvasive, and lacks ionic radiation. Its primary target group is the pediatric population where high image quality is obtained. It is highly accurate to detect ALCAPA and large coronary fistulae. It is also possible to visualize proximal coronary ostia and detect ACAOS,[33] but as age and body mass index increase the method becomes less accurate. Noteworthy is the discrepancy found between the 0.17% rate of ACAOS detected from a series of 2388 patients who underwent echocardiography[34] and the 1.07% rate found with coronary angiography.[2] This discrepancy implies that echocardiography is probably neither suitable nor reliable to detect ACAOS. Moreover, the acquired images do not have proper anatomic correlation with the anomalies and this modality is not recommended to rule out or even diagnose anomalies in the adult population.

Coronary magnetic resonance angiography is a noninvasive technique that allows three-dimensional reconstruction without using nephrotoxic agent or ionic radiation.[35] It is extremely supportive in investigating and evaluating coronary anomalies, especially in patients with joined congenital disease.[36] Its limitation is on visualizing the distal coronary course, therefore is not suitable in evaluating fistulae and coronary origination outside the sinuses.

Contrast-enhanced electron-beam tomography[37] has also been recommended. It offers excellent spatial resolution and identifies most anomalies of coronary course. The method offers high diagnostic accuracy with a low-radiation exposure estimated at 1.1 mSv.[38] Conversely, there is a risk for allergic reactions and nephrotoxic adverse events and the equipment is very costly.

Multidetector computed tomography (MDCT) is rapidly expanding on evaluating coronary artery disease. Several studies[39–41] have presented highly accurate results on detecting CAAs. Furthermore, when compared with conventional coronary angiography, MDCT has demonstrated superiority in evaluating the proximal origin and course of the anomalous vessel.[39,41] MDCT has an excellent spatial resolution with the ability to perform multiplanar reconstructions and volume rendering. On the other hand, the use of ionic agent and radiation exposure hamper the method especially in the young population for whom large-scaled screening programs should be considered.

CONCLUSIONS

CAAs are an infrequent finding in the general population. Their course is mainly benign, but certain entities are associated with severe prognosis. The population involved in sport and athletic activities is rapidly increasing. Sudden cardiac death is a public issue with tremendous consequences. Therefore, there is a need for a global network comprises healthcare specialists and scientists with government involvement to establish protocols, coordinate worldwide organizations, investigate the mechanisms, and educate physicians and most importantly the general public.

REFERENCES

1. Williams RA. The Historical Background of Sudden Death in Athletes. The Athlete and Heart Disease: Diagnosis Evaluation & Management. Philadelphia, PA: Lippincott Williams & Wilkins, 2000:1–8.
2. Angelini P. Villason S, Chan AV. Normal and anomalous coronary arteries in humans. In: Angelini P, ed. Coronary Artery Anomalies: A Comprehensive Approach. Philadelphia, PA: Lippincott Williams & Wilkins, 1999:27–150.

3. Baltaxe HA, Wixson D. The incidence of congenital anomalies of the coronary arteries in the adult population. Radiology 1977; 122(1):47–52.
4. Click RL, Holmes DR Jr, Vlietstra RE, et al. Anomalous coronary arteries: Location, degree of atherosclerosis and effect on survival—A report from the Coronary Artery Surgery Study. J Am Coll Cardiol 1989; 13(3):531–537.
5. Yamanaka O, Hobbs RE. Coronary artery anomalies in 126,595 patients undergoing coronary arteriography. Cathet Cardiovasc Diagn 1990; 21(1):28–40.
6. Ogden JA. Congenital anomalies of the coronary arteries. Am J Cardiol 1970; 25(4):474–479.
7. Roberts WC. Major anomalies of coronary arterial origin seen in adulthood. Am Heart J 1986; 111(5):941–963.
8. Angelini P, Velasco JA, Flamm S. Coronary anomalies: Incidence, pathophysiology, and clinical relevance. Circulation 2002; 105(20):2449–2454.
9. Greenberg MA, Fish BG, Spindola-Franco H. Congenital anomalies of the coronary arteries. Classification and significance. Radiol Clin North Am 1989; 27(6):1127–1146.
10. Corrado D, Basso C, Rizzoli G, et al. Does sports activity enhance the risk of sudden death in adolescents and young adults? J Am Coll Cardiol 2003; 42(11):1959–1963.
11. Angelini P, Walmsley RP, Libreros A, et al. Symptomatic anomalous origination of the left coronary artery from the opposite sinus of valsalva. Clinical presentations, diagnosis, and surgical repair. Tex Heart Inst J 2006; 33(2):171–179.
12. Angelini P. Coronary artery anomalies—Current clinical issues: Definitions, classification, incidence, clinical relevance, and treatment guidelines. Tex Heart Inst J 2002; 29(4):271–278.
13. Maron BJ, Thompson PD, Puffer JC, et al. Cardiovascular preparticipation screening of competitive athletes: Addendum: An addendum to a statement for health professionals from the Sudden Death Committee (Council on Clinical Cardiology) and the Congenital Cardiac Defects Committee (Council on Cardiovascular Disease in the Young), American Heart Association. Circulation 1998; 97(22): 2294.
14. Desmet W, Vanhaecke J, Vrolix M, et al. Isolated single coronary artery: A review of 50,000 consecutive coronary angiographies. Eur Heart J 1992; 13(12):1637–1640.
15. Dodge-Khatami A, Mavroudis C, Backer CL. Anomalous origin of the left coronary artery from the pulmonary artery: Collective review of surgical therapy. Ann Thorac Surg 2002; 74(3):946–955.
16. Wesselhoeft H, Fawcett JS, Johnson AL. Anomalous origin of the left coronary artery from the pulmonary trunk. Its clinical spectrum, pathology, and pathophysiology, based on a review of 140 cases with seven further cases. Circulation 1968; 38(2):403–425.
17. Angelini P, Flamm SD. Newer concepts for imaging anomalous aortic origin of the coronary arteries in adults. Catheter Cardiovasc Interv 2007; 69(7):942–954.
18. Eckart RE, Scoville SL, Campbell CL, et al. Sudden death in young adults: A 25-year review of autopsies in military recruits. Ann Intern Med 2004; 141(11):829–834.
19. Roberts WC, Siegel RJ, Zipes DP. Origin of the right coronary artery from the left sinus of valsalva and its functional consequences: Analysis of 10 necropsy patients. Am J Cardiol 1982; 49(4): 863–868.
20. Chaitman BR, Lesperance J, Saltiel J, et al. Clinical, angiographic, and hemodynamic findings in patients with anomalous origin of the coronary arteries. Circulation 1976; 53(1):122–131.
21. Angelini P. Coronary artery anomalies: An entity in search of an identity. Circulation 2007; 115(10):1296–1305.
22. Maron BJ, Zipes DP. Introduction: Eligibility recommendations for competitive athletes with cardiovascular abnormalities-general considerations. J Am Coll Cardiol 2005; 45(8):1318–1321.
23. Angelini P, Velasco JA, Ott D, et al. Anomalous coronary artery arising from the opposite sinus: Descriptive features and pathophysiologic mechanisms, as documented by intravascular ultrasonography. J Invasive Cardiol 2003; 15(9):507–514.
24. Chen M, Hong T, Huo Y. Stenting for left main stenosis in a child with anomalous origin of left coronary artery: Case report. Chin Med J (Engl) 2005; 118(1):80–82.
25. Tio RA, Van Gelder IC, Boonstra PW, et al. Myocardial bridging in a survivor of sudden cardiac near-death: Role of intracoronary doppler flow measurements and angiography during dobutamine stress in the clinical evaluation. Heart 1997; 77(3):280–282.
26. McNamara JJ, Gross RE. Congenital coronary artery fistula. Surgery 1969; 65(1):59–69.
27. Reagan K, Boxt LM, Katz J. Introduction to coronary arteriography. Radiol Clin North Am 1994; 32(3):419–433.
28. Angelini P. Coronary-to-pulmonary fistulae: What are they? What are their causes? What are their functional consequences? Tex Heart Inst J 2000; 27(4):327–329.
29. Liberthson RR, Sagar K, Berkoben JP, et al. Congenital coronary arteriovenous fistula. Report of 13 patients, review of the literature and delineation of management. Circulation 1979; 59(5):849–854.

30. Cheung DL, Au WK, Cheung HH, et al. Coronary artery fistulas: Long-term results of surgical correction. Ann Thorac Surg 2001; 71(1):190–195.
31. Kamiya H, Yasuda T, Nagamine H, et al. Surgical treatment of congenital coronary artery fistulas: 27 years' experience and a review of the literature. J Card Surg 2002; 17(2):173–177.
32. Bonello L, Com O, Gaubert JY, et al. Covered stent for closure of symptomatic plexus-like coronary fistula. Int J Cardiol 2006; 109(3):408–410.
33. Davis JA, Cecchin F, Jones TK, et al. Major coronary artery anomalies in a pediatric population: Incidence and clinical importance. J Am Coll Cardiol 2001; 37(2):593–597.
34. Frommelt PC, Berger S, Pelech AN, et al. Prospective identification of anomalous origin of left coronary artery from the right sinus of valsalva using transthoracic echocardiography: Importance of color Doppler flow mapping. Pediatr Cardiol 2001; 22(4):327–332.
35. Bunce NH, Lorenz CH, Keegan J, et al. Coronary artery anomalies: Assessment with free-breathing three-dimensional coronary MR angiography. Radiology 2003; 227(1):201–208.
36. Taylor AM, Thorne SA, Rubens MB, et al. Coronary artery imaging in grown up congenital heart disease: Complementary role of magnetic resonance and x-ray coronary angiography. Circulation 2000; 101(14):1670–1678.
37. Ropers D, Moshage W, Daniel WG, et al. Visualization of coronary artery anomalies and their anatomic course by contrast-enhanced electron beam tomography and three-dimensional reconstruction. Am J Cardiol 2001; 87(2):193–197.
38. Hunold P, Vogt FM, Schmermund A, et al. Radiation exposure during cardiac CT: Effective doses at multi-detector row CT and electron-beam CT. Radiology 2003; 226(1):145–152.
39. Shi H, Aschoff AJ, Brambs HJ, et al. Multislice CT imaging of anomalous coronary arteries. Eur Radiol 2004; 14(12):2172–2181.
40. Datta J, White CS, Gilkeson RC, et al. Anomalous coronary arteries in adults: Depiction at multi-detector row CT angiography. Radiology 2005; 235(3):812–818.
41. Schmitt R, Froehner S, Brunn J, et al. Congenital anomalies of the coronary arteries: Imaging with contrast-enhanced, multidetector computed tomography. Eur Radiol 2005; 15(6):1110–1121.

2 Practical uses of online quantitative coronary angiography

Kengo Tanabe

INTRODUCTION

Quantitative Coronary Angiography (QCA) has been established as the golden standard for coronary artery stenosis assessment because visual interpretation of coronary artery is erroneous when compared with QCA.[1–4] Visual assessment is a subjective evaluation with a large inter- and intraobserver variability. Angiographers tend to overestimate the severity of tight stenosis and underestimate the degree of mild ones. QCA has the advantage of being more reproducible in the assessment of coronary lesion severity; therefore, QCA has been widespread and utilized to estimate the efficacy of enormous percutaneous devices and pharmacological agents in important clinical scientific studies, especially for restenosis prevention trials.

With the advent of novel therapeutic interventional devises such as intravascular brachytherapy, radioactive stents, and drug-eluting stents, several new and unforeseen problems have emerged. In this circumstance, QCA had to be adapted to more complicated and complex situations related to the effect of the intervention on the angiographic appearance of the treated artery. For example, intracoronary radiation therapy has emerged as a promising modality to attenuate the neointimal hyperplasia after stent placement,[5,6] however, the use of radiation therapy has been limited by logistic requirements, late thrombosis, and the occurrence of stenosis in the segments adjacent to the stent (so called "edge stenosis").[7] Following brachytherapy, stent-based local drug delivery such as sirolimus- and paclitaxel-eluting stents was developed.[8,9] Sirolimus and paclitaxel have potent antiproliferative and antimigratory effects similar to that of intravascular brachytherapy. Based on the previous experience with brachytherapy, there were some concerns that sirolimus and paclitaxel might potentially behave the same way as brachytherapy, thus providing untoward effects, such as edge stenosis, on the vessel wall. Therefore, it was indispensable for QCA to include the segments adjacent to the stent in clinical trials to test the safety and feasibility of drug-eluting stents. Three coronary segments were subjected to quantitative angiography: in-stent, proximal edge, and distal edge segment (Figs. 2.1 and 2.2). The in-stent analysis encompassed the length of all stents used during the procedure. The proximal and distal edge segments included up to 5 mm length from the proximal and distal edge of the total segment treated with the implanted stents, respectively. Figure 2.3 shows one case of a drug-eluting stent with serial coronary angiography. The serial QCA analyses reveal no restenosis in the in-stent segment as well as that of the proximal and distal edge segments. In fact, utilizing this application of serial QCA analyses, many clinical prospective randomized trials[8–10] demonstrated that elution of sirolimus and paclitaxel not only inhibited neointimal hyperplasia within the stent, but also prevented edge restenosis previously seen in intravascular radiation therapy. Thus, the advent of drug-eluting stents has impacted interventional cardiology by dramatically decreasing neointimal growth and in-stent restenosis as compared to those of bare metal stents. QCA still remains as a golden standard to investigate the safety and efficacy of new generation of drug-eluting stents. However, given the fact that target lesion revascularization following implantation of the first generation of drug-eluting stents is rare in clinical trials, there is a question about performing online QCA during the procedure to further improve the safety and efficacy of the devices. In this chapter, I describe the application of online QCA in the era of drug-eluting stent.

ASSESSMENT OF GEOGRAPHIC MISS

Sirolimus-eluting stents have dramatically reduced restenosis, however, there is a small, but sizable number of patients who develop restenosis. Restenosis of the eluting stent is sometimes attributable to a mismatch of lesion and injured segments with the stent deployment sites (so-called geographical miss).[11] The term of geographic miss was first reported to describe the failure

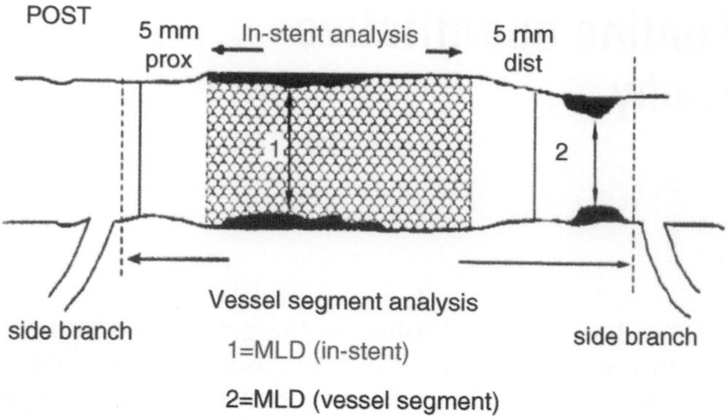

Figure 2.1 QCA methodology in the era of drug-eluting stents. Three coronary segments are subjected to QCA: in-stent, proximal edge, and distal edge segment. The in-stent analysis encompassed the length of an implanted stent. The proximal and distal edge segment included up to 5 mm length from the proximal and distal edge of the total segment treated with the stent, respectively.

to cover the injured or diseased segment with intravascular radiation therapy.[12] There was a four-fold increase in incidence of edge restenosis in patients with geographic miss compared to those without geographic miss. Recently, the STLLR trial has demonstrated that geographic miss is associated with an increased risk of target vessel revascularization (5.1% vs. 2.5%, $p = 0.025$) and myocardial infarction (2.4% vs. 0.8%, $p = 0.04$) at 1-year follow-up after implantation of sirolimus-eluting stents in daily clinical practice.[13] In addition, it is noteworthy that geographic miss occurred in as high as 66.5% of the patients. Two categories of geographic miss were defined in the STLLR trial: longitudinal geographic miss (Fig. 2.4) and axial geographic miss (Fig. 2.5). Longitudinal geographic miss was defined in cases in which the entire length of the injured segment or the entire length of the stenotic segment was not fully covered by the total length of the eluting stents. Axial geographic miss was defined in cases in which the ratio between the size of the largest balloon and the reference vessel diameter was <0.9 or >1.3. In fact, in the STLLR trial, the difference of target vessel revascularization rates between the patients with and without geographic miss was primarily driven by differences in the incidence of target vessel

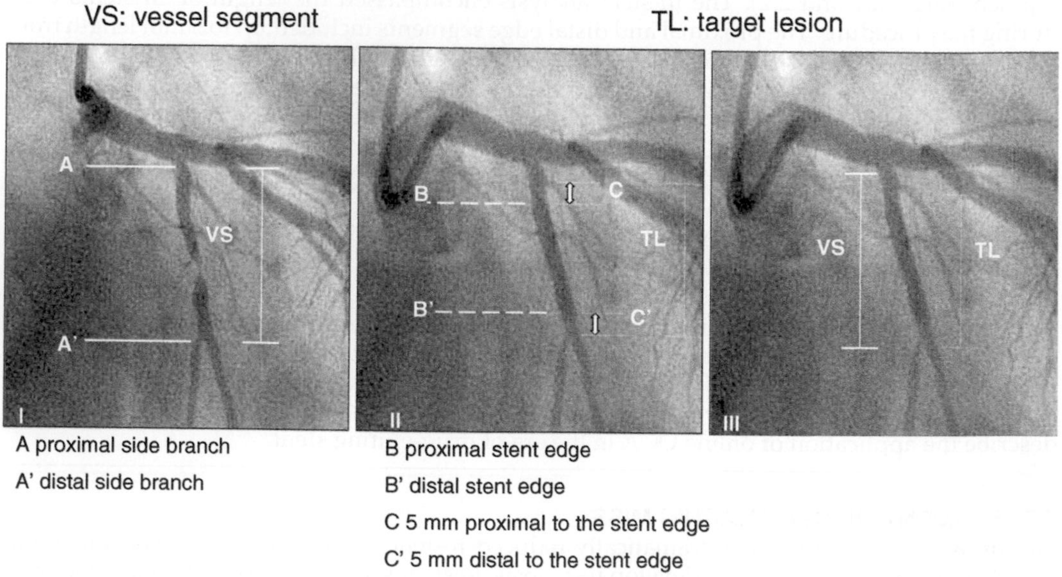

Figure 2.2 QCA of a case which has a tight stenosis in the left circumflex artery (I) and was successfully treated with a drug-eluting stent (II and III).

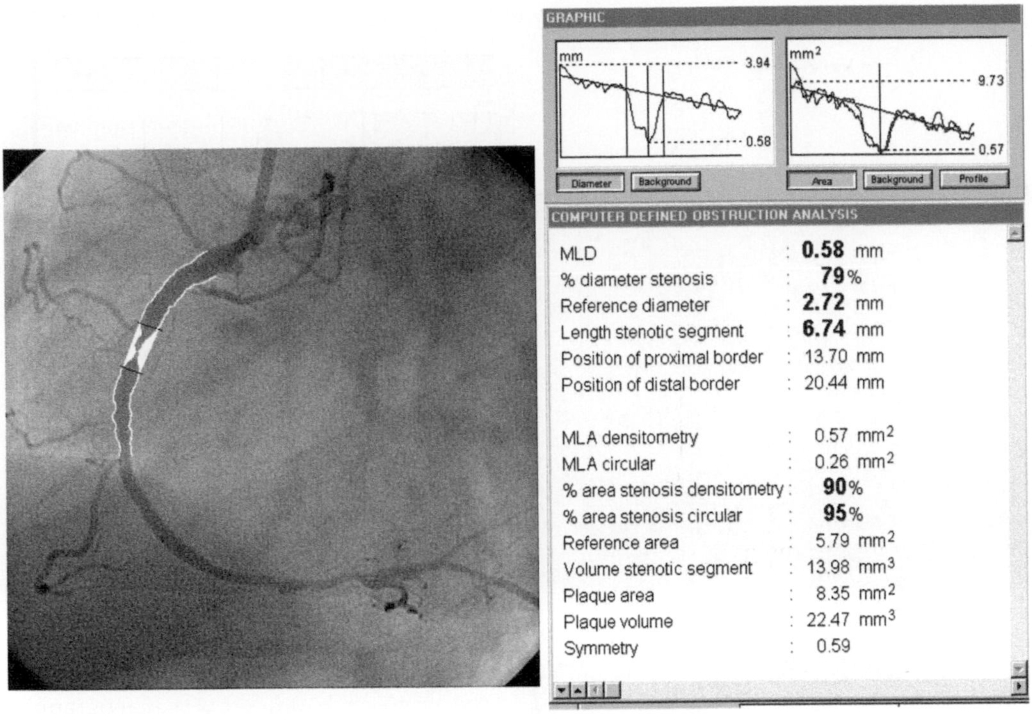
GRAPHIC
mm
3.94
0.58
mm2
9.73
0.57
Diameter
Background
Area
Background
Profile
COMPUTER DEFINED OBSTRUCTION ANALYSIS
MLD : 0.58 mm
% diameter stenosis : 79%
Reference diameter : 2.72 mm
Length stenotic segment : 6.74 mm
Position of proximal border : 13.70 mm
Position of distal border : 20.44 mm
MLA densitometry : 0.57 mm2
MLA circular : 0.26 mm2
% area stenosis densitometry : 90%
% area stenosis circular : 95%
Reference area : 5.79 mm2
Volume stenotic segment : 13.98 mm3
Plaque area : 8.35 mm2
Plaque volume : 22.47 mm3
Symmetry : 0.59

A

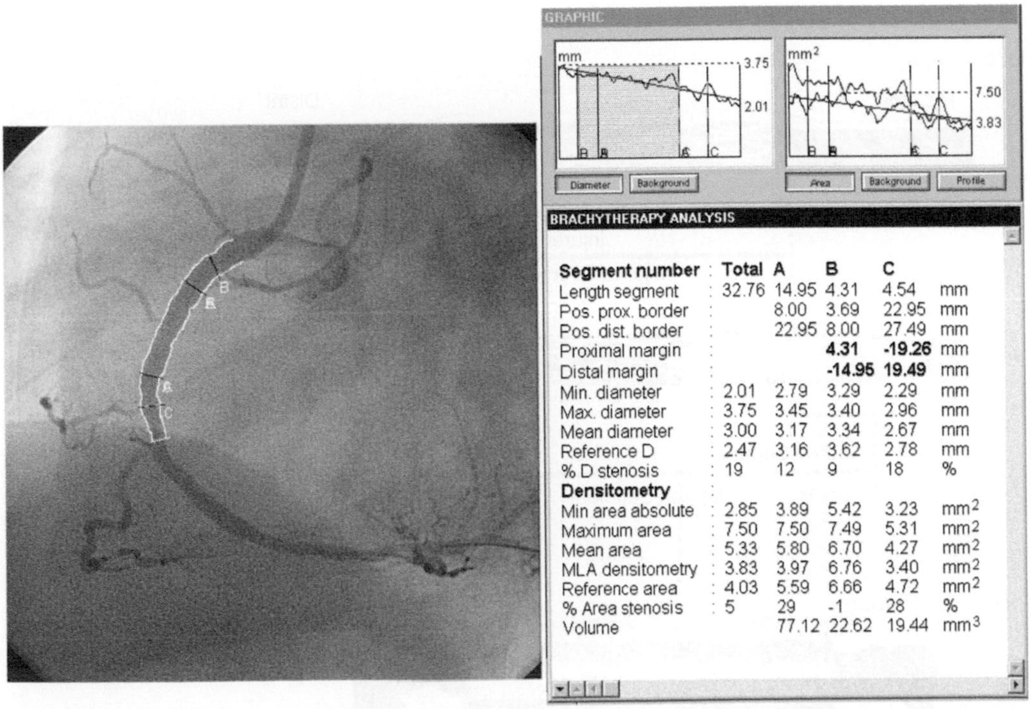
GRAPHIC
mm
3.75
2.01
mm2
7.50
3.83
Diameter
Background
Area
Background
Profile
BRACHYTHERAPY ANALYSIS
Segment number : Total A B C
Length segment : 32.76 14.95 4.31 4.54 mm
Pos. prox. border : 8.00 3.69 22.95 mm
Pos. dist. border : 22.95 8.00 27.49 mm
Proximal margin : 4.31 -19.26 mm
Distal margin : -14.95 19.49 mm
Min. diameter : 2.01 2.79 3.29 2.29 mm
Max. diameter : 3.75 3.45 3.40 2.96 mm
Mean diameter : 3.00 3.17 3.34 2.67 mm
Reference D : 2.47 3.16 3.62 2.78 mm
% D stenosis : 19 12 9 18 %
Densitometry :
Min area absolute : 2.85 3.89 5.42 3.23 mm2
Maximum area : 7.50 7.50 7.49 5.31 mm2
Mean area : 5.33 5.80 6.70 4.27 mm2
MLA densitometry : 3.83 3.97 6.76 3.40 mm2
Reference area : 4.03 5.59 6.66 4.72 mm2
% Area stenosis : 5 29 -1 28 %
Volume 77.12 22.62 19.44 mm3

B

Figure 2.3 Serial angiography to assess the efficacy of a drug-eluting stent. QCA analyses of the preprocedure angiogram (**A**), the postprocedure angiogram (**B**), and the follow-up angiogram (**C**) identify no restenosis in the in-stent segment as well as that of the proximal and distal edge segments.

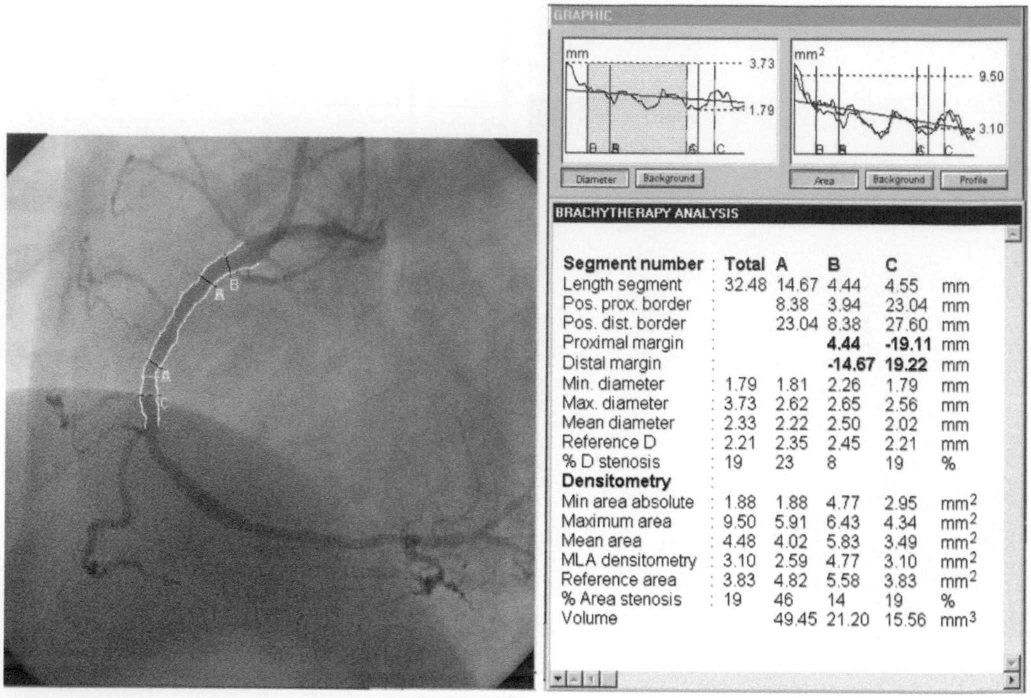

Segment number	Total	A	B	C	
Length segment	32.48	14.67	4.44	4.55	mm
Pos. prox. border		8.38	3.94	23.04	mm
Pos. dist. border		23.04	8.38	27.60	mm
Proximal margin			**4.44**	**-19.11**	mm
Distal margin			**-14.67**	**19.22**	mm
Min. diameter	1.79	1.81	2.26	1.79	mm
Max. diameter	3.73	2.62	2.65	2.56	mm
Mean diameter	2.33	2.22	2.50	2.02	mm
Reference D	2.21	2.35	2.45	2.21	mm
% D stenosis	19	23	8	19	%
Densitometry					
Min area absolute	1.88	1.88	4.77	2.95	mm^2
Maximum area	9.50	5.91	6.43	4.34	mm^2
Mean area	4.48	4.02	5.83	3.49	mm^2
MLA densitometry	3.10	2.59	4.77	3.10	mm^2
Reference area	3.83	4.82	5.58	3.83	mm^2
% Area stenosis	19	46	14	19	%
Volume		49.45	21.20	15.56	mm^3

Figure 2.3 (*Continued*)

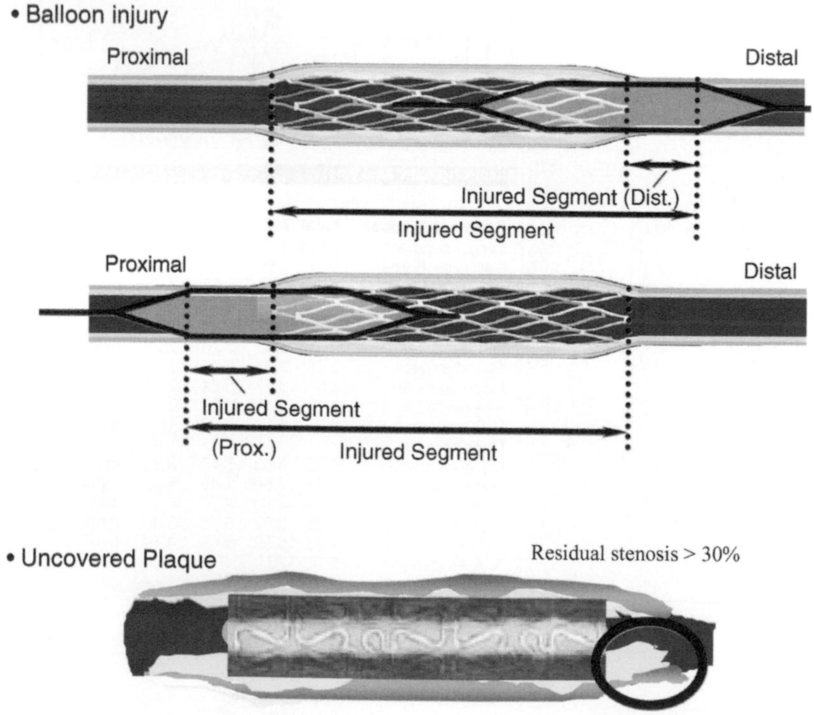

Figure 2.4 Definition of longitudinal geographic miss.

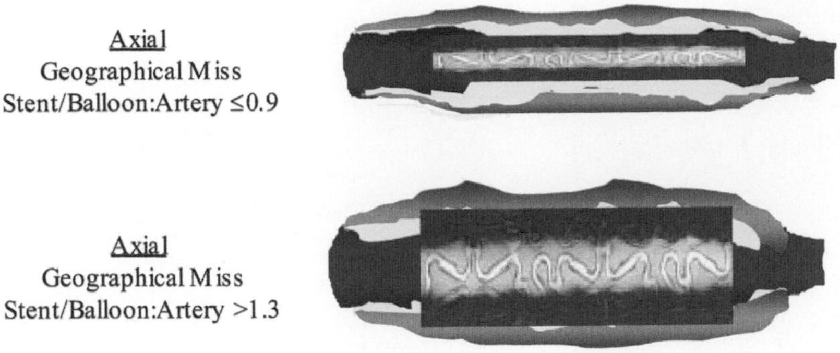

Figure 2.5 Definition of axial geographic miss.

revascularization between patients with and without longitudinal geographic miss (6.1% vs. 2.6%, $p = 0.001$). To note, rates of target vessel revascularization were similar between patients with and without axial geographic miss (4.2% vs. 4.3%, $p =$ NS). The incidence of myocardial infarction was also similar between patients with and without axial geographic miss. Therefore, it is considered that interventional operators should avoid longitudinal geographic miss. Of the longitudinal geographic miss observed in the STLLR trial, the miss was related to balloon injury in 53.7%, uncovered plaque in 32.4%, and both in 13.9% of the procedures. With regard to the sites, the miss was observed in the proximal edge in 30.5%, distal edge in 33.9%, and both edges in 23.1%. Of course, operators should avoid making balloon injury sites, which are not fully covered with drug-eluting stents by carefully looking at cine angiograms. Online QCA may help operators to avoid making the segments with uncovered plaque. Technicians and/or physicians should perform online QCA to check whether there are proximal or distal edge segments of which diameter stenosis was greater than 30% at postprocedure. This kind of attitude and analysis during the procedure may further improve the performance of drug-eluting stents.

ASSESSMENT OF ENDOTHELIAL DYSFUNCTION

The presence of paradoxical vasoconstriction induced by acetylcholine has been shown in coronary patients at sites of severe stenosis or moderate wall irregularities and in angiographic normal segments.[14,15] Coronary artery spasm after acetylcholine infusion has also been demonstrated in patients with variant angina. The assessment of the variability and severity of coronary spasm of variant angina over time has been performed by QCA.[16] With the widespread clinical application of coronary drug-eluting stents, the concern has been raised that drug-eluting stents may hamper endothelial function in the regions adjacent to the stents. Hofma et al. described endothelial dysfunction in the peri-stent segments after implantation of sirolimus-eluting stents using QCA with acetylcholine testing.[17] Recently, the author have experienced one patient who sometimes suffered from angina at rest at 8 months after implantation of two sirolimus-eluting stents in left main coronary artery to left anterior descending artery. His invasive coronary angiography showed no restenosis both in the in-stent segment and in the distal edge segment, however, intracoronary infusion of acetylcholine induced severe vasoconstriction in the regions distal to the sirolimus-eluting stents (Fig. 2.6). To note, less vasoconstriction was observed in his left circumflex artery. Online QCA was helpful to compare the severity of coronary spasm with acetylcholine between in the segments with and without the drug-eluting stents. He received additional vasoactive medications including calcium channel blocker and nitrates after the angiography. The medical therapy relieved his angina symptoms at rest. Clinicians should not overlook the potential risk of symptomatic coronary vasospasm after implantation of drug-eluting stents in relation to endothelial dysfunction. Acetylcholine infusion test assessed by QCA should be considered in case patients experience angina symptoms, although there is no angiographic restenosis.

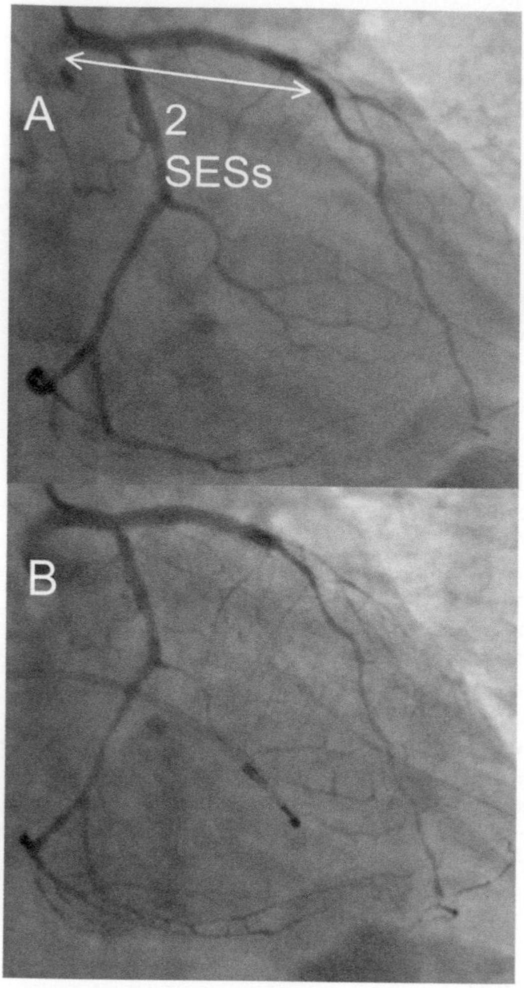

Figure 2.6 (**A**) No in-stent restenosis is observed in coronary angiography at 8 months following implantation of two sirolimus-eluting stents (SES) from left main coronary artery to left anterior descending coronary artery. (**B**) Acetylcholine infusion induces more severe vasoconstriction to acetylcholine in the distal segments adjacent to SESs when compared to left circumflex artery.

CONCLUSIONS

Online QCA during procedure might be helpful to assess and avoid longitudinal geographic miss with drug-eluting stents. It might also be useful to evaluate abnormal vasoconstriction after implantation of drug-eluting stents.

REFERENCES

1. DeRouen TA, Murray JA, Owen W. Variability in the analysis of coronary arteriograms. Circulation 1977; 55:324–328.
2. White CW, Wright CB, Doty DB, et al. Does visual interpretation of the coronary arteriogram predict the physiologic importance of a coronary stenosis? N Engl J Med 1984; 310:819–824.
3. Katritsis D, Lythall DA, Cooper IC, et al. Assessment of coronary angioplasty: Comparison of visual assessment, hand-held caliper measurement and automated digital quantitation. Cathet Cardiovasc Diagn 1988; 15:237–242.
4. Serruys PW, Foley DP, de Feyter P. Quantitative Coronary Angiography in Clinical Practice. Boston, MA: Kluwer Academic Publishers, 1994.
5. Waksman R, White RL, Chan RC, et al. Intracoronary gamma-radiation therapy after angioplasty inhibits recurrence in patients with in-stent restenosis. Circulation 2000; 101:2165–2171.
6. Leon MB, Teirstein PS, Moses JW, et al. Localized intracoronary gamma-radiation therapy to inhibit the recurrence of restenosis after stenting. N Engl J Med 2001; 344:250–256.
7. Albiero R, Nishida T, Adamian M, et al. Edge restenosis after implantation of high activity (32)P radioactive beta-emitting stents. Circulation 2000; 101:2454–2457.

8. Morice MC, Serruys PW, Sousa JE, et al. A randomized comparison of a sirolimus-eluting stent with a standard stent for coronary revascularization. N Engl J Med 2002; 346:1773–1780.
9. Colombo A, Drzewiecki J, Banning A, et al. Randomized study to assess the effectiveness of slow- and moderate-release polymer-based paclitaxel-eluting stents for coronary artery lesions. Circulation 2003; 108:788–794.
10. Serruys PW, Degertekin M, Tanabe K, et al. Vascular responses at proximal and distal edges of paclitaxel-eluting stents: Serial intravascular ultrasound analysis from the TAXUS II trial. Circulation 2004; 109:627–633.
11. Lemos PA, Saia F, Ligthart JM, et al. Coronary restenosis after sirolimus-eluting stent implantation: Morphological description and mechanistic analysis from a consecutive series of cases. Circulation 2003; 108:257–260.
12. Sabate M, Costa MA, Kozuma K, et al. Geographic miss: A cause of treatment failure in radio-oncology applied to intracoronary radiation therapy. Circulation 2000; 101:2467–2471.
13. Costa MA, Angiolillo DJ, Tannenbaum M, et al. STLLR Investigators. Impact of stent deployment procedural factors on long-term effectiveness and safety of sirolimus-eluting stents (final results of the multicenter prospective STLLR trial). Am J Cardiol 2008; 101(12):1704–1711.
14. Werns SW, Walton JA, Hsia HH, et al. Evidence of endothelial dysfunction in angiographically normal coronary arteries of patients with coronary artery disease. Circulation 1989; 79:287–291.
15. Ludmer PL, Selwyn AP, Shook TL, et al. Paradoxical vasoconstriction induced by acetylcholine in atherosclerotic coronary arteries. N Engl J Med 1986; 315:1046–1051.
16. Ozaki Y, Takatsu F, Osugi J, et al. Long-term study of recurrent vasospastic angina using coronary angiograms during ergonovine provocation tests. Am Heart J 1992; 123:1191–1198.
17. Hofma SH, van der Giessen WJ, van Dalen BM, et al. Indication of long-term endothelial dysfunction after sirolimus-eluting stent implantation. Eur Heart J 2006; 27:166–170.

3 Preintervention evaluation of chronic total occlusions

Hussein M. Ismail and Angela Hoye

INTRODUCTION

Chronic total coronary occlusions (CTO) represent approximately 10% of lesions treated by percutaneous coronary intervention (PCI).[1] CTOs are a common finding on diagnostic angiography; in one large registry, 52% of patients with significant coronary disease (defined as a coronary artery lesion with a diameter stenosis of >75%) had at least one CTO.[2] Importantly, the presence of a CTO affects the subsequent choice of therapy made by the physician, with the majority of such patients managed medically or referred for coronary bypass graft surgery.[2] This is likely to reflect the complex nature of these lesions and the perceived difficulty in treating them with PCI because of lower rates of success due to the inability to recanalize the lesion. However, the advancement of equipment particularly in wire technology, together with the adoption of specialized wiring techniques have improved PCI recanalization success rates in contemporary practice in many centers. Optimal angiographic images are vital in the assessment of CTO lesions to gain information of characteristics that deem the lesion suitable for a strategy of PCI.

THE IMPORTANCE OF CTO RECANALIZATION

Successful CTO PCI has been shown to improve patient symptoms and exercise capacity, and improve left ventricular function.[3] Large registry studies have also reported that successful PCI may improve long-term survival.[4–6] In a consecutive series of 874 CTO patients, Hoye et al. found a 5-year survival rate of 93.5% in those with successful PCI compared with only 88.0% following unsuccessful CTO PCI (HR, 1.86; 95% CI, 1.12–3.10; $p = 0.02$).

CTO assessment

Good-quality diagnostic coronary angiography is vital in assessing CTOs. In the absence of antegrade filling, the role of quantitative angiography is less important in an occluded vessel. It is important to try to identify patients most likely to benefit from attempted PCI of a CTO. Such an attempt is not without risk—registry data suggest that in patients whereby PCI is unsuccessful, the short-term mortality rate is 1% to 2%.[4–6] The assessment of a CTO must not be undertaken in isolation, and it is also important to assess the presence of other lesions—patients with multivessel disease and a complex CTO may be better considered for coronary artery bypass grafting (CABG) than PCI.

When treating a patient with a CTO, one of the first principles is the evaluation of viability. Viable myocardium has the potential for functional recovery after reperfusion therapy, whereas infarcted and nonviable myocardium has not. Thus, it is of great clinical importance to be able to distinguish viable from nonviable myocardium in order not to expose patients to unnecessary risks associated with revascularization procedures.[7] The presence of viability has been shown to be a predictor of long-term prognosis after revascularization.[8]

Diagnostic coronary angiography will determine the location of a CTO and the region of the left ventricle that it supplies. Left ventriculography undertaken at the time of diagnostic angiography may demonstrate that the CTO is associated with a regional wall movement abnormality. The absence of a wall movement abnormality is a sufficient evidence of myocardial viability to indicate consideration of revascularization. However, the presence of a regional wall movement abnormality with akinesia does not necessarily imply lack of viability. Information from the angiogram should in this case be combined with information obtained from noninvasive imaging methods. Viability may be assessed from a range of imaging modalities including contrast or stress echocardiography, nuclear perfusion imaging (single-photon emission computerized tomography (SPECT) scanning), contrast-enhanced magnetic resonance

Table 3.1 Factors to assess during diagnostic coronary angiography as possible predictors of the outcome of a subsequent percutaneous attempt of CTO recanalization

Factors thought to be possible predictors of unsuccessful CTO angioplasty
Duration of occlusion >3 months
Absolute occlusion (TIMI 0 flow through the occlusion)
Longer lesion length (especially if >15 mm)
Blunt stump
Side branch at the point of occlusion
Calcification
Presence of bridging collaterals
Presence of retrograde collaterals
Poor visualization of the distal vessel
Small caliber/diseased distal vessel
Tortuosity of the proximal vessel, especially if heavily diseased
Ostial location of the occlusion
Bifurcation present at the distal cap of the occlusion
Presence of multivessel disease

imaging, and PET (positron emission tomography) scanning. Patients with myocardial viability on dobutamine stress echocardiography have been shown to have better outcome with revascularization compared with medical therapy.[9,10] Recently, delayed contrast–enhanced magnetic resonance imaging (DE-MRI) has emerged as a new reference method for infarct characterization. By acquiring images after the injection of a gadolinium-based extracellular contrast agent, infarcted myocardium can be visualized and assessed accurately.[7] In patients with a CTO, preprocedural MRI scanning can predict the beneficial effect of revascularization on improvement in end-systolic left ventricular volume and ejection fraction.[11]

Angiographic predictors of successful CTO recanalization

Over the last 20 years, many factors have been suggested as predictors of whether subsequent angioplasty is likely to be successful or not (Table 3.1). Importantly, several of these proposed predictors relate to angiographic features of the CTO and should therefore be assessed during diagnostic catheterization. One strong predictor of procedural failure is the duration of occlusion; a true CTO is at least of 3 months duration which can be typically estimated from an index clinical event, such as a myocardial infarction or a change in anginal pattern with prolonged chest pain.[3]

Functional rather than absolute occlusions

Functional occlusions should be differentiated from true chronic total occlusions as they have a significantly higher angioplasty success rate. Indeed, in line with the recent guidance from the European CTO club, in contemporary practice, functional occlusions should probably be excluded from series of true CTOs.[12] Functional occlusions are lesions whereby there is slow antegrade (TIMI 1) flow through the occlusion but without complete opacification of the distal coronary bed. An example is shown in Figure 3.1. To determine whether a lesion is a true CTO, it is therefore important to take a long angiographic run and evaluate the image on a frame-by-frame basis—true CTOs will have no (TIMI 0) flow across the occlusion. In order to make a long angiographic run, coronary injection is made in the standard way using the usual volume of contrast, but acquisition is continued until the contrast clears.

Lesion length

Several studies have suggested that the length of the occlusion is an important predictor of procedural success.[13–18] As reported in the TOAST-GISE study, procedural failure is higher with a longer length of occlusion, especially if >15 mm, or if the lesion length is not measurable on diagnostic angiography because of an absence of antegrade filling.[16] An example of a long complex occlusion of the right coronary artery is shown in Figure 3.2. During diagnostic catheterization, in order to measure the occlusion length, it is important to take a long acquisition to allow time for the distal segment of the vessel to be filled through collaterals (Fig. 3.3). In some occlusions, the distal vessel can only be seen via filling from retrograde collaterals (see below). In this instance, use of simultaneous coronary injections should be

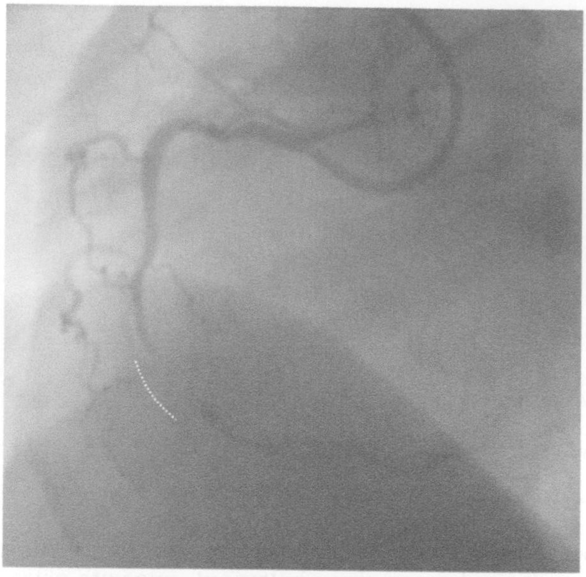

Figure 3.1 Example of a functional total occlusion in the mid-right coronary artery (RCA). Slow filling of the distal RCA was evident, however, careful analysis demonstrated evidence of TIMI 1 intraluminal flow through the "occlusion."

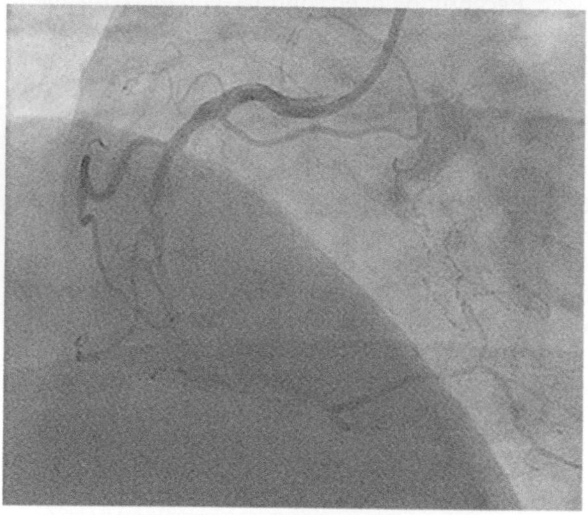

Figure 3.2 Long segment of occlusion starting from the mid-right coronary artery (RCA) up to the bifurcation of the distal RCA. This type of occlusion is significantly more difficult to recanalize than short occlusions such as that shown in Figure 3.4B.

utilized during angioplasty to assess the occlusion length and facilitate successful recanalization (Fig. 3.6C). The contralateral approach can be achieved by puncturing the same groin with 4 F or 5 F sheath and using 4 F or 5 F diagnostic catheters or more commonly by obtaining access from a radial approach or the other groin.

Stump morphology

A tapered as opposed to an abrupt morphology at the point of coronary occlusion has been shown by several investigators to predict a favorable angioplasty procedure outcome.[3] These investigators reported success rates with a tapered morphology of 68% to 88% versus 43% to 59% if the occlusion was abrupt ($p = 0.0001$). Diagnostic angiography should therefore evaluate the stump (Fig. 3.4), with the choice of view targeted to demonstrate the stump morphology clearly, particularly if hidden by the presence of side branches (Fig. 3.5).

Side branch at the point of occlusion

The presence of a side branch at the point of occlusion is a predictor of angioplasty failure, an example is shown in Figure 3.6.[3] This is likely to reflect the difficulty that may occur in penetrating the proximal cap of the occlusion that is often particularly tough; the angioplasty wire tends to take the path of least resistance and will prolapse into the branch vessel. A side

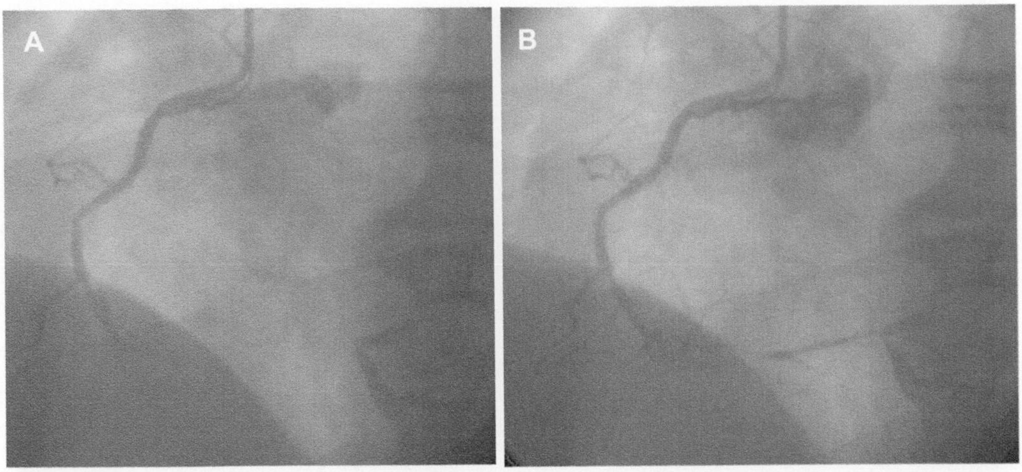

Figure 3.3 The importance of taking a long run is evident in these images of an occlusion of the right coronary artery (RCA). (**A**) A short run demonstrates an absence of antegrade flow indicating a complex occlusion. (**B**) A much longer acquisition was made and slow filling of the distal RCA was observed suggesting angioplasty is more likely to be successful.

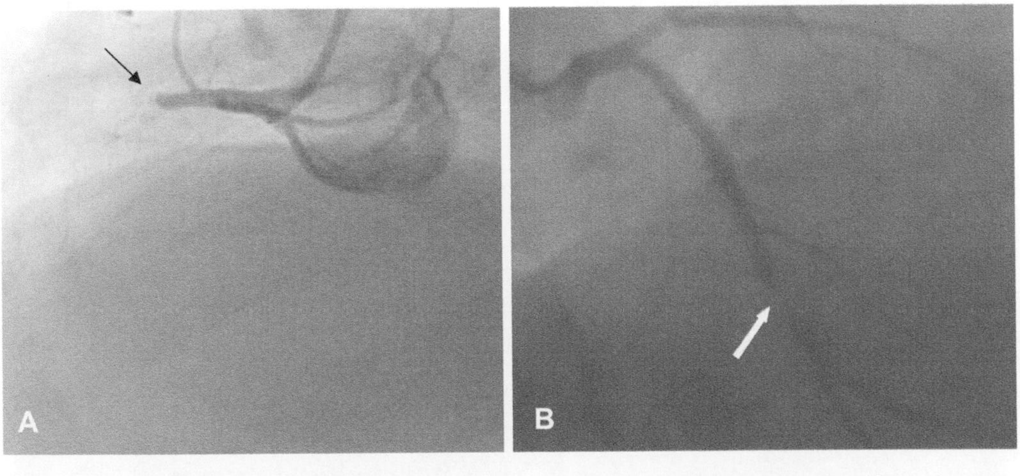

Figure 3.4 (**A**) Example of a complete chronic occlusion of the right coronary artery with a blunt, abrupt stump. (**B**) Example of a simpler occlusion of the circumflex artery with a tapered stump and short occlusion length.

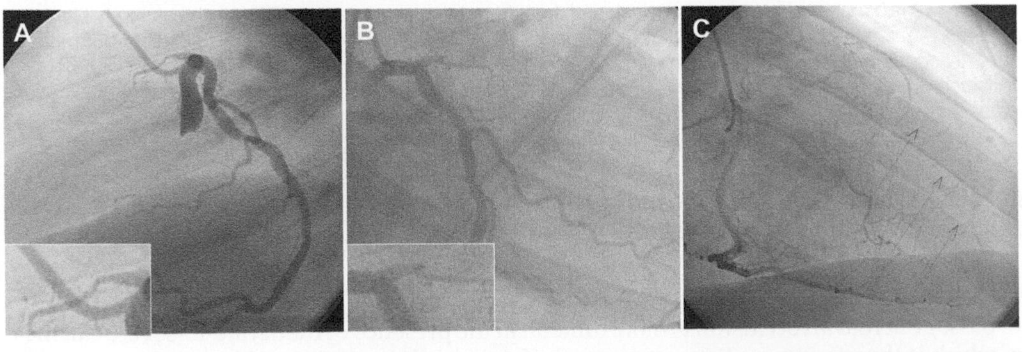

Figure 3.5 The importance of taking multiple views to visualize the point of occlusion. (**A**) The lateral view suggests a blunt stump with a side branch at the point of occlusion of the left anterior descending (LAD) artery (see inset). (**B**) The right anterior oblique (RAO) caudal view demonstrates that the occlusion is less complex—the stump is tapered and the side branch originates proximal to the point of occlusion (see inset). (**C**) Filling of the LAD distal to the occlusion is via retrograde collaterals (Rentrop grade 2) from the right coronary artery.

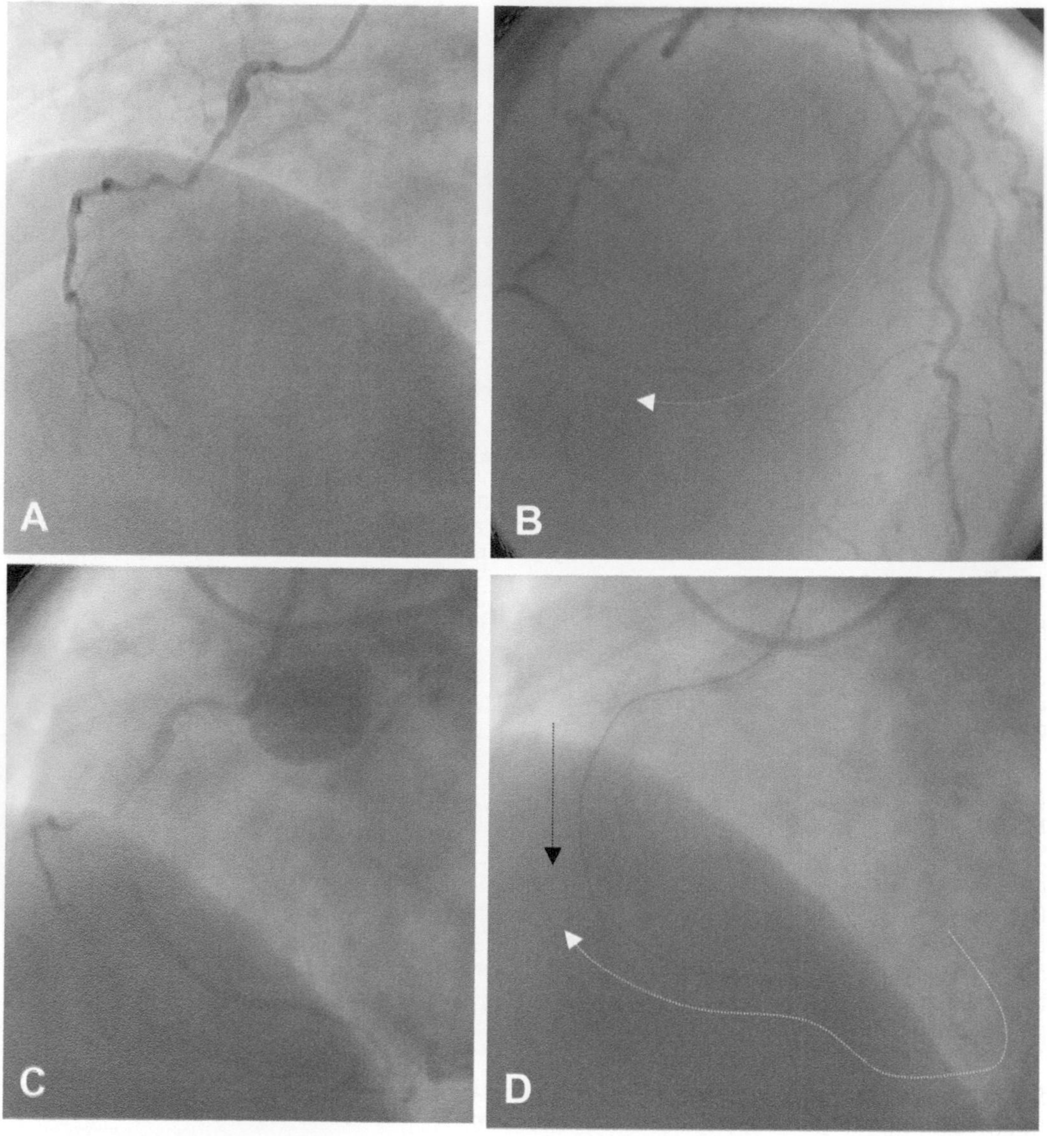

Figure 3.6 (**A**) Example of a complex occlusion of the mid-right coronary artery (RCA)—the stump is blunt and there is a sizeable side branch at the point of occlusion. (**B**) The distal RCA is filled via collaterals from the left anterior descending artery. A large septal vessel is evident that is relatively straight and is assessed in detail to be considered for use for CTO recanalization using a retrograde approach. (**C**) Simultaneous coronary injections made at the time of angioplasty can be used to better define the length of occlusion. (**D**) The occlusion was successfully recanalized using combined antegrade (*black arrow*) and retrograde (*white arrow*) approaches.

branch that originates just proximal to the stump does not pose the same problem and so the anatomy of the point of occlusion must be clearly visualized on angiography.

The presence of calcification

Wire passage across an occlusion is more difficult in the presence of moderate-to-severe calcification, which is therefore a predictor of unsuccessful angioplasty and should be evaluated during coronary angiography.[15–18] Recent studies have demonstrated that more detailed assessment of coronary calcification can be made on multislice computed tomography (MSCT)[17,19] and can predict the outcome of CTO angioplasty. The use of preprocedural MSCT to detail features of CTOs may facilitate a higher rate of successful CTO recanalization.[20]

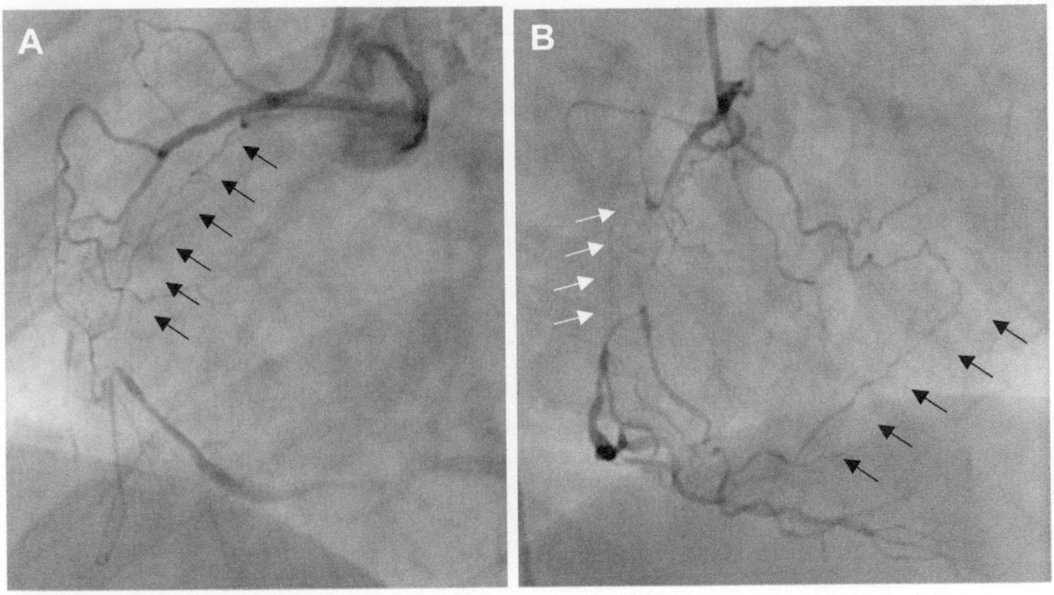

Figure 3.7 Example of a complex chronic total occlusion of the mid-right coronary artery (RCA): (**A**) LAO view and (**B**) RAO view. The stump is blunt with a side branch at the point of occlusion; the distal end of the occlusion occurs at a bifurcation. The distal vessel is filled via collateral vessels; two larger collaterals are evident (*black arrows*), with smaller vessels directly bridging the occlusion (*white arrows*). These bridging collaterals typically demonstrate "corkscrew" tortuosity.

Bridging collateral vessels

Histopathology studies demonstrate the presence of neovascularization with microvessels. These form of the vasa vasorum are seen in the adventitia and outer media and tend to run radially. If well developed, they are termed as bridging collaterals and may be seen angiographically (which has a resolution of ~250 μm). They "bridge" the occlusion and allow for anterograde opacification of the distal coronary bed (Fig. 3.7). They typically have a "corkscrew" appearance and their development appears to be proportional to the duration of occlusion. The presence of bridging collateral vessels is a strong predictor of procedural failure,[3] such vessels are friable and may perforate with an angioplasty wire relatively easily during attempted recanalization.

EVALUATION OF THE PROXIMAL PART OF THE OCCLUDED VESSEL

In addition to optimal imaging of the stump, evaluation of the proximal segment of the CTO vessel is very important, as it will help the operator to choose the proper guiding catheter. This is the first key to successful angioplasty—the guiding catheter should be coaxially oriented, and provide good stability and backup forces to facilitate wire crossing, balloon advancement, and subsequent stent implantation.

EVALUATION OF THE NONOCCLUDED VESSEL

The other coronary vessels should be evaluated for disease, as the presence of multivessel disease is a predictor of unsuccessful CTO angioplasty.[15,16] In addition, the other vessel should be evaluated for the presence of retrograde collaterals which provide cross-filling to the distal bed of the occluded vessel (Fig. 3.5c) (though it should be emphasized that the presence of retrograde collaterals does not necessarily indicate left ventricular viability). A long run is important to provide sufficient information regarding the quality of these collateral vessels, which can be graded according to the Rentrop classification (Table 3.2).[21]

Recently, good-quality retrograde collaterals have become more important due to the introduction of the retrograde technique to facilitate successful CTO recanalization.[22,23] Using this approach, the occlusion is reached retrogradely via a collateral channel, and this has been shown to increase the CTO angioplasty success rate.[24] Features of suitable retrograde

Table 3.2 The Rentrop classification of retrograde collaterals

Grade 0	No retrograde filling
Grade 1	Filling of side branches of the artery via collateral channels without visualization of the epicardial segment
Grade 2	Partial filling of the epicardial segment via collateral channels
Grade 3	Complete filling of the epicardial segment of the artery being dilated via collateral channels

collaterals include being a septal vessel of relatively good size, comparatively straight with a lack of corkscrewing and continuous to the distal part of the target vessel without interruption (Fig. 3.6). During angioplasty using the retrograde technique, this collateral vessel is wired using a hydrophilic floppy guidewire, which is advanced into the distal part of the occluded artery. This wire may then be substituted with a specialized CTO wire, and recanalization of the CTO is facilitated by retrograde crossing of the occlusion—in many complex CTOs this direction of wire passage is more likely to successfully cross the occlusion than the antegrade approach.

CONCLUSIONS

Chronic total occlusions are a relatively frequent finding during diagnostic coronary angiography. It is important that the lesion is well imaged, as this enables more optimal planning of the subsequent therapy. When undertaking optimal coronary angiography, at least two orthogonal views should be taken, and an appropriate angle should be chosen to ensure clear imaging of the occlusion, particularly the stump. Long acquisitions must be made of both the occluded vessel, and the non-occluded vessel to evaluate the presence, size, and course of retrograde collaterals. Detailed assessment of a CTO at the time of diagnostic coronary angiography will help to decide on the most appropriate treatment for the patient (revascularization with either angioplasty or bypass graft surgery). In addition, angiography provides important information to plan the strategy of CTO angioplasty such as the choice of guiding catheter, guidewire, and technique (such as an antegrade or retrograde approach) to facilitate an increased chance of procedural success.

REFERENCES

1. Delacretaz E, Meier B. Therapeutic strategy with total coronary artery occlusions. Am J Cardiol 1997; 79(2):185–187.
2. Christofferson RD, Lehmann KG, Martin GV, et al. Effect of chronic total coronary occlusion on treatment strategy. Am J Cardiol 2005; 95(9):1088–1091.
3. Puma JA, Sketch MH Jr, Tcheng JE, et al. Percutaneous revascularization of chronic coronary occlusions: An overview. J Am Coll Cardiol 1995; 26(1):1–11.
4. Suero JA, Marso SP, Jones PG, et al. Procedural outcomes and long-term survival among patients undergoing percutaneous coronary intervention of a chronic total occlusion in native coronary arteries: A 20-year experience. J Am Coll Cardiol 2001; 38(2):409–414.
5. Hoye A, van Domburg RT, Sonnenschein K, et al. Percutaneous coronary intervention for chronic total occlusions: The Thoraxcenter experience 1992–2002. Eur Heart J 2005; 26(24):2630–2636.
6. Aziz S, Stables RH, Grayson AD, et al. Percutaneous coronary intervention for chronic total occlusions: Improved survival for patients with successful revascularization compared to a failed procedure. Catheter Cardiovasc Interv 2007; 70(1):15–20.
7. Engblom H, Arheden H, Foster JE, et al. Myocardial infarct quantification: Is magnetic resonance imaging ready to serve as a gold standard for electrocardiography? J Electrocardiol 2007; 40(3): 243–245.
8. Rizzello V, Poldermans D, Schinkel AF, et al. Long term prognostic value of myocardial viability and ischaemia during dobutamine stress echocardiography in patients with ischaemic cardiomyopathy undergoing coronary revascularisation. Heart 2006; 92(2):239–244.
9. Afridi I, Grayburn PA, Panza JA, et al. Myocardial viability during dobutamine echocardiography predicts survival in patients with coronary artery disease and severe left ventricular systolic dysfunction. J Am Coll Cardiol 1998; 32(4):921–926.

10. Meluzin J, Cerny J, Frelich M, et al. Prognostic value of the amount of dysfunctional but viable myocardium in revascularized patients with coronary artery disease and left ventricular dysfunction. Investigators of this multicenter study. J Am Coll Cardiol 1998; 32(4):912–920.
11. Kirschbaum SW, Baks T, Van Den Ent M, et al. Evaluation of left ventricular function three years after percutaneous recanalization of chronic total coronary occlusions. Am J Cardiol 2008; 101(2):179–185.
12. di Mario C, Werner G, Sianos G, et al. European perspective in the recanalisation of chronic total occlusions (CTO): Consensus document from the EuroCTO Club. Eurointervention 2007; 3:30–43.
13. Maiello L, Colombo A, Gianrossi R, et al. Coronary angioplasty of chronic occlusions: Factors predictive of procedural success. Am Heart J 1992; 124(3):581–584.
14. Tan KH, Sulke N, Taub NA, et al. Determinants of success of coronary angioplasty in patients with a chronic total occlusion: A multiple logistic regression model to improve selection of patients. Br Heart J 1993; 70(2):126–131.
15. Noguchi T, Miyazaki MS, Morii I, et al. Percutaneous transluminal coronary angioplasty of chronic total occlusions. Determinants of primary success and long-term clinical outcome. Catheter Cardiovasc Interv 2000; 49(3):258–264.
16. Olivari Z, Rubartelli P, Piscione F, et al. Immediate results and one-year clinical outcome after percutaneous coronary interventions in chronic total occlusions: Data from a multicenter, prospective, observational study (TOAST-GISE). J Am Coll Cardiol 2003; 41(10):1672–1678.
17. Mollet NR, Hoye A, Lemos PA, et al. Value of preprocedure multislice computed tomographic coronary angiography to predict the outcome of percutaneous recanalization of chronic total occlusions. Am J Cardiol 2005; 95(2):240–243.
18. Tanaka HKM, Inoue K, Goto T. Predictors of procedural failure in chronic total occlusion. J Am Coll Cardiol 2005; 45(3 Suppl. 1):62 A.
19. Yokoyama N, Yamamoto Y, Suzuki S, et al. Impact of 16-slice computed tomography in percutaneous coronary intervention of chronic total occlusions. Catheter Cardiovasc Interv 2006; 68(1):1–7.
20. Kaneda H, Saito S, Shiono T, et al. Sixty-four-slice computed tomography-facilitated percutaneous coronary intervention for chronic total occlusion. Int J Cardiol 2007; 115(1):130–132.
21. Rentrop KP, Cohen M, Blanke H, et al. Changes in collateral channel filling immediately after controlled coronary artery occlusion by an angioplasty balloon in human subjects. J Am Coll Cardiol 1985; 5(3):587–592.
22. Ozawa N. A new understanding of chronic total occlusion from a novel PCI technique that involves a retrograde approach to the right coronary artery via a septal branch and passing of the guidewire to a guiding catheter on the other side of the lesion. Catheter Cardiovasc Interv 2006; 68(6):907–913.
23. Mitsudo K. The how and why of chronic total occlusion part one: How to treat CTOs. Eurointervention 2006; 2:375–381.
24. Saito S. Different strategies of retrograde approach in coronary angioplasty for chronic total occlusion. Catheter Cardiovasc Interv 2008; 71(1):8–19.

4 Evaluation of myocardial perfusion

Claudia P. Hochberg and C. Michael Gibson

INTRODUCTION

Epicardial coronary artery patency has been the primary outcome measure of coronary angiography and intervention. Strategies to improve the effectiveness of both fibrinolytic and percutaneous interventional therapies have relied on these angiographic measures to assess treatment efficacy and outcome. Despite this reliance on epicardial patency there is significant variability in morbidity and mortality among patients with "full" restoration of coronary artery blood flow or TIMI grade 3 flow. The realization that restoration of epicardial flow is necessary but not sufficient has led to the evaluation of the myocardial microvasculature and reperfusion downstream as a more accurate predictor of clinical outcome and treatment efficacy.[1,2] The goal of this chapter is to review the methods used to directly and indirectly evaluate myocardial perfusion.

TIMI FLOW GRADES (TFGs)

For the past 20 years, epicardial blood flow as measured by the Thrombolysis in Myocardial Infarction (TIMI) flow grade classification scheme has been used to evaluate coronary blood flow in acute coronary syndromes (Table 4.1).[1] It has become the benchmark comparator in trials to analyze the angiographic outcomes of epicardial reperfusion strategies, and the association of TFGs with clinical outcomes and mortality has been well documented.[2] High rates of TIMI grade 3 flow approaching 100% after primary percutaneous intervention (PCI) have been reported when a "3 cardiac cycles to fill the artery" definition is applied. However, when assessed more rigorously, rates of TIMI grade 3 flow may in fact be substantially lower at approximately 80%.[3] Other confounding variables limit the use of TIMI 3 flow as the sole correlate of mortality. Infarct location is one such confounder. For example, the majority of TIMI grade 3 flow is observed in the right coronary artery (RCA), while the majority of TIMI grade 2 flow is observed in the left anterior descending (LAD) artery territory.[2] The differential between the mortality rate of inferior myocardial infarctions (MI) and anterior wall myocardial infarctions may therefore account for some of the improved outcomes among patients with TIMI grade 3 flow.[2] Use of more precise angiographic measures such as the TIMI frame count support the notion that improved epicardial flow is associated with improved clinical outcomes, however, the magnitude of the clinical improvement associated with TIMI grade 3 flow may have been overestimated. An additional variable that complicates the association of TFG with mortality is the nonlinearity of TFGs. Far greater clinical improvement is seen with re-establishment of TIMI grade 2 flow from TIMI grade 0/1 flow than is seen in progress from grade 2 to grade 3 flow.

Restoration of epicardial flow does not necessarily lead to restoration of tissue level or microvascular perfusion,[4] suggesting that "not all TIMI grade 3 flow is created equally." Impaired tissue perfusion can persist despite restoration of epicardial flow and its assessment can provide important diagnostic and prognostic information. Perfusion of the myocardium can be assessed directly by the myocardial blush grade (MBG), TIMI Myocardial Perfusion Grade (TMPG), coronary clearance frame count or digital subtraction angiography or can be assessed indirectly by quantitative measurements of epicardial flow rates with use of corrected TIMI frame counts. Beyond epicardial flow, myocardial perfusion has been shown to be an independent predictor of outcome.[5]

DIRECT METHODS OF MEASURING MYOCARDIAL PERFUSION

TIMI myocardial perfusion grade (TMPG) and myocardial blush grade (MBG)

Direct measurement of myocardial perfusion provides important diagnostic and prognostic information, as impaired tissue perfusion may persist despite restoration of epicardial flow. Two methods of direct measurement of myocardial perfusion are the TMPG and the MBG. In

Table 4.1 Definitions of the TFG and TMPG systems

Grade	Characteristics
TFG, a grading system for epicardial coronary flow	
0	No perfusion; no antegrade flow beyond the point of occlusion
1	Penetration without perfusion; the contrast material passes beyond the area of obstruction but "hangs up" and fails to opacify the entire coronary bed distal to the obstruction for the duration of the cine run
2	Partial reperfusion; the contrast material passes across the obstruction and opacifies the coronary bed distal to the obstruction. However, the rate of entry of contrast into the vessel distal to the obstruction and/or its rate of clearance from the distal bed is perceptibly slower than its entry into and/or clearance from comparable areas not perfused by the culprit vessel (e.g., the opposite coronary artery or coronary bed proximal to the obstruction)
3	Complete perfusion; antegrade flow into the bed distal to the obstruction occurs as promptly as into the bed proximal to the obstruction, and the clearance of the contrast material from the involved bed is as rapid as from an uninvolved bed in the same vessel or the opposite artery
TMPG, a grading system for myocardial perfusion	
0	Dye fails to enter the microvasculature; there is either minimal or no ground glass appearance ("blush") or opacification of the myocardium in the distribution of the culprit artery indicating lack of tissue level perfusion
1	Dye slowly enters but fails to exit the microvasculature; there is the ground glass appearance ("blush") or opacification of the myocardium in the distribution of the culprit lesion that fails to clear from the microvasculature, and dye staining is present on the next injection (~30 sec between injections)
2	Delayed entry and exit of dye from the microvasculature; there is the ground glass appearance ("blush") or opacification of the myocardium in the distribution of the culprit lesion that is strongly persistent at the end of the washout phase (i.e., dye is strongly persistent after 3 cardiac cycles of the washout phase and either does not diminish or only minimally diminishes in intensity during washout)
3	Normal entry and exit of dye from the microvasculature; there is the ground glass appearance ("blush") or opacification of the myocardium in the distribution of the culprit lesion that clears normally, and it is either gone or only mildly/moderately persistent at the end of the washout phase (i.e., dye is gone or only mildly/moderately persistent after 3 cardiac cycles of the washout phase and noticeably diminishes in intensity during washout phase), similar to that in an uninvolved artery; blush that is of only mild intensity throughout the washout phase but fades minimally is also classified as grade 3

Source: Adapted from Ref. 6.

the TMPG system (Table 4.1), TMPG 0 represents minimal or no myocardial blush; in TMPG 1, dye stains the myocardium, and this stain persists on the next injection; in TMPG 2, dye enters the myocardium but washes out slowly so that it is strongly persistent at the end of the injection; and in TMPG 3, there is normal entrance and exit of dye in the myocardium (Fig. 4.1).[6] Another method of assessing myocardial perfusion on the angiogram is the MBG developed by van't Hof et al.[7] The MBG is an index that defines the intensity of contrast opacity of the infarcted area compared to the contralateral or ipsilateral noninfarct-related artery. In contrast, the TMPG is an index that defines not only the intensity of blushing but also focuses on the rate of clearance of contrast opacity. A grade of 0 (no blush) and a grade of 3 (normal blush) are the same in the TMPG and MBG systems. Thus, normal perfusion in the myocardium carries a score of 3 in both TMPG and MBG systems, and a closed muscle carries a score of 0 in both systems.[6]

TMPG has been shown to be a multivariate predictor of mortality in acute STEMI, independent of flow in the epicardial artery, age, blood pressure, and heart rate.[5] TIMI grade 2/3 flow, reduced corrected TIMI frame count (CFTC) and an open microvasculature (TMPG 2/3) were all associated with an improved 2-year survival.[5] Thus, the TMPG adds additional long-term prognostic information to the conventional epicardial TFG and CTFC. Compared to patients who achieve both TIMI grade 3 flow and TMPG 3, patients in whom epicardial flow is restored (TIMI grade 3 flow) whose microvasculature fails to open (TMPG 0/1) have a seven-fold increase in mortality. Achievement of TIMI grade 3 flow in both the artery and the myocardium is associated with mortality under 1% (Fig. 4.1).[5] In a recent analysis of the PROTECT-TIMI 30 study, an abnormal post-PCI TMPG was the strongest correlate of death, MI, or an ischemic event within 48 hours in patients with NSTEMI undergoing PCI[8] (Fig. 4.2).

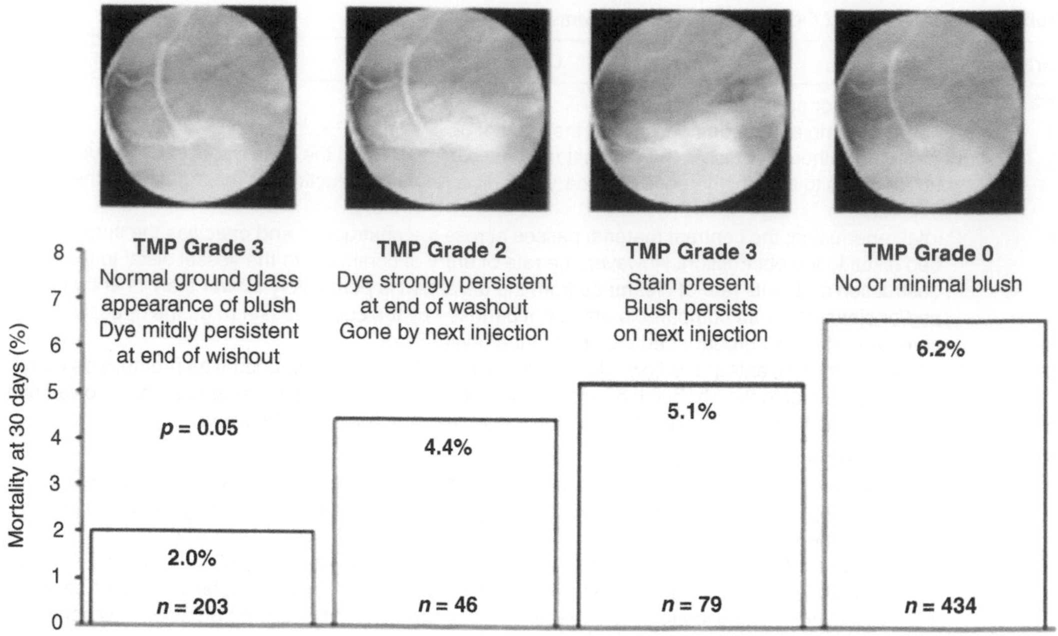

Figure 4.1 The TMPG assesses tissue level perfusion using the angiogram and is a multivariate predictor of mortality in acute MI. The TMPG permits risk stratification even within epicardial TIMI grade 3 flow. Despite achieving epicardial patency with normal TIMI grade 3 flow, those patients whose microvasculature fails to open (TMPG 0/1) have a persistently elevated mortality of 5.4% at 30 days. In contrast, those patients with both TIMI grade 3 flow in the epicardial artery and TMPG 3 have mortality under 1% [0.7% (1/137) vs. 4.7% (15/318); $p = 0.05$ using Fisher's exact test for TMPG 3 vs. grades 0, 1, and 2]. *Source*: Adapted from Ref. 6.

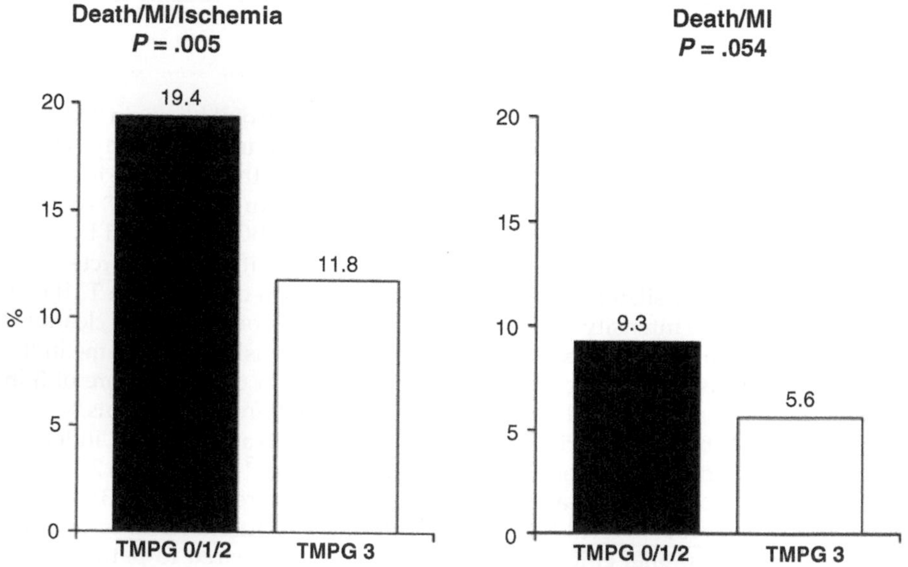

Figure 4.2 Association of TMPG after PCI with rates of adverse events. *Source*: Adapted from Ref. 8.

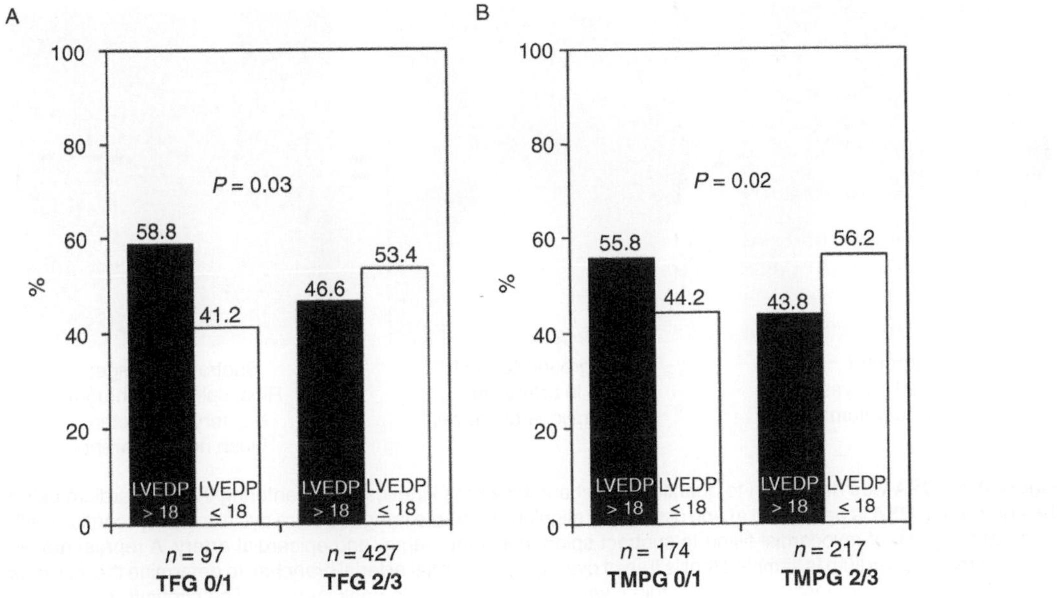

Figure 4.3 Percentage of patients with elevated LVEDP in relation to epicardial flow and microvascular perfusion. (**A**) LVEDP and artery patency. The percentage of patients with elevated LVEDP is shown by TFG strata (TFG 0/1 = closed artery, TFG 2/3 = open artery). (**B**) LVEDP and myocardial perfusion. The percentage of patients with elevated LVEDP is shown by TMPG strata (TMPG 0/1 = closed myocardium, TMPG 2/3 = open myocardium). *Abbreviations*: TFG, TIMI flow grade; TMPG, TIMI Myocardial Perfusion Grade. *Source*: Adapted from Ref. 9.

Impaired myocardial perfusion on the angiogram has also been associated with higher left ventricular end-diastolic pressure[9] (Fig. 4.3) and the presence of overt congestive heart failure on presentation. Among patients presenting with cardiogenic shock, a restoration of normal myocardial perfusion is associated with improved survival.

Similar to what has been observed in STEMIs, in UA/NSTEMIs, TMPG 0/1 flow is associated with elevated troponin T and I both pre- and post-PCI and levels were higher among patients with TMPG 0/1 compared with TMPG 2/3.[10] TMPG 0/1 was independently associated with elevations of cardiac troponin independent of the epicardial TFG, the severity of the stenosis or the presence of thrombus in the vessel. Importantly, TMPG 0/1 was associated with increased risk of death or MI at 6 months.[10] Similarly, TMPG 0/1/2 perfusion following PCI is associated with a nearly 10-fold rise in the risk of creatine kinase (CK)–MB elevations in patients with UA/NSTEMI, as well as a higher risk of adverse clinical outcomes at 1 year.[11] These findings implicate a pathophysiological link between impaired myocardial perfusion, the release of markers of myonecrosis (both pre- and post-PCI), and adverse clinical outcomes.

Both MBG and TMPG are subjective measures of myocardial perfusion. In addition to these qualitative assays, two quantitative measures have been developed.

Coronary clearance frame count (CCFC)

In an effort to remove observer bias from the qualitative assessment of myocardial perfusion, quantitative methods of assessments, such as CCFC, have been described. To use the CCFC, the number of cineframes required for dye to clear a standardized distal landmark in the artery is calculated. In this index, the number "0" represents the first frame in which the contrast medium is seen to be cleared from the ostium of the artery of interest (at least 70% of the width of the artery has been washed free of contrast medium) and the "final frame" is that in which the contrast begins to be cleared from the standardized distal landmark proposed by the TIMI Group (the first branch of the posterolateral artery for the RCA; the most distal branch of the obtuse marginal branch for the circumflex system; and in the LAD, the distal bifurcation). The CCFC is defined as the difference between the values of these two frame counts. In one study, the CCFC has been shown to correlate with both the TMPG and the MBG.[12]

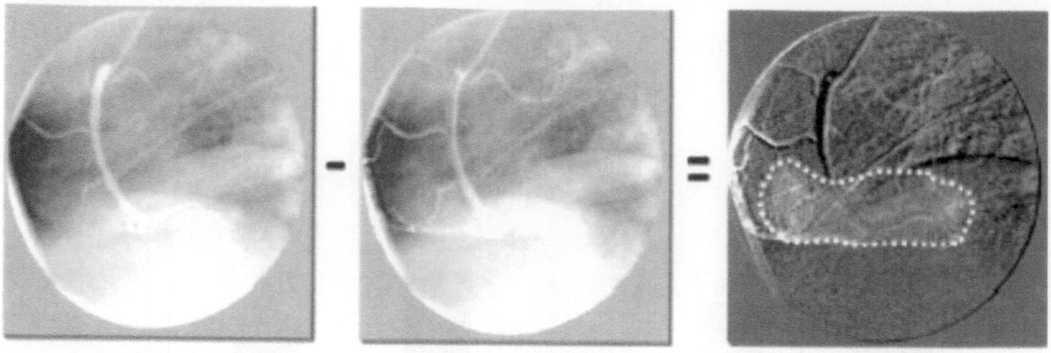

Figure 4.4 DSA was developed to quantitatively characterize the kinetics of dye entering the myocardium using the angiogram. DSA is performed at end diastole by aligning cineframe images before dye fills the myocardium with those at the peak of myocardial filling to subtract spine, ribs, diaphragm, and epicardial artery. A representative region of the myocardium is sampled that is free of overlap by epicardial arterial branches to determine the increase in the Gray-scale brightness of the myocardium when it first reached its peak intensity. The circumference of the myocardial blush is measured using a handheld planimeter. The number of frames required for the myocardium to first reach its peak brightness is converted into time (sec) by dividing the frame count by 30. In this way, the rate of rise in brightness (Gy/sec) and the rate of growth of blush (cm/sec) can be calculated. *Source*: Adapted from Ref. 6.

Digital subtraction angiography

To quantitatively characterize the kinetics of dye entering the myocardium using the angiogram, digital subtraction angiography (DSA) has been utilized to estimate the rate of brightness (Gy/sec) and the rate of growth of blush (cm/sec). DSA is performed at end diastole by aligning cineframe images before dye fills the myocardium with those at the peak of myocardial filling to subtract spine, ribs, diaphragm, and epicardial artery (Fig. 4.4). A representative region of the myocardium is sampled that is free of overlap by epicardial arterial branches to determine the increase in the Gray-scale brightness of the myocardium at peak intensity. The circumference of the myocardial blush is measured using a handheld planimeter. The number of frames required for the myocardium to reach peak brightness is converted into time by dividing the frame count by 30.[6]

INDIRECT METHODS OF MEASURING MYOCARDIAL PERFUSION

The corrected TIMI frame count

The TFG classification has been extraordinarily useful in assessing the success of reperfusion strategies and identifying patients at higher risk for poor outcomes in acute coronary syndromes for the past two decades. Despite its widespread use, it is not without limitations.[2] A more objective and precise index of coronary blood flow called the CTFC can be used to overcome some of the limitations of TFG. To use CTFC, the number of cineframes required for dye to reach standardized distal landmarks is counted (Fig. 4.5).[2,5] In the first frame used for TIMI frame counting, a column of dye touches both borders of the coronary artery and moves forward (Fig. 4.5).[2] In the last frame, dye begins to enter (but does not necessarily fill) a standard distal landmark in the artery. These standard distal landmarks are as follows: in the RCA, the first branch of the posterolateral artery; in the circumflex system, the most distal branch of the obtuse marginal branch, which includes the culprit lesion in the dye path; and in the LAD, the distal bifurcation, which is also known as the "moustache," "pitchfork" or "whale's tail" (Fig. 4.5). These frame counts are corrected for the longer length of the LAD by dividing by 1.7 to arrive at the CTFC.[2]

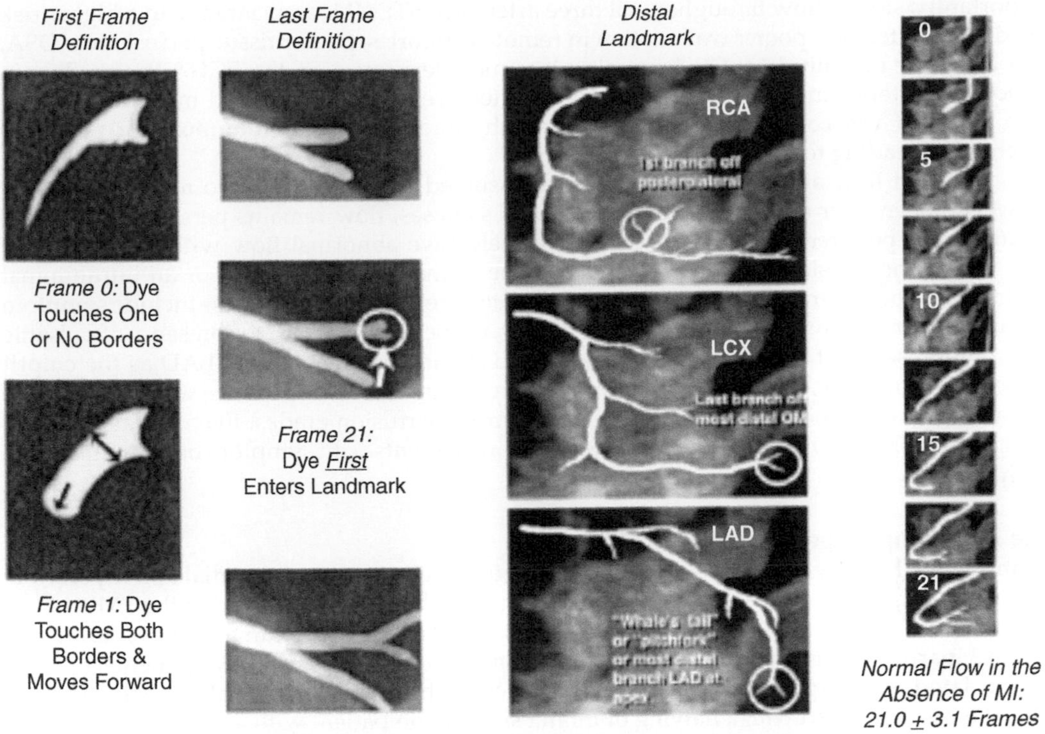

Figure 4.5 TIMI frame-counting method. In the first frame (*lower left panel*), a column of near or fully concentrated dye touches both borders of the coronary artery and moves forward. In the last frame (*second column*), dye begins to enter (but does not necessarily fill) a standard distal landmark in the artery. These standard distal landmarks are as follows: the first branch of the posterolateral artery in the RCA (*third column, top panel*); in the circumflex system, the most distal branch of the obtuse marginal branch that includes the culprit lesion in the dye path (*third column, middle panel*); and in the LAD the distal bifurcation, which is also known as the moustache, pitchfork, or whale's tail (*third column, bottom panel*). *Source*: Adapted from Ref. 6.

The CTFC is a quantitative measurement of epicardial flow rather than a qualitative assessment and it is highly reproducible.[2] It should be noted that if an epicardial artery is occluded, then a frame count of 100 is imputed. A normal CTFC is 21 frames and despite extensive physiologic variability and operator technique there is only a 3.1-frame standard deviation among patients with normal flow. The 95% confidence interval extends from >14 to <28 frames (7). Faster than normal flow is defined as CTFC <14 frames and constitutes what we now term "TIMI grade 4 flow."[2] Several variables, both technical and physiologic, do impact the CTFC such as the use of a power injector, dye injection at the beginning of diastole and an increase in the heart rate by 20 beats per minute. These factors all significantly decrease the CTFC whereas nitrate administration increases the CTFC.[13]

The CTFC is related to a variety of clinical outcomes.[2,5,14] Flow in the infarct related artery in survivors is significantly faster than in patients who die and mortality rates increase by 0.7% for every 10-frame rise in CTFC ($p < 0.001$).[14] Likewise, in patients with unstable angina (UA) or non–ST-elevation MI (NSTEMI), the post-PCI culprit flow among survivors is significantly faster than among those patients who died.[15] Rapid flow is associated with good clinical outcomes. None of the patients in the TIMI studies who have had a CTFC <14 died by 30 days.[14] Lastly, the CTFC is associated with lower rate of restenosis.[15]

Until recently, it was assumed that flow in nonculprit arteries in the setting of acute coronary syndromes was "normal." However, the CTFC in uninvolved arteries in acute STEMI (30.5 frames) is in fact 40% slower than normal (21 frames; $p < 0.001$).[2] In STEMI, adjunctive and rescue PCI restores flow in culprit vessels that is nearly identical to that of nonculprit arteries but this flow remains slower than normal.[6] PCI of the culprit lesion is also associated with improvements in the nonculprit artery after the intervention in both STEMI and UA/NSTEMI.[6]

Importantly, slower flow throughout all three arteries in STEMI is associated with a higher risk of adverse outcomes, poorer wall motion in remote territories, poorer tissue perfusion on DSA, and a greater magnitude of ST depression in remote territories on the ECG.[6] Poorer flow in nonculprit arteries may be the result of more extensive necrosis in shared microvasculature, or a result of vasoconstriction mediated through either a local neurohumoral or paracrine mechanism leading to an overall worse outcome.[6]

Delayed flow after fibrinolysis has been assumed to be secondary to residual stenosis. However, even after adjunctive PCI and relief of stenoses, flow remains persistently delayed to 26 frames poststent, and 34% of stented vessels have abnormal flow with a CTFC ≥28.[3] This persistence of slow flow is probably not due to the residual stenosis or an intraluminal obstruction but rather due to other factors that influence epicardial flow. These include symptom duration prior to arrival, the presence of collaterals, the percent stenosis, the presence of pulsatile flow, the presence of thrombus in the vessel, and the involvement of the LAD as the culprit vessel.[3] For instance, prolonged symptoms to treatment times in patients with ST segment elevation MI are associated with impaired myocardial perfusion grades. Even in patients with TFG 3, the CTFC at 60 minutes trended higher among patients with symptom onset to treatment >4 hours.

The angiographic perfusion score (APS)

A simplified, broadly applicable angiographic metric that integrates epicardial and myocardial perfusion assessments is needed. The APS is the sum of the TFG (0–3) added to the TMPG (0–3) before and after PCI (total possible grade of 0–12).[16] Failed perfusion can be defined as an APS of 0 to 3; partial perfusion, 4 to 9; and full perfusion, 10 to 12.[16] Among STEMI patients, the APS is associated with larger SPECT infarct sizes and with the incidence of death or MI. Partial or full APS are associated with a halving of infarct size and no patient with a full APS died.[16] The integration of epicardial and tissue level perfusion to arrive at a single angiographic variable that is associated with infarct size and 30-day death or MI, may prove valuable in clinical risk stratification.

THERAPIES TO IMPROVE MYOCARDIAL PERFUSION

Vasodilators

There are few randomized trials looking at the efficacy of vasodilator therapy in improving myocardial perfusion. One small trial evaluated high-dose intracoronary adenosine (100 μg during each intracoronary injection) and demonstrated that adenosine was associated with improved echocardiographic and clinical outcomes.[17] Adenosine administration may be associated with bradycardia and the placement of a temporary pacing wire should be considered (Table 4.2). In the randomized VAPOR (VAsodilator Prevention Of no-Reflow) trial, intragraft

Table 4.2 Agents used to treat impaired myocardial perfusion[a]

	Dose	Side effects
Adenosine	100 μg IC to a total dose of 4000 μg. Half-life is 6 sec. Adenosine can be repeatedly administered when pulse and blood pressure normalize	Bradycardia, hypotension, difficulty in breathing
Verapamil	200 μg IC as a single dose to a total of 1000 μg (1 mg)	Bradycardia, hypotension
Diltiazem	200 μg IC as a single dose to a total dose of 1000 μg (1 mg) IC	Bradycardia, hypotension
Nicardipine	200 μg IC as a single dose to a total dose of 1000 μg (1 mg) IC	Lower incidence of bradycardia, hypotension with this vasoselective agent
Nitroprusside[b]	100 μg IC as a single dose to a total dose of 1000 μg (1 mg) IC	Lower incidence of bradycardia, hypotension

[a]Administration of these agents is not listed as an approved indication in the package insert (i.e., off label use).
[b]Median dose was 200 μg IC in the Hillegass study (19)
Source: Adapted from Ref. 21.

verapamil (200 μg IC) was associated with a reduction in no-reflow during saphenous vein graft PCI. Care must be taken in administration, as verapamil administration can be associated with decreased contractility and bradycardia.[18] Intracoronary nitroprusside administration at a median dose of 200 μg produces improved CTFCs among patients with no-reflow and may also be associated with a lower incidence of hypotension and bradycardia.[19]

Glycoprotein (GP) IIb/IIIa inhibitors

A substudy of the Intergrillin and Tenecteplase in Acute Myocardial Infarction (INTEGRITI) trial looking at the impact of combination reperfusion therapy with reduced-dose tenecteplase and eptifibatide compared with full-dose lytic on ST segment recovery and angiographic measures of reperfusion demonstrated a trend toward improvement in TFGs, TMPG, and CTFC across the dosing regimens as compared with full-dose tenecteplase.[20] Another substudy of INTEGRITI looking at the association between platelet receptor occupancy (RO) after eptifibatide and myocardial perfusion in patients with STEMI showed a higher percent RO in patients with TMPG 2/3 than those with delayed or no perfusion (TMPG 0/1).[20] These results taken cumulatively suggest that combination reperfusion with fibrinolysis and GP IIb/IIIa inhibitors are associated with improved angiographic measures of myocardial perfusion.

FUTURE DIRECTIONS

While the last 25 years has been the era of the "open artery hypothesis" there is growing recognition that epicardial artery patency is necessary but not sufficient to assure good clinical outcomes. Clearly, the best outcomes are present when both epicardial and myocardial perfusion are restored. We must now incorporate the evaluation of myocardial perfusion into our clinical practice as both a measure of treatment efficacy and as a predictor of clinical outcome. We must shift the paradigm away from relying solely on "coronary angiography" towards the emerging technique of "myocardial angiography" where we assess both epicardial and myocardial perfusion.

REFERENCES

1. The thrombolysis in myocardial infarction (TIMI) trial. Phase I findings. TIMI Study Group. N Engl J Med 1985; 312:932–936.
2. Gibson CM, Cannon CP, Daley WL, et al. TIMI frame count: A quantitative method of assessing coronary artery flow. Circulation 1996; 93:879–888.
3. Gibson CM, Murphy S, Menown IB, et al. Determinants of coronary blood flow after thrombolytic administration. TIMI Study Group. Thrombolysis in Myocardial Infarction. J Am Coll Cardiol 1999; 34:1403–1412.
4. Ito H, Tomooka T, Sakai N, et al. Lack of myocardial perfusion immediately after successful thrombolysis. A predictor of poor recovery of left ventricular function in anterior myocardial infarction. Circulation 1992; 85:1699–1705.
5. Gibson CM, Cannon CP, Murphy SA, et al. Relationship of the TIMI myocardial perfusion grades, flow grades, frame count, and percutaneous coronary intervention to long-term outcomes after thrombolytic administration in acute myocardial infarction. Circulation 2002; 105:1909–1913.
6. Gibson CM, Schomig A. Coronary and myocardial angiography: Angiographic assessment of both epicardial and myocardial perfusion. Circulation 2004; 109:3096–3105.
7. van't Hof AW, Liem A, Suryapranata H, et al. Angiographic assessment of myocardial reperfusion in patients treated with primary angioplasty for acute myocardial infarction: Myocardial blush grade. Zwolle Myocardial Infarction Study Group. Circulation 1998; 97:2302–2306.
8. Gibson CM, Kirtane AJ, Morrow DA, et al. Association between thrombolysis in myocardial infarction myocardial perfusion grade, biomarkers, and clinical outcomes among patients with moderate- to high-risk acute coronary syndromes: Observations from the randomized trial to evaluate the relative PROTECTion against post-PCI microvascular dysfunction and post-PCI ischemia among antiplatelet and antithrombotic agents—Thrombolysis in Myocardial Infarction 30 (PROTECT-TIMI 30). Am Heart J 2006; 152:756–761.
9. Kirtane AJ, Bui A, Murphy SA, et al. Association of epicardial and tissue-level reperfusion with left ventricular end-diastolic pressures in ST-elevation myocardial infarction. J Thromb Thrombolysis 2004; 17:177–184.

10. Wong GC, Morrow DA, Murphy S, et al. Elevations in troponin T and I are associated with abnormal tissue level perfusion: A TACTICS-TIMI 18 substudy. Treat angina with aggrastat and determine cost of therapy with an invasive or conservative strategy-Thrombolysis in Myocardial Infarction. Circulation 2002; 106:202–207.
11. Gibson CM, Murphy SA, Marble SJ, et al. Relationship of creatine kinase-myocardial band release to Thrombolysis in Myocardial Infarction perfusion grade after intracoronary stent placement: An ESPRIT substudy. Am Heart J 2002; 143:106–110.
12. Perez de Prado A, Fernandez-Vazquez F, Cuellas-Ramon JC, et al. Coronary clearance frame count: A new index of microvascular perfusion. J Thromb Thrombolysis 2005; 19:97–100.
13. Abaci A, Oguzhan A, Eryol NK, et al. Effect of potential confounding factors on the thrombolysis in myocardial infarction (TIMI) trial frame count and its reproducibility. Circulation 1999; 100:2219–2223.
14. Gibson CM, Murphy SA, Rizzo MJ, et al. Relationship between TIMI frame count and clinical outcomes after thrombolytic administration. Thrombolysis In Myocardial Infarction (TIMI) Study Group. Circulation 1999; 99:1945–1950.
15. Gibson CM, Dotani MI, Murphy SA, et al. Correlates of coronary blood flow before and after percutaneous coronary intervention and their relationship to angiographic and clinical outcomes in the RESTORE trial. Randomized Efficacy Study of Tirofiban for Outcomes and REstenosis. Am Heart J 2002; 144:130–135.
16. Gibson CM, Murphy SA, Morrow DA, et al. Angiographic perfusion score: An angiographic variable that integrates both epicardial and tissue level perfusion before and after facilitated percutaneous coronary intervention in acute myocardial infarction. Am Heart J 2004; 148:336–340.
17. Marzilli M, Orsini E, Marraccini P, Testa R. Beneficial effects of intracoronary adenosine as an adjunct to primary angioplasty in acute myocardial infarction. Circulation 2000; 101:2154–2159.
18. Michaels AD, Appleby M, Otten MH, et al. Pretreatment with intragraft verapamil prior to percutaneous coronary intervention of saphenous vein graft lesions: Results of the randomized, controlled vasodilator prevention on no-reflow (VAPOR) trial. J Invasive Cardiol 2002; 14:299–302.
19. Hillegass WB, Dean NA, Liao L, et al. Treatment of no-reflow and impaired flow with the nitric oxide donor nitroprusside following percutaneous coronary interventions: Initial human clinical experience. J Am Coll Cardiol 2001; 37:1335–1343.
20. Gibson CM, Jennings LK, Murphy SA, et al. Association between platelet receptor occupancy after eptifibatide (integrilin) therapy and patency, myocardial perfusion, and ST-segment resolution among patients with ST-segment-elevation myocardial infarction: an INTEGRITI (Integrilin and Tenecteplase in Acute Myocardial Infarction) substudy. Circulation 2004; 110:679–684.
21. Gibson CM. Has my patient achieved adequate myocardial reperfusion? Circulation 2003; 108:504–507.

5 Challenges in the assessment of bifurcation lesions

Yves Louvard, Kamaldeep Chawla, Thierry Lefèvre, and Marie-Claude Morice

Coronary bifurcation lesions are currently the subject of considerable attention because of their frequency and because their management by PCI treatment with bare metal stents, especially drug-eluting stents, has not yet been adequately codified.[1–3] PCI is associated with lower success rate and higher risk of complication and its midterm outcome is poorer compared to that of nonbifurcated lesions.

Most of the related studies are nonrandomized and are characterized by numerous imperfections, namely, variable definitions of bifurcation lesions, absence of detailed description of the heterogeneous techniques used, absence of outcome analysis by intention to treat, and above all, absence of accurate description of highly variable and frequently complex lesions.

The European Bifurcation Club (EBC)[4] recently proposed the following definition:

> A coronary bifurcation lesion is a coronary artery narrowing occurring adjacent to, and/or involving the origin of a significant side branch. A significant side branch is a branch that you don't want to lose in the global context of a particular patient (symptoms, location of ischemia, branch responsible for symptoms or ischemia, viability, collateralizing vessel, left ventricular function . . .)

Description of coronary stenosis is still mostly based on angiographic findings and qualitative analysis (presence or absence of bifurcations, calcifications, thrombus) or quantitative data for certain parameters (quantitative coronary angiography or QCA).

However, in the setting of coronary bifurcation lesions, QCA generates a considerable dilemma in the absence of any standardized method. Indeed, the analysis methods used in straight lesions lead to erroneous results when applied to bifurcation lesions.

The first bifurcation analysis package (MEDIS QVA-CMS V6.0) was introduced in 2003; however, in clinical research consensus on reporting of the relevant data has not been established until today.

The purpose of this chapter based on the work of the EBC[5,6] is to outline the limitations and pitfalls of conventional analysis and propose a new standard approach for the analysis and the reporting of angiographic findings in coronary bifurcation lesions. This comes as a complement to the designation and classification of bifurcation lesions and the accurate description and classification of currently used stenting techniques elaborated by the EBC. The objective is to improve the quality of studies involving this controversial subject by allowing the comparison of well-defined and homogeneous groups of coronary bifurcation lesions treated by means of accurately described techniques using the same stents.

PATTERN OF CORONARY ARTERY RAMIFICATION

The function of coronary circulation is to ensure a continuous blood flow to the cardiac muscular tissue according to its needs. The coronary arterial system is composed of epicardial arteries (EPCA) ("distributing" vessels with a lower branching rate), which run along the external surface of the myocardium and branch off into intramyocardial coronary arteries, which penetrate into the myocardium (IMCA) ("delivering" vessels with a higher branching rate). The asymmetric branching pattern of the coronary arterial tree is complex and generates millions of capillary loops, which feed the myocardium.[7]

For EPCA, coronary artery branching complies with the fractal geometry pattern and its self-similarity principle.[8] Diameter relation between the mother branch and the daughter branches are governed by Murray's law: D^3 mother = D^3 daughter 1 + D^3 daughter 2 (Ref. 9).

There is a linear relationship between the flow and the diameter of the EPCA.[10] Flow distribution in a bifurcation corresponds to the flow continuity formula, which is analogous to Murray's law for diameters. This allows constant velocity to be maintained in EPCA (as the total cross-sectional area).[11] The length of an EPCA is proportional to its initial diameter.[10] The diameter and/or flow and/or length of each epicardial vessel account(s) for its importance. A simplified expression of Murray's law was proposed and validated in humans[12]: D mother = (D daughter 1 + D daughter 2) × 0.68. This formula is very useful in practice when the diameter of one of the three segments of a bifurcation cannot be measured (occluded vessel, absence of proximal reference like in diffuse left main stenosis). The self-similar branching pattern is discrete at the connection between the EPCA and IMCA.[13] In IMCA there is a transition between the proximal segment, where constant flow velocity is maintained, and distal segments, where flow velocity is reduced in order to ensure a prolonged transit time allowing exchanges.

The number of ultimate branches (arteriovenous loops) is proportional to the initial diameter of each epicardial arterial branch. This allows the definition of a myocardial infarction index for each individual branch, connecting the proximal diameter of a vessel with the myocardial mass in jeopardy in cases of vessel occlusion.[8] All these findings provide direct evidence of a structure–function relation of the coronary circulation.[10]

CORONARY FLOW AND ATHEROSCLEROSIS

The coronary atherosclerosis process amenable to interventional cardiology treatment is mainly observed in EPCA and possibly in the proximal segment of septal branches. There is a clear relationship between certain flow characteristics in these arteries and the formation of atheroma.[14,15] Flow linearity and velocity are not constant in EPCA. Coronary artery flow is pulsatile and reaches the left coronary artery during diastole; flow is inverted during systole. Friction exerted on the artery wall (wall shear stress or WSS) is proportional to the flow velocity. Consequently, friction is minimal during systole.

Flow disturbances occurring in bifurcations account for the high frequency of coronary lesions observed in the vicinity of bifurcations. In bifurcations, flow is linear and its velocity high at the carina wall (flow divider), whereas it is reduced and turbulent close to the wall opposite to the carina in the proximal vessel and proximal segments of the two distal vessels.[16] This generates a high WSS on the artery wall, in the carina, and on the external side of the curves; however, WSS is considerably reduced in areas of turbulent flow and inside the curves. Atheroma builds up in low WSS areas (inverse relation between wall thickness and WSS)[15,16] (Fig. 5.1), whereas normal WSS is atheroprotective (decreased expression of vasoconstrictors, growth factors, inflammatory mediators, adhesion molecules, oxidants).[17] Some particular coronary geometries have been recognized as risk factors of atheroma formation.[15]

QUANTITATIVE CORONARY ANGIOGRAPHY[18]

Historically, assessment of coronary stenosis was made by visual estimate and expressed in percentage. This was an efficient method for moderate and tight stenoses, though leading to frequent over-estimation and significant interobserver variability (between 40% and 80%) in narrowings, which is the range where clinical significance may be difficult to establish. Visual analysis was then replaced by digital callipers combined with hand drawing of the vessel edges. Later, analogical/digital conversion of 35-mm films allowed semiautomatic analysis. Automatic vessel edge detection permitted practically operator-independent analysis.[19] Calibration was performed by means of a catheter of a known diameter (or measured with a micrometer) and then according to measured diameter of the contrast-filled catheter, or even better by using isocentric calibration.

Although relatively unreliable immediately after PTCA outside stents, densitometric analysis was proposed in order to solve the issue raised by eccentric stenoses. Three-dimensional reconstruction of coronary arteries has been tested during the past 15 years; this is a very promising method for bifurcation analysis and helps overcome the issues of eccentric stenoses, foreshortening, as well as angle and curve measurements.

Since the advent of coronary interventional cardiology, digital angiography has been used in the selection of patients (vessel diameter, lesion length) and during procedures with on-line QCA (balloon sizing) to document the quality of immediate and follow-up outcome or

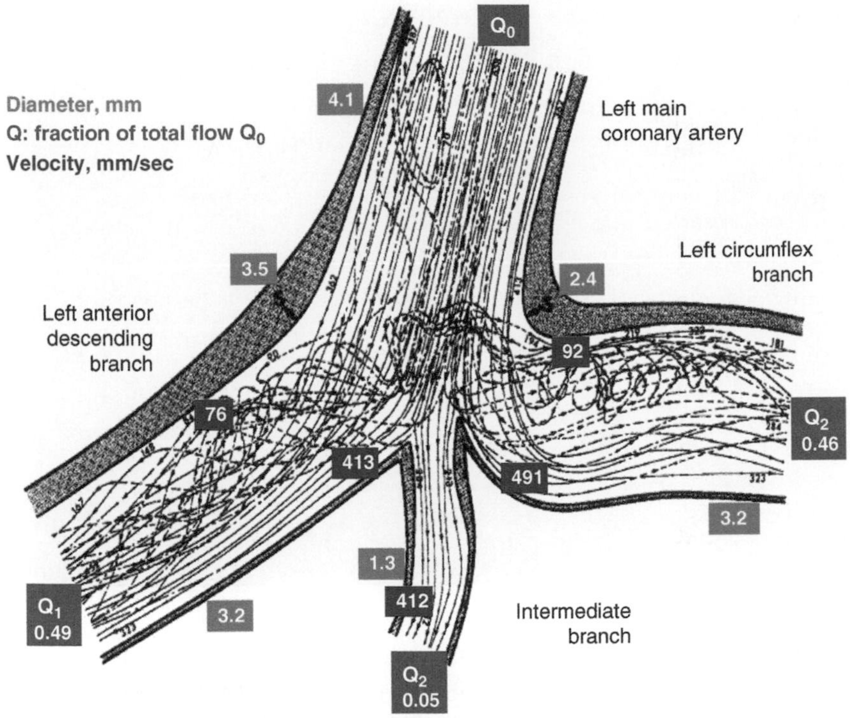

Figure 5.1 A true left main trunk trifurcation perfused with microparticles, showing (*i*) a flow proportional to branch diameter in each distal branches, (*ii*) high-velocity linear flow close to the carenas, (*iii*) turbulent and slow flow opposite to the carenas inducing low wall shear stress, and (*iv*) wall thickness is increased in front of low wall shear stress. *Source*: Adapted from Ref. 16.

off-line QCA for computerized, objective, and reproducible measurements of coronary luminal dimensions [i.e., iterative measurements of MLD for quantification of acute and midterm results and evaluation of late lumen loss (LLL].

Methods

For optimal QCA, the areas to be studied should be placed in the center of the screen in order to avoid edge distortion (this is no more true with "flat panel" technology). Vasomotor tonus should be suppressed by injection of nitrates and the same contrast medium or osmolarity should be used to ensure accurate comparisons. Side branches should be used to precisely define the segment to be analyzed. Manual correction of automatic edge detection must be avoided, and the analyzed image must be recorded at the end of diastole in order to avoid blurring and systolic compression. Eccentric lesions raise a difficult issue. One way of solving this problem is to perform an average of two analyses in two orthogonal views, which is very difficult to achieve without foreshortening or overlapping. This implies that the tightest segment of the stenosis is equally visible in the same location in both views. In practice, a single view is frequently the best available solution, namely, the view showing the tightest part of the lesion.

The software provides automated contour detection of the arterial lumen within the start and end positions defined by the operator. Subsequently, the degree of stenosis is calculated from the MLD measurement and the interpolated reference diameter. In the poststenting phase, the same measurements are taken out in the same view (MLD, reference diameter, and degree of stenosis) and once again during follow-up with similar conditions. The difference between pre- and postprocedural MLD accounts for the acute gain (AG), and the difference between postprocedural MLD and MLD at follow-up represents the late lumen loss, considered in the era of antirestenosis strategies as a precise measurement of neointimal proliferation and a surrogate of target lesion revascularization (TLR).[20,21] Recently, Costa et al.[22] raised the issue of MLD relocation between pre- and postprocedural and even more between postprocedural

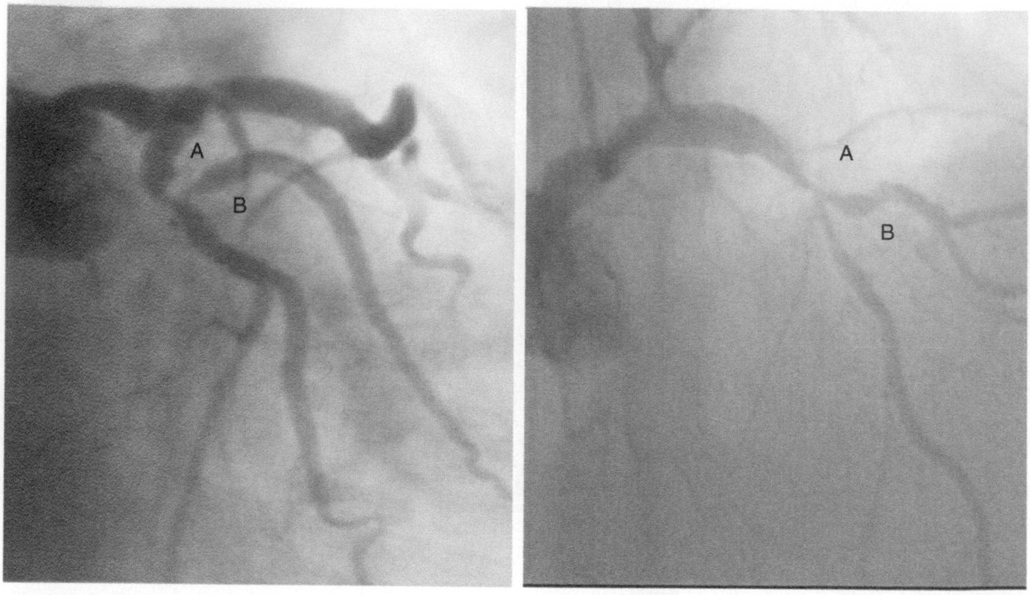

Figure 5.2 Angles of a bifurcation (from EBC).

and follow-up analysis outcome. Between pre- and post-procedure, the MLD location moves within the analyzed segment, most frequently from stented area to distal edge (in 65–70% of cases). This relocation is related to vessel tapering. At follow-up, MLD shifts frequently in the direction of the stent, with a higher frequency in BMS compared to DES. MLD relocation may also occur within the stent between postprocedure and follow-up measurement. The relocation phenomenon results frequently in an underestimation of AG and LLL. One may solve this problem by means of a multisegment analysis by dividing the analyzed vessel segment, the lesion, and/or the stent into subsegments equal in length. Between the completion of the procedure and follow-up, maximal LLL (in the subsegment where LLL is maximal) may be defined as well as mean LLL (by averaging LLL in all segments) and matched LLL (in the segment with MLD at follow-up). Maximal LLL seems to be the most accurate predictor of target lesion revascularization.

Other quantifiable values such as bifurcation angles (Fig. 5.2) and stenosis length may be measured by QCA. Measurement of angle A (or angle of access to the side branch) allows a precise assessment of the expected difficulties in accessing the side branch with guidewires, balloons and stents before and after stent placement in the main branch (parent vessel). This angle is increased significantly by the insertion of a guidewire in the side branch.[4] Angle B between two distal branches, when acute, is an angiographic predictor of side branch occlusion during initial stenting of the main branch across the side branch ostium.[1] The angle between the two branches has a prognostic value following bifurcation lesion stenting. This prognostic value may vary according to the techniques used.[23]

Pitfalls and limitations of QCA in the analysis of bifurcation lesions

Selection of appropriate angiographic views is essential in order to perform PTCA whether the lesion is located in a bifurcation or not. For bifurcation treatment the "working" view is selected according to the following parameters: optimal visualization of the stenosis, minimal foreshortening, and reduction of X-ray exposure. An additional view, if possible orthogonal, is useful, even in the stenting era, in order to confirm the quality of the results achieved and especially the absence of edge dissection. In the presence of a bifurcation lesion, it is almost always impossible to achieve visualization of the three (or more) arterial segments in the same projection without foreshortening (reliable length measurement). It is often possible to obtain an accurate view of two segments in the same projection. However, the ostium of the side branch, which, from a technical and clinical viewpoint, is the most debatable site of the bifurcation, may often be

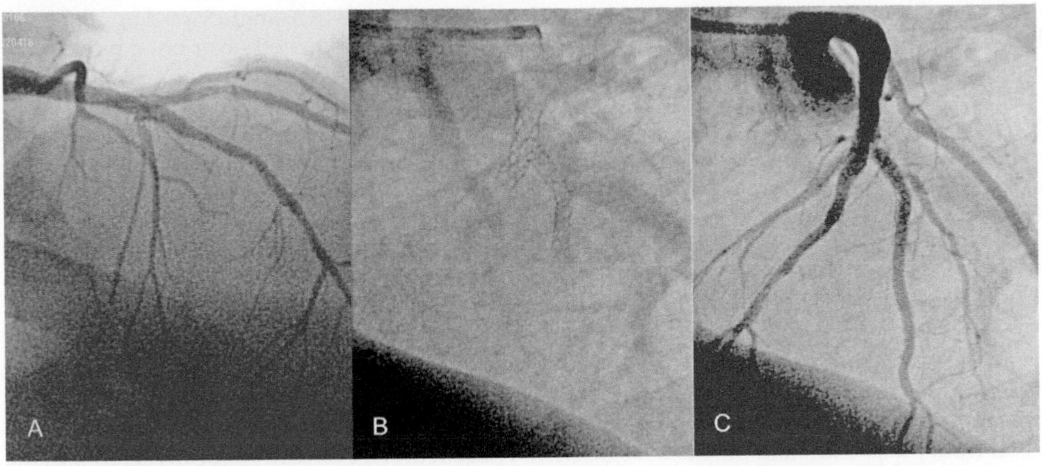

Figure 5.3 Influence of the incidence on diagnosis of restenosis. (**A**) AP + cranial was the working incidence during the procedure in this LAD/Diagonal bifurcation: no restenosis at FU angio. (**B**) T stenting technique with drug eluting stents without gap in LAO + cranial projection. (**C**) Tight restenosis in diagonal branch ostium in LAO + cranial projection.

visualized only in one or two nonorthogonal projections (LAO cranial and LAO caudal, for instance, for LAD diagonal bifurcation). In the orthogonal view, the ostium of the side branch is frequently hidden by the main branch. Consequently, analysis of two bifurcation branches is frequently carried out using a single view where the narrowings are the tightest but the optimal view may vary from one branch (proximal and distal main vessel) to another (side branch). Furthermore, potential restenosis is not always visible in the same view as in the initial analysis (change in branch angles) (Fig. 5.3).

Main branch analysis: By using nondedicated software, automated edge detection of the main branch is usually performed across the side branch. Lumen detection is usually accurate and reproducible and MLD location is well established.

In the presence of several or long lesions, MLD is frequently located in the most distal area (step-down phenomenon) (Fig. 5.4). This does not pose any problems in the absence of

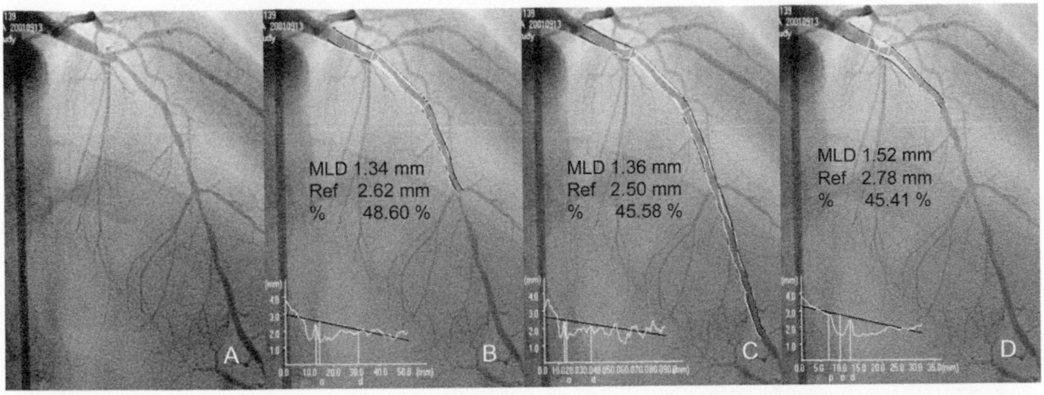

Figure 5.4 LAD/diagonal bifurcation; QCA of main vessel (proximal and distal). (**A**) LAD1, LAD2, Diag1, Medina 1,1,1 bifurcation lesion. (**B**) Automatic lumen design from main proximal vessel to main distal vessel. Only one reference (linear) function is defined. The MLD is automatically positioned at the beginning of the main distal vessel (1.34 mm), where the reference is clearly overestimated (2.62 mm), increasing the stenosis degree (48.6%). (**C**) While including more distal main vessel in the analyzed segment to get more "normal" vessel, the reference diameter at the level of the MLD is reduced (2.5 mm). (**D**) The MLD (1.52 mm) is manually moved to the stenosis immediately proximal to the diagonal where the reference diameter is clearly underestimated (2.78 mm) with, as a consequence, an underestimation of the stenosis (45.78%) clinically more important (two distal branches). This stenosis in fact is certainly tighter than the distal one.

branching, because the clinical consequences of multiples lesions in a single vessel involve only this vessel. If the analyzed segment involves a significant branch, whether or not a bifurcation lesion, the MLD location may have different clinical implications, depending on its localization in either the proximal or distal main branch and depending on the size of the side branch (Murray's law). The software calculates a single reference function for the proximal and distal main branch. This is not consistent with the law of branching inherent in biological trees, which implies that the tapering toward the distal end of a normal vessel is related to the presence of collateral branches. The diameter of the two branches between two side branches is invariable and its tapering is proportional with the diameter of each individual side branch. With a nondedicated software, the reference diameter of the main branch is underestimated in the segment proximal to the side branch and overestimated distal to the side branch (and the difference is more pronounced in the immediate proximity of the bifurcation). Any lesion located in the main branch immediately proximal to the side branch is overestimated and any lesion located in the immediate distal segment is underestimated. Furthermore, by varying start and end points of the automated edge detection, one may shift the location of the tightest lesion from the proximal to the distal segment in relation to the bifurcation (or inversely). In the presence of stenosis proximal and distal to the side branch, these mechanisms contribute to the shifting of the lesion from the proximal to the distal main branch (with less clinical relevance).

Side branch analysis: QCA of the side branch is even more complex (Fig. 5.5). Automated design of the side branch from the ostium in the presence of a proximal lesion results in an increasing elevation of the reference diameter function, especially when there is not a long distal segment without overlapping available. This may lead to an underestimation of the proximal stenosis. One way of solving this issue is to construct the vessel and reference profile by including the proximal vessel in the automated design, which runs counter to Murray's law to an even greater extent than the construction of a single main vessel. The reference diameter of the side branch lesion is then interpolated between two normal areas, one of which is in the proximal segment of the main branch. This increases the reference diameter and the degree of SB stenosis even more as the difference in diameter between the two vessels is larger.

Furthermore, it has been shown[24] that the provisional side branch stenting strategy, after main branch stenting across the side branch, results in the degree of stenosis in the ostium being overestimated compared to fractional flow reserve measurements[25] (suggested explanations are a combination of angiographic artifacts such as "halo" phenomenon and "slitlike" stenosis, inability to obtain a true orthogonal view, local edema of the SB ostium, alterations

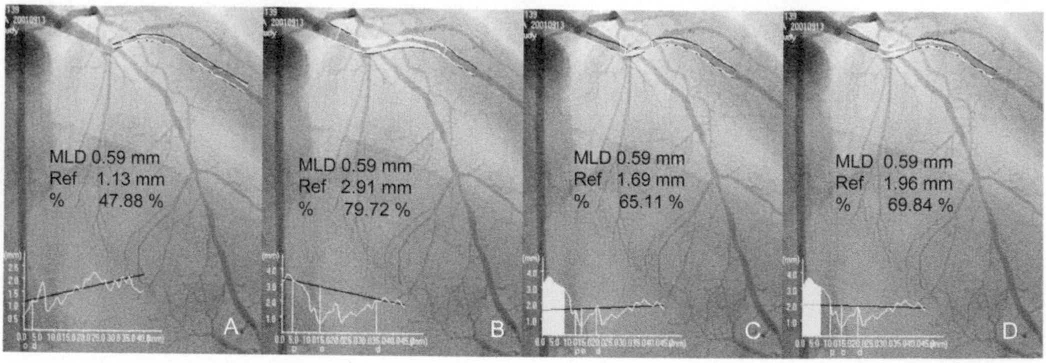

Figure 5.5 QCA of the side branch of bifurcation (LAD diagonal). (**A**) Automatic design of the lumen from diagonal ostium: the reference diameter function is increasing and the stenosis is moderate. (**B**) Automatic design from main proximal vessel: same MLD, but the reference is overestimated and the stenosis very tight. (**C**) Flagging off of a part of the proximal vessel results in a slightly increasing reference diameter function. (**D**) Flagging off slightly less than proximal vessel results in a reference diameter function that fits well with the distal diagonal branch "normal" vessel (solution close to the operator chosen reference diameter: maximal diameter distal to the stenosis). Notice that even these last solutions are wrong as per the Murray's law because there is a significant side branch taking off distal to the stenosis from the proximal diagonal branch: the diagonal reference diameter is underestimated.

of flow dynamics, etc.). Conversely, when double stenting strategies are implemented, QCA underestimates systematically the degree of stenosis in the side branch compared to IVUS.[26]

The fact that each of the three segments of a bifurcation has its own reference diameter precludes the use of a single LLL for the whole lesion. Moreover, with DES, the MLD tends to shift from the main branch to the side branch regardless of the initial lesion, number of stents, and technique used (important LL = small vessel restenosis and low MACE rate).

HOW TO IMPROVE QCA OF CORONARY BIFURCATION LESIONS?

Multisegmental analysis

Even though bifurcation stenosis is usually regarded as a single entity and described as the presence of a significant lesion in at least one of the three segments, the precise location of the lesion(s) in the various segments has an influence on the prognosis, stenting technique, and immediate and midterm treatment outcomes.[27] The distinction between the main branch (segments proximal and distal to the side branch) and the side branch (single segment) does not permit the adequate description of the clinical significance of the lesion (a tight stenosis of the main branch segment distal to the side branch does not involve the same amount of myocardium than a tight proximal lesion, especially if the side branch is large). Distinguishing between the main distal branch and the side branch of a coronary bifurcation may be difficult, for instance, in the midcircumflex artery and distal right coronary artery, which may have equally significant distal vascular beds. The numerous coronary bifurcation classifications available[28] reflect the need for an accurate description of lesion distribution in the three segments of the bifurcation. In order to avoid arbitrary description, classification must be made on the basis of significant lesions (>50%) even if the presence of two moderate lesions in two iterative segments may constitute a significant lesion.

The EBC has recommended the Medina classification[29] (Fig. 5.6), which gathers all information contained in previously published classification and can be easily memorized.

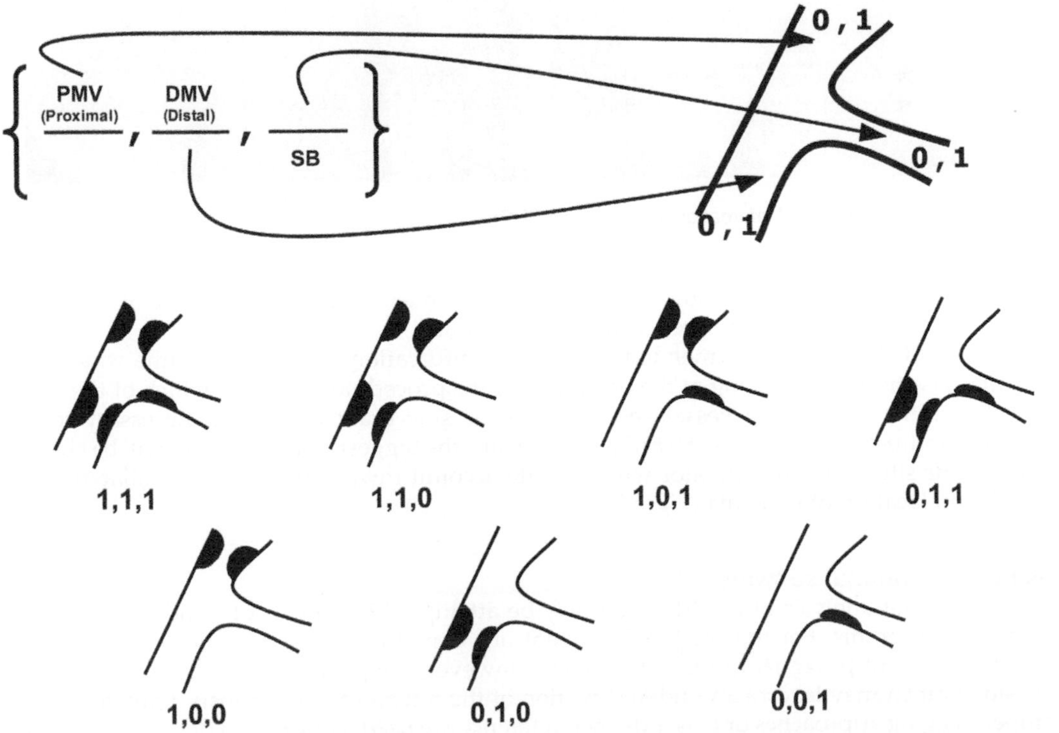

Figure 5.6 Medina classification. Based on QCA measured stenosis degree, either a 1 or a 0 fills the spaces depending the presence or absence a $\geq$ 50% stenosis (from A. Medina).

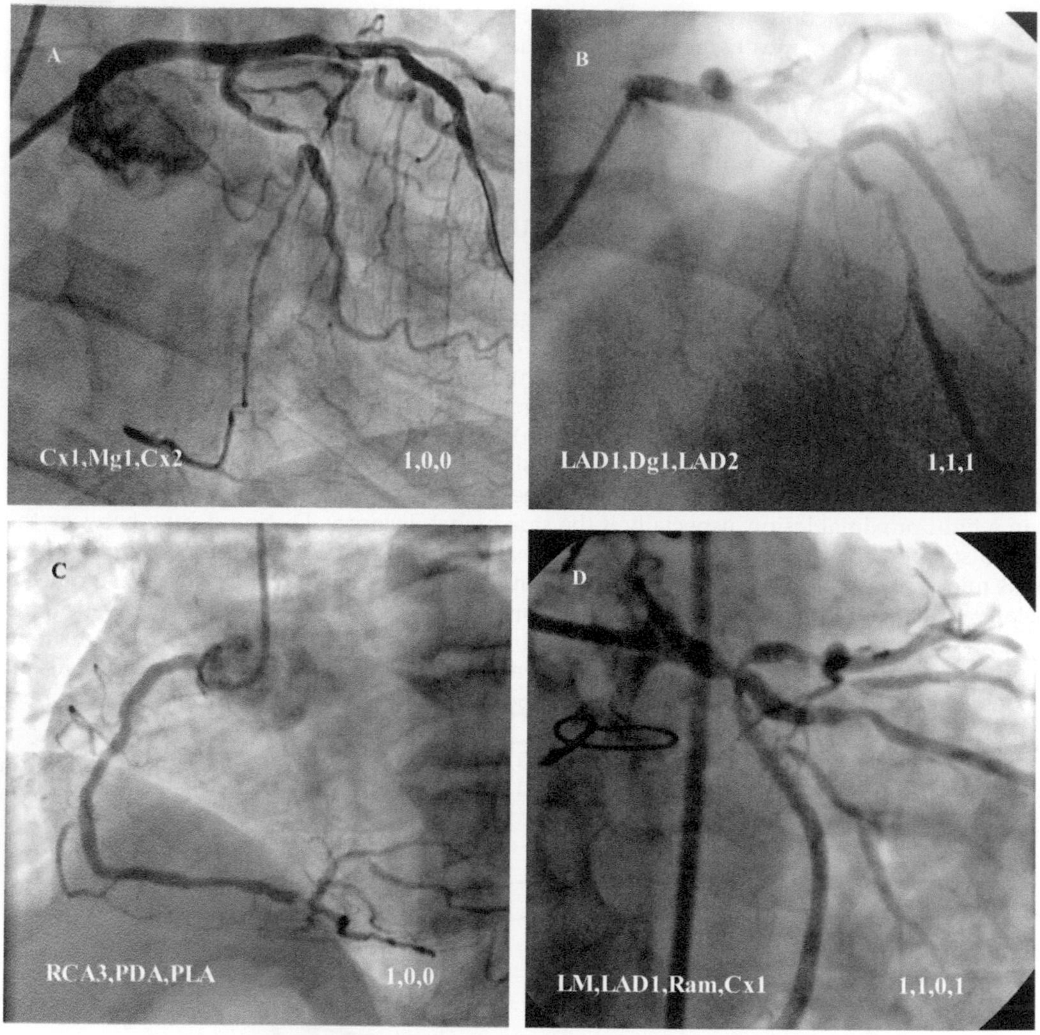

Figure 5.7 Denomination of bifurcation lesions (from EBC).

Furthermore, classification should be completed by means of QCA of each of the three segments, each with its own reference diameter function.

The EBC has also recommended to name the bifurcation lesion in the same way as the Medina classification, allowing at the beginning of the procedure to choose which of the distal branches is the main distal vessel and which is the side branch, which is necessary for an intention-to-treat analysis of any technique. Normally, the biggest/longest vessel will be chosen, but in some situations the operator will take into account myocardial viability, collateralizing vessel, and location of ischemia (Fig. 5.7).

Using conventional software

Multisegmental analysis of a bifurcation may be attempted by means of nondedicated computerized programs. For the proximal segment of the main branch, this entails constructing only the segment proximal to the side branch. However, the presence of a lesion proximal to the side branch may lead to an underestimation of the reference and stenosis diameter unless proper flagging approaches or a user defined reference are used. Automated design of the distal segment in the presence of a post–side branch lesion may lead to a similar result, especially if the segment available for analysis is short.

Another solution is to construct the two segments of the main branch, and analyze each individual segment while flagging off the other segment. The purpose of "flagging" a particular portion of a segment is to exclude that portion in the calculation of the reference diameter function. This tool has been shown to work very efficiently. The only drawback is that it makes the analysis semiautomatic or user dependent. With respect to the side branch, especially when the difference in diameter with the proximal main branch is important, the best solution is to use the maximal distal diameter (user defined reference) as a reference diameter in the absence of branching (constant reference diameter along the whole segment) and in the presence of a short lesion (Fig. 5.5).

New dedicated software

The common principle of new softwares is to propose automated and fast analysis of all the three segments of a bifurcation, with a diameter function, MLD definition, and calculation of stenosis degree for each individual segment. They also allow measurement of lesion length and angles between segments.

The MEDIS Qangio XA V8.0 software with the bifurcation analysis option can be used[30] (for coronary and peripheral application) (Fig. 5.8) to start up the bifurcation analysis. The user has to select one of the two bifurcation models that represents the bifurcation's vessel morphology best: (*i*) a new two-section model (for T-shaped bifurcations) and (*ii*) an improved three-section model (for Y-shaped bifurcations). Both these models have the advantage of combining the proximal and two distal vessel segments with the carinal segment (i.e., the actual bifurcation, which is defined by an automatically determined proximal delimiter and the first diameters of the two distal vessel segments), which results in a total of two and three sections, respectively. This way, the user can obtain specific and optimal analysis data about the bifurcation morphology present and the relevant stenting technique.

The user needs to place three pathline points in the image to define the arterial bifurcation segment for the analysis: one in the proximal vessel segment and one in each of the two distal vessel segments. Subsequently, two pathlines are detected followed by the automated detection of all the arterial contours of the bifurcation by using the MEDIS' minimum cost algorithm.[31] Additionally, the position of the carinal point (defining the border between the two distal vessel segments) on the middle contour will be automatically determined. This carinal point is needed by both models so that it can take into account the theory that a lesion does not emerge at the position of the carinal point because of existing high WSS. When needed, a semiautomatic

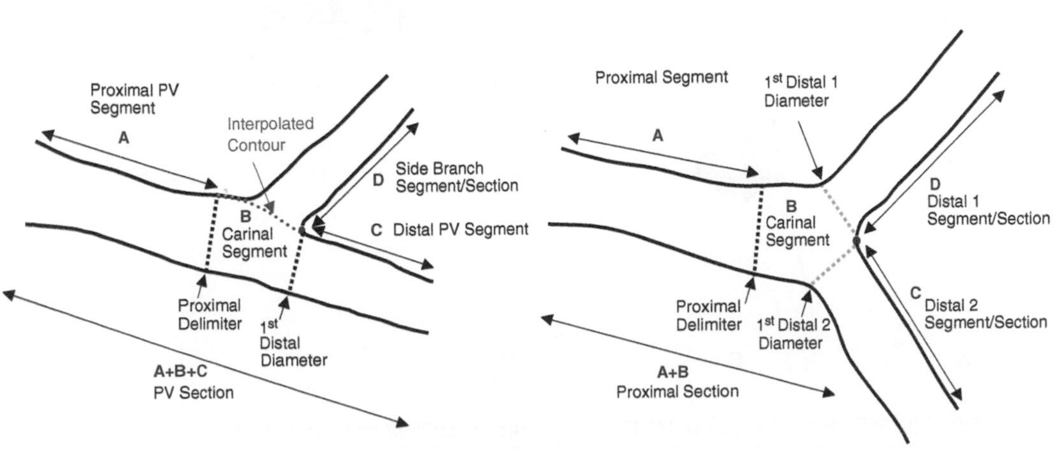

Figure 5.8 The MEDIS software. Schematic drawing of (**A**) the two-section model and (**B**) the three-section model explaining the used terminology. For each model, four segments that represent the building blocks of the models are generated by the MEDIS software. Combined according the model used, (**A**) the two-sections model consists of two sections [the parent vessel (PV) section and the side branch section] and (**B**) the three-section model consists of three sections (the proximal section, the distal 1 section and the distal 2 section). *Source*: Courtesy of MEDIS.

(repositioning of carinal point or adding an attraction point) or manual contour correction can be carried out.

In the next step, the arterial and reference diameter functions are derived for each section. The arterial diameters represent the shortest distances between the vessel walls, while at the same time being perpendicular to the local direction of the centerline; this is in accordance with the blood flow principles. In the two-section model this means that two arterial diameter functions are derived: one for the proximal to distal parent vessel segment (by means of an interpolated contour crossing the side branch ostium) and one for the side branch segment. In the three-section model this means that three arterial diameter functions are derived: one for the proximal (including the carinal segment) segment, one for the distal 1 segment, and one for the distal 2 segment. In both the two- and three-section models the interpolated reference diameter functions are based on each of the segments separately. This is accomplished by means of an iterative regression technique, which excludes the influence of minor lesions or ectatic coronary segments and the carinal segment. By this approach, it is assured that these reference diameter functions are based only on the arterial diameters outside of the carinal segment. Additionally, the reference diameter function of the carinal segment is based on the reconstruction of a smooth transition between the proximal and distal reference contours, thereby providing an optimal representation of this important segment. As a result, the two-section model will display two diameter functions and the three-section model three.

Finally, the MLD is determined for each section and compared with the corresponding reference diameter in order to determine the maximal percentage diameter stenosis for each section. In addition, extended edge-segment analyses are provided based on the user-defined positions of stent markers, allowing in-stent, in-lesion, stent edge, and ostial edge segment analysis within each of the three vessel segments (Fig. 5.10).

The new CAAS PIE MEDICAL software (Fig. 5.9)[32] allows the analysis of bifurcations. The program starts with the designation of three points delineating the segment to be analyzed

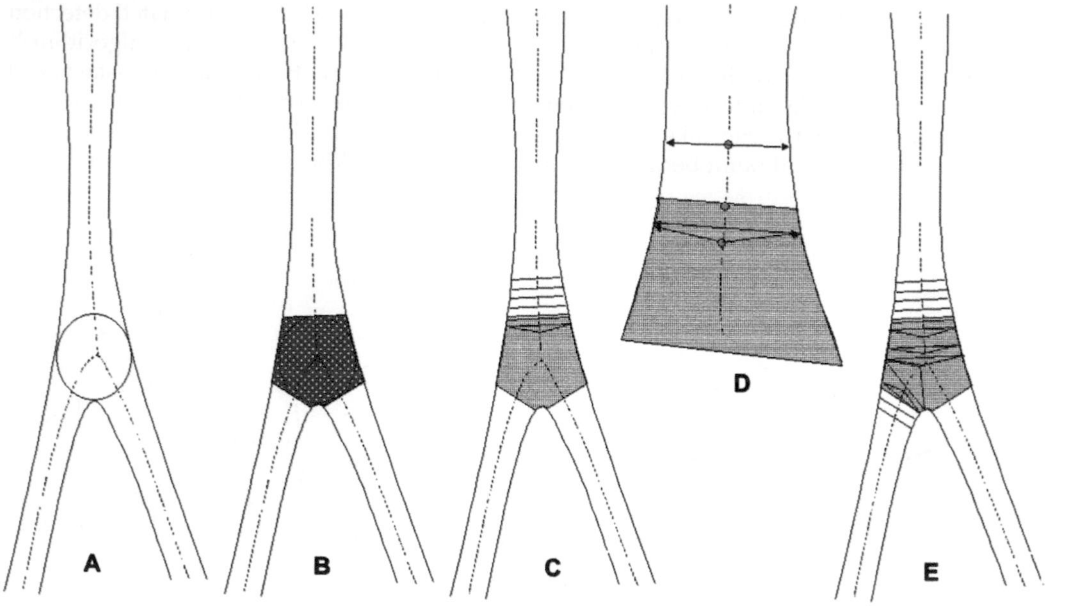

Figure 5.9 The PIE Medical software. (**A**) Design of three centerlines and point of bifurcation (POB). (**B**) POB relocation (center of circle) and polygon of confluence (POC). (**C**) Measurement of diameter outside the POC and perpendicular to centerline. (**D**) Diameter measurement inside the POC. (**E**) Distal to the POB measurement of diameters jump from proximal main vessel to distal branches. (**F**) Diameter measurements (stenosis in the side branch). Diameter profiles from main proximal vessel to main distal vessel (**G**) and main proximal vessel to side branch (**H**). (**I**) Reference contour design outside (traditional CAAS system) and inside POC. (**J**) Reference and luminal diameter measurements in stenosis outside and inside POC. (**K**) Angles measurements. *Source*: Courtesy of P. Serruys and EuroIntervention.

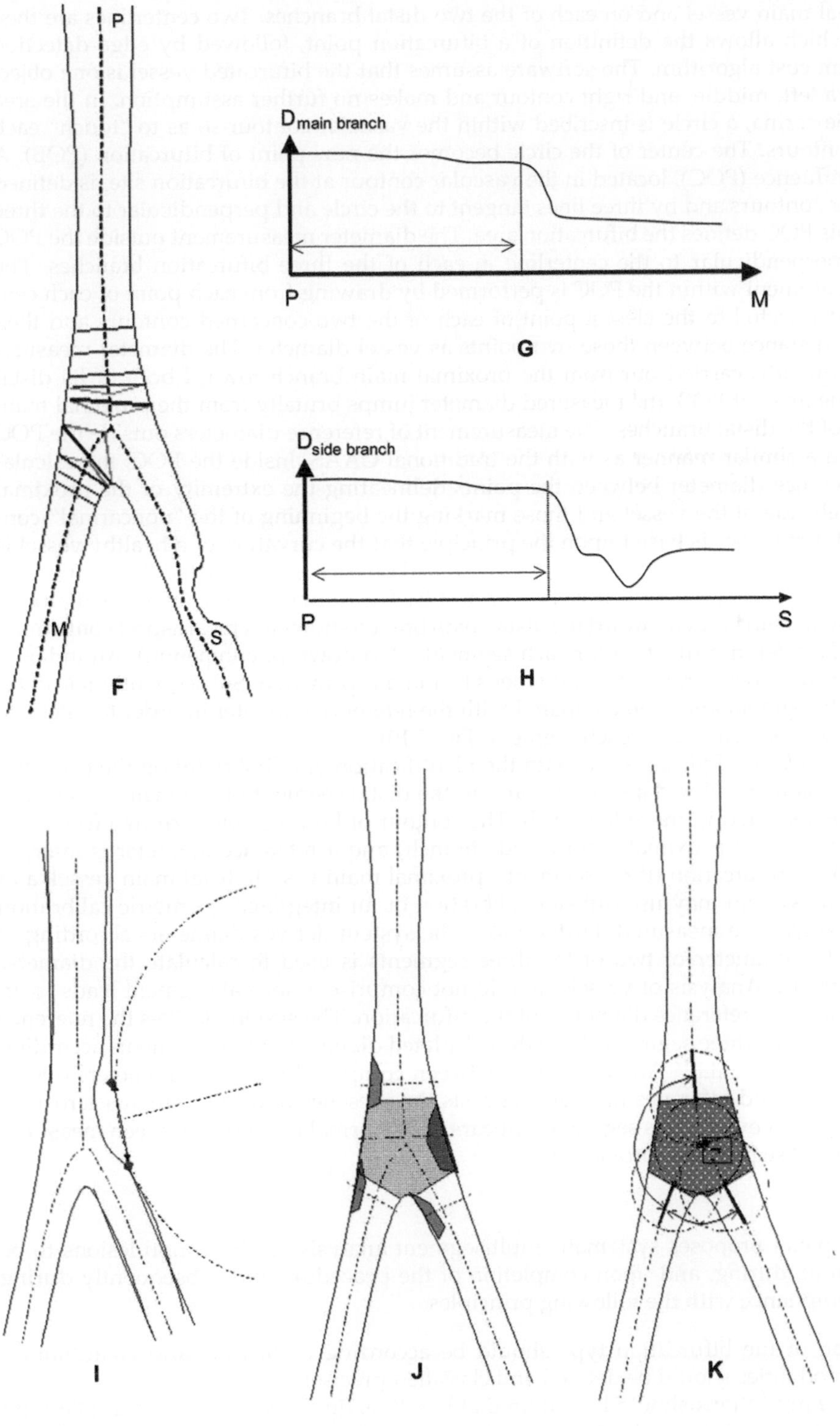

Figure 5.9 (*Continued*)

on the proximal main vessel and on each of the two distal branches. Two centerlines are then constructed, which allows the definition of a bifurcation point, followed by edge detection using minimum cost algorithm. The software assumes that the bifurcated vessel is one object delineated by a left, middle, and right contour and makes no further assumption. In the area proximal to the carina, a circle is inscribed within the vascular contour so as to "touch" each of the three contours. The center of the circle becomes the new point of bifurcation (POB). A polygon of confluence (POC), located in the vascular contour at the bifurcation site, is defined by the vascular contours and by three lines tangent to the circle and perpendicular to the three centerlines. This POC defines the bifurcation area. The diameter measurement outside the POC is performed perpendicular to the centerline in each of the three bifurcation branches. The diameter measurement within the POC is performed by drawing from each point of each centerline, a line connected to the closest point of each of the two concerned contours and then measuring the distance between those two points as vessel diameter. The diameter measurement is, consequently, carried out from the proximal main branch toward both of its distal branches. At the level of POB, the measured diameter jumps brutally from the proximal main branch to one of the distal branches. The measurement of reference diameters outside the POC is performed in a similar manner as with the traditional CAAS. Inside the POC, the calculation of the reference diameter between the points delineating the extremity of the proximal segment on each side of the vessel and those marking the beginning of the "noncarinal" contour of the distal branches is based upon the principle that the curvature of a healthy vessel is constant. A circle tangent to the two proximal and distal profiles is constructed therewith completing the missing part of the reference contour profile. The drawing of the reference diameter from the proximal main branch toward the distal main branch shows a typical aspect confirming the presence of a reference function for each segment (step-down phenomenon). An index of optimality according to Murray's law and Finet's formula is provided. Subsequently, a MLD is defined for each segment and then compared with the reference diameter in order to calculate a maximal stenosis percentage for each segment (Fig. 5.10).

The General Electric Software starts with the identification of a first point on the proximal segment of the main vessel and a second point on the distal segment of the main vessel, and this operation is repeated in the side branch. The contour of both vessels is drawn (proximal main to distal main and proximal main to side branch) and a reference diameter is interpolated for the whole bifurcation (three segments: proximal main vessel, distal main vessel, and side branch). The system may use catheter calibration or an integrated geometric calibration process.[33] The angles are measured. Furthermore, the system derives diameters according to Murray's law: the diameter of two of the three segments is used to calculate the diameter of the third segment. Analysis of vessels that do not comprise a normal segment leads to an underestimation of the reference diameters of the bifurcation. The system derives the reference diameter of each of the three segments from the calculated diameter of two segments according to Finet's validated formula.[12] Any difference between computed reference diameters (QCA) and the linearly derived reference measure suggests the presence of diffuse atherosclerosis in the proximal segment even if this segments appears to be normal (the ratio between measured proximal and distal segments is provided).

REPORTING

The EBC QCA panel proposes systematic multisegment analysis of bifurcation lesions to be undertaken before, during, and upon completion of the procedure and subsequently during follow-up in compliance with the following principles:

1. Classification of the bifurcation type should be according to Medina and co-authors.[29] Treatment modalities should be defined and classified precisely.
2. At least three projections should be acquired at baseline, final intervention, and follow-up angiography for optimal visualization of the lesion. Ideally, the quantitative analysis should be preformed in two views with no vessel overlap and minimal foreshortening.
3. The two-dimensional angulations between the parent vessel and the side branch should be reported in identical views even if the best way to measure angles is the use of three-dimensional reconstruction.[34]

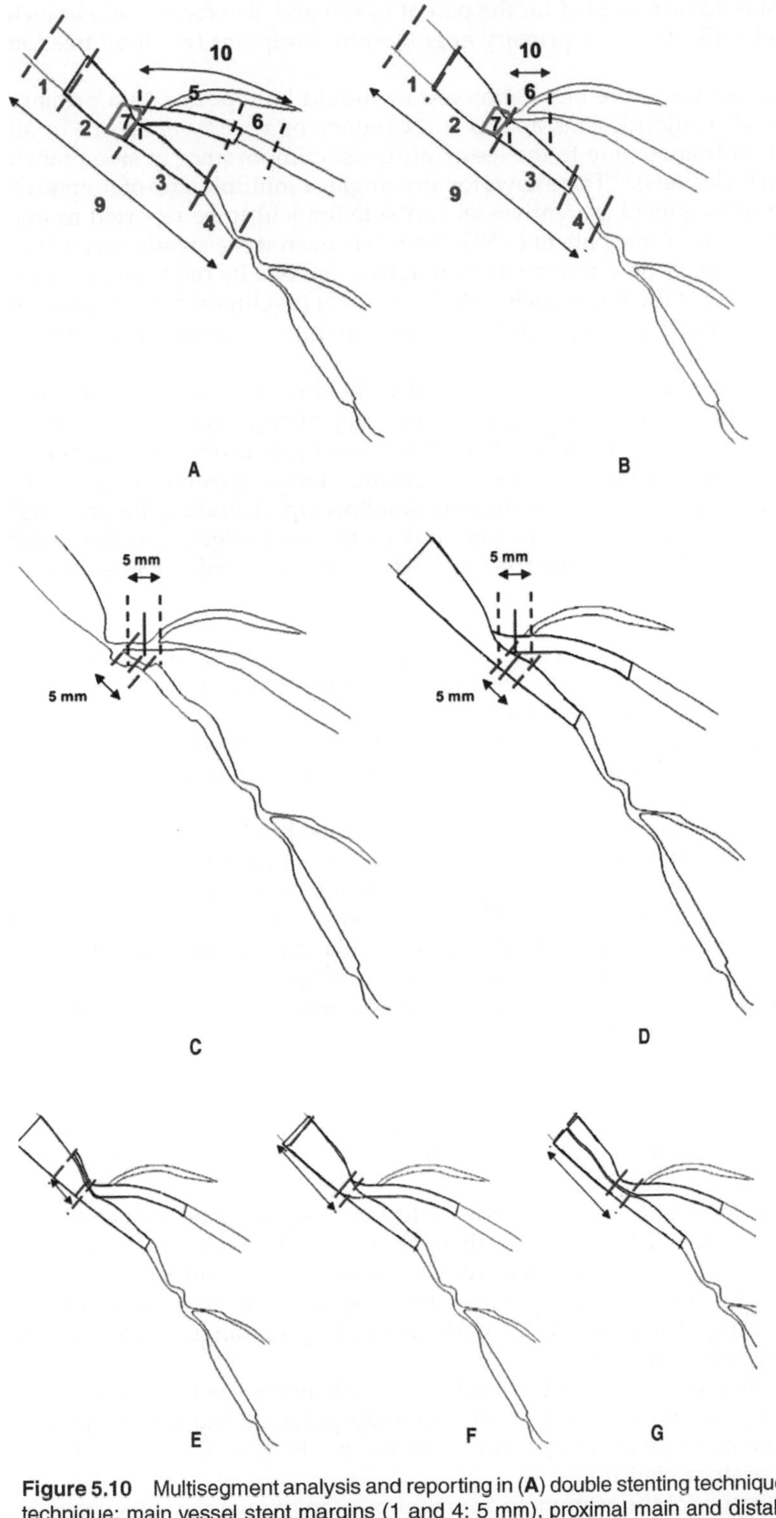

Figure 5.10 Multisegment analysis and reporting in (**A**) double stenting technique and (**B**) in main vessel stenting technique: main vessel stent margins (1 and 4: 5 mm), proximal main and distal main vessel in-stent (2 and 3), side branch in-stent (5) and margin (6) (5 mm or in case of single main vessel stenting site of balloon angioplasty), Carena segment (7), main vessel in-lesion (9), and side branch in-lesion (10). [*Source*: Adapted from Ref. 30.] Multisegmental analysis (**C**) before treatment, (**D**) after treatment and at FU. Distal branch ostial segment analysis on main vessel (4) and side branch (8). Multisegmental analysis: technical analysis. (**E**) Crushed stent segment, (**F**) stent double layer in Culotte technique, and (**G**) stent double barrel in SKS technique.

4. A single (re-)stenosis should be provided for the parent vessel and also for the side branch by using the Medina classification as a primary angiographic endpoint for all bifurcation trials.
5. An overall (re-)stenosis for the entire bifurcation lesion should be reported as a primary endpoint in left main bifurcation lesions and as a secondary or tertiary endpoint in all non–left main bifurcation lesions (due to the lesser prognostic importance of side branch restenosis in non–left main lesions).[25] This allows for any single or multiple sites of restenosis within a bifurcation lesion segment (parent vessel and side branch) to be reported as one for the bifurcation lesion and for the patient (>50% stenosis), even if the significance of the percentage in terms of coronary flow reserve limitation may have to be reinterpreted after analysis of the FFR especially in the side branch. It is obvious that the clinical consequences of the initial lesion, the acute result, and angiographic follow-up findings cannot be correlated with this definition.
6. A segmental analysis defined by Figure 5.10 performed at the time of postintervention and at follow-up (including LLL) would provide greater accuracy of angiographic parameters owing to minimal vessel taper and variation in reference vessel dimensions. This segmental analysis provides detailed insight into the location of residual stenosis postintervention and the precise location of treatment failure or restenosis at follow-up, including the proximal and distal stented segments, the 5-mm proximal and distal stent edges, and the ostial edges of the side branch and distal parent vessel. Additional segments of interest can be added to this scheme (such as stent overlap length, crush stent length, or gap areas), tailoring the analysis to the specific device and treatment strategy under investigation. In several treatment strategies, the two ostial edges correspond to the site of residual stenosis postprocedure (ostium of the distal main branch) and to the most frequent site of restenosis following DES implantation (ostium of the side branch).
7. Provided a segmental approach as described in Figure 5.10, the interpolated reference for each segment can reliably be used as the reference methodology of choice due to the minimal vessel taper of the focal segments of analysis.
8. Beyond reporting the results of the segmental analysis, the results should further be reported based on the target lesion location, the Medina bifurcation lesion classification, and on the specific treatment strategy of the bifurcation. There is currently no study available on the clinical impact of the Medina classification in the various lesion sites, at baseline, after the procedure, and during follow-up (symptoms, MACE, revascularization, induced ischemia). A hierarchical ranking of different Medina types by using serious clinical events would allow an evaluation of treatment efficacy: a 1,1,1 lesion becoming 0,0,1 after treatment is undoubtedly a better result than a 1,0,0.

CONCLUSIONS

Because of its wide availability, quantitative coronary angiography has still a major role in coronary bifurcation stenting in addition to other interesting assessment methods (IVUS, FFR) before, during, and after stenting.

QCA allows the classification of coronary bifurcation lesion types and their denomination (designation by the operator of the distal main branch and side branch), which constitutes an indispensable basis for prospective studies, randomized or not, analyzed by intention-to-treat, comparing various therapeutic options in comparable study populations. In such a context, QCA provides essential data that complement the Medina classification, angle degree, lesion length, and the presence of calcified segments.

On-line QCA may guide the operator in the selection of the balloon size for predilatation kissing balloons and stents. Certain lesion characteristics may preclude the use of specific techniques (Crush technique and open B angle). For example, the length of the side branch stenosis may influence the strategy choice.

Because of the fractal nature of the asymmetric branching of epicardial coronary arteries, the comparative analysis of the outcome of various stenting strategies for bifurcation lesions requires a multisegment analysis of the three bifurcation segments, each of these segments having a reference diameter function, in addition to in-stent and in-lesion analysis of each of the three segments.

The comparison of various stenting strategies requires that a technical analysis of the strategy used is conducted: ostial segment of the SB and distal main branch (gap, stent under-deployment), analysis of areas with double stent layer (Culotte, Crush)[35,36] or double lumen (simultaneous kissing stent or SKS)[37] regarding the relationships between those technical aspects and LLL (and related clinical events).

The use of recently developed dedicated software ensures the reliability of these analyses. In this specific context, only dedicated programs may guarantee the accurate assessment of anti-restenosis strategies by means of the segment analysis of late lumen loss.

New software can still be enhanced in order to comply with the following principles: minimal user interaction in the selection and processing of the coronary segments to be analyzed, minimal editing of the automatically determined results, short analysis time, providing highly accurate and precise results, with small systematic and random errors, and finally providing suitable reporting and data exchange mechanisms.[30]

REFERENCES

1. Louvard Y, Lefevre T, Morice MC. Percutaneous coronary intervention for bifurcation coronary disease. Heart 2004; 90:713–722.7
2. Steigen TK, Wiseth R, Erglis A, et. al. Randomized study on simple versus complex stenting of coronary artery bifurcation lesions: the Nordic bifurcation study. Nordic PCI Study Group. Circulation 2006; 114(18):1955–1961.
3. Tsuchida K, Colombo A, Lefèvre T, et al. The clinical outcome of percutaneous treatment of bifurcation lesions in multivessel coronary artery disease with the sirolimus-eluting stent: Insights from the Arterial Revascularization Therapies Study part II (ARTS II). Eur Heart J 2007; 28(4):433–442.
4. Louvard Y, Thomas M, Dzavik V, et al. Classification of coronary artery bifurcation lesions and treatments: Time for a consensus! Catheter Cardiovasc Interv 2008; 71(2):175–183.
5. Thomas M, Hildick-Smith D, Louvard Y, et al. Percutaneous coronary intervention for bifurcation disease. A consensus view from the first meeting of the European Bifurcation Club. EuroInterv 2006; 2:149–153.
6. Legrand V, Thomas M, Zelisko M, et al. Percutaneous coronary intervention of bifurcation lesions/state-of-the-art. Insights from the second meeting of the European Bifurcation Club. EuroInterv 2007; 9:144–149.
7. Kassab GS. Functional hierarchy of coronary circulation: Direct evidence of a structure-function relation. Am J Physiol Heart Circ Physiol 2005; 289(6):H2559–H2565.
8. Kamiya A, Takahashi T. Quantitative assessments and morphological and functional properties of biological trees based on their fractal nature. J Appl Physiol 2007; 102(6):2315–2323.
9. Murray CD. The physiological principle of minimum work. I. The vascular system and the cost of blood volume. Proc Nat Acad Sci USA 1926; 12:207–214.
10. Kassab GS. Scaling laws of vascular trees: Of form and function. Am J Physiol Heart Circ Physiol 2006; 290(2):H894–H903.
11. Zhou Y, Kassab GS, Molloi S. On the design of the coronary arterial tree: A generalization of Murray's law. Phys Med Biol 1999; 44(12):2929–2945.
12. Finet G GM, Perrenot B, Rioufol G, et al. Fractal geometry of arterial coronary bifurcations. A quantitative coronary angiography and intravascular ultrasound analysis. EuroInterv 2007; 3: 490–498.
13. Tanaka A, Mori H, Tanaka E, et al. Branching patterns of intramural coronary vessels determined by microangiography using synchrotron radiation. Am J Physiol Heart Circ Physiol 1999; 276:H2262–H2267.
14. Malek AM, Alper SL, Izumo S. Hemodynamic shear stress and its role in atherosclerosis. JAMA 1999; 282(21):2035–2042.
15. Zhu H, Friedman MH. Relationship between the dynamic geometry and wall thickness of a human coronary artery. Arterioscler Thromb Vasc Biol 2003; 23(12):2260–2265.
16. Asakura T, Karino T. Flow patterns and spatial distribution of atherosclerosis lesions in human coronary arteries. Circ Res 1990; 66:1045–1066.
17. Chatzizisis YS, Coskun AU, Jonas M, et al. Role of endothelial shear stress in the natural history of coronary atherosclerosis and vascular remodeling. Molecular, cellular, and vascular behavior. J Am Coll Cardiol 2007; 49:2379–2393.
18. Reiber JHC. Morphologic and densitometric quantitation of coronary stenoses; an overview of existing quantitation techniques. In: Reiber JHC, Serruys PW (eds) New Developments in Quantitative Coronary Arteriography. Dordrecht: Kluwer Academic Publishers, 1988; pp 34–88.

19. Reiber JHC, Serruys PW, Kooijman CJ, et al. Assessment of short-, medium-, and long-term variations in arterial dimensions from computer-assisted quantitation of coronary cineangiograms. Circulation 1985; 71:280–288.
20. Mauri L OE, Kuntz RE. Late loss in lumen diameter and binary restenosis for drug-eluting stent comparison. Circulation 2005; 111(25):3435–3442.
21. Pocock SJ, Lansky AJ, Mehran R, et al. Angiographic surrogate endpoints in drug-eluting stent trials: A systematic evaluation based on individual patient data from eleven randomized controlled trials. JACC 2008; 51(1):23–32.
22. Costa MA, Sabate M, Angiolillo DJ, et al. Relocation of minimal luminal diameter after bare metal and drug-eluting stent implantation: incidence and impact on angiographic late loss. Catheter Cardiovasc Interv 2007;69(2):181–188.
23. Dzavik VKR, Ivanov J, Ing DJ, et al. Predictors of long-term outcome after crush stenting of coronary bifurcation lesions: importance of the bifurcation angle. Am Heart J 2006; 152(4):762–769.
24. Lefevre T, Louvard Y, Morice MC, et al. Stenting of bifurcation lesions: A rational approach. J Interv Cardiol 2001; 14:573–585.
25. Koo B-K, Kang H-J, Youn T-J, et al. Physiologic assessment of jailed side branch lesions using fractional flow reserve. J Am Coll Cardiol 2005; 46:633–637.
26. Costa RA, Mintz GS, Carlier SG, et al. Bifurcation coronary lesions treated with the "crush" technique: An intravascular ultrasound analysis. J Am Coll Cardiol 2005; 46(4):599–605.
27. Lefevre T, Morice MC. Influence of technical strategies on the outcome of coronary bifurcation stenting. EuroInterv 2005; 1:31–37.
28. Movahed MR. Coronary artery bifurcation lesion classifications, interventional techniques and clinical outcome. Expert Rev Cardiovasc Ther 2008; 6(2):261–274.
29. Medina A, Suarez de Lezo J, Pan M. A new classification of coronary bifurcation lesions. Rev Esp Cardiol 2006; 59(2):183.
30. Lansky A, Tuinenburg J, Costa M, et al. European Bifurcation Angiographic Sub-Committee. Quantitative angiographic methods for bifurcation lesions: A consensus statement from the European Bifurcation Group. Catheter Cardiovasc Interv 2009; 73(2):258–266.
31. Reiber JH vd Zwet P, Koning G, von Land CD, et al. Accuracy and precision of quantitative digital coronary arteriography: Observer-, short-, and medium-term variabilities. Cathet Cardiovasc Diagn 1993; 28(3):187–198.
32. Ramcharitar S, Onuma Y, Aben JP, et al. A novel dedicated quantitative coronary analysis methodology for bifurcation analysis. EuroInterv 2008; 3:553–557.
33. Vaillant R G-HL, Lienard J. A new calibration approach for quantification application in the cath lab. CARS Int Congress Ser 2004; 1268:1040–1044.
34. Dvir D, Marom H, Assali A, et al. Bifurcation lesions in the coronary arteries: Early experience with a novel 3-dimensional imaging and quantitative analysis before and after stenting. EuroIntervention 2007; 3:(1):95–99.
35. Chevalier B, Glatt B, Royer T, et al. Placement of coronary stents in bifurcation lesions by the "culotte" technique. Am J Cardiol 1998; 82(8):943–949.
36. Colombo A, Stankovic G, Orlic D, et al. Modified T-stenting technique with crushing for bifurcation lesions: immediate results and 30-day outcome. Catheter Cardiovasc Interv. 2003; 60(2):145–151.
37. Sharma SK, Choudhury A, Lee J, et al. Simultaneous kissing stents (SKS) technique for treating bifurcation lesions in medium-to-large size coronary arteries. Am J Cardiol 2004; 94(7):913–917.

6 The vulnerable plaque and angiography

John A. Ambrose and Usman Javed

INTRODUCTION

The vulnerable plaque is usually defined as that plaque which is prone to thrombosis and/or disruption, and it is the immediate precursor to acute ST–elevation myocardial infarction. Such a lesion also precedes in many to most cases of non–ST-elevation myocardial infarction and unstable angina. However, the definition of non–ST-elevation myocardial infarction now includes any elevation of troponin and there are many other reasons for an increase in troponin other than the presence, development, or progression of a narrowing in the epicardial coronary arteries. These include heart failure, atrial fibrillation or other tachyarrhythmias, prolonged hypotension and renal failure amongst others.

Based on autopsy data from patients dying after myocardial infarction or with sudden coronary death in which a coronary thrombosis was present, the underlying mechanism for thrombus formation is either disruption of the fibrous cap of a so-called thin-capped fibroatheroma (TCFA) or superficial erosion of a non–thin-capped plaque.[1] These are usually referred to as thrombosed plaque. What does the vulnerable plaque prior to a myocardial infarction then look like? Well the answer is simple. We do not know for sure. This is because the natural history of the TCFA and other potential lesions that might be responsible for a future myocardial infarction (presumed "vulnerable plaques") as of yet has not been documented. Many techniques can identify in vivo the TCFA. However, determining which one will progress to a future coronary event can only be demonstrated in natural history studies in which all TCFA's and other potential lesions are sequentially followed to determine which ones under which circumstances progress to an acute myocardial infarction. Until these studies are published, one is left uncertain about the utility of noninvasive or invasive modalities to predict the site of a future adverse event and more importantly about the necessity of intervening on these presumed "vulnerable plaques" prior to the development of the event.[2]

What might then the role of angiography be? This chapter discusses the ability of angiography to identify thrombosed plaque, the immediate cause of myocardial infarctions, and its potential to identify in some cases the presumed vulnerable plaque.

THROMBOSED PLAQUE

The culprit lesion

Before a discussion on the angiographic features of thrombosed plaque, it is necessary to discuss the most underappreciated concept that contributed to our understanding of thrombosed plaque and ultimately that of vulnerable plaque. This concept is that of the culprit lesion, which when simply put is the lesion responsible for the syndrome. Early angiographic data in unstable angina failed to differentiate it from stable coronary syndromes based upon the number of diseased vessels or percent diameter stenosis. The most likely reason for this was that the culprit lesion was not evaluated in these studies. In patients with single-vessel disease and an acute coronary syndrome, it is usually very easy to find the culprit lesion, as it is the significant stenosis present in that vessel. Only when one began to assess the qualitative aspects of this lesion was it apparent that unstable angina and stable angina were different.[3–5] On the other hand, in patients with multivessel disease, a single culprit lesion may be identifiable in only about 50% of individuals. Obviously, if there are multiple lesions that are significantly stenosed, it can be impossible to find a single culprit.

Another mechanism for finding the culprit lesion has been the evaluation of serial angiographic findings. If a patient had a prior angiogram and then presents with an acute coronary syndrome, one can often see significant progression of at least one site or the appearance of a new lesion on angiography. This lesion is likely the culprit lesion. In other cases, analysis of the angiographic film along with the electrocardiographic or left ventricular findings may help distinguish a culprit lesion even in multivessel disease. It was this process that allowed Ambrose et al. to evaluate the qualitative angiographic features of the unstable or thrombosed plaque both in unstable angina as well as in non–Q-wave myocardial infarction.[6,7] Furthermore, it was serial analysis of coronary lesions in studies by Ambrose et al. and Little et al. that developed the concept that most ST-elevation myocardial infarctions as well as a majority of patients presenting with unstable angina or non–Q-wave myocardial infarction arise from lesions that had <50% diameter stenosis on a prior angiogram.[6,8]

Clinical plaque progression

As mentioned above, it is now believed that most ST-elevation myocardial infarctions arise from lesions that before the event did not have a significant diameter stenosis. It is this finding which has been largely responsible for the efforts now placed on vulnerable plaque detection. If the lesion is not severe, are there particular aspects of the lesion that cannot be determined by angiography alone that make it more prone to rupture and/or thrombosis? It has also been established, based on pathologic analysis in pressure-fixed coronary arteries as well as by utilizing intravascular ultrasound, that most "normal" segments of the coronary tree as shown by angiography contain atherosclerotic plaque in patients who have risk factors for coronary artery disease or who have lesions in other vessels.[9,10] Yet, nonobstructive lesions, those <50% diameter stenosis, angiographically leading to myocardial infarction are not small lesions. These lesions are often large and well developed but the process of positive remodeling allows the lumen to be maintained, while the plaque, which is often eccentric, grows outward into the vessel wall.[11]

While these concepts of myocardial infarction and unstable angina developing from nonobstructive lesions were first proposed 20 years ago, more recent data substantiate these earlier findings. Glaser et al. reported the findings of an NHLBI dynamic registry.[12] A total of 3747 PCI (percutaneous coronary intervention) lesions were analyzed. Out of these, 216 patients required additional nontarget lesions PCI for clinical plaque progression at 1 year. Of these, 2/3 presented with an acute coronary syndrome either being new onset unstable angina or nonfatal myocardial infarction. The mean stenosis of the progressed lesion was 41.8% at the initial angiogram and 83.9% at the second angiogram. The majority of lesions requiring subsequent PCI were <75% in severity at the time of the initial PCI, whereas only 13.4% of lesions greater than 70% on the initial angiogram required PCI on subsequent studies. These data are similar to the previously reported angiographic data in the 1980 s, which found that 12% of ST-elevation myocardial infarction arose from obstructive (>70%) lesions.[13] Similar data exist for unstable angina and non–Q-wave infarction indicating that the culprit lesion often originates from nonobstructive plaques as seen on a prior angiogram.[7] Pathologic studies also support this concept in that most TCFAs found at autopsy are not significantly obstructed plaques.[14]

Initially, the concept that myocardial infarction arose from the nonobstructive (less than severely stenosed) lesions was met with a great deal of skepticism. However, when one considers the pathophysiology of coronary artery disease and supply/demand physiology, it makes sense. If a lesion acutely is blocked off by a thrombus, there is an acute reduction in supply and collateral vessels may not be able to immediately perfuse that area. Only severe chronic lesions would be expected to acutely develop collaterals. These patients are rare in acute ST–elevation myocardial infarction. Thus, a severely stenosed lesion that occludes acutely is less likely to cause myocardial infarction than a nonobstructive one. Nevertheless, based on data from the Coronary Artery Surgery Study (CASS) registry, Alderman et al. showed that on serial angiographic studies, it was the severely stenosed lesions that were more likely to progress to total occlusion.[15] However, no clinical information was presented in that study. They also showed that while a higher percentage of severely stenosed lesions progressed to 100% occlusion, there were many more nonobstructive lesions. While their progression rate to total occlusion was smaller, the fact that there were so many indicated that most of the total occlusions even in this study originated from lesions that originally were not severely stenosed. This is consistent with the observation from other studies that only when there is a sudden and large reduction in lumen diameter will there be a clinical event. The type of event will depend on how much ischemia has developed and what is the supply/demand ratio. If supply is completely cutoff acutely, ST-elevation infarction is likely if the occlusion persists. When a severely stenosed lesion progresses, total occlusion will be clinically silent or may result in only a transient episode of ischemia.

Angiographic features of thrombosed plaque

As mentioned previously, coronary thrombosis on a disrupted or eroded plaque is the main cause of most ST elevation myocardial infarctions as well as in the majority of cases of unstable angina or non–ST-elevation myocardial infarction. To understand the contribution of angiography, one needs to consider the topic of morphologic analysis of lesion. The original description of the angiographic morphology of coronary plaques was performed by Levin and Fallon.[16] In this autopsy series of patients dying after myocardial infarction or after coronary bypass grafting, 73 localized, subtotaled stenoses were studied with postmortem angiography and then analyzed histologically. Angiographic analysis of pressure-fixed segments divided these lesions into type I or type II lesions. Type I lesions were lesions described as having smooth borders, an hour-glass configuration, and no intralumenal lucencies, while type II lesions were eccentric with irregular borders and intraluminal lucencies. On histologic analysis, only 12% of type I angiographic lesions were complicated which was defined pathologically as containing plaque rupture, plaque hemorrhage or superimposed partially occluded thrombi, while 79% of type II lesions were complicated histologically. This study suggested an association between the angiographic morphology and histologic complexity of the lesions. However, clinical data were lacking.

The clinical data were reported in the 1980 s by Ambrose et al.[3] Angiographic correlates were made between plaque morphology and clinical presentation. In a retrospective analysis of 110 patients presenting with either stable or unstable angina, the morphology of the culprit lesions were blindly assessed. If a culprit lesion could be identified with a >50% luminal stenosis, the culprit lesion was divided into four different morphologic types: (1) symmetric or concentric narrowing, (2) eccentric type I (asymmetric narrowing with smooth boarders and a smooth neck), (3) eccentric type II (asymmetric narrowing with irregular boarders and/or a narrow neck with overhanging edges), and (4) multiple irregular lesions. Type II eccentric lesions were frequently encountered in patients with unstable angina and were present in about 70% of culprit lesions, while only 16% of culprit lesions in stable angina contained an eccentric type II lesion. In subsequent studies, the classification was simplified into simple versus complex lesions.[17] Complex lesions included any lesion that had irregular boarders, overhanging edges, ulcerations or filling defects (Fig. 6.1). These were seen in the majority of patients presenting with an acute coronary syndrome whether it was unstable angina or non–Q-wave infarction. These angiographic observations were confirmed more recently with angioscopy. In a combined angiographic/angioscopic study, Waxman et al. found that type II eccentric lesions and complex

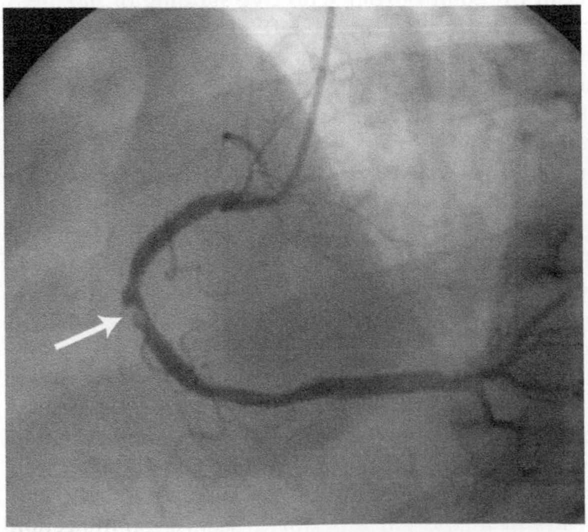

Figure 6.1 Injection of the RCA in the LAO projection. In its mid-portion, there is an eccentric, ulcerated lesion with a filling defect (*arrow*). The patient presented with NSTEMI.

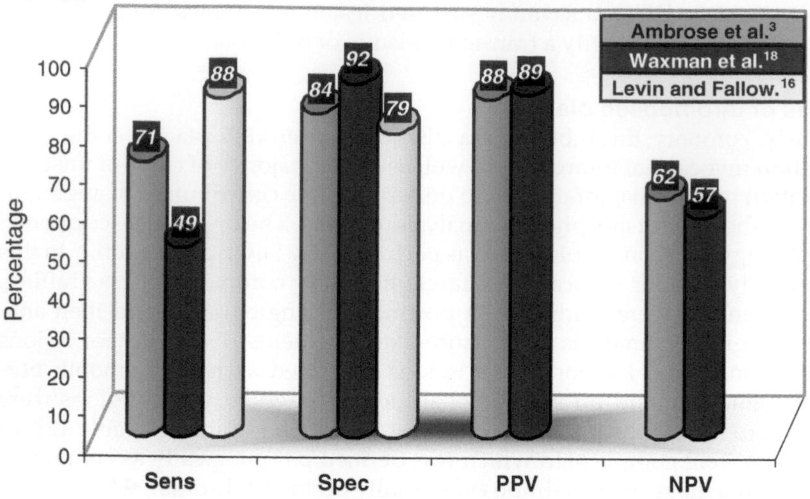

Figure 6.2 Type II eccentric (complex) lesions correlate with clinical presentation of unstable angina,[3] with plaque disruption and/or intracoronary thrombus on angioscopy,[18] and with complicated histology on postmortem angioscopy.[16] Sensitivity (Sens), specificity (Spec), positive predictive value (PPV), and negative predictive value (NPV) where applicable are given.

lesions were strongly associated with disrupted plaques and/or thrombus by angioscopy with positive predictive values of about 90%[18] (Fig. 6.2).

While myocardial infarctions are no longer classified as Q or non-Q wave but rather ST and non-ST elevation, these angiographic observations are still relevant. In these initial studies, only lesions that were <100% occluded were analyzed. The angiographic features of totally occluded lesions was first described by DeWood et al.[19] They analyzed patients with an acute Q-wave myocardial infarction (presenting with ST-segment elevation) and showed that within the first 4 hours of myocardial infarction, angiographically 87% of culprit arteries were totally occluded. These occluded lesions could be easily identified at angiography. There was dye staining of the lesion most likely related to infiltration of contrast into the thrombus. At surgery, thrombus could be extracted from the coronary artery. Of course, the era of thrombolytic therapy has taught us much about the coronary thrombus. Totally occluded lesions with dye staining or haziness can be recanalyzed with intracoronary or intravenous thrombolytic therapy and then subsequently in other studies by angioplasty. Thus, in a totally occluded lesion, the most common feature of a thrombosed plaque is an irregular border with dye staining or haziness. Following successful opening of a thrombosed artery with thrombolytic therapy, it is usual to find residual lesions that are severely stenosed, irregular, and/or ulcerated with filling defects at distal or even proximal to the site of the occlusion which represent residual thrombus.[20] In fact, recent data indicates that the site of the total coronary occlusion is often proximal to the most severe lesion in the vessel.[21] This is most likely related to the fact that once the vessel occludes and flow is interrupted, the thrombus will form and propagate proximally up to the location of the nearest side branch in the vessel.

Another angiographic observation of recanalyzed lesions in myocardial infarction was that of ulceration of the infarct-related lesion as described by Wilson et al.[22] However, the first angiographic analysis of STEMI patients was made by Brown et al.[20] In analyzing angiograms early after thrombolysis, they were able to show a distinct translucency in the vessel at the site of occlusion superimposed on a less-conspicuous plaque. The plaque was generally only 50% to 60% obstructive, while the translucency was felt to represent partially lysed and residual thrombus that was superimposed on the atherosclerotic plaque.

There is another important feature of myocardial infarction and the thrombosed plaque that is related to the location of these lesions within the epicardial coronary arteries. Gotsman et al. evaluated the angiographic location of culprit lesions in 308 patients presenting with ST-elevation myocardial infarction from a lesion in the left anterior descending artery who received thrombolytic therapy.[23] Coronary angiography was performed 1 week after presentation and a majority of stenoses were found to be proximal to or at a bifurcation in the vessel. Gibson et al. utilizing angiographic data from the TIMI trials found that 75% of culprit lesions in acute myocardial infarction were located within 60 mm from the origin in the three major coronary arteries, with the median distance from the vessel ostium to the end of culprit lesion being 43 mm.[24] Wang et al. also demonstrated the preferential relationship of plaque rupture with its proximity to the vessel ostium.[25] In this series of 208 patients with STEMI, for each 10 mm increase in distance from the ostium, the risk of a coronary occlusion was decreased by 13% in the right coronary artery (RCA), 26% in the left circumflex coronary artery (LCx), and 30% in the left anterior descending artery (LAD) ($p < 0.001$ for all). This clustered and nonuniform distribution of coronary thromboses was supported by the fact that 50% of such lesions occurred within the first 25 mm of the LAD or the LCx and 45 mm of the RCA. When taking into account the infarct-related vessel, 44% of culprit lesions occurred in the RCA, 39% in the LAD, and 16% in the LCx (Figs. 6.3–6.5). Based upon the above evidence, the proximal coronary tree appears more susceptible to occlusive thromboses and symptomatic acute coronary syndromes.

Therefore, qualitative analysis of culprit coronary lesions at angiography has been very useful in differentiating patients presenting with an acute coronary syndrome in whom significant coronary artery disease is present from stable coronary syndromes. This is the thrombosed plaque. If the artery is patent with <100% stenosis, the acute coronary syndrome culprit lesion is usually severe (≥70% diameter stenosis) and the lesion is often eccentric with either irregular borders, ulcerations, and/or filling defects—a so-called complex lesion. In totally occluded lesions, the common denominator for thrombus is the presence of filling defects with dye staining and/or a hazy or irregular border to the total occlusion. Total coronary occlusion of the culprit lesion is uncommon in unstable angina and usually present with ST elevation infarction at presentation. In non–ST-elevation infarction myocardial infarction, the incidence of total coronary occlusions varies probably between 20% and 40% based on data originally obtained from patients presenting with non–Q-wave infarction.[7,26]

There are, however, significant limitations to this approach. Morphologic analysis of coronary plaques can only be done properly if multiple angiographic projections of the coronary artery are taken in orthogonal views that minimize foreshortening of the vessel as well as the overlap of branch points. Without this, a lesion may look simple in one view as the ulceration or irregularity may not be visible unless the orthogonal view has been taken (Fig. 6.6). It should be noted that this morphologic classification of lesions is different from the modified ACC/AHA classification system for lesion morphology.[27] The later was a classification system proposed to determine the appropriateness and risk of a lesion at the time of balloon angioplasty. In most recent articles on coronary intervention, the complex lesion referred to is based upon the ACC/AHA classification and not the morphological classification of Ambrose et al. However, all qualitative analyses have shortcomings and are limited with angiography. Angiography does not assess the vessel wall but only the luminal surface. It is this limitation of angiography that has been the major impetus to the development of new techniques for assessing the plaque and ultimately its histology/biochemistry.

ANGIOGRAPHY AND THE VULNERABLE PLAQUE

Given the above limitations of angiography what can we say about its ability to identify vulnerable plaque? The whole discussion is complicated by the fact that the exact characteristics of a vulnerable plaque are unknown due to the lack of natural history studies as outlined in the first section in this chapter. While ST-elevation myocardial infarctions are concentrated in the proximal portions of the coronary artery and/or perhaps at a branch point, their precise location can be detected angiographically. If the vulnerable plaque turns out to be a TCFA with an intact fibrous cap (based on natural history), angiography is unlikely to be able to find its precise location in a vessel without a significant obstruction.

On the other hand, the best indicator of vulnerable plaque could be an already disrupted but clinically silent plaque.[2] If an asymptomatic plaque rupture of a TCFA preceded symptomotology, it is conceivable that angiography could detect at least some of these lesions. A complex lesion on angiography, by the definition of Ambrose et al., is a very specific although less-sensitive indicator of plaque disruption and/or thrombus formation as previously

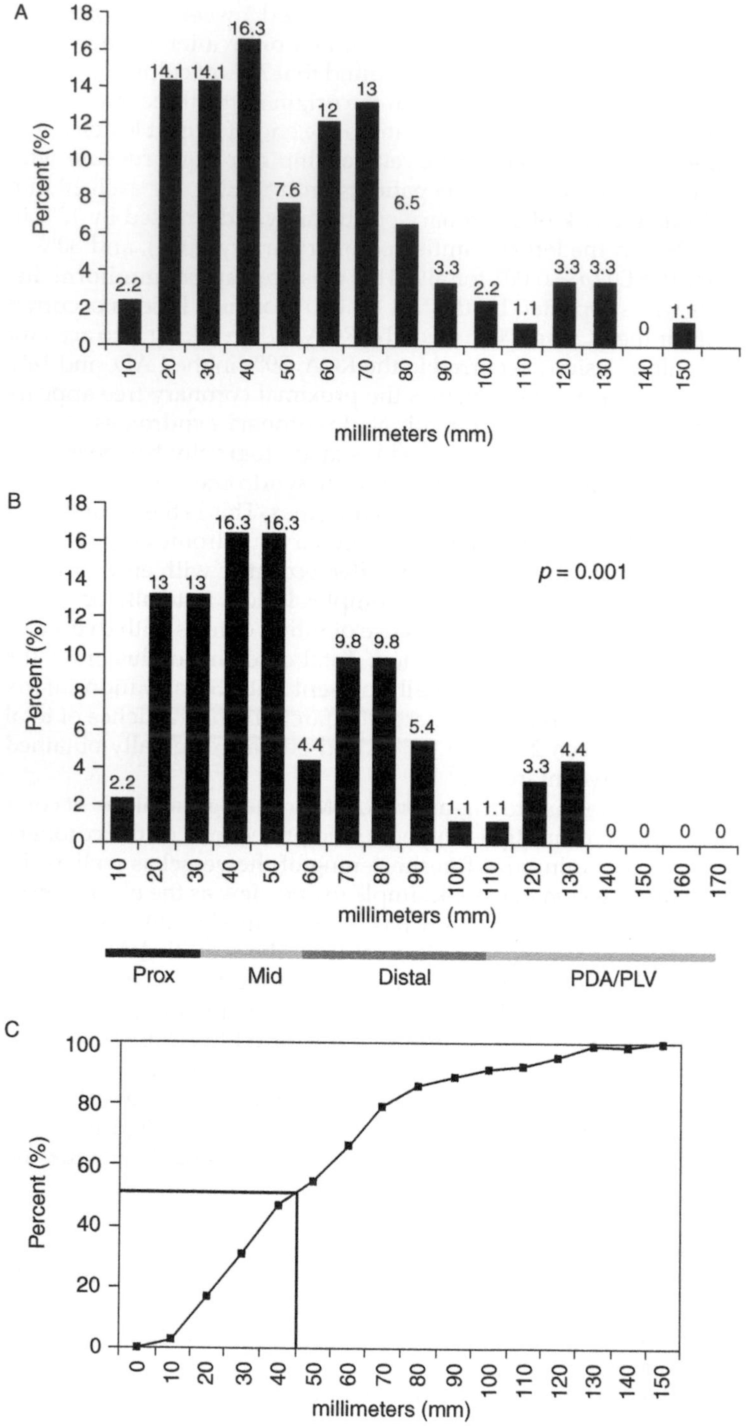

Figure 6.3 RCA analysis: (**A**) ostium analysis of distribution of acute coronary occlusions, (**B**) normalized segment analysis of acute coronary occlusions, and (**C**) cumulative frequency distribution curve that demonstrates the cumulative frequency of thrombotic locations from ostium of RCA. *Source*: Adapted from Ref. 25.

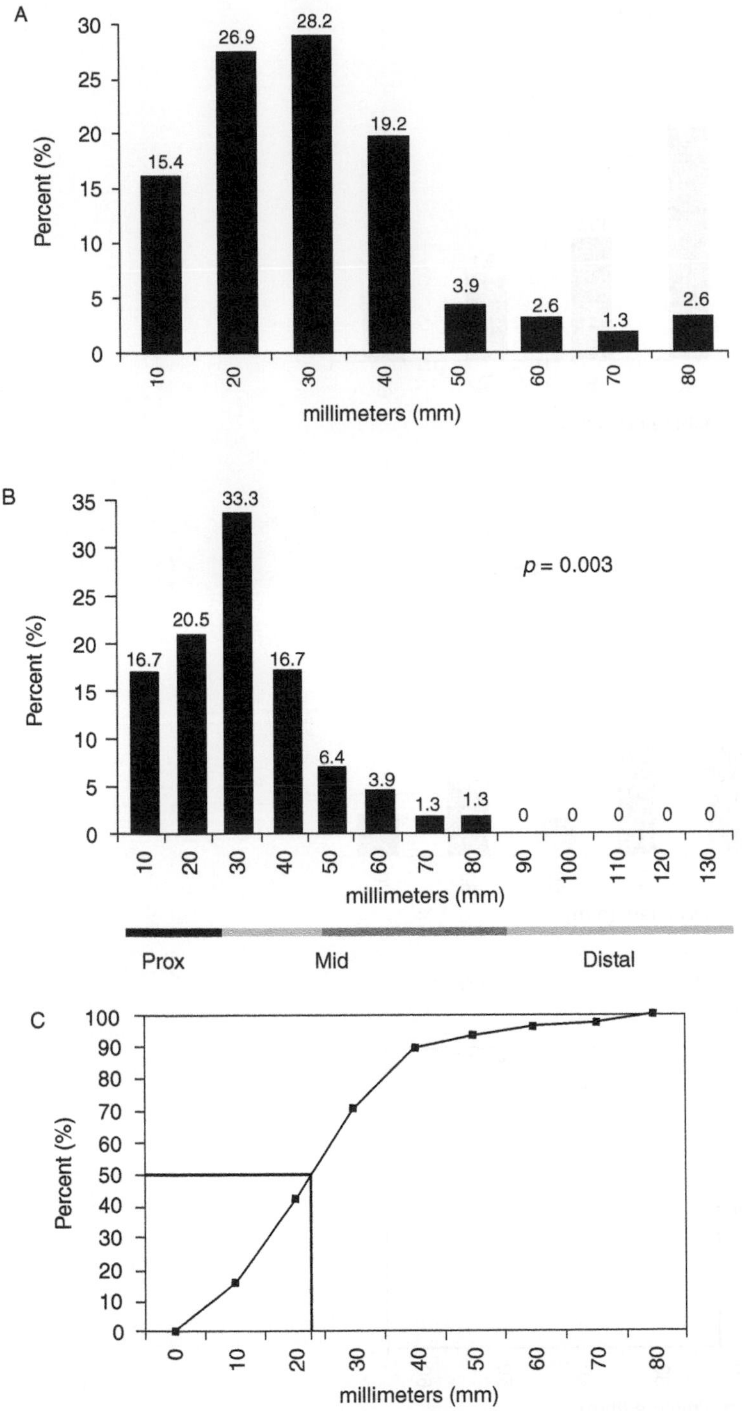

Figure 6.4 LAD analysis: (**A**) ostium analysis of distribution of acute coronary occlusions, (**B**) normalized segment analysis of acute coronary occlusions, and (**C**) cumulative frequency distribution curve that demonstrates the cumulative frequency of thrombotic locations from ostium of LAD. *Source*: Adapted from Ref. 25.

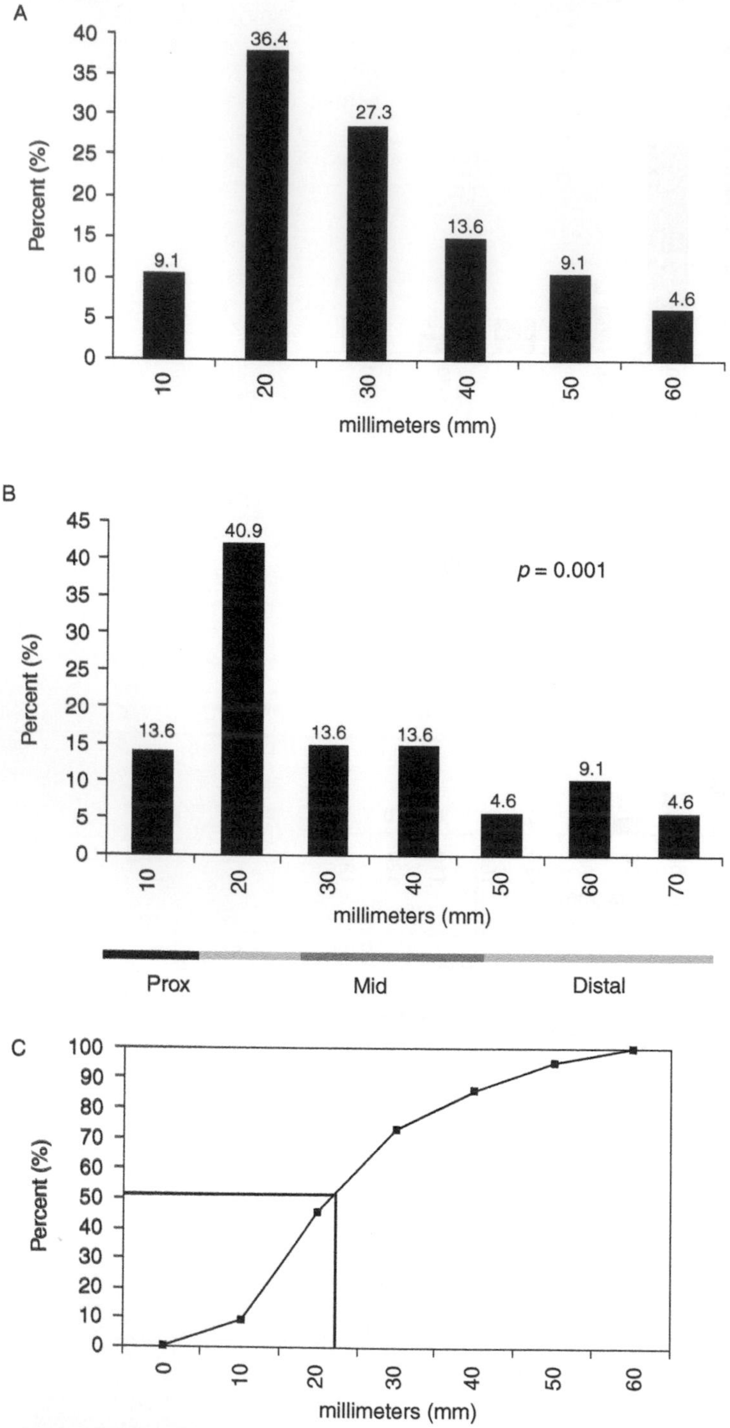

Figure 6.5 LCx analysis: (**A**) ostium analysis of distribution of acute coronary occlusions, (**B**) normalized segment analysis of acute coronary occlusions, and (**C**) cumulative frequency distribution curve that demonstrates the cumulative frequency of thrombotic locations from ostium of LCx. *Source*: Adapted from Ref. 25.

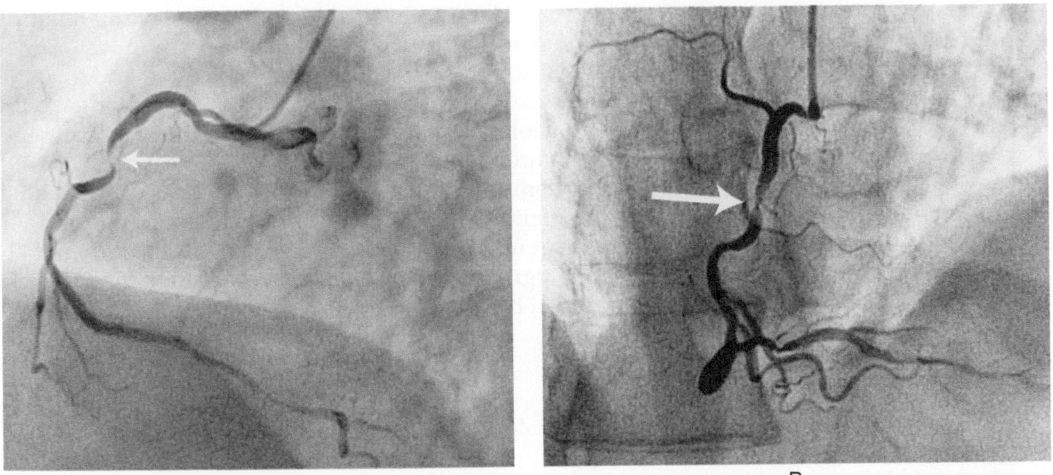

Figure 6.6 (**A**) A tight stenosis (*arrow*) at the junction of proximal and mid-RCA is seen in the LAO projection. In the RAO projection (**B**), the same stenosis is seen. There is a distinct lucency distal to the narrowest portion in the lesion (*arrow*). This lucency in a vessel without angiographic calcification likely represents intracoronary thrombus. This patient presented with NSTEMI.

discussed. Prior studies support the possible association of lesion complexity with angiographic progression and coronary events. Chester et al. studied 222 patients with chronic stable angina who where awaiting angioplasty.[28] The angioplasty was done during a subsequent hospitalization (a median interval of 7 months later) and these less than total occlusions underwent repeated angiography immediately before coronary intervention. Complex lesions had a 14% incidence of progression usually with clinical symptoms in comparison to only 4% of the smooth lesions ($p < 0.02$). Although these data were published before the use of more potent antiplatelet and statin therapy, they indicate the potential danger of these complex lesions. Likewise, Goldstein et al. found that multiple complex lesions present on angiography during ST-elevation myocardial infarction have a bad prognosis. Nearly 40% of patients had multiple complex lesions with one or more additional complex lesions other than the infarct-related culprit vessel.[29] Those with multiple complex lesions were more likely to undergo repeat or a second intervention of the noninfarct related lesion or required coronary bypass on follow up compared to patients with a single complex lesion. Finally, in a small retrospective study of patients with angiogram performed before and after myocardial infarction, Dacanay et al. found that eccentric and irregular plaques with moderate stenosis on the initial angiogram were associated with Q-wave myocardial infarction on follow up angiography at the same site as the original blockage.[30] Of course, the ultimate ability of angiography to predict "vulnerable plaques" will only be determined by natural history studies such as the PROSPECT trial.

In addition to lesion morphology, there are other data suggesting that plaque geometry as determined at angiography contributes to predicting a future myocardial infarction. Ledru et al. compared angiograms before and after myocardial infarction.[31] On the initial angiogram, the culprit lesions leading to a future myocardial infarction had different anatomic features including the fact that they were more symmetrical and had steeper outflow angles compared to controls. Coronary arteries undergo a continuous cyclic bending during each cardiac cycle, which may predispose proximal lesions (where the degree of bending appears to be greater) to subsequent plaque disruption.[32] It must be mentioned that none of these discussions address myocardial infarctions that occur due to plaque erosion and subsequent thrombus formation. This represents about one-third of myocardial infarctions as detected at autopsy.[33] In these individuals, hypercoagulability of the blood is probably the primary factor. It is unlikely that even the most advanced and sophisticated techniques that asses the anatomy and composition of the plaque including the thickness of the fibrous cap and the volume of the lipid pool could accurately detect the site of these future infarctions.

In conclusion, coronary angiography can identify thrombosed plaques. Its potential for identifying vulnerable plaques that are the site of future myocardial infarction is limited. However, its potential might improve, if proper natural history studies are carried out and are able to identify certain angiographic aspects that predispose a particular lesion in an individual with certain risk factors to progress and be responsible for an acute coronary syndrome. At present, it is known that ST-elevation myocardial infarction tends to occur in proximal segments of the coronary artery at or near bifurcations. Complex lesion morphology (in a lesion with only mild or moderate obstruction) given its specificity for the presence of plaque disruption and/or thrombus might detect the site of a subsequent infarction in some cases, although further analyses are required. Finally, whether other angiographic techniques such a CT angiography may add to this knowledge will only be determined by subsequent studies.

REFERENCES

1. Kolodgie FD, Virmani R, Burke AP, et al. Pathologic assessment of the vulnerable human coronary plaque. Heart 2004; 90:1385–1391.
2. Ambrose JA. In search of the "vulnerable plaque". Can it be localized and will focal regional therapy ever be an option for cardiac prevention? J Am Coll Cardiol 2008; 22; 51:1539–1542.
3. Ambrose JA, Winters SL, Stern A, et al. Angiographic morphology and the pathogenesis of unstable angina pectoris. J Am Coll Cardiol 1985; 5:609–616.
4. Ambrose JA, Winters SL, Arora RR, et al. Coronary angiographic morphology in myocardial infarction: A link between the pathogenesis of unstable angina and myocardial infarction. J Am Coll Cardiol 1985; 6:1233–1238.
5. Ambrose JA, Dangas G. Unstable angina: Current concepts of pathogenesis and treatment. Arch Intern Med 2000; 160(1):25–37.
6. Ambrose JA, Tannenbaum MA, Alexopoulos D, et al. Angiographic progression of coronary artery disease and the development of myocardial infarction. J Am Coll Cardiol 1988; 12:56–62.
7. Ambrose JA, Hjemdahl-Monsen CE, Borrico S, et al. Angiographic demonstration of a common link between unstable angina pectoris and non-Q-wave acute myocardial infarction. Am J Cardiol 1988; 61:244–247.
8. Little WC, Constantinescu M, Applegate RJ, et al. Can coronary angiography predict the site of a subsequent myocardial infarction in patients with mild-to-moderate coronary artery disease? Circulation 1988; 78:1157–1166.
9. Virmani R, Kolodgie FD, Burke AP, et al. Lessons from sudden coronary death: A comprehensive morphological classification scheme for atherosclerotic lesions. Arterioscler Thromb Vasc Biol 2000; 20;1262–1275.
10. Schoenhagen P, Ziada KM, Kapadia SR, et al. Extent and direction of arterial remodeling in stable versus unstable coronary syndromes: An intravascular ultrasound study. Circulation 2000; 101;598–603.
11. Glagov S, Weisenberg E, Zarins CK, et al. Compensatory enlargement of human atherosclerotic coronary arteries. N Engl J Med 1987; 316:1371–1375.
12. Glaser R, Selzer F, Faxon DP, et al. Clinical progression of incidental, asymptomatic lesions discovered during culprit vessel coronary intervention. Circulation 2005; 111:143–149.
13. Falk E, Shah PK, Fuster V, et al. Coronary plaque disruption. Circulation 1995; 92:657–671.
14. Kolodgie FD, Virmani R, Burke AP, et al. Pathologic assessment of the vulnerable human coronary plaque. Heart 2004; 90:1385–1391.
15. Alderman EL, Corley SD, Fisher LD, et al. Five-year angiographic follow-up of factors associated with progression of coronary artery disease in the Coronary Artery Surgery Study (CASS). J Am Coll Cardiol 1993; 22:1141–1154.
16. Levin DC, Fallon JT. Significance of the angiographic morphology of localized coronary stenoses: Histopathologic correlations. Circulation 1982; 66:316–320.
17. Dangas G, Mehran R, Wallenstein S, et al. Correlation of angiographic morphology and clinical presentation in unstable angina. J Am Coll Cardiol 1997; 29:519–525.
18. Waxman S, Mittleman MA, Zarich SW, et al. Plaque disruption and thrombus in Ambrose's angiographic coronary lesion types. Am J Cardiol 2003; 92:16–20.
19. DeWood MA, Spores J, Notske RN, et al. Prevalence of total coronary occlusion during the early hours of transmural myocardial infarction. N Engl J Med 1980; 303:897–902.
20. Brown BG, Gallery CA, Badger RS, et al. Incomplete lysis of thrombus in the moderate underlying atherosclerotic lesion during intracoronary infusion of streptokinase for acute myocardial infarction: Quantitative angiographic observations. Circulation 1986; 73:653–661.

21. Takumi T, Lee S, Hamasaki S, et al. Limitation of angiography to identify the culprit plaque in acute myocardial infarction with coronary total occlusion utility of coronary plaque temperature measurement to identify the culprit plaque. J Am Coll Cardiol 2007; 50:2197–2203.
22. Wilson RF, Holida MD, White WC, et al. Quantitative angiographic morphology of coronary stenoses leading to myocardial infarction or unstable angina. Circulation 1986; 73:286–293.
23. Gotsman M, Rosenheck S, Nassar H, et al. Angiographic findings in the coronary arteries after thrombolysis in acute myocardial infarction. Am J Cardiol 2002; 70:715–723.
24. Gibson CM, Kirtane AJ, Murphy SA, et al. Distance from the coronary ostium to the culprit lesion in acute ST-elevation myocardial infarction and its implications regarding the potential prevention of proximal plaque rupture. J Thromb Thrombolysis 2003; 15:189–196.
25. Wang JC, Normand SL, Mauri L, et al. Coronary artery spatial distribution of acute myocardial infarction occlusions. Circulation 2004; 110:278–284.
26. DeWood MA, Stifter WF, Simpson CS, et al. Coronary arteriographic findings soon after non-Q-wave myocardial infarction. N Engl J Med 1986; 315:417–423.
27. Guidelines for percutaneous transluminal coronary angioplasty. A report of the American College of Cardiology/American Heart Association Task Force on Assessment of Diagnostic and Therapeutic Cardiovascular Procedures (Subcommittee on Percutaneous Transluminal Coronary Angioplasty). J Am Coll Cardiol 1988; 12:529–545.
28. Chester MR, Chen L, Kaski JC, et al. The natural history of unheralded complex coronary plaques. J Am Coll Cardiol 1996; 28:604–608.
29. Goldstein JA, Demetriou D, Grines CL, et al. Multiple complex coronary plaques in patients with acute myocardial infarction. N Engl J Med 2000; 343:915–922.
30. Dacanay S, Kennedy HL, Uretz E, et al. Morphological and quantitative angiographic analyses of progression of coronary stenoses. A comparison of Q-wave and non-Q-wave myocardial infarction. Circulation 1994; 90:1739–1746.
31. Ledru F, Theroux P, Lesperance J, et al. Geometric features of coronary artery lesions favoring acute occlusion and myocardial infarction: A quantitative angiographic study. J Am Coll Cardiol 1999; 33:1353–1361.
32. Stein PD, Hamid HS, Shivkumar K, et al. Effects of cyclic flexion of coronary arteries on progression of atheroscelrosis. Am J Cardiol 1994; 73:431–437.
33. Farb A, Burke AP, Tang AL, et al. Coronary plaque erosion without rupture into a lipid core. A frequent cause of coronary thrombosis in sudden coronary death. Circulation 1996; 93:1354–1363.

7 Merits and limitations of IVUS for the evaluation of ambiguous lesions

Philippe L.-L'Allier and Jean-Claude Tardif

INTRODUCTION

When performing coronary angiography to assess the extent and severity of coronary artery disease, clinicians are often faced with lesions that cannot be easily classified as significant or not (i.e., flow limiting and responsible for inducible myocardial ischemia). Typically, a cutoff value of 50% angiographic luminal narrowing is used for this purpose, based on animal studies (and human clinical correlations), showing functional significance at that level of severity. Because such determination is crucial for clinical decision making and because there is significant inter- and intraobserver variability in this assessment, it is necessary to understand and appropriately use complementary diagnostic tools in many circumstances. Intravascular ultrasound (IVUS), a catheter-based technique, allows cross-sectional imaging of coronary vessels and precise visualization of both the lumen and the vessel wall. Owing to its excellent sensitivity and its very close correlation with histopathology, IVUS is considered the most accurate coronary imaging modality in vivo. It is therefore frequently used to evaluate angiographically ambiguous lesions in the catheterization laboratory.

DEFINITION OF AMBIGUOUS LESIONS

So-called ambiguous or intermediate lesions relate to the uncertainty surrounding the anatomopathologic correlation with the angiographic image and physiological significance of lesions, respectively. Limitations of angiography in this regard are well known and understood. They include underestimation of the true lesion severity owing to unrecognized disease in the reference segment and inability to find optimal and orthogonal projections for a given segment or lesion. Therefore, lesions yielding >40% and <70% angiographic diameter stenosis typically fall in the intermediate category, especially when the determination of lesion severity is visual and ad hoc (Fig. 7.1). Left main, ostial, bifurcation, tandem, and ectatic/aneurismal lesions, as well as hazy, thrombotic, and ruptured/dissected lesions are frequently considered ambiguous.

IVUS TECHNIQUE AND SAFETY

IVUS is performed over a 0.014 in. guidewire using 2.5F to 3.5F catheters with miniaturized transducers at their tips and requires full anticoagulation. Mechanical (rotational) and solid-state (multielements) designs are available (similar reproducibility and small differences in measurements have been reported).[1,2] A tradeoff between the higher spatial resolution of higher frequencies and deeper penetration of lower frequencies needs to be considered. Currently, 40 and 45 MHz catheters appear to offer the best compromise. Intracoronary nitroglycerin (150–300 μg) should be administered (unless contraindicated) before IVUS examination to minimize dynamic fluctuations in vasomotor tone. It is recommended that the guiding catheter be disengaged from the coronary ostium to allow adequate IVUS evaluation of the aorto-ostial junction when appropriate. In this situation, it is important to position the guiding catheter (in the aorta) in the prolongation of the long axis of the proximal segment of the vessel to avoid geometric distortion associated with IVUS probe obliquity (Fig. 7.2). The transducer is then pulled back mechanically (preferred, 0.5 mm/sec) or manually. A detailed running audio commentary describing the location of the transducer is extremely useful for off-line analyses. Such a procedure typically takes 10 to 15 minutes when performed following a diagnostic angiogram.

The safety of IVUS examination is well established. Recently, we reported the results of a multicenter study evaluating the safety of IVUS in nontransplant, nonintervened, atherosclerotic coronary arteries.[3] Acute complications were extremely rare and we identified the most frequent acute side effect of IVUS to be reversible coronary spasm (1.9%). There was a single

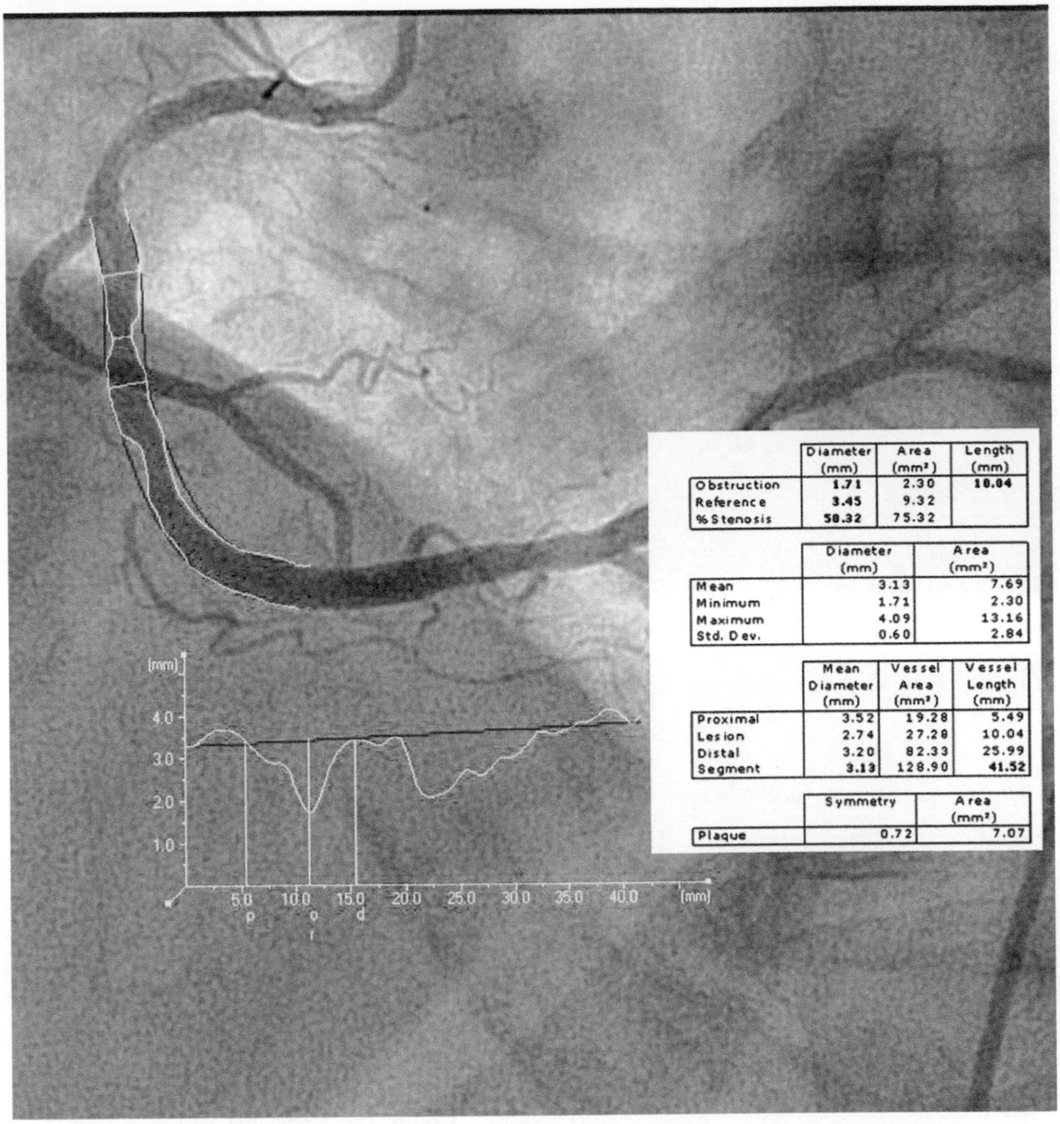

Figure 7.1 Intermediate lesion by angiography. Quantitative coronary angiographic (QCA) measurements confirm a 50.32% diameter stenosis.

occurrence of coronary acute closure (0.2%) that was easily treated percutaneously, and follow-up angiography showed no residual stenosis. We recommend meticulous catheter preparation (especially flushing of the inner lumen of the IVUS catheter to remove any residual air) immediately before entering the guiding catheter and very slow/steady advancement and retrieval of the catheter inside the coronary arteries to allow it to "find" the path of least resistance. The later recommendation is especially important when performing IVUS in tortuous and calcified vessels (because of the very short over-the-wire segment of IVUS catheters and absent hydrophilic coating). Furthermore, it is important to realize that IVUS catheters tend to be large in relation to the inner lumen of 6F guiding catheters, making the likelihood of aspirating air into the guiding catheter during rapid advancement much higher (Venturi effect).

Concerns about damage to the endothelium and long-term deleterious effect on disease progression were also addressed in this study. When IVUS-related arteries were compared with non-IVUS arteries, the coronary change score, the increase in angiographic percent diameter stenosis, and the overall incidence of lesion progression (all measured by quantitative coronary

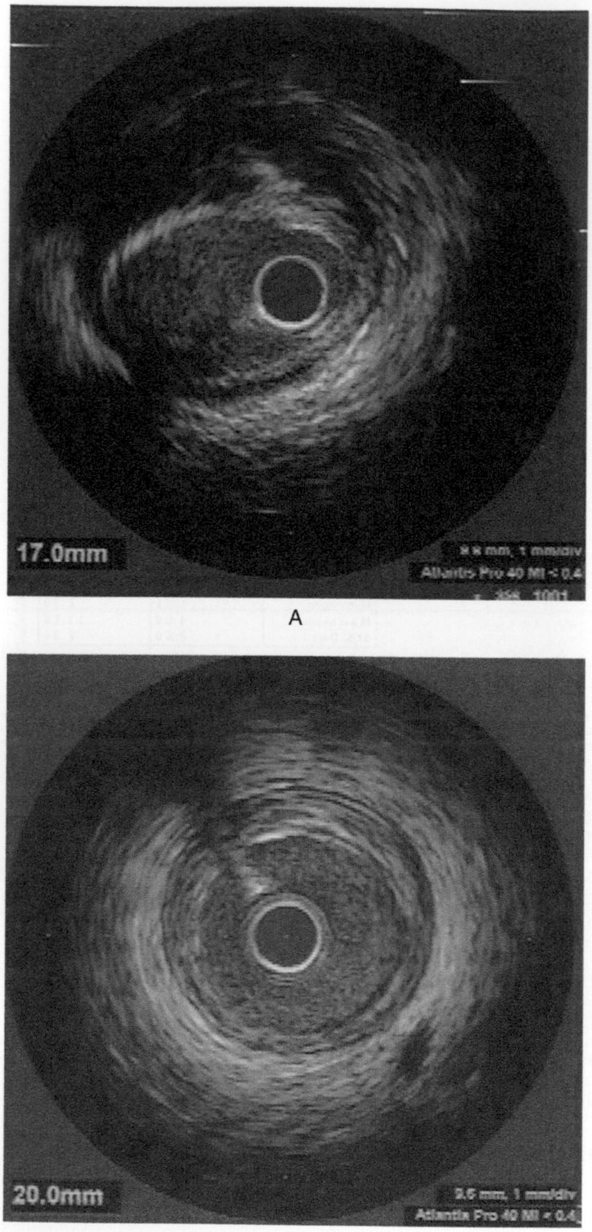

Figure 7.2 Geometric distortion caused by intravascular ultrasound probe obliquity. **(A)** IVUS probe at an angle with the vessel lumen (obliquity) creating an artifact (*oval lumen*). **(B)** IVUS probe ideally positioned perpendicular to the vessel lumen (*appropriately circular lumen*).

angiography) did not differ at 18 to 24 months follow-up. Other studies have also documented the safety of IVUS in a variety of clinical settings.

CLINICAL DECISION MAKING BASED ON IVUS ASSESSMENT

IVUS allows accurate determination of lumen dimensions [minimum lumen diameter (MLD) and surface (MLA)], vessel dimensions [external elastic membrane (EEM)], percent diameter (PDS) and area stenosis (PAS), atherosclerotic plaque surface volume, and vessel remodeling (Fig. 7.3). These parameters have been correlated with physiological measurements and can be used in clinical decision making. IVUS also provides insight into plaque composition (echolucent-soft, echodense-fibrotic, calcified, and mixed) and potential vulnerability (e.g., echolucent central core and thin fibrous cap) (Fig. 7.4).[4–6] While there is theoretical merit to treat lesions based on their suspected vulnerability or propensity to rupture and cause clinical events,

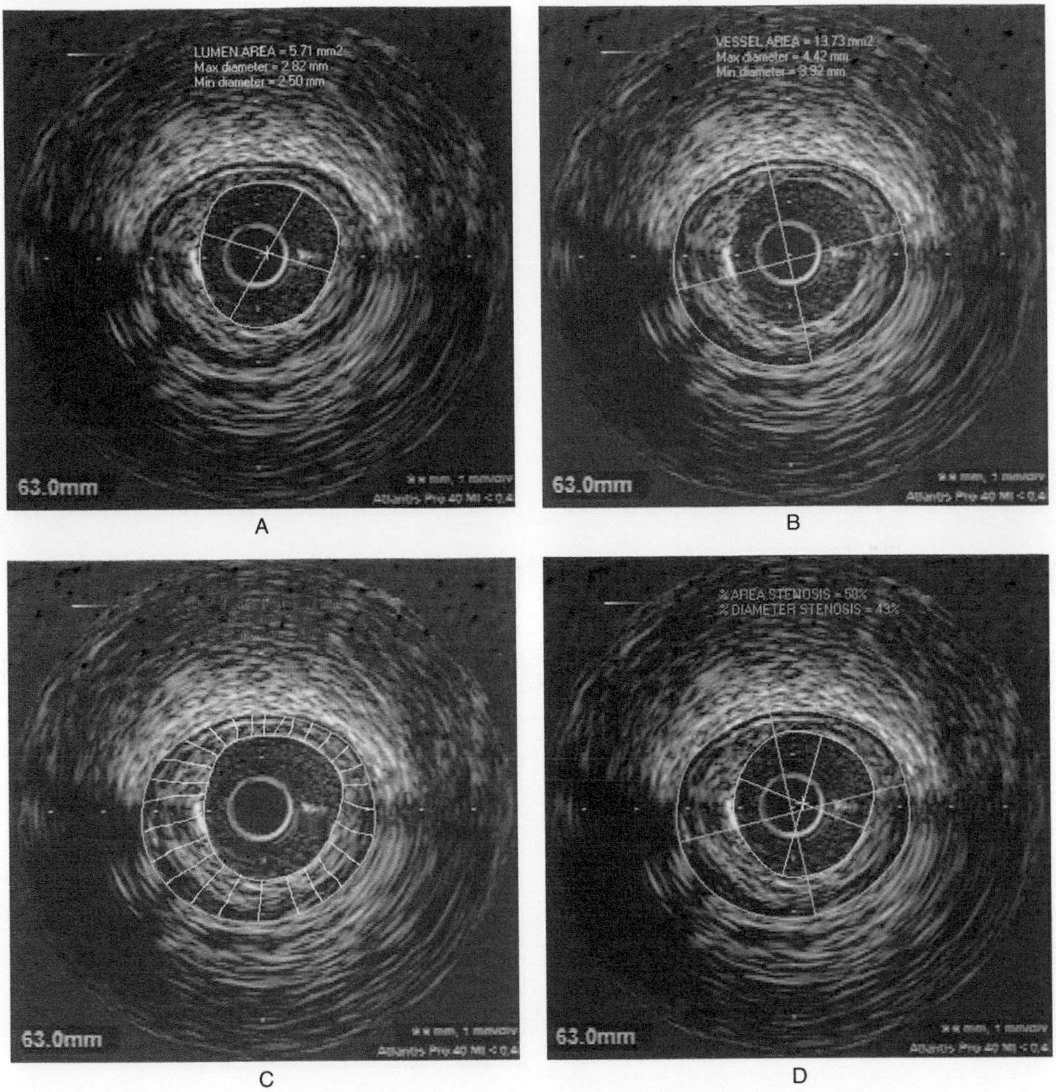

Figure 7.3 Intravascular ultrasound-derived lumen and vessel dimensions—(**A**) lumen dimensions: diameter (MLD; *straight yellow lines*) and cross-sectional area (MLA; *circular yellow line*); **(B)** vessel dimensions: diameter (*straight green lines*) and area (EEM; *circular green line*); **(C)** plaque area (vessel area minus lumen area; *shaded area*). (**D**) Percent diameter stenosis (PDS) and percent area stenosis (PAS) are obtained by [(vessel diameter−MLD)/vessel diameter] and [(vessel area−MLA)/vessel area], respectively.

such a strategy has not yet been validated. In order to realize the full potential of this technique in clinical decision making, it is therefore necessary to be able to derive reliable quantitative measurements from the ultrasound images. This requires expertise and proficiency.[7]

The angiographic significance cutoff of 50% luminal diameter stenosis corresponds to approximately 75% luminal area stenosis by IVUS. Although IVUS provides strictly anatomical information, correlations with functional assessment modalities do exist. In native coronary arteries, IVUS MLD, MLA, and PAS have all been compared to fractional flow reserve (FFR) or nuclear perfusion imaging as gold standards for functional significance. Of those measurements, MLA is often preferred because of its accuracy and reproducibility. An optimal MLA cutoff value of ≤ 4.0 mm^2 was identified in two separate studies using FFR <0.75 and reversible deficit on nuclear perfusion imaging studies (MIBI; methoxyisobutyl isonitrile stress), respectively, with very good sensitivity and specificity (Table 7.1).[8,9] Another study found the optimal MLA

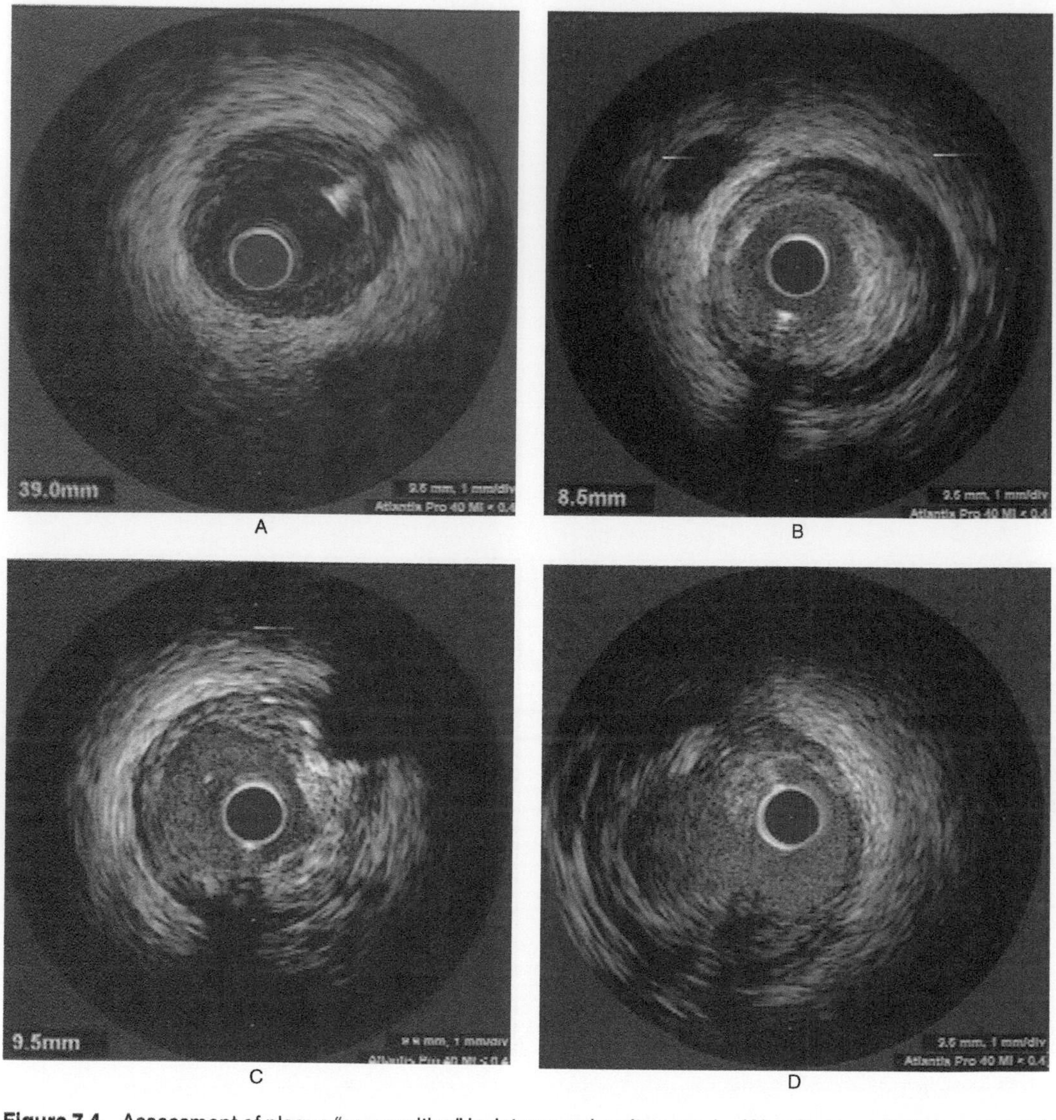

Figure 7.4 Assessment of plaque "composition" by intravascular ultrasound—(**A**) soft plaque (echolucent; bright spot at 8 o'clock is the guidewire), (**B**) fibrotic plaque (echobright without acoustic shadowing between 2- and 4-o'clock; bright spot at 7-o'clock is the guidewire), (**C**) calcified plaque (echobright with acoustic shadowing identified by the asterisk at 8-o'clock), and (**D**) ruptured plaque (echolucent central cavity and thin overlying residual fibrous cap as seen at 4-o'clock). Mixed plaques are frequently encountered.

cutoff value to be <3.0 mm^2.[10] Similar findings were reported for MLD by IVUS (cutoff value <1.8 mm) and PAS (cutoff values $<73\%$, $<70\%$, and $<60\%$). Combining criteria (e.g., MLA and PAS or MLA and MLD) increase specificity. Therefore, IVUS-derived anatomical parameters (especially MLA) correlate well with physiological significance in native coronary arteries and can be used to guide clinical decision making.

FOCUS ON SPECIFIC LESION SUBSETS

Left main coronary artery stenosis

The accurate characterization of left main coronary artery (LMCA) stenoses is crucial because of the associated poor long-term outcome when a significant lesion is present and left unrevascularized, and because of the premature closure of grafts when coronary artery bypass

Table 7.1 Comparison of quantitative IVUS with FFR/SPECT in native coronary arteries

IVUS criteria		FFR/SPECT	Sens/Spec	References
MLA	≤4.0 mm^2	<0.75	92/56	(9)
		Reversible deficit	88/90	(8)
	<3.0 mm^2	<0.75	83/92	(10)
MLD	≤1.8 mm	<0.75	100/70	(9)
PAS	>0.70	<0.75	100/68	(9)
	>0.60	<0.75	92/88	(10)
	≥0.73	Reversible deficit	84/81	(8)

Abbreviations: MLA, mimimun lumen area by IVUS; MLD, minimum lumen diameter by IVUS; PAS, percent area stenosis; FFR, fractional flow reserve; SPECT, single-photon emission computed tomography imaging (nuclear); Sens, sensitivity; Spec, specificity.

graft (CABG) surgery is performed in the absence of a significant LMCA lesion (and other vessels). Despite the fact that angiographic inter- and intraobserver variability is highest for LMCA (even when quantitative methods are used), the significance of an LMCA stenosis typically modulates the choice of the revascularization modality (percutaneous vs. surgical approach). Ostial LMCA lesions are particularly difficult to assess angiographically. Furthermore, disease in other coronary vessels is often present when the LMCA is abnormal, and noninvasive testing cannot easily distinguish the respective contributions of the left anterior descending artery (LAD) and left circumflex artery (LCx) against that of the LMCA. The need for lesion-specific diagnostic modalities is therefore especially important when LMCA is implicated. The use of IVUS in this setting has been studied (Table 7.2), and IVUS criteria have been correlated with clinical events. A single study has correlated IVUS criteria with both clinical events and FFR in the specific context of angiographically ambiguous LMCA lesions. Jasti et al. have reported excellent correlations between IVUS MLD ($r = 0.79$, $p < 0.0001$) or IVUS MLA ($r = 0.74$, $p < 0.0001$) and FFR in 55 patients.[11] An IVUS MLD cutoff value of ≤2.8 mm had a sensitivity of 93% and a specificity of 98% for an FFR <0.75, while an IVUS MLA cutoff value of ≤5.9 mm^2 had a sensitivity of 93% and a specificity of 95% for the same value of FFR. In that study, 38-month survival was not significantly different in patients with FFR <0.75 who underwent revascularization compared with those with FFR ≥0.75 who were treated medically (indirectly MLA > 5.9 mm^2 or MLD > 2.8 mm). The authors concluded that a decision-making strategy based on validated IVUS criteria in patients with ambiguous LMCA was safe and superior to angiography. Other studies corroborating these findings are available.[12–14]

Table 7.2 Quantitative IVUS predictors of clinical events in patients with intermediate left main coronary artery stenosis

IVUS criteria		Event-free survival	Follow-up (mo)	References
MLA	≤5.9 mm^2	100% with surgical therapy[a]	38	(11)
MLD	≤2.8 mm			
MLD	>3.0 mm	97%	12	(12)
	2.5–3.0 mm	84%		
	2.0–2.5 mm	76%		
	2.0 mm	40%		
MLA	<7.5 mm^2	49.9% with medical therapy and 79.2% with revascularization[b]	36	(13)

[a]Versus 90% 38-month event-free survival when MLA > 5.9 mm^2 and MLD > 2.8 mm and patients were maintained on medical therapy alone (p = NS).
[b]Versus 88.4% event-free survival when patients with MLA ≥ 7.5 mm^2 were maintained on medical therapy (p = NS).
Abbreviations: MLA, minimum lumen area by IVUS; MLD, minimum lumen diameter by IVUS.

Bifurcation lesions

Bifurcating vessels present a particular imaging challenge because of the complexity of such an anatomy (three-dimensional relationship between main and side branches). Angiography is inaccurate in the significant proportion of patients in whom adequate visualization of the true bifurcation (both branches plus the side branch origin in two perpendicular planes) is impossible to obtain. Although no dedicated three-dimensional IVUS reconstruction software is available for bifurcation lesions, it is nevertheless possible to obtain important and unique anatomical details in bifurcations by performing IVUS in the main branch alone or main branch and side branch sequentially. For example, Badak et al. have characterized patterns of plaque distribution at bifurcation sites according to side branch take-off angle in the cross-sectional plane[15]; and Costa et al. were able to identify by IVUS that the main mechanism of restenosis at the origin of side branches after "crush" stenting was chronic stent underexpansion that was not identifiable by angiography.[16] Bifurcation lesions of uncertain severity or restenosis at bifurcation sites thus represent another diagnostic application of IVUS. We recommend the use of the same IVUS criteria for "significance" in respective branches as those described in Table 7.1.

Ostial lesions

There is little data available for the specific evaluation of coronary ostial lesions by IVUS.[12,14,17,18] Lesions involving the aorto-ostial junction still represent an angiographic challenge. It is our experience that these lesions can usually be discriminated by IVUS using the usual criteria (Table 7.1) and that in most cases, the ostium is either severely diseased or very mildly so. As mentioned above, catheter obliquity is frequent when the proximal segment of a vessel is at a significant angle with the coronary ostium. It is therefore very important to position the guiding catheter as parallel as possible to the long axis of the ostial segment (Fig. 7.2). It is also frequent to find asymmetrical ostia with a fraction of the very proximal portion of the vessel being opposed to the open aorta. The optimal choice of frame is crucial in these circumstances and must include a circular (as opposed to oval) vessel over 360°.

Tandem lesions

Tandem lesions represent a limitation of IVUS in the assessment of ambiguous lesions. While IVUS can provide detailed information regarding individual lesions, there is no method available to integrate the cumulative physiological effects of multiple lesions within a given vessel. IVUS therefore has a limited role in this situation outside the determination of the most severe lesion and individual lesion characteristics.

Ectatic vessels

IVUS can accurately distinguish between true aneurysms (intact vessel wall), false aneurysms (loss of vessel wall integrity but rupture prevented by perivascular tissue), and complex plaques (ruptured plaques or spontaneous/unhealed dissections).[19,20] Furthermore, IVUS allows accurate identification and measurement of reference segment dimensions and true vessel size at the lesion site. These very important data are often elusive by angiography and we believe that IVUS is extremely valuable in ectatic/aneurysmal vessel to determine significance and optimize stenting procedures. We recommend the use of the usual MLA and MLD criteria (Table 7.1) for functional assessment.

In-stent restenosis

IVUS has modulated our current understanding of the clinical problem of in-stent restenosis by illustrating the underlying mechanism of disease. IVUS has made a major contribution in identifying chronic stent underexpansion (versus true vessel size) as the primary mechanism of restenosis in a significant proportion of patients (rather than excessive neointimal proliferation). In addition, quantitative volumetric assessment of in-stent neointimal proliferation has been used extensively to compare stent types. More recently, IVUS was used to document the vascular healing process following drug-eluting stent placement in vivo.[21] When in-stent restenosis is of intermediate severity angiographically, we recommend the use of the same IVUS criteria as for de novo lesions to discriminate between stenoses that are significant and not.[22]

Diffusely diseased vessels

When objective ischemia is documented (e.g., dynamic ECG changes, reversible deficit on nuclear perfusion imaging, or stress echocardiography) and diffuse disease without any severe, focal stenosis is found on angiography, IVUS interrogation of the corresponding coronary artery is helpful to localize the most severe lesion.[23] The same IVUS criteria then apply for determination of significance (Table 7.1) and the appropriateness of revascularization in this context.

Miscellaneous lesions

In most circumstances where atypical angiographic images are found, IVUS can complement angiography and is very helpful to clarify the anatomy. For example, IVUS was performed in a right internal mammary artery graft to the LAD to assess an ambiguous lesion; an extrinsic compression of the graft by an ascending aorta aneurysm was documented (Fig. 7.5). Therefore,

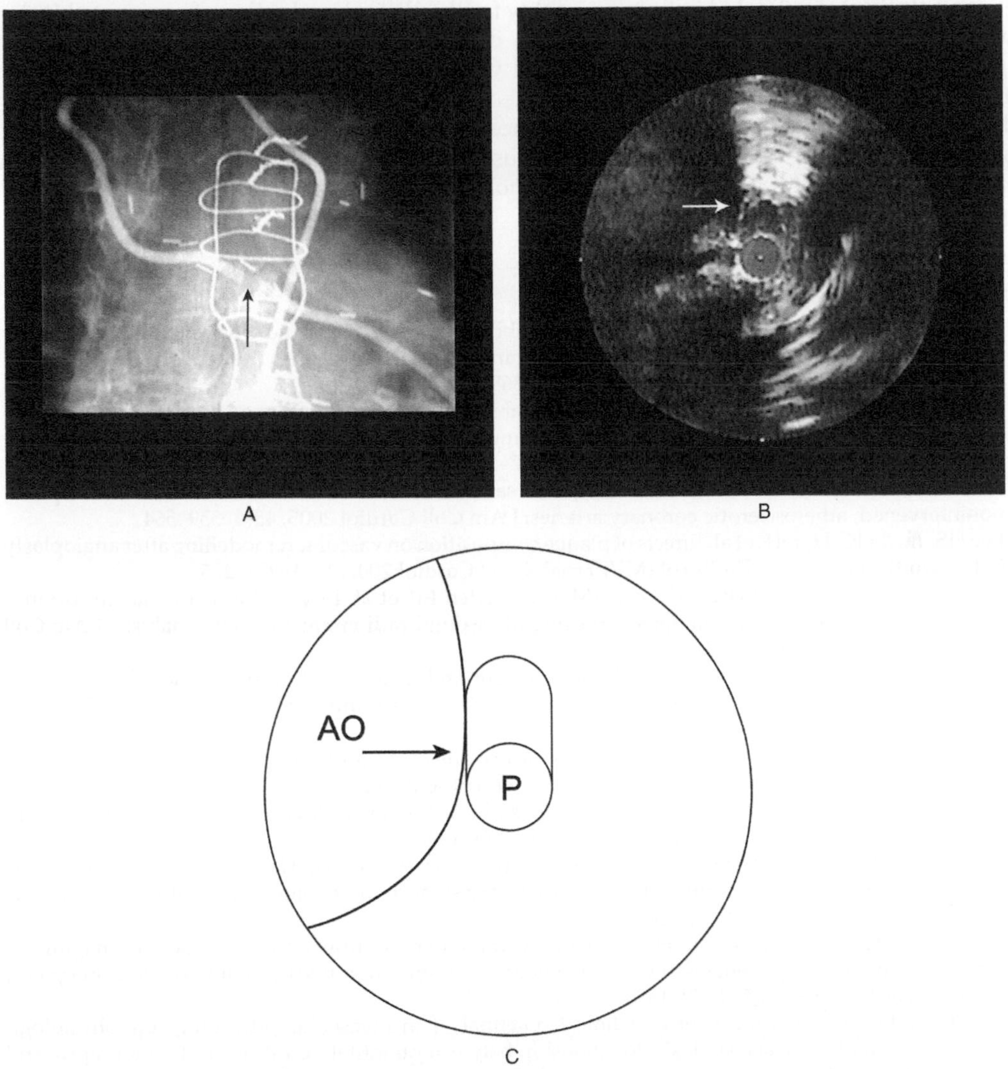

Figure 7.5 Intravascular ultrasound diagnosis of right internal mammary coronary bypass compression by an ascending aortic aneurysm. (**A**) Angiography of the right internal mammary artery graft (RIMA). The arrow points to the severe stenosis in the mid-portion of the graft. (**B**) Intravascular ultrasound at the site of severe RIMA stenosis (arrow in the aorta pointing to the compressed RIMA graft. MLA was 3.1 mm^2 and MLD 1.19 mm. Blood speckle was present in the vascular structure compressing the RIMA graft. (**C**) Schematic representation of the anatomy (AO, ascending aorta; P, IVUS probe; arrow, compressed RIMA graft).

a low threshold for its use is appropriate in clinical practice. A word of caution is needed for the use of IVUS in degenerated vein grafts due to the risk of distal embolization. There are no validated IVUS criteria for the functional significance of vein graft lesions. Thrombotic lesions present a challenge, and it is indeed often impossible to distinguish with certainty thrombus from soft atheroma with IVUS. Angiography and IVUS can again complement each other in this setting since contrast injection may often be helpful in the identification of coronary thrombus.

There are limitations to the use of IVUS in this context, which include difficult delivery of the catheter distal to the target lesion in some circumstances (e.g., calcified, tortuous, small vessels) and the unknown impact of specific anatomies on physiology (e.g., tandem lesions, very long lesions).

CONCLUSIONS

IVUS is a helpful and validated imaging modality for the clinical evaluation of angiographically ambiguous or intermediate lesions. It provides clinicians with high-resolution tomographic images of the vessel wall and lumen that yield very accurate and reproducible quantitative measurements of MLA, MLD, and PAS. Validated criteria incorporating these measurements are highly correlated with physiologic significance of single native coronary lesions, including those in the LMCA. In addition, IVUS data are useful for guidance of percutaneous interventional procedures and to clarify the anatomopathologic correlation of ambiguous angiographic images.

REFERENCES

1. Tardif JC, Bertrand OF, Mongrain R, et al. Reliability of mechanical and phased-array designs for serial intravascular ultrasound examinations—Animal and clinical studies in stented and non-stented coronary arteries. Int J Card Imaging 2000; 16(5):365–375.
2. Schoenhagen P, Sapp SK, Tuzcu EM, et al. Variability of area measurements obtained with different intravascular ultrasound catheter systems: Impact on clinical trials and a method for accurate calibration. J Am Soc Echocardiogr 2003; 16(3):277–284.
3. Guedes A, Keller PF, L'Allier PL, et al. Long-term safety of intravascular ultrasound in nontransplant, nonintervened, atherosclerotic coronary arteries. J Am Coll Cardiol 2005; 45(4):559–564.
4. Lee HS, Tardif JC, Harel F, et al. Effects of plaque composition on vascular remodelling after angioplasty in the MultiVitamins and Probucol (MVP) trial. Can J Cardiol 2002; 18(3):271–275.
5. Rodriguez-Granillo GA, Garcia-Garcia HM, Mc Fadden EP, et al. In vivo intravascular ultrasound-derived thin-cap fibroatheroma detection using ultrasound radiofrequency data analysis. J Am Coll Cardiol 2005; 46(11):2038–2042.
6. Schoenhagen P, Ziada KM, Kapadia SR, et al. Extent and direction of arterial remodeling in stable versus unstable coronary syndromes: An intravascular ultrasound study. Circulation 2000; 101(6): 598–603.
7. Mintz GS, Nissen SE, Anderson WD, et al. American College of Cardiology Clinical Expert Consensus Document on Standards for Acquisition, Measurement and Reporting of Intravascular Ultrasound Studies (IVUS). A report of the American College of Cardiology Task Force on Clinical Expert Consensus Documents. J Am Coll Cardiol 2001; 37(5):1478–1492.
8. Briguori C, Anzuini A, Airoldi F, et al. Intravascular ultrasound criteria for the assessment of the functional significance of intermediate coronary artery stenoses and comparison with fractional flow reserve. Am J Cardiol 2001; 87(2):136–141.
9. Nishioka T, Amanullah AM, Luo H, et al. Clinical validation of intravascular ultrasound imaging for assessment of coronary stenosis severity: Comparison with stress myocardial perfusion imaging. J Am Coll Cardiol 1999; 33(7):1870–1878.
10. Takagi A, Tsurumi Y, Ishii Y, et al. Clinical potential of intravascular ultrasound for physiological assessment of coronary stenosis: Relationship between quantitative ultrasound tomography and pressure-derived fractional flow reserve. Circulation 1999; 100(3):250–255.
11. Jasti V, Ivan E, Yalamanchili V, et al. Correlations between fractional flow reserve and intravascular ultrasound in patients with an ambiguous left main coronary artery stenosis. Circulation 2004; 110(18):2831–2836.
12. Abizaid AS, Mintz GS, Abizaid A, et al. One-year follow-up after intravascular ultrasound assessment of moderate left main coronary artery disease in patients with ambiguous angiograms. J Am Coll Cardiol 1999; 34(3):707–715.

13. Fassa AA, Wagatsuma K, Higano ST, et al. Intravascular ultrasound-guided treatment for angiographically indeterminate left main coronary artery disease: A long-term follow-up study. J Am Coll Cardiol 2005; 45(2):204–211.
14. Sano K, Mintz GS, Carlier SG, et al. Assessing intermediate left main coronary lesions using intravascular ultrasound. Am Heart J 2007; 154(5):983–988.
15. Badak O, Schoenhagen P, Tsunoda T, et al. Characteristics of atherosclerotic plaque distribution in coronary artery bifurcations: An intravascular ultrasound analysis. Coron Artery Dis 2003; 14(4): 309–316.
16. Costa RA, Mintz GS, Carlier SG, et al. Bifurcation coronary lesions treated with the "crush" technique: An intravascular ultrasound analysis. J Am Coll Cardiol 2005; 46(4):599–605.
17. Iyisoy A, Ziada K, Schoenhagen P, et al. Intravascular ultrasound evidence of ostial narrowing in nonatherosclerotic left main coronary arteries. Am J Cardiol 2002; 90(7):773–775.
18. Sano K, Mintz GS, Carlier SG, et al. Intravascular ultrasonic differences between aorto-ostial and shaft narrowing in saphenous veins used as aortocoronary bypass grafts. Am J Cardiol 2006; 97(10): 1463–1466.
19. Maehara A, Mintz GS, Ahmed JM, et al. An intravascular ultrasound classification of angiographic coronary artery aneurysms. Am J Cardiol 2001; 88(4):365–370.
20. Shimada Y, Courtney BK, Nakamura M, et al. Intravascular ultrasonic analysis of atherosclerotic vessel remodeling and plaque distribution of stenotic left anterior descending coronary arterial bifurcation lesions upstream and downstream of the side branch. Am J Cardiol 2006; 98(2):193–196.
21. Escolar E, Mintz GS, Popma J, et al. Meta-analysis of angiographic versus intravascular ultrasound parameters of drug-eluting stent efficacy (from TAXUS IV, V, and VI). Am J Cardiol 2007; 100(4): 621–626.
22. Malekianpour M, Rodes J, Cote G, et al. Value of exercise electrocardiography in the detection of restenosis after coronary angioplasty in patients with one-vessel disease. Am J Cardiol 1999; 84(3): 258–263.
23. Rodes-Cabau J, Candell-Riera J, Angel J, et al. Relation of myocardial perfusion defects and nonsignificant coronary lesions by angiography with insights from intravascular ultrasound and coronary pressure measurements. Am J Cardiol 2005; 96(12):1621–1626.

8 An in-depth insight of intravascular ultrasound for coronary stenting

Pareena Bilkoo and Khaled M. Ziada

Over the last two decades, intravascular ultrasound (IVUS) imaging has played a pivotal role in optimizing the technique of coronary stenting as it is currently practiced. In the early 1990s, two major limitations to coronary stenting seemed to prevent interventional cardiologists from adopting it on a large scale. The first was dramatic acute and subacute stent thrombosis and the need for intense anticoagulation, and the second was the slower paced process of stent restenosis. IVUS imaging was crucial in teaching the interventional cardiology community about the limitations of stenting techniques and subsequently provided the basis for the technical modifications that resulted in markedly improved results. That, coupled with better understanding of the role of antiplatelet therapy, eventually led to the explosive growth of coronary stenting as it is performed today. With the introduction of drug-eluting stents (DES), IVUS imaging was again instrumental in understanding the mechanisms of markedly improved restenosis rates and possible mechanisms of the resurgent stent thrombosis problem.

LESSONS LEARNED FROM INITIAL IVUS OBSERVATIONS

In the early 1990s, IVUS imaging of coronary stents immediately after implantation revealed that the technique of stent deployment utilized at that time frequently resulted in suboptimal expansion, which in turn led to imperfect apposition of the stent struts to the arterial wall. Early experience with IVUS imaging of stents led to the hypothesis that acute or subacute stent thrombosis may be secondary to hemodynamic factors caused by asymmetric stent expansion or inadequate apposition of the struts to the vessel wall.[1] In a study of 63 patients, IVUS imaging revealed inadequate expansion and/or strut apposition in 52 (80%) patients. Additional inflations using higher pressures or larger balloons led to significant improvements in the procedural results.[2] In other studies, IVUS imaging was used to evaluate the technique of Palmaz-Schatz stent deployment using the prepackaged delivery system. Following inflations at nominal pressures, stent underexpansion was quite common.[3] Importantly, in these studies, angiographic examination of the stented segment failed to identify the inadequate deployment that was evident with IVUS imaging (Fig. 8.1).

The major refinements in the technique of stenting, most notably higher pressure postdilatations coupled with dual antiplatelet therapy, were described in the seminal work of Colombo et al.[4] In this study of 359 patients, IVUS imaging was performed after angiographic appearance was optimized. Despite the angiographic appearance, IVUS definition of optimal expansion was noted in only 30% of cases. Subsequent interventions to optimize stent expansion included higher pressure inflations and upsizing postdilatation balloon (Fig. 8.2). At the end of the study, the average inflation pressure was approximately 15 atm and the average balloon-to-artery ratio slightly exceeded 1.1. Patients in whom the IVUS-guided definition of optimal stent expansion was achieved were placed on dual antiplatelet therapy with no warfarin therapy. The outcomes represented a significant improvement over the standards at that time: IVUS-guided optimal expansion was achieved in 96% and 2 months rate of stent thrombosis or occlusion was a mere 1.5%.[4]

Routine use of the high-pressure technique, dual antiplatelet therapy, and IVUS optimization, stent thrombosis has become a very rare occurrence. In a large registry including 7000 patients undergoing de novo stent placement over a 10-year period, subacute stent thrombosis was documented in 27 (0.4%) patients.[5] When compared to a matched control group, stent thrombosis patients were more likely to have longer lesions and angiographic evidence of thrombus at baseline. Prestent IVUS imaging revealed less calcification in this group compared to controls, suggesting that plaques with higher lipid and cellular content may be more at risk. In stents that subsequently developed subacute thrombosis, expansion was suboptimal in 78%,

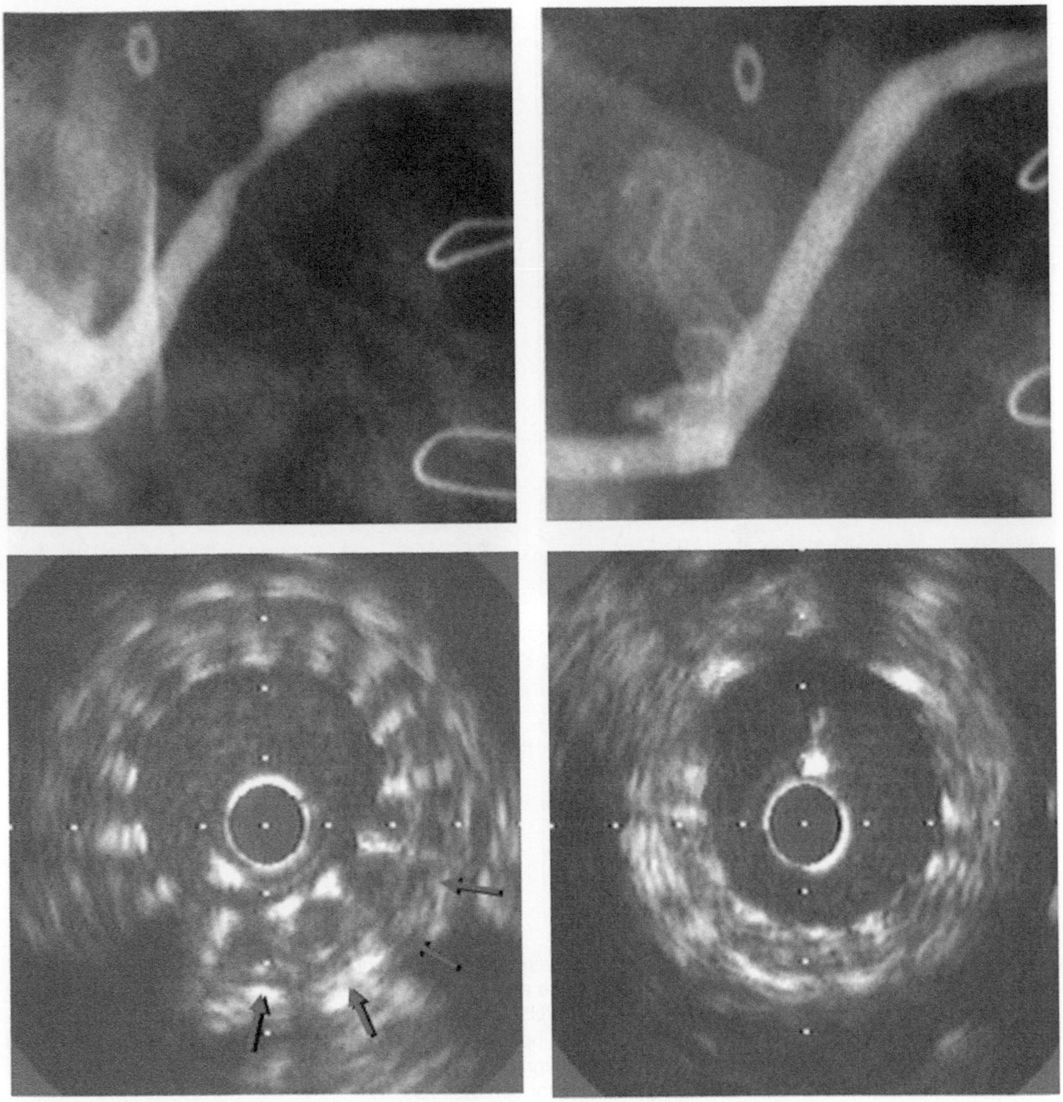

Figure 8.1 Lessons learned from early IVUS observations. Using standard angioplasty techniques of the early 1990s, a Palmaz-Shatz stent was used to treat this vein graft lesion (*upper left*). After using a 4-mm balloon at 10 atm, the angiographic result is excellent (*upper right*), but IVUS imaging reveals a markedly underdeployed stent with a whole quadrant of strut mal-apposition (*lower left, arrows*). Using a 5-mm balloon for postdilatation results in complete strut apposition (*lower right*).

peri-stent dissections were seen in 17%, and 4% had evidence of tissue prolapse. In about half of the cases of stent thrombosis, a combination of these findings were documented at the end of the original procedures, suggesting that subacute stent thrombosis is a multifactorial process and is significantly influenced by both lesion characteristics and procedural result.

UNDERSTANDING MECHANISMS OF IN-STENT RESTENOSIS

Restenosis following balloon angioplasty results from both an exaggerated neointimal proliferation and a process of "shrinkage" or negative arterial remodeling.[6] Following coronary stenting, restenosis is almost solely due to neointimal proliferation. In other words, stents have the ability to withstand the process of negative remodeling such that this process of shrinkage of the external elastic membrane does not play a major role in restenosis. In a serial study of 115 lesions treated with Palmaz-Schatz stents, Hoffmann et al. examined IVUS images obtained

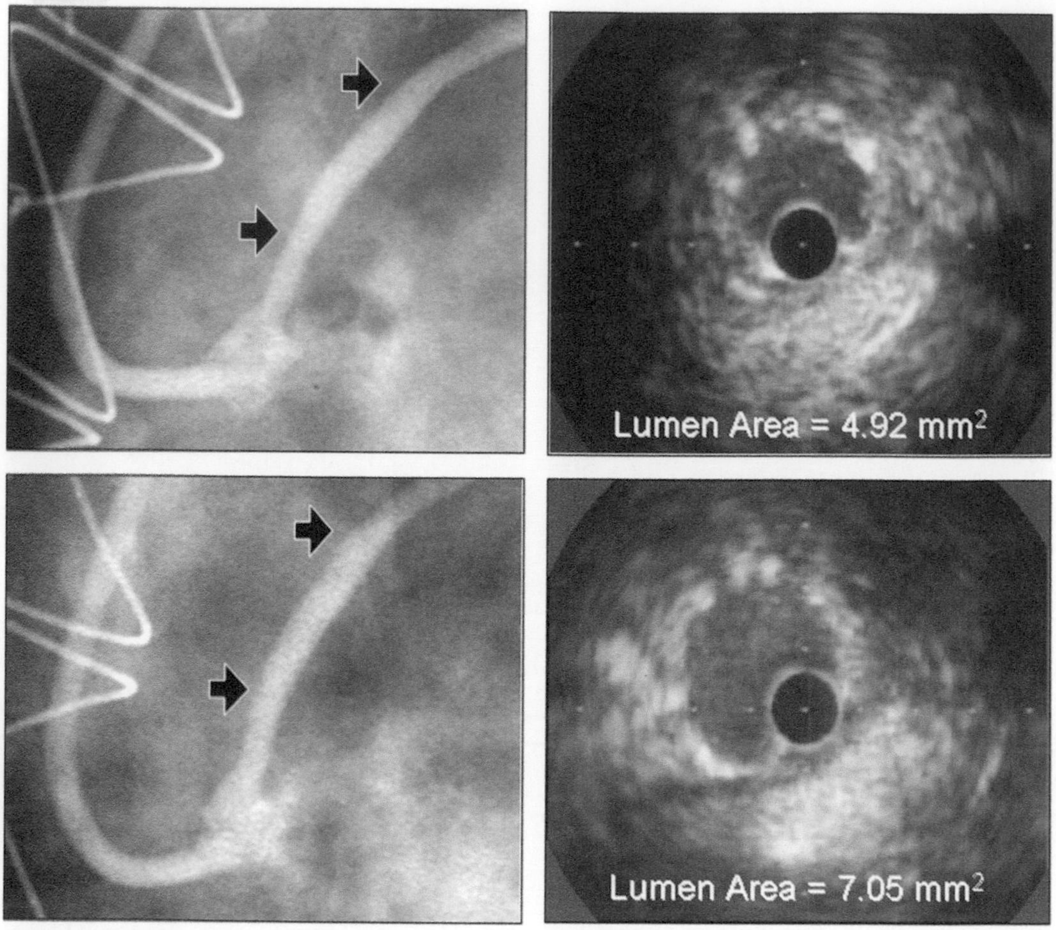

Figure 8.2 IVUS guidance of stent optimization. Even with routine high-pressure stenting, there is a small incidence of suboptimal expansion. In this example, the angiogram of the stented segment appears satisfactory after stent implantation (*black arrows, upper left*), but IVUS imaging reveals a small stent lumen area, significantly smaller than the reference vessel (*upper right*). After upsizing the balloon, the difference in the angiogram is very subtle (*lower left*), but IVUS imaging confirms a significantly (>25%) enlarged lumen area (*lower right*). As discussed later, the lumen area is the strongest predictor of restenosis.

immediately after stent implantation and at an average of 5.4 ± 3.8 months later.[7] Angiographic restenosis was noted in 36 lesions. Follow-up IVUS imaging demonstrated that arterial remodeling and stent recoil were minimal; late lumen loss and restenosis were the result of neointimal hyperplasia within the stent lumen. Immediate and follow-up stent areas averaged 10.5 and 10.3 mm^2, respectively. However, immediate and follow-up lumen areas averaged 10.5 and 7.5 mm^2, respectively, demonstrating that late lumen loss within the stented segment is caused by neointimal hyperplasia. Late lumen loss was directly proportionate to acute lumen gain and stents tend to have larger acute lumen gain compared to angioplasty alone.

Despite the central role of neointimal hyperplasia in stent restenosis, it is important to understand that stent underexpansion at the time of implantation is another major contributor to the increased risk of stent restenosis. In cases in which the acute lumen gain is modest, even modest degrees of neointimal hyperplasia will result in significant encroachment on the stent lumen. Although the prevalence of significant underexpansion was dramatically reduced with routine high-pressure stenting, there remains a small percentage of stent restenosis cases in which underexpansion is the primary mechanism of luminal compromise (Fig. 8.3).

In a large registry of 1706 patients with 2343 lesions, several clinical, angiographic, and IVUS criteria were identified as predictors of stent restenosis.[8] At 6 months, 24% of the patients

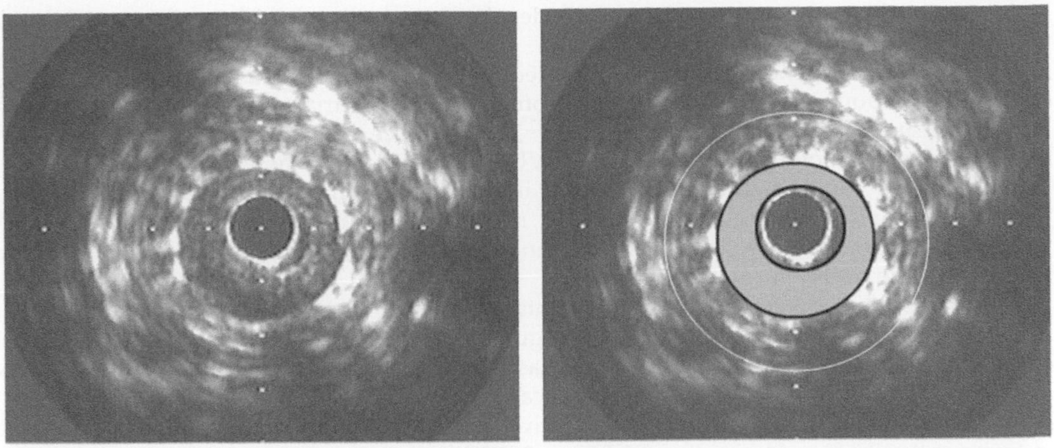

Figure 8.3 In-stent restenosis. The image (*left panel*) was obtained after a patient presented with recurrent symptoms 8 months after stent implantation. The stent area (*marked by the echodense struts*) has not changed, confirming that these stents are resistant to negative remodeling and will not recoil over time. There is significant intimal hyperplasia within the stent (*gray area*), leaving a very small lumen area around the IVUS catheter in the center. In addition, there is a significant discrepancy between the size of the vessel (*right panel, white circle*) and the size of the stent (*marked by the echodense struts*), suggesting that the stent expansion was suboptimal during the original procedure.

had angiographic restenosis. In patients who underwent IVUS-guided stenting, the acute lumen gain was larger and the final lumen diameter was significantly larger (3.2 vs. 3.0 mm; $p < 0.0001$). This resulted in a significantly reduced restenosis rate (24% vs. 29%; $p = 0.03$). In addition to clinical and angiographic variables, several IVUS findings can predict restenosis. These included a smaller stent lumen diameter or area and a smaller reference vessel size. Thus, it was proposed that routine use of IVUS guidance results in optimized expansion, larger stent dimensions, and a lower incidence of restenosis.

IVUS CRITERIA FOR OPTIMAL STENT EXPANSION OF BARE-METAL STENTS

Several observational studies have advocated the use of specific IVUS criteria to define optimal stent expansion based on angiographic and/or clinical outcome.[8–12] The general consensus among those studies is that minimum in-stent lumen dimensions are the most important predictors of restenosis. Minimum stent area <5 or 6 mm^2 was associated with the highest rates of restenosis and need for repeat revascularization (Fig. 8.4). Obviously, the lumen area within the stented segment was directly determined by the reference vessel size, explaining the relatively

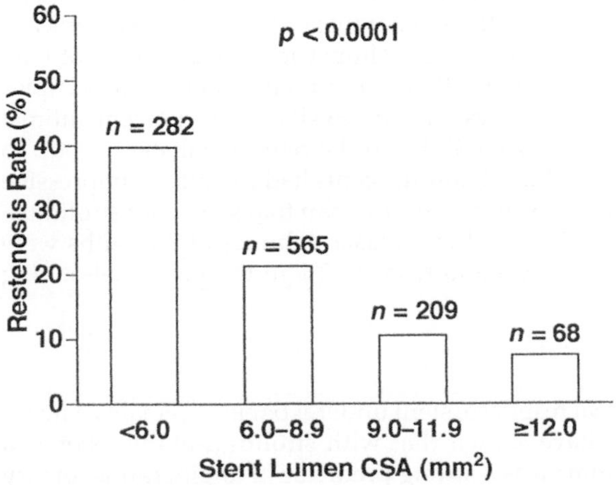

Figure 8.4 Impact of minimum stent lumen area on the rate of restenosis. The relationship is what has traditionally been known as "bigger is better." There is a near doubling of restenosis rate when the area is <6 mm^2. *Source*: Adapted from Ref. 8.

higher rates of restenosis in smaller vessels despite the achievement of excellent procedural results in the majority of cases.[12]

The potential advantages of IVUS-guided bare-metal stenting have been evaluated in several nonrandomized registries[13–17] and some randomized trials.[18–20] A meta-analysis of many of these studies has also been published.[21] The incidence of death and nonfatal myocardial infarction during follow-up was unaltered by IVUS guidance in all of these studies. IVUS-guided stenting is traditionally associated with larger in-stent lumen dimensions as a result of higher pressure and/or balloon upsizing. Despite that, reduction in binary restenosis and rates of target vessel revascularization were not consistent, and were observed more in the registries than in the randomized trials.

In the study by Schiele et al., 155 patients undergoing coronary stenting were randomized to IVUS guidance versus angiographic guidance. IVUS imaging was performed in the angiography arm, but only to document measurements and not to guide further intervention. As expected, the minimum lumen area was 20% larger in the IVUS-guided stenting arm. However, at 6 months, there was a 22% relative reduction in angiographic binary restenosis in favor of the IVUS-guidance arm (22.5% vs. 28.8%), but that was not statistically significant ($p = 0.25$). Because of the very small size of the study, no less than 50% reduction in restenosis would have yielded a statistically significant result. OPTICUS, the largest reported randomized trial on the comparison of IVUS-guided versus angiography-guided stenting showed similar binary restenosis rates (24.5% and 22.8%; $p = 0.68$) and similar target vessel revascularization rates at follow-up although acute gain was significantly higher in the IVUS-guided lesions.[19] OPTICUS specifically included patients with lesions ≤25 mm in length and vessels ≥2.5 mm in diameter.

Another randomized study, TULIP,[20] investigated the possible role of IVUS in stenting long (≥20 mm) coronary stenoses. Binary restenosis and ischemia-driven target lesion revascularization were less common with IVUS guidance as compared to angiography guidance (23% vs. 46%; $p = 0.008$ and 4% and 14%; $p = 0.037$, respectively). Stent length, number of stents per patient, final balloon size, and postintervention minimal luminal diameter were all greater in the IVUS-guided group. Additionally, a stent minimal luminal area >55% of the average reference vessel's cross-sectional area has been found to be the most appropriate single criterion in terms of frequency of achievement and increasing the probability of freedom from restenosis for non–DES.[11] The positive impact of IVUS guidance in this study (as opposed to the results of OPTICUS) may imply that IVUS guidance can reduce restenosis in patients who are at a particularly higher risk for it, for example, smaller vessels or longer lesions.

ROLE OF IVUS IMAGING IN THE ERA OF DES

Efficacy of DES in reducing restenosis

With more widespread use of DES, and the subsequent reduction in the absolute rates of restenosis, the potential advantage of IVUS guidance to reduce restenosis has become less significant. Observations from early IVUS studies with DES demonstrated the marked efficacy of these devices in suppressing intimal hyperplasia. IVUS volumetric measurements of bare metal stents 6 months after implantation have shown that neointimal hyperplasia occupies about 30% of the stent volume.[22] In the IVUS analysis of the SIRIUS trial, percent intimal hyperplasia volumes at 9 months were reduced from 33.4% in the bare-metal stent group to 3.1% in sirolimus-eluting stents ($p < 0.001$).[23] Paclitaxel-eluting stents had a similarly impressive reduction in neointimal hyperplasia, although less in magnitude than that seen with sirolimus-eluting stents. In the TAXUS-IV trial, percent intimal hyperplasia volumes at 9 months were reduced from 29.4% in the bare-metal stent controls and from 12.2% in the paclitaxel-eluting stent group ($p < 0.001$).[24]

Optimal expansion criteria

Despite the effective suppression of neointimal response, stent underexpansion remains a major cause of restenosis with DES. Two studies have shown that with sirolimus-eluting stents, a postprocedural minimum stent area of <5 mm^2 was a strong predictor of angiographic binary restenosis. Minimal lumen area of <4 mm^2 at follow-up[25,26] is generally an indicator of a hemodynamically significant lesion.[27] Thus, it is thought that higher inflation (>18 atm) pressures may be needed in selected patients to achieve a minimum acceptable stent area and therefore to prevent DES restenosis.[26]

In addition, DES underexpansion can be a predisposing factor to the dreaded complication of stent thrombosis. In a small case-control study of 13 patients with DES thrombosis, IVUS analyses showed the majority of the thrombosed stents (11 out of 14) had a minimum stent area of <5.0 mm^2. Compared to the matched controls, thrombosed stents had larger reference segment plaque burden and greater occurrences of edge dissections. Nonetheless, it is important to note that five patients with stent thrombosis prematurely discontinued clopidogrel therapy; one discontinued both aspirin and clopidogrel.[28]

DES strut mal-apposition

With heightened awareness and concern about stent thrombosis, the clinical impact of strut mal-apposition may be more significant than in the bare-metal stent era, and a lower threshold for IVUS examination may be justifiable after stenting. Incomplete apposition of DES struts has been reported[29,30] and stent apposition may be a major determinant of freedom from subacute stent thrombosis with DES. In a small retrospective study of patients who returned with late DES thrombosis, the prevalence of strut mal-apposition was 77%, compared to 12% in a control group of DES patients whose stents were imaged at 8 months during routine follow-up and who did not have stent thrombosis. The highly statistically significant difference suggests that strut mal-apposition may have a major role in precipitating this catastrophic complication.[31]

Strut mal-apposition is not always a residual finding caused at the time of stent implantation. The phenomenon of late strut mal-apposition has also been described in patients who have IVUS documentation of adequate apposition at the time of the procedure, but develop mal-apposition on follow-up IVUS imaging (Fig. 8.5). That phenomenon has been described to occur in approximately 5% of bare-metal stents, but did not appear to have any clinical consequences.[32] Late mal-apposition has increased in prevalence with the use of DES. In a recent analysis of 705 lesions in 557 patients, the incidence was 12% in the overall population, with a higher prevalence in patients with longer stents, those who received DES in the context of acute myocardial infarction or after chronic total occlusion.[33] Yet, in this series, there was no evidence of increased clinical events in this subset of patients for a period of 10 months after the identification of late strut mal-apposition. These findings suggest that strut mal-apposition is of particular concern in situations in which there is difficulty in selecting an appropriate stent size, for example, in long and diffusely diseased segments, myocardial infarction angioplasty, chronic total occlusions or in case of a large vessel size-mismatch between proximal and distal reference segments. While it is not definitive that this phenomenon is related to DES late thrombosis, it is prudent to optimize stent expansion and apposition with IVUS guidance in these situations.

MANAGEMENT OF STENT RESTENOSIS

IVUS imaging has provided an important perspective to study the mechanisms of restenosis following the use of various interventional devices including stents.[7,34,35]

IVUS studies have demonstrated that about 20% of restenotic stents were underexpanded (defined as an in-stent minimal luminal area <80% of average reference luminal area) probably at the time of their implantation.[36] Stent underexpansion is also a major contributing factor in the restenosis of DES.[26] Proper balloon dilatations based on IVUS measurements may lead to an improved lumen area in these types of restenotic lesions. Additionally, the exact localization of the restenotic site represents an important variable in deciding among treatment options. If restenosis is within the stent, higher-pressure inflation can be effective. Conversely, this strategy may not be appropriate to treat restenosis occurring primarily in the unstented reference segments.

In cases of adequately expanded stents, intimal hyperplasia within the stent struts is the primary mechanism of restenosis. In such cases, brachytherapy or re-stenting with DES are the available options of percutaneous therapy. In a randomized trial of 396 patients with

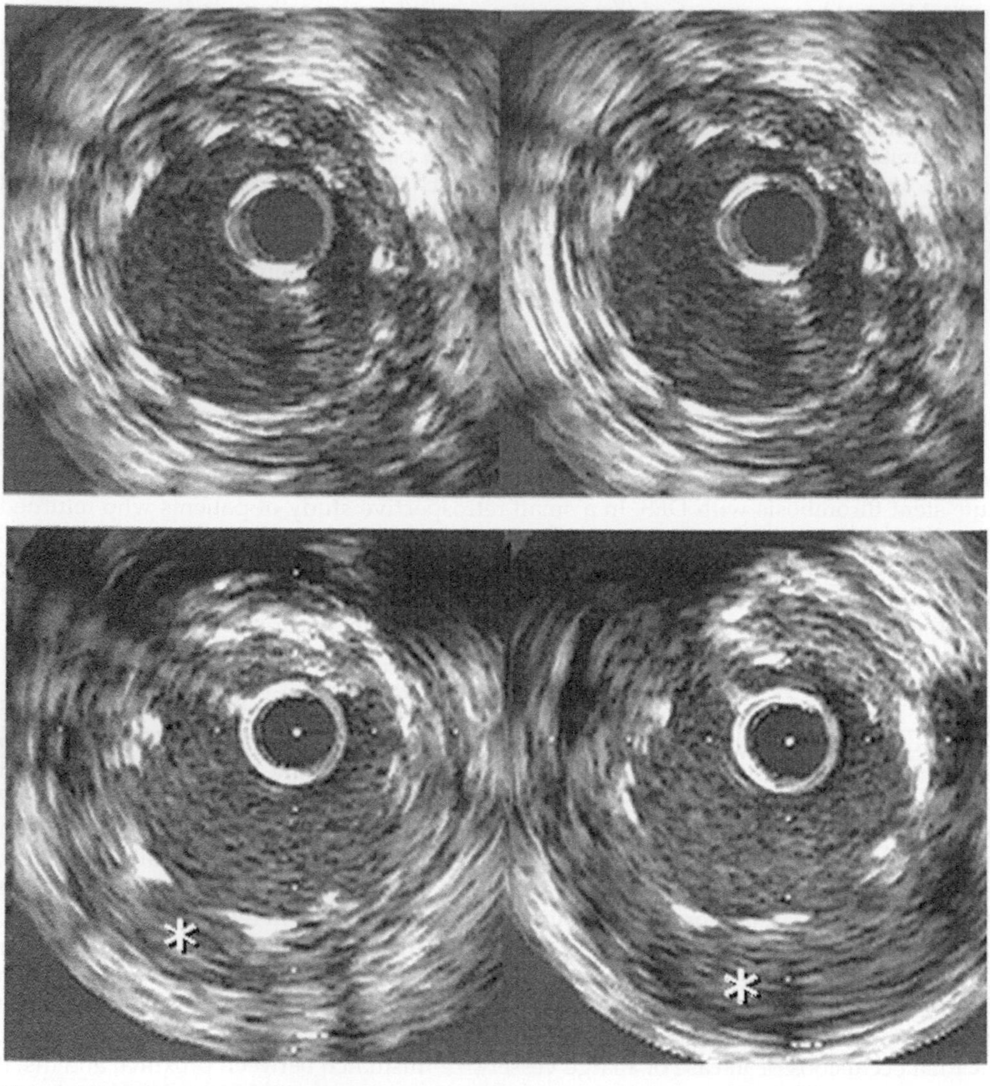

Figure 8.5 Late strut mal-apposition with DES. Two images obtained at the end of a sirolimus-eluting stent implantation procedure (*top*) and two matched images obtained after 6 months (*bottom*). The postimplantation IVUS shows optimal stent expansion and strut apposition, but on follow-up, there are large areas of late stent mal-apposition most prominently indicated by the white asterisk (*). There has been an increase in cross-sectional area of the artery from 17.8 to 28.9 mm^2, but the stent area (8.8 mm^2) has not changed. *Source*: Adapted from Ref. 22.

bare-metal stent restenosis, treatment with paclitaxel-eluting stents was more effective than brachytherapy in reducing major adverse events, primarily by reducing the need for target vessel revascularization.[37] Another randomized trial of 300 patients with bare-metal stent restenosis demonstrated that sirolimus-eluting stents may be more effective in this subset of patients than paclitaxel-eluting stents. The angiographic restenosis rate at 6 months was significantly reduced with both DES types compared to balloon angioplasty alone. In a secondary analysis, the binary restenosis and target vessel revascularization were reduced with sirolimus-eluting stents compared to paclitaxel-eluting stents (Fig. 8.6).[38]

Although the use of debulking devices such as rotational atherectomy or laser ablation makes theoretical sense in these cases, randomized trials have shown that these therapies are not superior to simple balloon angioplasty for treatment of in-stent restenosis.[39,40]

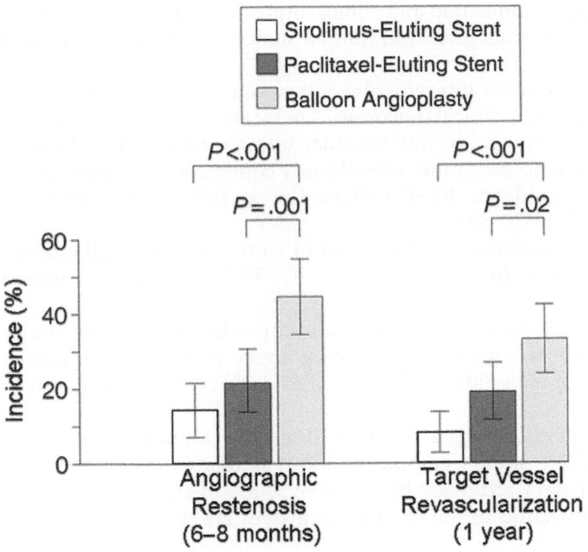

Figure 8.6 Angiographic restenosis and target vessel revascularization after treatment of bare-metal in-stent restenosis. Both types of DES outperformed balloon angioplasty, with sirolimus-eluting stents demonstrating slightly better outcomes. *Source*: Adapted from Ref. 38.

REFERENCES

1. Goldberg SL, Colombo A, Nakamura S, et al. Benefit of intracoronary ultrasound in the deployment of Palmaz-Schatz stents. J Am Coll Cardiol 1994; 24(4):996–1003.
2. Nakamura S, Colombo A, Gaglione A, et al. Intracoronary ultrasound observations during stent implantation. Circulation 1994; 89(5):2026–2034.
3. Kiemeneij F, Laarman G, Slagboom T. Mode of deployment of coronary Palmaz-Schatz stents after implantation with the stent delivery system: An intravascular ultrasound study. Am Heart J 1995; 129(4):638–644.
4. Colombo A, Hall P, Nakamura S, et al. Intracoronary stenting without anticoagulation accomplished with intravascular ultrasound guidance. Circulation 1995; 91(6):1676–1688.
5. Cheneau E, Leborgne L, Mintz GS, et al. Predictors of subacute stent thrombosis: Results of a systematic intravascular ultrasound study. Circulation 2003; 108(1):43–47.
6. Nissen SE, Yock P. Intravascular ultrasound: Novel pathophysiological insights and current clinical applications. Circulation 2001; 103(4):604–616.
7. Hoffmann R, Mintz GS, Dussaillant GR, et al. Patterns and mechanisms of in-stent restenosis. A serial intravascular ultrasound study. Circulation 1996; 94(6):1247–1254.
8. Kasaoka S, Tobis JM, Akiyama T, et al. Angiographic and intravascular ultrasound predictors of in-stent restenosis. J Am Coll Cardiol 1998; 32(6):1630–1635.
9. de Jaegere P, Mudra H, Figulla H, et al. Intravascular ultrasound-guided optimized stent deployment. Immediate and 6 months clinical and angiographic results from the multicenter ultrasound stenting in Coronaries Study (MUSIC Study). Eur Heart J 1998; 19(8):1214–1223.
10. Hoffmann R, Mintz GS, Mehran R, et al. Intravascular ultrasound predictors of angiographic restenosis in lesions treated with Palmaz-Schatz stents. J Am Coll Cardiol 1998; 31(1): 43–49.
11. Moussa I, Moses J, Di Mario C, et al. Does the specific intravascular ultrasound criterion used to optimize stent expansion have an impact on the probability of stent restenosis? Am J Cardiol 1999; 83(7):1012–1017.
12. Ziada KM, Kapadia SR, Belli G, et al. Prognostic value of absolute versus relative measures of the procedural result after successful coronary stenting: Importance of vessel size in predicting long-term freedom from target vessel revascularization. Am Heart J 2001; 141(5):823–831.
13. Albiero R, Rau T, Schluter M, et al. Comparison of immediate and intermediate-term results of intravascular ultrasound versus angiography-guided Palmaz-Schatz stent implantation in matched lesions. Circulation 1997; 96(9):2997–3005.
14. Blasini R, Neumann FJ, Schmitt C, et al. Restenosis rate after intravascular ultrasound-guided coronary stent implantation. Cathet Cardiovasc Diagn 1998; 44(4):380–386.
15. Fitzgerald PJ, Oshima A, Hayase M, et al. Final results of the Can Routine Ultrasound Influence Stent Expansion (CRUISE) study. Circulation 2000; 102(5):523–530.

16. Choi JW, Goodreau LM, Davidson CJ. Resource utilization and clinical outcomes of coronary stenting: A comparison of intravascular ultrasound and angiographical guided stent implantation. Am Heart J 2001; 142(1):112–118.
17. Orford JL, Denktas AE, Williams BA, et al. Routine intravascular ultrasound scanning guidance of coronary stenting is not associated with improved clinical outcomes. Am Heart J 2004; 148(3):501–506.
18. Schiele F, Meneveau N, Vuillemenot A, et al. Impact of intravascular ultrasound guidance in stent deployment on 6-month restenosis rate: A multicenter, randomized study comparing two strategies—with and without intravascular ultrasound guidance. RESIST Study Group. REStenosis after IVUS guided STenting. J Am Coll Cardiol 1998; 32(2):320–328.
19. Mudra H, di Mario C, de Jaegere P, et al. Randomized comparison of coronary stent implantation under ultrasound or angiographic guidance to reduce stent restenosis (OPTICUS Study). Circulation 2001; 104(12):1343–1349.
20. Oemrawsingh PV, Mintz GS, Schalij MJ, et al. Intravascular ultrasound guidance improves angiographic and clinical outcome of stent implantation for long coronary artery stenoses: Final results of a randomized comparison with angiographic guidance (TULIP Study). Circulation 2003; 107(1):62–67.
21. Casella G, Klauss V, Ottani F, et al. Impact of intravascular ultrasound-guided stenting on long-term clinical outcome: A meta-analysis of available studies comparing intravascular ultrasound-guided and angiographically guided stenting. Catheter Cardiovasc Interv 2003; 59(3):314–321.
22. Mintz GS, Weissman NJ. Intravascular ultrasound in the drug-eluting stent era. J Am Coll Cardiol 2006; 48(3):421–429.
23. Moses JW, Leon MB, Popma JJ, et al. Sirolimus-eluting stents versus standard stents in patients with stenosis in a native coronary artery. N Engl J Med 2003; 349(14):1315–1323.
24. Weissman NJ, Koglin J, Cox DA, et al. Polymer-based paclitaxel-eluting stents reduce in-stent neointimal tissue proliferation: A serial volumetric intravascular ultrasound analysis from the TAXUS-IV trial. J Am Coll Cardiol 2005; 45(8):1201–1205.
25. Sonoda S, Morino Y, Ako J, et al. Impact of final stent dimensions on long-term results following sirolimus-eluting stent implantation: Serial intravascular ultrasound analysis from the sirius trial. J Am Coll Cardiol 2004; 43(11):1959–1963.
26. Fujii K, Mintz GS, Kobayashi Y, et al. Contribution of stent underexpansion to recurrence after sirolimus-eluting stent implantation for in-stent restenosis. Circulation 2004; 109(9):1085–1088.
27. Briguori C, Anzuini A, Airoldi F, et al. Intravascular ultrasound criteria for the assessment of the functional significance of intermediate coronary artery stenoses and comparison with fractional flow reserve. Am J Cardiol 2001; 87(2):136–141.
28. Okabe T, Mintz GS, Buch AN, et al. Intravascular ultrasound parameters associated with stent thrombosis after drug-eluting stent deployment. Am J Cardiol 2007; 100(4):615–620.
29. Serruys PW, Degertekin M, Tanabe K, et al. Intravascular ultrasound findings in the multicenter, randomized, double-blind RAVEL (RAndomized study with the sirolimus-eluting VElocity balloon-expandable stent in the treatment of patients with de novo native coronary artery Lesions) trial. Circulation 2002; 106(7):798–803.
30. Degertekin M, Serruys PW, Tanabe K, et al. Long-term follow-up of incomplete stent apposition in patients who received sirolimus-eluting stent for de novo coronary lesions: An intravascular ultrasound analysis. Circulation 2003; 108(22):2747–2750.
31. Cook S, Wenaweser P, Togni M, et al. Incomplete stent apposition and very late stent thrombosis after drug-eluting stent implantation. Circulation 2007; 115(18):2426–2434.
32. Hong MK, Mintz GS, Lee CW, et al. Incidence, mechanism, predictors, and long-term prognosis of late stent malapposition after bare-metal stent implantation. Circulation 2004; 109(7):881–886.
33. Hong MK, Mintz GS, Lee CW, et al. Late stent malapposition after drug-eluting stent implantation: An intravascular ultrasound analysis with long-term follow-up. Circulation 2006; 113(3):414–419.
34. Painter JA, Mintz GS, Wong SC, et al. Serial intravascular ultrasound studies fail to show evidence of chronic Palmaz-Schatz stent recoil. Am J Cardiol 1995; 75(5):398–400.
35. Lemos PA, Saia F, Ligthart JM, et al. Coronary restenosis after sirolimus-eluting stent implantation: Morphological description and mechanistic analysis from a consecutive series of cases. Circulation 2003; 108(3):257–260.
36. Castagna MT, Mintz GS, Leiboff BO, et al. The contribution of "mechanical" problems to in-stent restenosis: An intravascular ultrasonographic analysis of 1090 consecutive in-stent restenosis lesions. Am Heart J 2001; 142(6):970–974.
37. Stone GW, Ellis SG, O'Shaughnessy CD, et al. Paclitaxel-eluting stents vs vascular brachytherapy for in-stent restenosis within bare-metal stents: The TAXUS V ISR randomized trial. JAMA 2006; 295(11):1253–1263.

38. Kastrati A, Mehilli J, von Beckerath N, et al. Sirolimus-eluting stent or paclitaxel-eluting stent vs balloon angioplasty for prevention of recurrences in patients with coronary in-stent restenosis: A randomized controlled trial. JAMA 2005; 293(2):165–171.
39. Sharma SK, Kini A, Mehran R, et al. Randomized trial of rotational atherectomy versus balloon angioplasty for diffuse in-stent restenosis (ROSTER). Am Heart J 2004; 147(1):16–22.
40. vom Dahl J, Dietz U, Haager PK, et al. Rotational atherectomy does not reduce recurrent in-stent restenosis: Results of the angioplasty versus rotational atherectomy for treatment of diffuse in-stent restenosis trial (ARTIST). Circulation 2002; 105(5):583–588.

9 Intravascular ultrasound guidance of stent deployment

Ricardo A. Costa, J. Ribamar Costa, Jr., Daniel Chamié, Dimytri A. Siqueira, and Alexandre Abizaid

INTRODUCTION

The advent of coronary stents into clinical practice resulted in lower rates of restenosis and superior long-term outcomes compared to balloon angioplasty.[1,2] However, the initial experience with coronary stenting in the early 1990s was associated with elevated incidence of acute and subacute stent thrombosis, vigorous antiplatelet/anticoagulant therapeutic regimen, and relatively high rates of restenosis and vessel revascularization; therefore, it became limited to a narrow subset of patients in the early years.[3,4] It was Colombo's pioneering work with intravascular ultrasound (IVUS) guidance for stent deployment with high pressure that deeply impacted the way to perform contemporary percutaneous coronary intervention (PCI), allowing stents to evolve into the most widespread modality for treatment of coronary artery disease (CAD).[5] Although IVUS has never been consistently proved to optimize routine stent implantation, it continued to play a pivotal role for understanding CAD as well as assessing the mechanisms of PCI failure.[6] Specifically, serial IVUS examinations have been demonstrated that "suboptimal" stent implantation is one of the main causes associated with stent thrombosis and restenosis.[7,8] In the current era, drug-eluting stents (DES) have shown an overall marked efficacy and superiority compared to bare-metal stents (BMS) in reducing neointimal hyperplasia and restenosis, and therefore, the need for repeat revascularization.[9,10] Importantly, several IVUS studies still demonstrate that "optimal" stent implantation with adequate stent expansion remains one of the most important factor impacting acute and long-term success after DES.[11,12]

In this chapter, an overview is provided including the major contributions of IVUS for the development of stent implantation techniques, stressing the role of this invasive image modality for optimization of stent deployment.

IVUS-GUIDED OPTIMAL STENT IMPLANTATION

Several previous studies were performed to address the clinical impact of optimal IVUS-guided stent deployment in the BMS era, but the conflicting results of these studies along with a variety of definitions for optimal stent deployment (also the economic burden of the routine use of IVUS catheters) prevented this image modality to become the gold standard to guide stent implantation.

The first prospective evaluation of the effect of optimal BMS expansion, according to a specific IVUS definition, was the Multicenter Ultrasound Stenting In Coronaries (MUSIC) trial.[13] Table 9.1 summarizes the rigid IVUS criteria introduced by the MUSIC study. Following the MUSIC trial, several other studies compared the clinical outcomes of PCI with stent implanted under angiography versus IVUS guidance (Table 9.1). In the OPTimization with Intravascular Coronary UltraSound to Reduce Stent Restenosis (OPTICUS) trial, 550 patients were randomized to either IVUS-guided or angiography-guided BMS implantation, and there were no significant differences in both angiographic and clinical outcomes at mid- and late follow-up.[14] Following this, there was the REStenosis after Intravascular Ultrasound STenting (RESIST) trial,[15] which randomized 155 patients into two groups after successful stent implantation: one was group A with no further balloon postdilatation ($n = 76$) and the other was group B ($n = 79$) with systematic additional balloon postdilatation until achievement of IVUS criterion for stent expansion of minimum stent cross-sectional area (CSA) becomes $\geq$80% of the reference-lumen CSA. In RESIST, despite no differences in restenosis rates at 6 months, a cost-effectiveness at 18 months demonstrated that the cumulative medical costs were nearly equivalent between both

Table 9.1 Optimal IVUS criteria for stent implantation in clinical series with BMS

Study	Design	*N*	Inclusion criteria	Primary endpoint	Angiographic optimal criteria for stent implant	IVUS optimal criteria for stent deployment/ expansion	Optimal IVUS criteria achieved	Postprocedural adjunctive therapy	Angio FU	RS	Clinical FU TLR[a]	MACE	Early ST[b]	Late ST[c]
MUSIC	Prospective, multicenter, nonran- domized, single arm	161	Lesion ≤15 mm in native vessel ≥3.00 mm	Safety and feasibility of IVUS-guided optimized stent deployment	Final residual stenosis <20%	Complete stent apposition In-stent MLA ≥90% of the average reference-lumen area, or ≥100% of lumen area of the reference-lumen area with the lowest lumen area. If in-stent MLA >9.0 mm^2: in-stent MLA ≥80% of average reference-lumen area, or ≥90% of lumen area of the reference-lumen area with the lowest lumen area Symmetric stent expansion: MLD-to-maximum LD ≥0.7	79.6%	Aspirin 100 mg daily if optimal IVUS criteria achieved; or combination of aspirin 100 mg daily plus acenocouramol[d] (INR 2.5–3.5) for 3 months	144 pts, at 6 mo	9.7%	7.0%	12.1%	1.3%	0.6% (?)

(*Continued*)

Table 9.1 Optimal IVUS criteria for stent implantation in clinical series with BMS (*Continued*)

Study	Design	*N*	Inclusion criteria	Primary endpoint	Angiographic optimal criteria for stent implant	IVUS optimal criteria for stent deployment/ expansion	Optimal IVUS criteria achieved	Postprocedural adjunctive therapy	Angio FU	RS	Clinical FU TLR[a]	MACE	Early ST[b]	Late ST[c]
RESIST	Prospective, multicenter, randomized comparison of stent deployment with vs. without IVUS guidance	155	Lesion <15 mm in native vessel ~3.00 mm. Randomization after optimal angiographic results was achieved	Restenosis rates at 6-month angiographic FU	Final residual stenosis <20%	Stent expansion >80%. Stent expansion defined as the ratio of intrastent minimal CSA to the average of the proximal and distal reference-lumen CSA	79.8% (in the IVUS-guided group)	Aspirin 250 mg plus thienopyridine (ticlopidine 250-mg Bid) for 1 mo	144 pts, at 6 mo	22.5% vs. 28.8%, $p = 0.25$				
OPTICUS	Prospective, multicenter, randomized comparison of IVUS- vs. angiography-guided stenting	550	Lesion ≤25 mm in native vessel ≥2.50 mm	Restenosis rates, MLD, and percent DS at >6-month angiographic FU	Final residual stenosis <10%	Same as in the MUSIC trial (above)	56.1% (in the IVUS-guided group)	Aspirin ≥100 mg indefinitely plus thienopyridine (ticlopidine 250 mg BID) for 4 wk	468 pts	24.5% vs. 22.8%, $p = 0.68$	RR, 1.04; 95% CI, 0.64–1.67; $p = 0.87$	15.8% vs. 18.6%, p = NS	-	-

[a]Includes both re-intervention and CABG.
[b]Events occurring within 30 days postprocedural.
[c]Events occurring >30 days postprocedural.
[d]Intravenous heparin was maintained immediately postprocedural until therapeutic level of acenocouramol was achieved.

Abbreviations: CI, confidence interval; CSA, cross-sectional area; DS, diameter stenosis; INR, International Normalized Ratio; IVUS, intravascular ultrasound; LD, lumen diameter; MACE, major adverse cardiac events; MLA, minimum lumen area; MLD, minimum lumen diameter; MUSIC, Multicenter Ultrasound Stenting In Coronaries; NS, not significant; OPTICUS, OPTimization with Intravascular Coronary UltraSound to Reduce Stent Restenosis; RESIST, REStenosis after Intravascular Ultrasound STenting; RR, relative risk; RS, angiographic binary restenosis; ST, stent thrombosis; TLR, target lesion revascularization.

strategies. This was because the higher acute cost of IVUS catheter usage was partially offset by the cost for additional revascularization procedures in the angiographic-guided group. Overall major adverse cardiac events (MACE) (death, myocardial infarction, unstable angina, or lesion revascularization) occurred in 37% in the control group versus 25% in the IVUS group).[16] Finally, the Angiography versus IVUS-Directed Stent Deployment (AVID) was a larger study randomizing 759 patients to IVUS- versus angiography-guided PCI. Overall, there was a nonsignificant trend for improved 12-month target lesion revascularization (TLR) (Table 9.1). However, for native vessels >2.5 mm, TLR was significantly lower in the IVUS-guided group (4.9% vs. 10.8%, $p = 0.02$). Similar results were found when considering saphenous vein grafts: 5.1% TLR in IVUS-guided group versus 20.8% in angiography-guided group ($p = 0.03$).[17]

The main limitations of the trials described above included the relatively small number of patients in most of the series, with consequent statistical underpower to demonstrate significant benefit regarding angiographic and clinical endpoints. Therefore, to address this issue, Casella et al. conducted a meta-analysis of all published studies comparing IVUS-guided to angiographically guided stenting.[18] From 7 original studies reports, 2 abstracts, and 35 reviews or editorial articles, 9 studies were found suitable to be included in the meta-analysis comprising 5 randomized trials (RESIST, OPTICUS, AVID, SIPS, and TULIP). Primary end point was a composite of death and nonfatal myocardial infarction (MI), as considered in every single study. Secondary end points were MACE, the individual cardiac events, as well as angiographic parameters at all study endpoints. Overall, 2972 patients were included. At 6 months, the composite endpoint of death and nonfatal MI was similar for both strategies (4.1% for angiographic-guided vs. 4.5% with IVUS-guided stenting; however, IVUS-guided stenting demonstrated significant reduction in overall MACE [odds ratio (OR), 0.79; confidence interval (CI) 95%, 0.64–0.98; $p = 0.03$], and 38% reduction on probability of TVR (OR, 0.62; CI 95%, 0.49–0.78; $p < 0.001$). In addition, patients with IVUS-guided stenting had significantly less restenosis (OR, 0.75; CI 95%, 0.60–0.94; $p = 0.01$).

Although it was generally accepted that larger final stent areas would be associated with lower rates of adverse events, it was never possible to reach a definite IVUS measure that could be applicable to most lesion subsets. Currently ongoing, the angiographic versus IVUS optimization (PRAVIO) study has been designed to compare the long-term clinical outcomes of patients treated with the deployment of DES guided by angiography versus IVUS. This study will use a novel criteria proposed to define optimal stent implantation: minimum lumen area (MLA) ≥70% of the nominal balloon CSA used to dilate a specific segment of the stent. Importantly, in this study, the noncompliant balloon used for postdilatation will be sized according to the average (maximum and minimum diameter) of the media-to-media diameter at the following points: (1) distal in-stent segment, (2) proximal in-stent segment, and (3) site of in-stent maximal narrowing. Alternatively, a final lumen CSA >9.0 mm^2 will also be considered adequate.[19]

UNDERSTANDING MECHANISMS OF STENT FAILURE

Given that in-stent restenosis is largely determined by the degree of intimal hyperplasia, it is reasonable to propose that larger lumens at the end of the procedure should translate into lower rates of clinically significant restenosis ("the bigger is better" theory). This hypothesis was evaluated in the Can Routine Ultrasound Influence Stent Expansion (CRUISE) trial.[20] In this study, an increment in final stent CSA resulted in a significant decrease in TLR rates at 9 months (CSAs of 4.0–5.9 mm^2 vs. 6.0–6.9 mm^2 vs. 7.0–8.9 mm^2 vs. >9.0 mm^2 were associated to TLR rates of 27% vs. 19% vs. 12% vs. 4%, respectively). In this study, a final CSA equal to 6.5 mm^2 after BMS was the cutoff threshold that predict TLR at follow-up.

With DES, once an effective drug inhibits most of the neointimal hyperplasia, the relative effect of stent underexpansion may have greater impact on DES failure.[21] In the IVUS substudy of the SIRIUS trial, the value of MSA >5.0 mm^2 for the overall cohort and >4.5 mm^2 for vessels with reference diameter <2.80 mm [by quantitative coronary angiography (QCA)] were the thresholds that best predicted adequate patency at follow-up with sirolimus-eluting stents (SES), defined as minimum lumen cross-sectional area >4 mm^2. The positive predictive value of the IVUS stent dimensions was 90%.[11] In this analysis, MSA values >6.5 mm^2 and >6.0 mm^2 were found to be the thresholds with BMS for the overall cohort and smaller vessels, respectively. Furthermore, a publication by Hong et al. investigated the IVUS predictors of angiographic restenosis after SES.[10] In this study, IVUS-guided SES implantation was performed in 670 lesions ($N = 550$) in native coronary vessels (saphenous vein grafts, in-stent restenosis, and bifurcations were excluded), and angiographic follow-up was available in 81.1% of lesions. Restenosis (3.9%) was associated with smaller vessel size ($p = 0.02$), smaller final and follow-up minimum lumen diameter (MLD) ($p = 0.02$ and <0.001, respectively), longer lesion length ($p < 0.001$), lower stent-to-lesion (length) ratio ($p < 0.001$), greater number of stents implanted ($p < 0.001$), longer stent length by IVUS ($p < 0.001$), stent underexpansion ($p = 0.001$), and smaller final MSA ($p = 0.001$). Multivariate independent predictors of angiographic restenosis included stent length, as assessed by IVUS (OR, 1.029; 95% CI, 1.002–1.056; $p = 0.035$), and final MSA (OR, 0.568; 95% CI, 0.387–0.888; $p = 0.012$). Importantly, an MSA of 5.5 mm^2 and IVUS-measured stent length of 40 mm were identified as cutoff thresholds that best predicted restenosis after SES. A significant relationship was observed between these two variables ($r = -0.273$, $p < 0.001$), with the highest restenosis rate (17.7%) found in the subset of lesions with >40 mm stent length (by IVUS) and <5.5 mm^2 MSA. The lowest restenosis rate (0.4%) was found amongst the subset of lesions including <40 mm stent length and final MSA ≥5.5 mm^2.[22] Similarly, Takebayashi et al. reported an association between restenosis after SES implantation and stent underexpansion (mean MSA in lesions with restenosis = 4.5 ± 1.7 mm^2; 67% of restenotic lesions with MSA <5.00 mm^2).[23] Thus, stent underexpansion appears to be the main mechanism of DES restenosis.

Regarding stent thrombosis following DES, both early and late (and very late) events were assessed in two studies. In the first study by Fujii et al. including 15 subacute stent thromboses after SES (median time 14 days), it was demonstrated that (1) MSA was significantly lower in the thrombosis group (4.3 ± 1.6 mm^2 vs. 6.2 ± 1.9 mm^2 in control; $p < 0.001$), (2) stent expansion was smaller in SES thromboses group (65 ± 18% vs. 85 ± 14%; $p < 0.001$), (3) significant residual reference segment stenosis (defined as MLA < 4.00 mm^2 and "plaque burden" >70%) was common in thromboses group (67% vs. 9%; $p < 0.001$), and (4) independent predictors of stent thrombosis were stent underexpansion ($p = 0.03$) and significant residual reference segment stenosis ($p = 0.02$).[12] In the other study, Cook et al. reported a series of 13 patients with very late stent thrombosis (mean time = 630 days) after DES, and compared with IVUS findings with controls ($n = 144$). By IVUS, stent experiencing thrombosis had longer total stent length (34.6 ± 22.4 mm vs. 18.6 ± 9.5 mm; $p < 0.001$), and decreased stent expansion (68 ± 19% vs. 81 ± 18%; $p = 0.04$). Stent expansion was associated with severely calcified segments, and the incidence of stent "malapposition" was significantly increased in stent thromboses patients (77% vs. 12%; $p < 0.001$).[24] These findings reinforce the importance of adequate stent expansion at implantation.

PRACTICAL RECOMMENDATIONS FOR OPTIMAL STENT DEPLOYMENT

In the absence of a clearly standardized approach, we present a practical algorithm that focuses on optimized stent expansion and completes stent apposition to the vessel wall at implant, which may be applicable to either BMS and DES (Table 9.2). Overall, the final stent CSA can be optimized by appropriate stent sizing using preintervention IVUS followed by adjunct balloon postdilatation at high pressure guided by iterative IVUS. In addition, we discuss below some specific situations in which IVUS guidance may optimize stent deployment.

Stent sizing

Undersizing stent diameters relative to the target vessel diameter is perhaps the most frequent reason for suboptimal stent deployment. In patients with severe and diffuse disease, the choice of the correct stent size by angiographic means only is often difficult and very frequently leads to a inadequate balloon-to-artery ratio during stent deployment (<1.0).[25,26] Also, in some situations including subocclusive stenosis, the distal vessel may be underperfused and appears artificially small, and in this case, direct stenting may result in stent undersizing. Thus, IVUS imaging may contribute for the PCI strategy including appropriate stent sizing.

Optimal pressure for stent deployment

Stent manufacturers provide a compliance chart developed to predict minimum stent diameter (MSD) and area related to nominal balloon inflation pressure, which interventional cardiologists routinely rely on to optimize stent diameter according to inflation pressure during PCI. However, these charts are based on in vitro measurements (in air or water) and do not reflect the intrinsic

Table 9.2 Practical recommendations for optimal stent deployment

Recommendations	Considerations
1. Perform preintervention IVUS to assess stenosis severity, measure reference vessel size, and lesion length (Fig. 9.1)	(a) Proximal reference is the image slice within the same segment as the target lesion that has the largest lumen and the smallest plaque burden. It is important to visualize the entire vessel proximal to the target site to determine the extent of the plaque burden and the presence of calcium. Calcification causes the vessel to be rigid and noncompliant. This may provide great information on the need to select bulky devices (e.g., atherectomy catheter) and performing or not, direct stenting. Typical measures that are used for device sizing are maximum and mean lumen diameter, mean mid-wall diameter, and mean EEM diameter. (b) Lesion length is the distance between the proximal and distal reference sites. Length measurements are performed using a motorized transducer pullback (typical 0.5 or 1 mm/sec). It is not possible with manual catheter pullback. Unlike angiography, length measurements are less affected by tortuosity, bends or foreshortening. (c) In the stent era, assessment of lesion morphology is less important than it was previously, as stent implantation tends to minimize the impact of lesion morphology on the acute and chronic results of percutaneous intervention.
2. Select stent size using maximum reference-lumen diameter, whether proximal or distal to the lesion[a]	(a) This approach is the simplest and, perhaps, the most reliable. In general, results in upsizing by 0.75 mm (on average) compared with angiography. (b) Other approach is to use mean mid-wall measurements. In general, it results in upsizing by 0.85 mm. (c) Full reference and lesion-site EEM diameters probably should not be used for stent sizing, especially with high-pressure inflations, once it is more likely to cause complications such as dissections and perforations.
3. Select stent length based on the distance between proximal and distal references	This approach may be adjusted to accommodate the planned procedure. The length may need to be shortened to avoid jailing a side branch or "lengthened" to cover this branch deliberately.
4. Determine the optimum stent CSA assuming the least residual stenosis	Considering reference-lumen dimensions and the final lumen CSA, assuming a final 0% residual stenosis. (a) Ideally, IVUS guidance should result in 0% final stenosis, but this is often not achievable. (b) Inflating a stent according to the package label does not reliably result in the final stent diameter indicated[27,28]
5. Implant the stent according to conventional techniques	Best recommended technique for DES implant includes: adequate stent sizing, full lesion coverage from distal "normal" to proximal "normal" reference segments, final angiographic result with the absence or minimal residual stenosis—high-pressure balloon postdilatation performed inside the stent (balloon length shorter than stent length) is strongly recommended if significant residual stenosis is present.

(*Continued*)

Table 9.2 Practical recommendations for optimal stent deployment (*Continued*)

Recommendations	Considerations
6. Repeat IVUS to assess minimum stent CSA (Fig. 9.2)	(a) If minimum stent CSA is adequate, stop. (b) If minimum stent CSA is inadequate, perform additional higher pressure inflations, if necessary, using a balloon with larger diameter. (c) If there is malapposition, select a balloon sized to the distance between the nonapposed intimas and inflate at low pressure.
7. Check to make sure that there are no complications (Fig. 9.3)	

[a]Distal reference lumen may be preferable, especially in situations of vessel tapering.

conditions found in a diseased coronary vessels. An IVUS study by Costa Jr. et al. demonstrated that only 3.8% of BMS achieve >90% of the predicted MSD, and only 24.6% achieved >80% of the predicted MSD.[27] Such results occurred independently of manufacturer, stent length and diameter, and deployment pressure. Later, the same group reported a similar analysis with DES and demonstrated that stent underexpansion was also common with first generation DES. In this analysis, SES achieved mean 75% of the predicted MSA, and PES achieved mean 79.9% of the predicted MSA. Also, 24% of SES and 28% of PES did not achieve a final MSA >5.0 mm^2.[28] Thus, in the context of both DES failures, such findings are critical and highlight the potential usefulness of IVUS on improving clinical outcomes by optimizing stent deployment and stent expansion.

Heavily calcified lesions

PCI of calcified lesions has been associated with acute complications (dissections, perforations) and also stent underexpansion.[29–31] A study by Vavuranakis et al. evaluated 27 lesions with significant calcification, and an optimal stent expansion ≥90% of the average proximal and distal reference-lumen CSAs were adopted. By IVUS, the mean arc of calcium was 181 ± 60°, and after stent implant (mean pressure = 16 atm), 63% did not meet adequate stent expansion. In this study, underexpanded lesions had further balloon postdilatation at a mean pressure equal to 19.5 atm; however, adequate proposed criteria for stent expansion was obtained in only 59% of this subset.[31] In such lesions, the use of debulking devices (rotational atherectomy) and aggressive balloon postdilatation should be considered, and IVUS may be helpful to define the best strategy for a successful procedure.

Lesions with large plaque burden

The primary mechanism of lumen enlargement after stenting is known to be arterial expansion (accounting for approximately 70% of luminal gain) rather than plaque reduction (6–34%).[26,32] Yoon et al.[31] assessed a series of lesions treated with BMS investigate by IVUS at postprocedural. Mean deployment pressure of the stents was 12.8 atm and optimal angiographic result was found in 92%. However, using the MUSIC criteria, stents were fully expanded in only 37.8%; importantly, lesions with larger "plaque burden" (>50%) were associated with a significant lower rate of successful stent expansion compared to those with only mild "plaque burden."[33]

Aorto-ostial lesion location

In aorto-ostial lesions, precise stent positioning is required to cover the entire lesion and prevent exaggerated protrusion out to the aorta. Regarding left main (LM) lesions, angiography may mislead the correct interpretation, therefore, preintervention IVUS should be mandatory to define the real severity of lesion (ostial and shaft location) and should also clarify whether the distal bifurcation is involved or not (an important predictor of outcomes).[21] Regarding the procedure, a recent study by **Park et al.** demonstrated significant improvement in outcomes in patients undergoing IVUS-guided LM stenting compared to angiography-guided procedures, including superior long-term survival.[34]

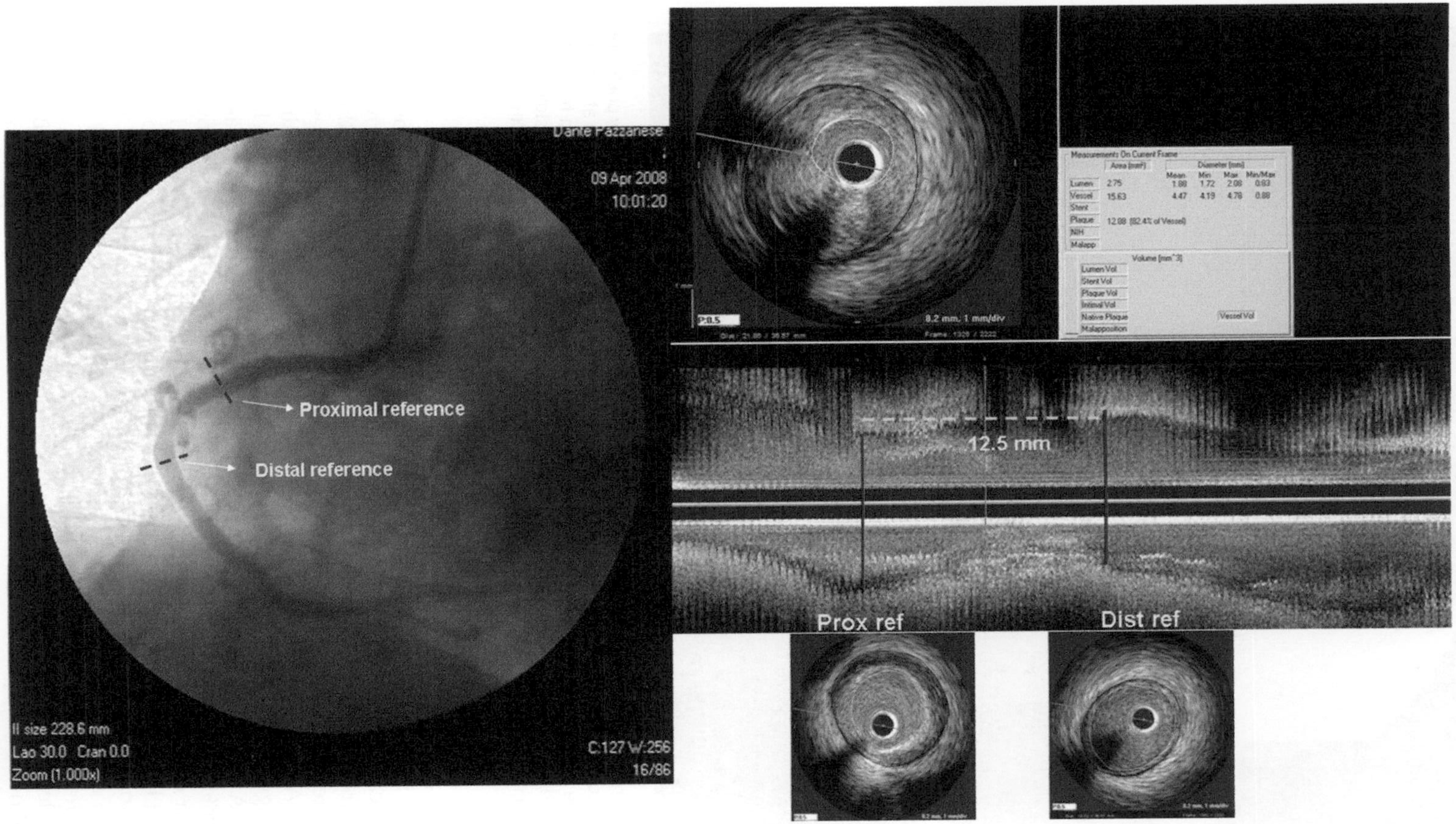

Figure 9.1 Use of IVUS to guide PCI. In the angiography (*left*), we can appreciate the presence of a severe stenosis in the mid-portion of the RCA. IVUS was used to define the proximal and distal reference segment and therefore lesion length. Notice that reference segment does not mean "normal" or "free of disease" segment as seen in proximal reference of this example. However, the references should be free of "significant" plaque burden that could impair normal coronary flow. IVUS also allows the assessment of lesion severity. In this example, we have a minimum in-lesion area of 2.75 mm^2 (minimum lumen diameter of 1.7 mm and plaque burden of 82%). It is also possible to (roughly) evaluate plaque characteristics by IVUS. For instance, in this case, we have a very eccentric, positively remodeled plaque, containing predominantly fibrous-fatty tissue. For the selection of the stent diameter, we used the minimum lumen diameter at the smallest lumen reference (in this specific case, it was selected the proximal reference where the minimum lumen diameter was 3.4 mm). With the use of motorized pullback (0.5 mm/sec), it was also possible to determine lesion length from "normal-to-normal" segment (12.5 mm). In our routine practice, we try to pick a stent 20% to 30% longer than the diseased segment to avoid "edge effect." For this case, our choice was a Diver^{TM} stent 3.5 × 15 mm, directly deployed at 10 atm.

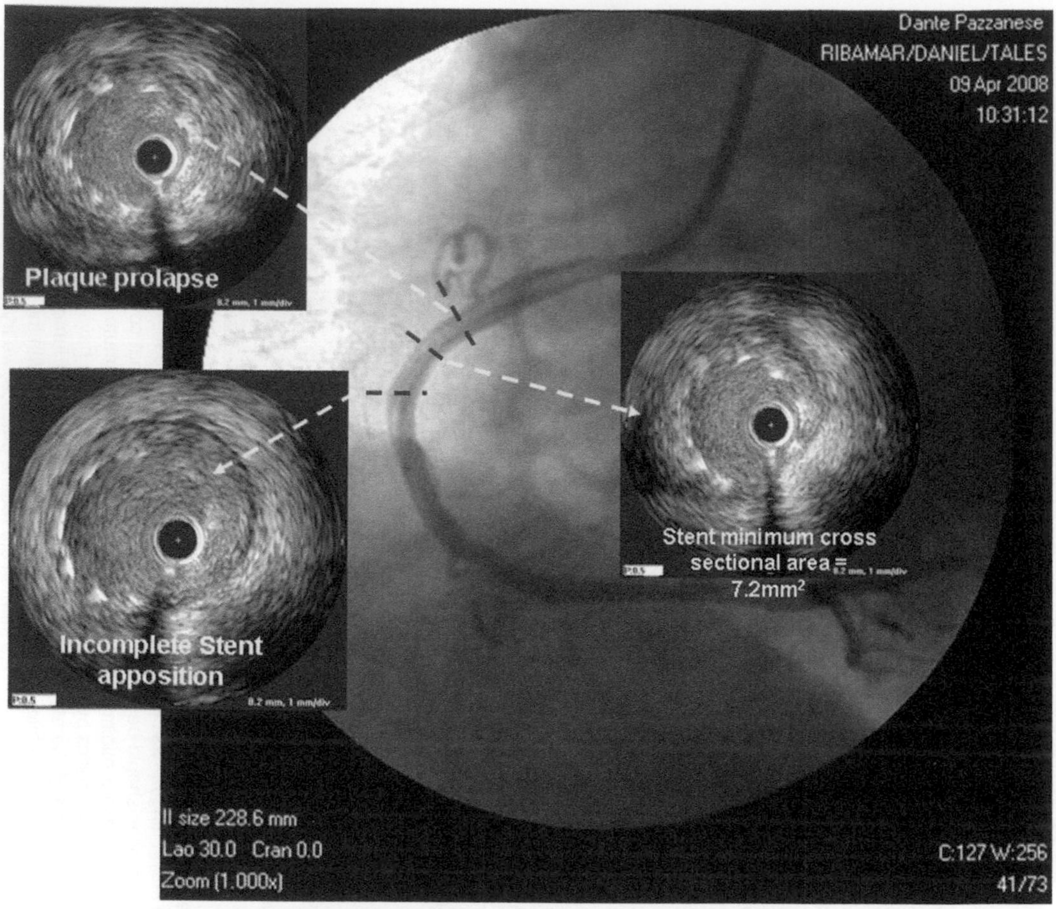

Figure 9.2 Angiographic result of the Driver™ stent implanted in the mid-RCA. IVUS done immediately poststent deployment showed (1) incomplete stent apposition at the distal edge, (2) considerable plaque prolapse at the mid to proximal segment of the stent, and (3) in-stent minimum cross-sectional area of 7.2 mm^2 (although relatively large; considering vessel dimensions, we could expect a minimum area around 9.0 to 9.5 mm^2). Postdilatation with noncompliant Quantum Maverick™ balloon (3.5 × 12 mm at 22 atm) was proceeded to optimize the result.

Bifurcation lesions

Preintervention IVUS imaging may be helpful to determine the degree of side branch (SB) involvement, whether it is not diseased, or diseased but not stenotic, or stenotic; at postprocedural, IVUS imaging can determine whether the SB has been compromised (after provisional stenting) or whether there is adequate stent expansion (if SB stented).[21] It is of notice that relatively high rates of restenosis still occur systematically at the SB ostium location, regardless of the technical approach.[35] A study by **Costa et al.** reported a series treated with crush stenting with SES. Important findings in this study included: (1) the MSA was found at the SB ostium location in 68%; (2) an SB MSA <5.00 mm^2 was found in 76%, and an SB MSA <4.00 mm^2 was found in 44% (90% and 55% when considering only non–LM bifurcations); and (3) significant SB stent underexpansion compared to the parent vessel (PV) (stent expansion 79.9 ± 12.3% in SB vs. 92.1 ± 16.6% in PV; $P = 0.02$).[36] At 6 months clinical follow-up (available in 35 patients), SB restenosis was found in six lesions (all at the ostium location), and was associated with SB stent underexpansion at baseline.[37] Conversely, a series by **Colombo et al.** reported in-stent restenosis of 20% in the SB at 6 months (all at the ostium location). IVUS imaging at follow-up in four restenotic SB lesions demonstrated evidence of incomplete coverage of the SB ostium associated with focal neointimal proliferation.[38] The crush technique was designed, in part, to overcome incomplete coverage of the SB ostium. However, a study by Costa found incomplete crush (incomplete apposition of the PV or SB stent strus against the PV wall proximal to the

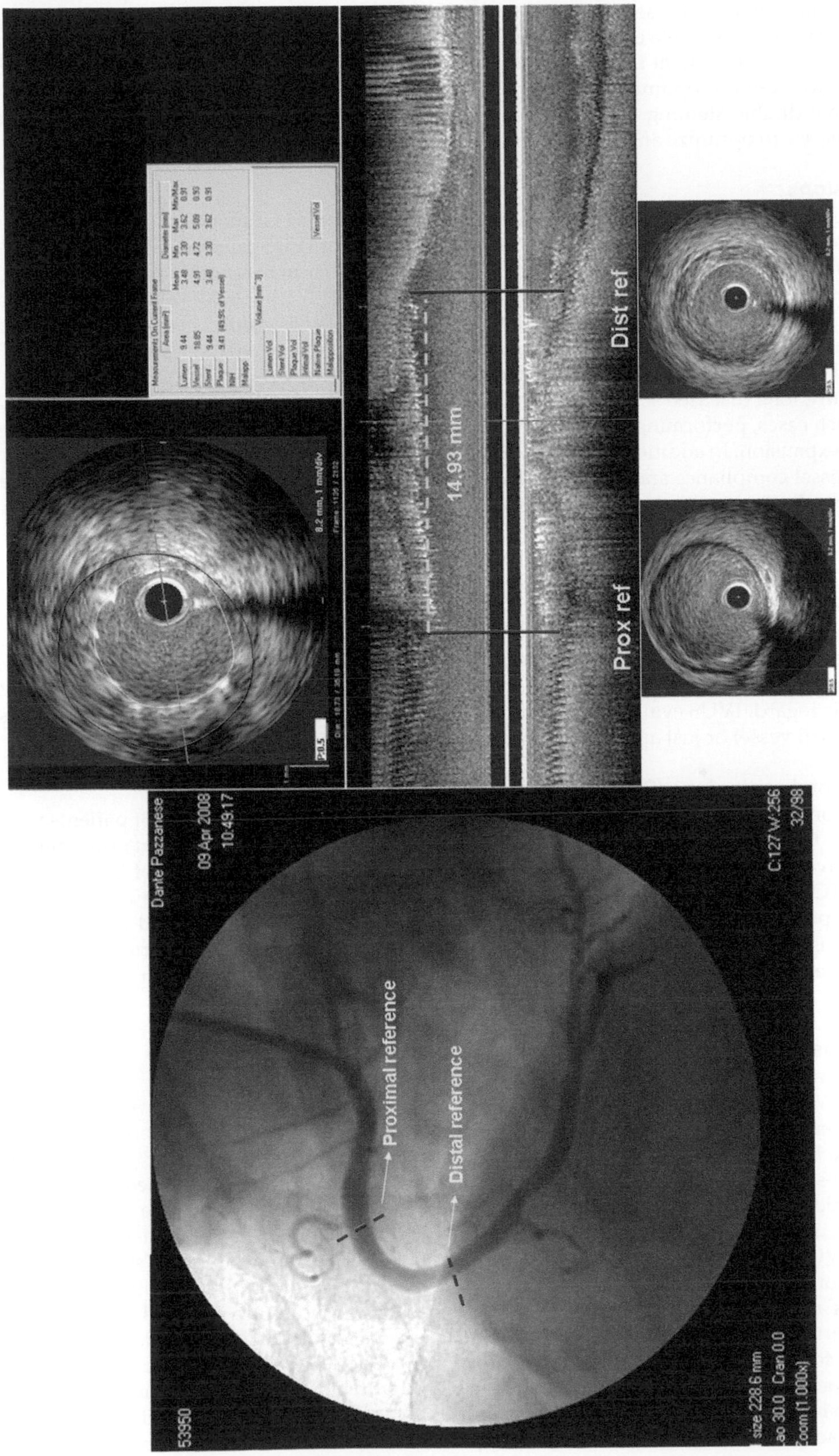

Figure 9.3 IVUS done after stent postdilatation showed: (1) resolution of the stent incomplete apposition at distal edge, (2) reduction in the amount of prolapsed material, and (3) increase of 30% in in-stent minimum lumen area (final MCSA of 9.4 mm^2). Importantly, stent-edge evaluation did not show dissections, significant residual stenosis or any other complications.

carina) in the majority of cases (>60%),[36] which could affect drug delivery and thereby restenosis. Importantly, incomplete crush was associated with lower balloon pressure in the SB during FKB ($p = 0.04$) and SB stent underexpansion ($p = 0.04$).[36,39] Finally, in the INSIDE I trial, IVUS guidance was used to optimize stent implant in bifurcations, and preliminary results demonstrated that double-stenting techniques may be necessary in larger SB with longer and more severe disease to optimize angiographic results.[40]

Long lesions

The Thrombocyte Activity Evaluation and Effects of Ultrasound Guidance in Long Intracoronary Stent Placement (TULIP) study addressed the benefits of IVUS guidance versus angiography guidance for the treatment of long coronary lesions (>20 mm in length). The IVUS-guided group demonstrated more stents per patient (1.4 ± 0.6 vs. 1.1 ± 0.4; $p < 0.001$) and longer stented length (42 ± 11 mm vs. 35 ± 11 mm; $p = 0.001$); at 6 months, IVUS-guided group demonstrated less restenosis (23% vs. 45%; $p = 0.008$), lower TLR (4% vs. 14%; $p = 0.037$), and lower MACE (6% vs. 20%; $p = 0.01$), this benefit persisted up to 1-year follow-up (12% vs. 27%; $p = 0.026$).[41] Importantly, long diseased segments are often associated with small vessels and diabetes mellitus. In such cases, performing IVUS during procedure can be especially valuable in optimizing the stent expansion. In addition, when multiple stents are needed, the overlapping segment may reduce vessel compliance and prevent adequate expansion at that portion, as well as produce incomplete stent apposition beneath the overlapping area. For these reasons, a systematic post-dilatation of the long stent, especially at the overlapping segment, with high-pressure inflations and/or larger balloon is strongly recommended.[26]

Small vessels

Despite the marked efficacy of DES demonstrated in small coronaries, small vessel size is still a major predictor of restenosis in the DES era.[9,10,42,43] Thus, it seems reasonable that optimization of stent implantation in this subset is crucial to long-term results. IVUS can play an important role in this regard. IVUS evaluation can accurately assess if an angiographically small vessel is really a small vessel or just appear as a consequence of diffuse disease.

Chronic total occlusions (CTO)

These lesions are frequently encountered at diagnostic angiography (up to 52% of patients with CAD).[44,45] CTO recanalization is still a challenge for the interventionalist. Some preliminary studies have suggested that IVUS can guide operator for optimal penetration of the proximal cap of CTO.[46,47] After crossing the proximal fibrous cap of the occlusion, the most difficult step is to penetrate the distal cap and re-enter the true lumen at the distal end of the lesion, and IVUS is useful for identifying the site where the wire has gone from the true to the false lumen, assessing the length, depth, and circumferential extent of the false lumen caused by the guidewire.

In-stent restenosis

Stent underexpansion appears to be the main mechanism of DES restenosis.[21–23,48] Importantly, previous IVUS studies have suggested that stent dimensions do not change over time; thus, optimal stent expansion at implantation is required in order to prevent this phenomenon.[49,50] It has also been speculated that strut fractures may contribute to DES failure.[51] The reduced rates of in-stent restenosis in DES has allowed more complex lesions to be treated with longer stents, which may become vulnerable to mechanical forces, particularly at hinge points within the vessel, and this may lead to strut fracture or stent deformation.[52] To confirm, strut fracture requires IVUS identification of stent struts seen at implantation that are no longer seen at follow-up. It is not clear to what extent strut fracture occurs with DES or BMS, or whether DES strut fracture is a common cause of restenosis. Thus, prospective studies are required to investigate this. Nevertheless, IVUS identification of the mechanisms involved (Figs. 9.4–9.6) in ISR may be critical for treatment strategy as well as procedure guidance as focal ISR associated to stent underexpansion may be successfully treated by PTCA with a balloon properly sized inflated at high-pressure to improve lumen and expansion, whereas DES ISR associated with drug failure or stent fracture may need a more complex approach.[53–55]

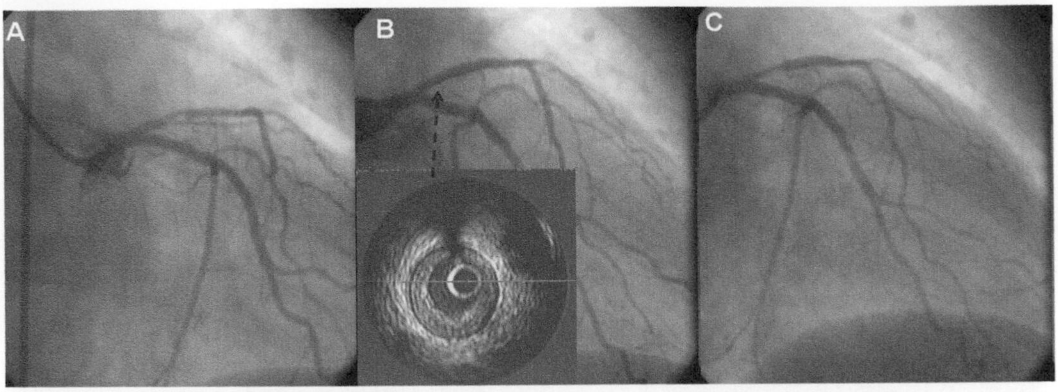

Figure 9.4 Incomplete lesion coverage. The example illustrates a typical "edge" restenosis case. This patient had a lesion in the proximal LAD coronary (panel A) treated with a 3.0 × 18 Cypher™ stent (angiography; panel B). IVUS done immediately after the DES implantation (IVUS; panel B) demonstrated the presence of at least moderated residual stenosis at the proximal edge of the stent. Four months later, patient had recurrence of angina symptoms and the angiogram confirmed a proximal edge restenosis (panel C).

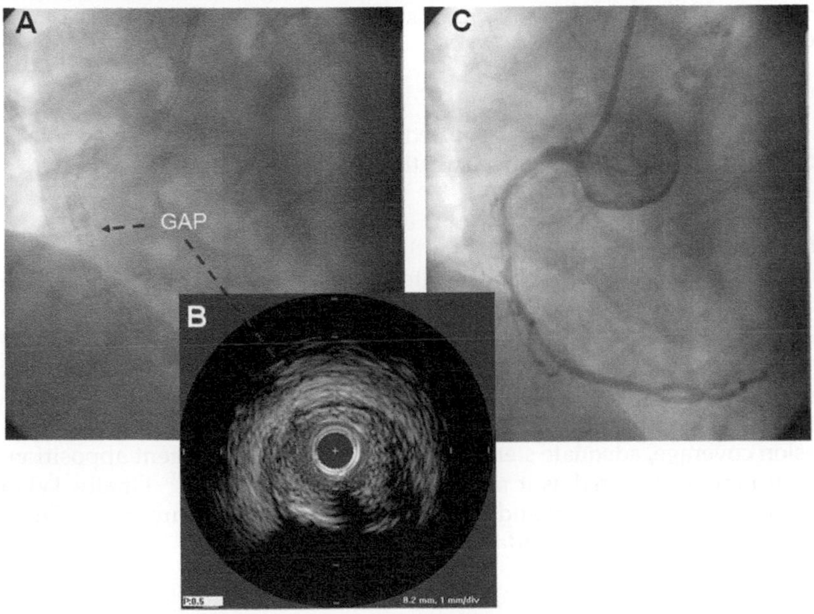

Figure 9.5 "Gap" between stents as a cause of restenosis. An important aspect when deploying multiple stents to treat a long lesion is to make sure that they will have a segment of overlapping. In this example, two Endeavor™ stents (3.5 × 24 mm and 3.0 × 30 mm) were deployed to treat a long lesion in the RCA (angiography; panel A). IVUS done immediately after the procedure evidenced a "gap" between the stents with moderate-to-severe uncovered plaque (IVUS; panel A). Three months later, patient returned with clinical restenosis (panel B).

Stent thrombosis

Stent underexpansion has been associated with thrombosis with both BMS and DES.[12] Recent studies have also suggested an association between late-acquired incomplete stent apposition (ISA) and very late stent thrombosis.[24] Two mechanisms of late-acquired ISA have been proposed including (1) positive arterial remodeling with increase in external-elastic membrane out of proportion to the increase in persistent plaque and media and (2) a decrease in plaque and media due to dissolution of jailed thrombus or plaque debris (i.e., patients undergoing primary stent implantation for acute myocardial infarction).[56,57] While high-pressure inflation may

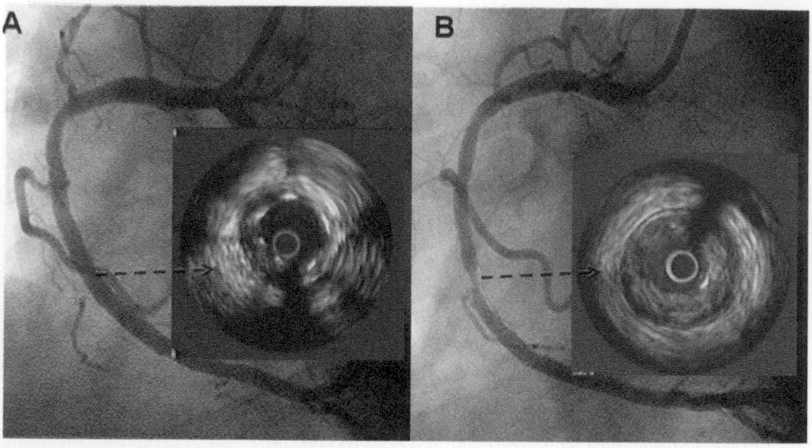

Figure 9.6 Stent fracture. In this case, a long Cypher stent (3.0 × 33) was deployed in the mid-RCA (angiography; panel A). IVUS done right after the procedure demonstrated a good stent apposition, expansion, and complete lesion coverage, with no sign of fracture (IVUS; panel A). Eight months later, this patient had recurrence of angina symptoms. Angiography confirmed the restenosis in the mid-to-distal portion of the stent, at the level of a coronary bend (panel B). IVUS done at that time showed a complete separation of the stent struts (fracture; panel B). This phenomenon has been more frequently described after stainless steel stent deployment for the treatment of tortuous/angulated segments, especially in the RCA.

improve stent expansion,[26] the treatment for late-acquired ISA is still unknown. Nevertheless, IVUS may be critical to identify the underlying mechanistic cause of stent thrombosis.

FINAL CONSIDERATIONS

Although stent underexpansion has been clearly associated with DES failure, even with BMS implantation, high-pressure inflation with IVUS guidance to ensure adequate stent expansion has been shown to reduce restenosis and thrombosis.[18,23,58,59] Since stent underexpansion is common finding with BMS and DES, IVUS-guided DES implantation may improve MSA and stent expansion, especially in more complex subsets.[28,41,60] IVUS may provide accurate assessment of stenosis severity, lesion length, and vessel size, and may also optimize stenting technique including full lesion coverage, adequate stent expansion, and complete stent apposition; therefore, it should be strongly considered as it may also improve outcomes.[21] Finally, IVUS imaging remains the best method to identify and exclude causes of DES failure.[12,22,51] Thus, IVUS assessment of DES failures should be mandatory in all cases.

REFERENCES

1. Serruys PW, de Jaegere P, Kiemeneij F, et al. A comparison of balloon-expandable stent implantation with balloon angioplasty in patients with coronary artery disease. Benestent Study Group. N Engl J Med 1994; 331(8):489–495.
2. Macaya C, Serruys PW, Ruygrok P, et al. Continued benefit of coronary stenting versus balloon angioplasty: One-year clinical follow-up of Benestent Trial. Benestent Study Group. J Am Coll Cardiol 1996; 27(2):255–261.
3. Carrozza JP, Jr., Kuntz RE, Levine MJ, et al. Angiographic and clinical outcome of intracoronary stenting: immediate and long-term results from a large single-center experience. J Am Coll Cardiol 1992; 20(2):328–337.
4. Nath FC, Muller DW, Ellis SG, et al. Thrombosis of a flexible coil coronary stent: frequency, predictors and clinical outcome. J Am Coll Cardiol 1993; 21(3):622–627.
5. Colombo A, Hall P, Nakamura S, et al. Intracoronary stenting without anticoagulation accomplished with intravascular ultrasound guidance. Circulation 1995; 91(6):1676–1688.
6. Nissen SE, Yock P. Intravascular ultrasound: Novel pathophysiological insights and current clinical applications. Circulation 2001; 103(4):604–616.

7. Cheneau E, Leborgne L, Mintz GS, et al. Predictors of subacute stent thrombosis: results of a systematic intravascular ultrasound study. Circulation 2003; 108(1):43–47.
8. Blessing E, Hausmann D, Sturm M, et al. Incomplete expansion of Palmaz-Schatz stents despite high-pressure implantation technique: impact on target lesion revascularization. Cardiology 1999; 91(2):102–108.
9. Moses JW, Leon MB, Popma JJ, et al. Sirolimus-eluting stents versus standard stents in patients with stenosis in a native coronary artery. N Engl J Med 2003; 349(14):1315–1323.
10. Stone GW, Ellis SG, Cox DA, et al. A polymer-based, paclitaxel-eluting stent in patients with coronary artery disease. N Engl J Med 2004; 350(3):221–231.
11. Sonoda S, Morino Y, Ako J, et al. Impact of final stent dimensions on long-term results following sirolimus-eluting stent implantation. Serial intravascular ultrasound analysis from the sirius trial. J Am Coll Cardiol 2004; 43(11):1959–1963.
12. Fujii K, Carlier SG, Mintz GS, et al. Stent underexpansion and residual reference segment stenosis are related to stent thrombosis after sirolimus-eluting stent implantation: An intravascular ultrasound study. J Am Coll Cardiol 2005; 45(7):995–998.
13. de Jaegere P, Mudra H, Figulla H, et al. Intravascular ultrasound-guided optimized stent deployment. Immediate and 6 months clinical and angiographic results from the Multicenter Ultrasound Stenting in Coronaries Study (MUSIC Study). Eur Heart J 1998; 19(8):1214–1223.
14. Mudra H, Di Mario C, de Jaegere P, et al. Randomized comparison of coronary stent implantation under ultrasound or angiographic guidance to reduce stent restenosis (OPTICUS Study). Circulation 2001; 104(12):1343–1349.
15. Schiele F, Meneveau N, Vuillemenot A, et al. Impact of intravascular ultrasound guidance in stent deployment on 6-month restenosis rate: A multicenter, randomized study comparing two strategies—with and without intravascular ultrasound guidance. RESIST Study Group. REStenosis after Ivus guided STenting. J Am Coll Cardiol 1998; 32(2):320–328.
16. Schiele F, Meneveau N, Seronde MF, et al. Medical costs of intravascular ultrasound optimization of stent deployment. Results of the multicenter randomized 'REStenosis after Intravascular ultrasound STenting' (RESIST) study. Int J Cardiovasc Intervent 2000; 3(4):207–213.
17. Russo RJ, Attubato MJ, Davidson CJ, et al. Angiography versus intravascular ultrasound-directed stent placement: Final results from AVID (abstract). Circulation 1999; 100(Suppl. 1): I234.
18. Casella G, Klauss V, Ottani F, et al. Impact of intravascular ultrasound-guided stenting on long-term clinical outcome: A meta-analysis of available studies comparing intravascular ultrasound-guided and angiographically guided stenting. Cathet Cardiovasc Interv 2003; 59(3):314–321.
19. Gerber RT, Latib A, Ielasi A, et al. Defining a new standard for IVUS optimized drug eluting stent implantation: the PRAVIO study. Catheter Cardiovasc Interv 2009; 74(2):348–356.
20. Fitzgerald PJ, Oshima A, Hayase M, et al. Final results of the Can Routine Ultrasound Influence Stent Expansion (CRUISE) study. Circulation 2000; 102(5):523–530.
21. Mintz GS, Weissman NJ. Intravascular ultrasound in the drug-eluting stent era. J Am Coll Cardiol 2006; 48(3):421–429.
22. Hong MK, Mintz GS, Lee CW, et al. Intravascular ultrasound predictors of angiographic restenosis after sirolimus-eluting stent implantation. Eur Heart J 2006; 27(11):1305–1310.
23. Takebayashi H, Kobayashi Y, Mintz GS, et al. Intravascular ultrasound assessment of lesions with target vessel failure after sirolimus-eluting stent implantation. Am J Cardiol 2005; 95(4):498–502.
24. Cook S, Wenaweser P, Togni M, et al. Incomplete stent apposition and very late stent thrombosis after drug-eluting stent implantation. Circulation 2007; 115(18):2426–2434.
25. Briguori C, Tobis J, Nishida T, et al. Discrepancy between angiography and intravascular ultrasound when analysing small coronary arteries. Eur Heart J 2002; 23(3):247–254.
26. Romagnoli E. Sangiorgi GM, Cosgrave J, et al. Drug-eluting stenting: the case for post-dilation. JACC Cardiovasc Interv 2008; 1(1):22–31.
27. de Ribamar Costa J, Jr, Mintz GS, Carlier S, et al. Intravascular ultrasonic assessment of stent diameters derived from manufacturer's compliance charts. Am J Cardiol 2005; 96(1):74–78.
28. de Ribamar Costa J, Jr, Mintz GS, Carlier S, et al. Intravascular ultrasound assessment of drug-eluting stent expansion. Am Heart J 2007; 153(2):297–303.
29. Wilensky RL, Selzer F, Johnston J, et al. Relation of percutaneous coronary intervention of complex lesions to clinical outcomes (from the NHLBI Dynamic Registry). Am J Cardiol 2002; 90(3):216–221.
30. Ramana RK, Arab D, Joyal D, et al. Coronary artery perforation during percutaneous coronary intervention: incidence and outcomes in the new interventional era. J Invasive Cardiol 2005; 17(11):603–605.
31. Vavuranakis M, Toutouzas K, Stefanadis C, et al. Stent deployment in calcified lesions: can we overcome calcific restraint with high-pressure balloon inflations? Cathet Cardiovasc Interv 2001; 52(2):164–172.

32. Mintz G. Intracoronary Ultrasound. New York, NY: Taylor & Francis. 2005.
33. Yoon SC, Laskey WK, Assadourian A, et al. Assessment of contemporary stent deployment using intravascular ultrasound. Cathet Cardiovasc Interv 2002; 57(2):150–154.
34. Park SJ, Kim YH, Park DW, et al. Impact of Intravascular Ultrasound Guidance on Long-Term Mortality in Stenting for Unprotected Left Main Coronary Artery Stenosis. Circ Cardiovasc Imaging 2009; 2:167–177.
35. Costa RA, Moussa ID. Percutaneous treatment of coronary bifurcation lesions in the era of drug-eluting stents. Minerva Cardioangiol 2006; 54(5):577–589.
36. Costa RA, Mintz GS, Carlier SG, et al. Bifurcation coronary lesions treated with the "crush" technique: An intravascular ultrasound analysis. J Am Coll Cardiol 2005; 46(4):599–605.
37. Costa RA, Mintz GS, Carlier S, et al. Impact of Final Lumen Dimensions on Restenosis After Crush Drug-Eluting Stent Implantation for Bifurcation Lesions. J Am Coll Cardiol 2005; 45:66. Suppl II (abstract).
38. Colombo A, Moses JW, Morice MC, et al. Randomized study to evaluate sirolimus-eluting stents implanted at coronary bifurcation lesions. Circulation 2004; 109(10):1244–1249.
39. Costa RA, Mintz GS, Carlier S. Reply letter: Bifurcation coronary lesions treated with the "crush" technique - An intravascular ultrasound analysis J Am Coll Cardiol 2006; 47(12):2567.
40. Costa RA. Imaging of the Main Vessel and the Side Branch with Different Stenting Bifurcation Treatment Approaches (INSIDE I and II Trials). Presented at: Transcatheter Cardiovascular Therapeutics (TCT) 2007. 2007:October 21, 2007; Washington, DC.
41. Oemrawsingh PV, Mintz GS, Schalij MJ, et al. Intravascular ultrasound guidance improves angiographic and clinical outcome of stent implantation for long coronary artery stenoses: final results of a randomized comparison with angiographic guidance (TULIP Study). Circulation 2003; 107(1): 62–67.
42. Ardissimo D, Cavallini C, Bramucci E, et al. Sirolimus-eluting vs. uncoated stents for prevention of restenosis in small coronary arteries: a randomized trial. JAMA 2004; 292(22):2727–2734.
43. Kastrati A, Dibra A, Mehilli J, et al. Predictive factors of restenosis after coronary implantation of sirolimus- or paclitaxel-eluting stents. Circulation 2006; 113(19):2293–2300.
44. Grantham JA, Marso SP, Spertus J, et al. Chronic total occlusion angioplasty in the United States. JACC Cardiovasc Interv 2009; 2(6):479–486.
45. Werner GS, Gitt AK, Zeymer U, et al. Chronic total coronary occlusions in patients with stable angina pectoris: impact on therapy and outcome in present day clinical practice. Clin Res Cardiol 2009; 98(7):435–441.
46. Cuneo A, Tebbe U. The management of chronic total coronary occlusions. Minerva Cardioangiol 2008; 56(5):527–541.
47. Furuichi S, Airoldi F, Colombo A. Intravascular ultrasound-guided wiring for chronic total occlusion. Catheter Cardiovasc Interv 2007; 70(6):856–859.
48. Fujii K, Mintz GS, Kobayashi Y, et al. Contribution of stent underexpansion to recurrence after sirolimus-eluting stent implantation for in-stent restenosis. Circulation 2004; 109(9):1085–1088.
49. Kim SW, Mintz GS, Lee KJ, et al. Repeated stenting of recurrent in-stent restenotic lesions: intravascular ultrasound analysis and clinical outcome. J Invasive Cardiol 2007; 19(12):506–509.
50. Sano K, Mintz GS, Carlier SG, et al. Treatment of restenotic drug-eluting stents: an intravascular ultrasound analysis. J Invasive Cardiol 2007; 19(11):464–468.
51. Kim EJ, Rha SW, Wani SP, et al. Coronary stent fracture and restenosis in the drug-eluting stent era: do we have clues of management? Int J Cardiol 2007; 120(3):417–419.
52. Shaikh F, Maddikunta R, Djelmami-Hani M, et al. Stent fracture, an incidental finding or a significant marker of clinical in-stent restenosis? Catheter Cardiovasc Interv 2008; 71(5):614–618.
53. Radke PW, Klues HG, Haager PK, et al. Mechanisms of acute lumen gain and recurrent restenosis after rotational atherectomy of diffuse in-stent restenosis: a quantitative angiographic and intravascular ultrasound study. J Am Coll Cardiol 1999; 34(1):33–39.
54. Rathore S, Kinoshita Y, Terashima M, et al. Sirolimus eluting stent restenosis: Impact of angiographic patterns and the treatment factors on angiographic outcomes in contemporary practice. Int J Cardiol 2009.
55. Alfonso F, Perez-Vizcayno MJ, Cruz A, et al. Treatment of patients with in-stent restenosis. EuroIntervention 2009; 5 Suppl D:D70–78.
56. Miyazawa A, Tsujino I, Ako J, et al. Characterization of late incomplete stent apposition: a comparison among bare-metal stents, intracoronary radiation and sirolimus-eluting stents. J Invasive Cardiol 2007; 19(12):515–518.
57. Sianos G, Papafaklis MI, Daemen J, et al. Angiographic stent thrombosis after routine use of drug-eluting stents in ST-segment elevation myocardial infarction: the importance of thrombus burden. J Am Coll Cardiol 2007; 50(7):573–583.

58. Bonello L, De Labriolle A, Lemesle G, et al. Intravascular ultrasound-guided percutaneous coronary interventions in contemporary practice. Arch Cardiovasc Dis 2009; 102(2):143–151.
59. Roy P, Steinberg DH, Sushinsky SJ, et al. The potential clinical utility of intravascular ultrasound guidance in patients undergoing percutaneous coronary intervention with drug-eluting stents. Eur Heart J 2008; 29(15):1851–1857.
60. Castagna MT, Mintz GS, Leiboff BO, et al. The contribution of "mechanical" problems to in-stent restenosis: An intravascular ultrasonographic analysis of 1090 consecutive in-stent restenosis lesions. Am Heart J 2001; 142(6):970–974.

10 A practical approach to IVUS for in-stent restenosis and thrombosis

Daniel H. Steinberg

INTRODUCTION

Despite the remarkable impacts that bare-metal and drug-eluting stents have made on coronary intervention, important limitations remain. From an efficacy standpoint, restenosis continues to occur in a substantial proportion of patients. With regard to safety, stent thrombosis remains our primary concern. While angiography alone is often adequate to diagnose and treat either condition, intravascular ultrasound (IVUS) can provide important insight into the underlying mechanisms and ultimately help guide treatment.

RESTENOSIS

In-stent restenosis refers to obstructive disease occurring within the stent or 5 mm proximal or distal to a previously placed stent. From a research perspective, the so-called "binary restenosis" in angiographic follow-up refers to 50% obstruction to flow, while clinically, restenosis typically implies that disease within (or around) a stent is sufficient to warrant treatment.

Based on IVUS studies, multiple mechanisms underlie the angiographic appearance of in-stent restenosis. The most common mechanism of restenosis is neointimal hyperplasia (Fig. 10.1), and this occurs in various patterns (Fig. 10.2).[1] Focal restenosis involves <10 mm of a stented segment. Diffuse restenosis involves >10 mm but remains within the stent. Proliferative restenosis involves >10 mm and extends beyond the stent edges.

Although it is the most common cause of restenosis, neointimal hyperplasia does not explain all cases. Castagna et al. reported on 1090 patients who underwent IVUS evaluation of in-stent restenosis prior to definitive treatment.[2] In this series, 25% of angiographic restesnosis cases were due to a mechanism other than neointimal hyperplasia (Fig. 10.3). Mechanical issues such as geographic miss were responsible for 4.9% of cases, and stent underexpansion (Fig. 10.4) was responsible for another 20%.[2]

These findings have important implications when considering treatment. Although vascular brachytherapy remains the only FDA-approved modality with which to treat in-stent restenosis, based on numerous registries and randomized trials, drug-eluting stents have emerged as the treatment of choice.[3,4] Indeed, drug-eluting stent implantation is technically simple and results in excellent long-term outcomes in patients with bare-metal stent restenosis. However, patients with drug-eluting stent restenosis may not fare as well when treated with repeat drug-eluting stent.[5] It is important to recognize that implanting another drug-eluting stent may place patients at elevated risk of recurrent restenosis thrombosis, especially if the mechanism of restenosis has nothing to do with tissue hyperplasia. In this regard, IVUS has particular relevance.

When IVUS analysis of angiographic in-stent restenosis demonstrates tissue hyperplasia, treatment can be based on the pattern of restenosis. If the pattern is focal (often the case in DES restenosis) then balloon angioplasty alone may be sufficient with regard to future revascularization. With diffuse restenosis (more common with bare-metal stents), the drug-eluting stents should be the treatment of choice. In proliferative restenosis, balloon angioplasty with adjunctive brachytherapy is a reasonable option.

When IVUS demonstrates a mechanism of restenosis other than in-stent neointimal hyperplasia, treatment must be tailored to the specific underlying issue. In cases of underexpansion, the treatment is simply high-pressure balloon inflation with IVUS guidance to maximize stent expansion; however, adjunctive therapies may be necessary. In cases of geographic miss, additional stents should be implanted to adequately cover the lesion.

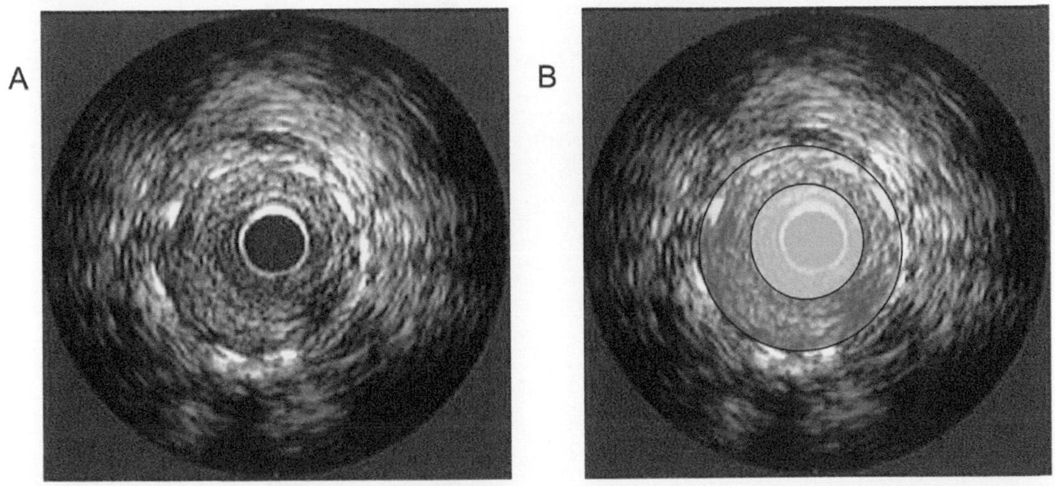

Figure 10.1 Neointimal hyperplasia: (**A**) IVUS image and (**B**) the border of the green circle denotes the stent borders. The yellow circle denotes the lumen. The green area represents neointimal hyperlasia.

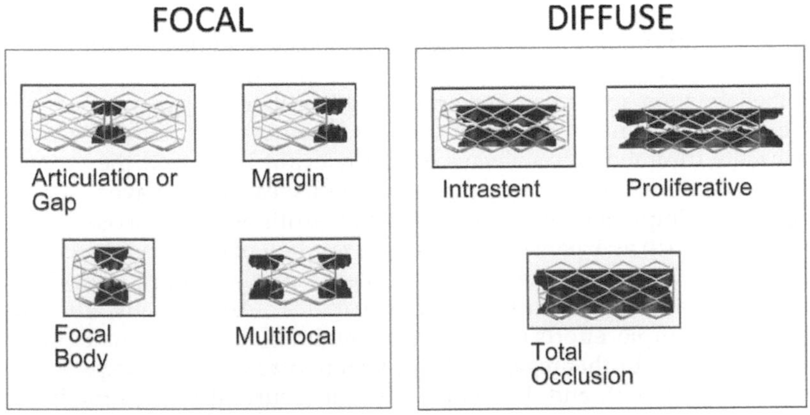

Figure 10.2 Patterns of restenosis. *Source*: Adapted from Ref. 1.

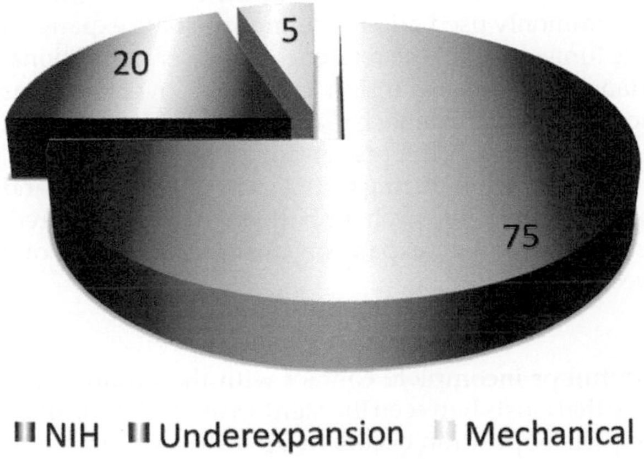

Figure 10.3 Mechanisms of in-stent restenosis. A total of 1090 lesions with in-stent restenosis were referred for treatment on which IVUS was performed. *Source*: Adapted from Ref. 2.

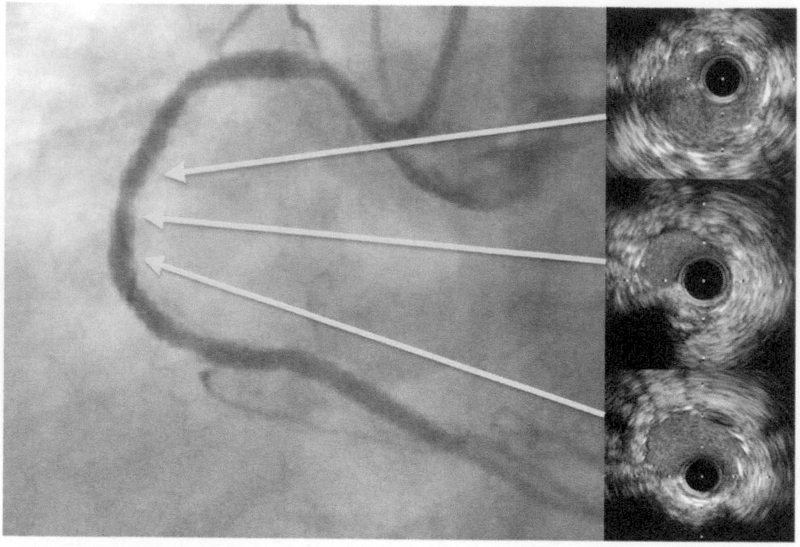

Figure 10.4 Angiographic appearance of in-stent restenosis in this case due to inadequate expansion with minimal tissue proliferation.

THROMBOSIS

The whirlwind of controversy surrounding very late stent thrombosis with drug-eluting stent has brought the long-term safety of percutaneous coronary intervention (PCI) to center stage. Certainly, delayed endothelialization and inflammation related to either the drug or polymer should remain the subject of intense research; however, stent thrombosis is not a new phenomenon. Acute and subacute thrombosis has always been a relevant issue, and the event is often due to mechanical (and therefore, preventable) factors.[6] For this reason, we have long proposed routine IVUS-guided stent implantation to optimize initial results and reduce risk factors associated with stent thrombosis such as expansion, apposition, residual plaque, and dissection.

Particularly important are concepts that the mortality of stent thrombosis approaches 20%, and once it occurs in a particular patient, the recurrence rate is up to 20%.[7] Additionally, while the causes of stent thromboses are multiple, efforts must focus on minimizing the potential impact of those causes that are modifiable. In this regard, IVUS plays two roles. IVUS helps reveal the causal mechanism, guide treatment, and, hopefully, prevent recurrent stent thrombosis. However, far more importantly, addressing the same principles during initial stent deployment can help prevent stent thrombosis altogether.[8]

Expansion

Stent expansion refers to the comparison of the minimum stent area and the reference lumen. Although various definitions exist, the most commonly used criteria define adequate expansion as a minimum stent area, 90% of the reference lumen (80% if the reference lumen cross-sectional area is greater than 9 mm^2).[9] The importance of stent expansion cannot be overstated, as inadequate stent expansion has been implicated in both restenosis[10] and thrombosis.[11]

Assuring optimal stent expansion is fundamental in the prevention of stent thrombosis. To ensure optimal stent expansion, high-pressure inflation during initial stent deployment, and if necessary, further high-pressure postdilation with a noncompliant balloon, may be required. In cases of thrombosis due (at least in part) to inadequate expansion, further expansion of a previously placed stent may help prevent recurrence.

Apposition

Apposition refers to the stent strut being in full or incomplete contact with the luminal wall (Fig. 10.5). Mechanistically, the potential space that exists between the stent struts and the intimal wall can lead to thrombus formation. Incomplete apposition occurs in up to 10% of cases, and its occurrence has been implicated in both subacute and late stent thrombosis.[6,12]

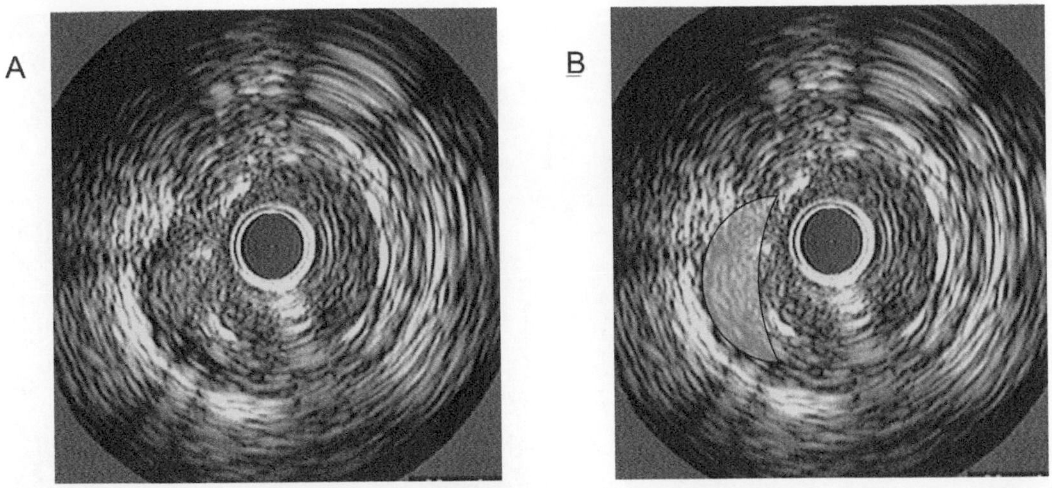

Figure 10.5 Incomplete stent apposition: (**A**) IVUS image and (**B**) the yellow-shaded area denotes incomplete stent apposition to the vessel wall.

When incomplete apposition is noted, either at the time of initial stent deployment or at the time of stent thrombosis, it can be easily treated with IVUS guidance. The space between the stent and the vessel wall should have low resistance. Therefore, a larger, compliant balloon at relatively low pressure can optimize apposition without significant impact on neighboring untreated vessel or the stent itself.

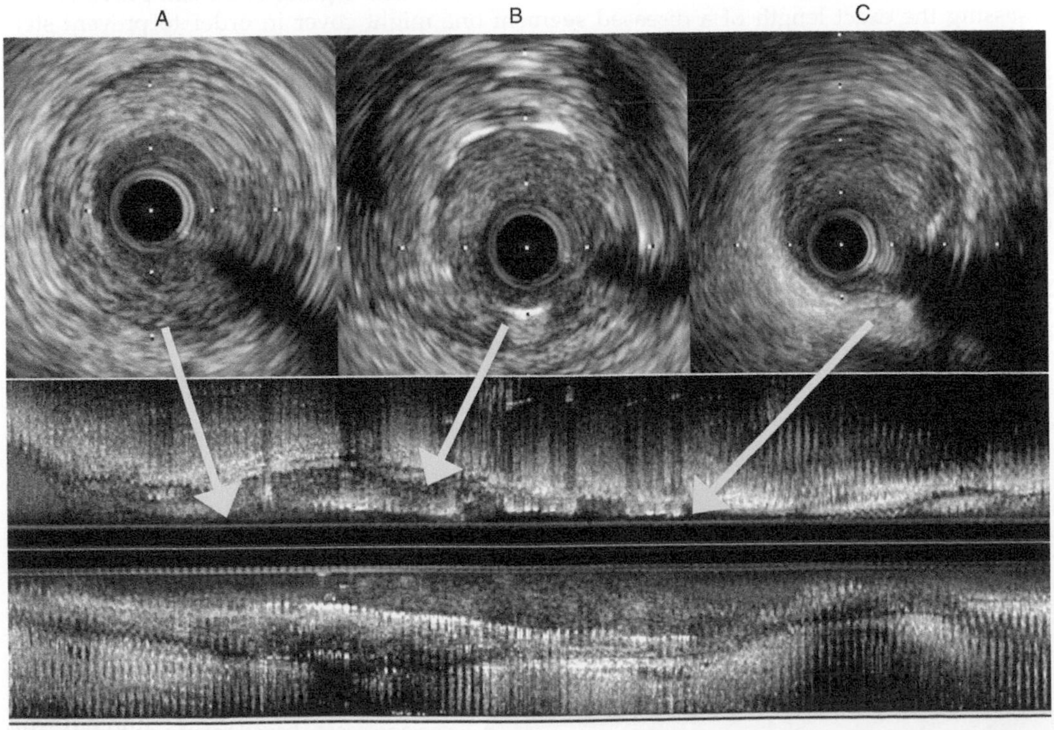

Figure 10.6 Stent thrombosis due to reference stenosis. (**A**) Proximal reference demonstrating greater than 70% area stenosis. (**B**) Thrombotic material within the stent. (**C**) Distal reference demonstrating greater than 70% area stenosis.

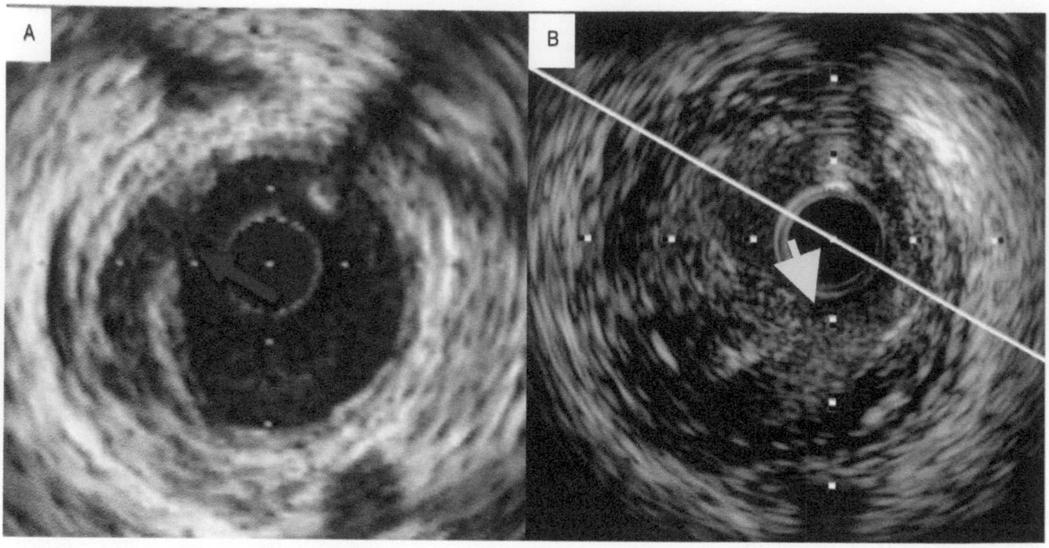

Figure 10.7 Dissection. (**A**) Intimal tear post without lumen obstrution. This lesion would require treatment. (**B**) Intimal tear with thrombus formation and lumen obstruction, which would require additional stent placement.

Residual plaque

Another important mechanism of thrombosis is significant disease at the proximal and distal edges of the stent. This may be especially true in the era of drug-eluting stents, where impaired inflow and/or outflow coupled with incompletely endotheliazed stent struts and delayed healing can pose additional risk for thrombosis.[13,14] Angiography often underestimates the true burden of disease within a vessel, and in that regard, IVUS can prove vital in assessing the exact length of a diseased segment one might cover in order to prevent stent thrombosis. Additionally, when assessing the cause of stent thrombosis, important stenosis affecting either inflow or outflow must be treated with additional stents in order to prevent recurrences (Fig. 10.6).

Lastly, complications occurring during the initial intervention are often important causes of stent thrombosis. These include dissection (Fig. 10.7), intramural hematoma (Fig. 10.8), and tissue prolapse (Fig. 10.9). While the exact incidence and magnitude of risk posed by each of these complications is not well known, numerous studies have implicated them in stent

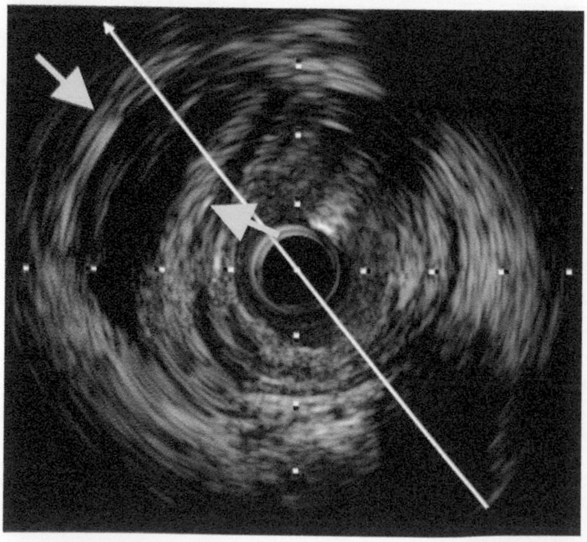

Figure 10.8 Intramural hematoma. Hypoechoic crescent-shaped defect outside the medial stripe (*yellow arrows*) compressing the vessel and causing clinically important luminal obstruction.

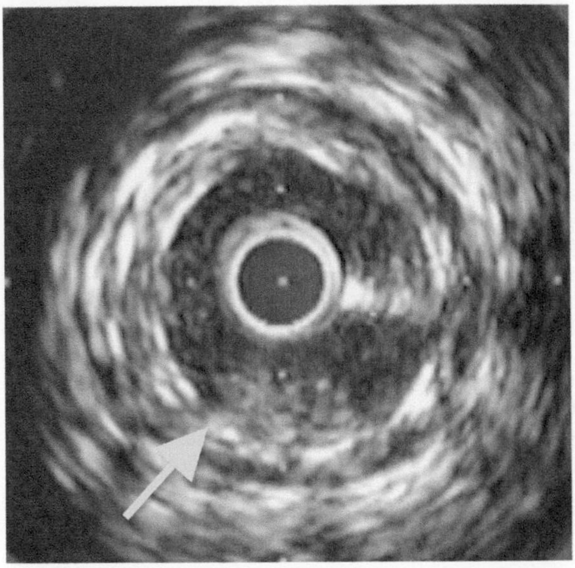

Figure 10.9 Plaque prolapse. In this example of a newly implanted stent, plaque (*arrow*) is seen prolapsing through the stent struts.

thrombosis.[6,15,16] Thus, monitoring for and addressing these complications at the time of initial PCI or on presentation of stent thrombosis is advisable.

In the event of stent thrombosis and the acute presentation often associated with it, common sense dictates that all efforts should focus on establishing adequate antegrade flow through the vessel. However, once flow is established, IVUS can be utilized to assess a mechanistic cause of thrombosis and ultimately prevent a recurrent event. Ideally, this is done a few days after the acute presentation once the patient is stabilized on optimal medial therapy.

SUMMARY

Restenosis and thrombosis remain the two drawbacks of PCI. While angiography is often sufficient to guide treatment of both restenosis and thrombosis, it is limited in scope. IVUS provides significantly more information and allows one to assess the proximal and distal references, expansion, apposition, and complications that lead to restenosis and stent thrombosis. Routine IVUS use during initial stent implantation may help reduce the incidence of restenosis and thrombosis, and tailored treatment geared toward the underlying mechanism may help significantly reduce their recurrence.

REFERENCES

1. Mehran R, Dangas G, Abizaid AS, et al. Angiographic patterns of in-stent restenosis: Classification and implications for long-term outcome. Circulation 1999; 100(18):1872–1878.
2. Castagna MT, Mintz GS, Leiboff BO, et al. The contribution of "mechanical" problems to in-stent restenosis: An intravascular ultrasonographic analysis of 1090 consecutive in-stent restenosis lesions. Am Heart J 2001; 142(6):970–974.
3. Holmes DR Jr, Teirstein P, Satler L, et al. Sirolimus-eluting stents vs vascular brachytherapy for in-stent restenosis within bare-metal stents: The SISR randomized trial. JAMA 2006; 295(11): 1264–1273.
4. Stone GW, Ellis SG, O'Shaughnessy CD, et al. Paclitaxel-eluting stents vs vascular brachytherapy for in-stent restenosis within bare-metal stents: The TAXUS V ISR randomized trial. JAMA 2006; 295(11):1253–1263.
5. Whan Lee C, Kim SH, Suh J, et al. Long-term clinical outcomes after sirolimus-eluting stent implantation for treatment of restenosis within bare-metal versus drug-eluting stents. Catheter Cardiovasc Interv 2008; 71(5):594–598.
6. Cheneau E, Leborgne L, Mintz GS, et al. Predictors of subacute stent thrombosis: Results of a systematic intravascular ultrasound study. Circulation 2003; 108(1):43–47.
7. Chechi T, Vecchio S, Vittori G, et al. ST-segment elevation myocardial infarction due to early and late stent thrombosis: A new group of high-risk patients. J Am Coll Cardiol 2008; 51(25):2396–2402.

8. Roy P, Steinberg DH, Sushinsky SJ, et al. The potential clinical utility of intravascular ultrasound guidance in patients undergoing percutaneous coronary intervention with drug-eluting stents. Eur Heart J 2008; 29(15):1851–1857.
9. de Jaegere P, Mudra H, Figulla H, et al. Intravascular ultrasound-guided optimized stent deployment. Immediate and 6 months clinical and angiographic results from the Multicenter Ultrasound Stenting in Coronaries Study (MUSIC Study). Eur Heart J 1998; 19(8):1214–1223.
10. Fujii K, Mintz GS, Kobayashi Y, et al. Contribution of stent underexpansion to recurrence after sirolimus-eluting stent implantation for in-stent restenosis. Circulation 2004; 109(9):1085–1088.
11. Okabe T, Mintz GS, Buch AN, et al. Intravascular ultrasound parameters associated with stent thrombosis after drug-eluting stent deployment. Am JCardiol 2007; 100(4):615–620.
12. Cook S, Wenaweser P, Togni M, et al. Incomplete stent apposition and very late stent thrombosis after drug-eluting stent implantation. Circulation 2007; 115(18):2426–2434.
13. Joner M, Finn AV, Farb A, et al. Pathology of drug-eluting stents in humans: Delayed healing and late thrombotic risk. J Am Coll Cardiol 2006; 48(1):193–202.
14. van Beusekom HM, Saia F, Zindler JD, et al. Drug-eluting stents show delayed healing: Paclitaxel more pronounced than sirolimus. Eur Heart J 2007; 28(8):974–979.
15. Moussa I, Di Mario C, Reimers B, et al. Subacute stent thrombosis in the era of intravascular ultrasound-guided coronary stenting without anticoagulation: Frequency, predictors and clinical outcome. J Am Coll Cardiol 1997; 29(1):6–12.
16. Uren NG, Schwarzacher SP, Metz JA, et al. Predictors and outcomes of stent thrombosis: An intravascular ultrasound registry. Eur Heart J 2002; 23(2):124–132.

11 Pharmacological intervention trials

Paul Schoenhagen and Ilke Sipahi

INTRODUCTION

Atherosclerosis and its complications including myocardial infarction and stroke is a major health problem in most parts of the world. Early prevention, including lifestyle/diet modification and pharmacological treatment of risk factors, will allow reducing the associated morbidity and mortality.

Novel pharmacological interventions for cardiovascular prevention are emerging and need to be carefully tested before incorporation into clinical practice. However, demonstrating efficacy is increasingly difficult, as the incremental benefit against established background treatment is relatively small. Therefore, pharmacological intervention trials with traditional mortality endpoints require large patient populations and long observation times. Intermediate or surrogate endpoints have the potential to guide and accelerate the development of the most promising approaches, which then eventually are tested in large clinical outcome studies. For therapies affecting low-density lipoprotein cholesterol (LDL-C) and high-density lipoprotein cholesterol (HDL-C), the role of these lipid markers as intermediate endpoints has been demonstrated in multiple trials.

Atherosclerosis imaging endpoints allow serial assessment of atherosclerotic plaque burden with relatively small patient populations and short follow-up.[1] The validity of this approach as an intermediate endpoint in progression/regression trials is best documented for carotid ultrasound (carotid intima-media thickness; CIMT) and coronary intravascular ultrasound (IVUS).[2,3] In these studies, the change in plaque burden has been concordant with reduction of mortality endpoint in similar designed clinical studies.[4] Atherosclerosis imaging trials already have significant impact on clinical decision making, for example, supporting more aggressive lipid-lowering treatment with the goal of atherosclerotic plaque regression. At the same time, negative studies have had significant impact on the drug development programs of compounds that appeared promising in animal and preclinical models.[5–7]

ATHEROSCLEROSIS IMAGING WITH IVUS

Using IVUS, the internal ultrasound reflection from the vessels wall/plaque and the strong signal reflected from the intima and external elastic membrane (EEM) allows identification, characterization, and quantification of atheroma.[8] Atherosclerosis imaging with IVUS has enhanced our understanding of the atherosclerotic disease process, including insights into progression of plaque burden, remodeling, and plaque vulnerability. IVUS has confirmed results from histologic studies that coronary atherosclerosis is commonly present at an early stage and progresses silently over long periods of time. This subclinical progression of accumulating atherosclerotic plaque is associated with outward, expansive remodeling of the arterial wall, initially maintaining luminal dimensions.[9] Paradoxically, IVUS studies demonstrated that expansive remodeling is associated with lesion inflammation and plaque instability and confirmed the hypothesis that plaque-stabilizing therapy is associated with constrictive remodeling.[10,11]

IVUS has been extensively validated for application in progression/regression trials. Initial quantitative IVUS studies examined the progression of plaque area at matched single cross-sectional lesion sites (Fig. 11.1). However, the reproducibility of this analysis approach is limited by the difficulties to exactly match individual sites. Accordingly, volumetric analysis approaches integrating consecutive plaque area measurements at 0.5- to 1-mm intervals along long vessel segments were developed in dedicated core laboratories (Fig. 11.2). In pharmacologic intervention trials "change in plaque volume" in a long coronary segment is the primary endpoint. Because the entire segment rather than individual sites are matched at baseline and follow-up, assessment of small percent changes in atheroma volume is possible with considerable statistical power.[1,3]

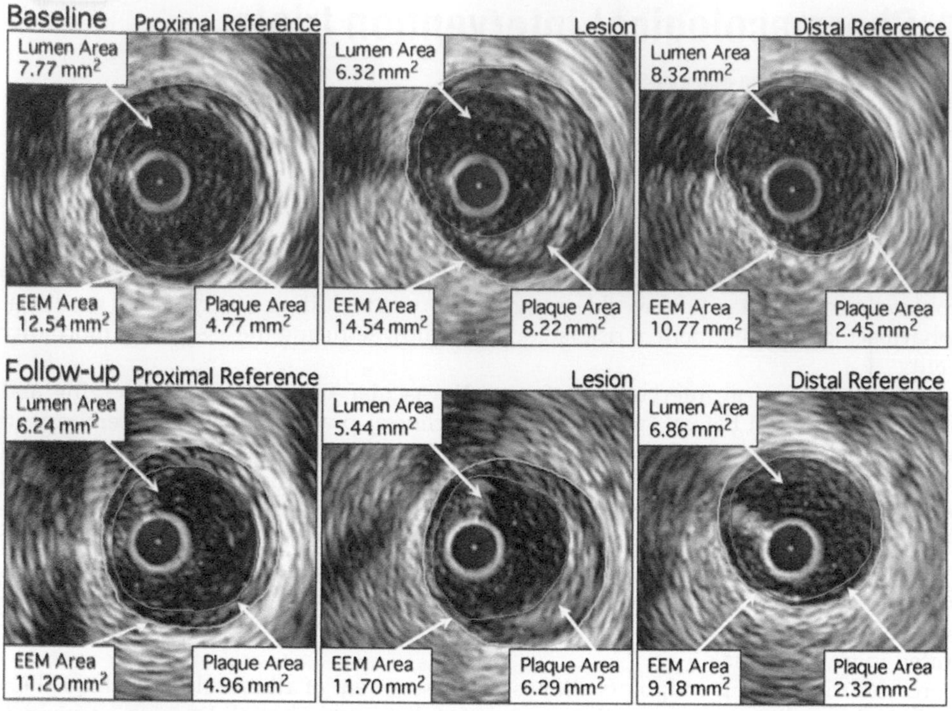

Figure 11.1 This figure demonstrates an example of a lesion with plaque regression and concomitant constrictive remodeling. Initial IVUS studies evaluated single lesions sites. While this provides important insights into the atherosclerotic disease process, matching of individual lesions is a limitation for serial studies. *Source*: Adapted from Ref. 11.

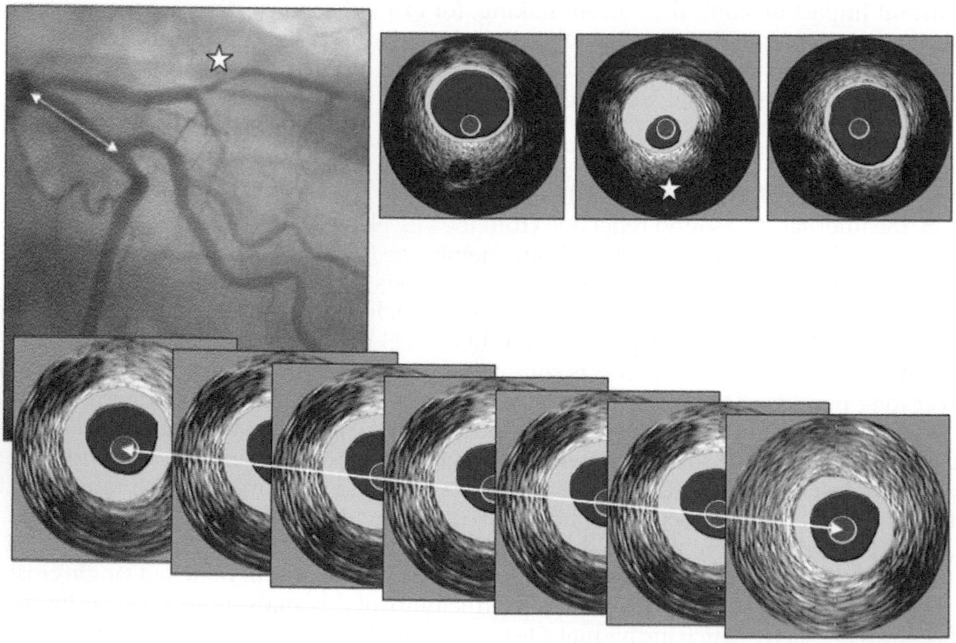

Figure 11.2 Because of the limitations of matching individual lesions, serial progression trials use plaque burden in long segments as the primary endpoint. This figure demonstrates the IVUS methodology. The highly stenotic lesion in the left anterior descending artery (LAD) is described by the worst lesion site and adjacent reference sites (*upper row of images*). The plaque burden in the angiographically mildly diseased left circumflex artery (LCx) is assessed by the evaluation of multiple adjacent cross sections.

In the typical trial design, patients undergoing angiography and percutaneous coronary intervention (PCI) for clinical indications are enrolled, and IVUS is performed in the nonculprit vessel (Fig. 11.2). An arterial segment of at least 30-mm length, without significant stenosis, is selected for evaluation. Identifiable geographic landmarks such as arterial side branches are selected to define the proximal and distal fiduciary points of the segment of interest. Following administration of heparin and intracoronary nitroglycerin, a guidewire is subselectively placed in the target vessel. A motor drive progressively withdraws the transducer at a speed of 0.5 mm/sec, acquiring images throughout the length of the arterial segment. Calculation of total atheroma volume (TAV) within the segment of interest is performed by summation of the plaque areas from each image (*n*) using the equation:

$$\mathrm{TAV} = \sum_{n} (\mathrm{EEM_{area}} - \mathrm{Lumen_{area}})$$

In order to account for the variability in the length of the target arterial segment evaluated in different subjects, TAV is "normalized" to median number of images in the entire study population using the equation:

$$\mathrm{TAV_{Normalized}} = \frac{\sum (\mathrm{EEM_{area}} - \mathrm{Lumen_{area}})}{\text{Number of images in pullback}} \times \text{Median number of images in cohort}$$

Alternatively, calculation of percent atheroma volume (PAV) takes into account plaque dimensions as a proportion of the EEM:

$$\mathrm{PAV} = \frac{\sum (\mathrm{EEM_{area}} - \mathrm{Lumen_{area}})}{\sum (\mathrm{EEM_{area}})} \times 100$$

It has become apparent that PAV is the measure with the smallest coefficient of variability.

Secondary IVUS endpoints include atheroma volume within the 10-mm segments that contain the greatest and the least amount of plaque at baseline, mean maximal plaque thickness throughout the segment, and the percentage of cross sections with a maximal plaque thickness greater than 0.5 mm.

RESULTS OF VOLUMETRIC PROGRESSION/REGRESSION TRIALS

Multicenter, randomized trials collectively demonstrate either arrest of progression or actual regression during intensive lipid-modifying therapy with statin medications (Fig. 11.3). In a 12-month, open-label trial, plaque volume progression and changes in plaque echogenicity during lipid-lowering therapy were examined in 131 patients.[12] A total of 131 patients were randomized. After 12 months, mean LDL-C was reduced to 86 mg/dL in the atorvastatin group and to 140 mg/dL in the usual care group. Mean absolute plaque volume showed a nonsignificantly smaller increase in the atorvastatin group (atorvastatin $1.2 \pm 30.4\ \mathrm{mm}^3$, usual care $9.6 \pm 28.1\ \mathrm{mm}^3$; $p = 0.191$). The hyperechogenicity index (a marker of fibrous tissue) of the plaque increased to a larger extent for the atorvastatin group than for the usual care group ($p = 0.021$).

In the Reversal of Atherosclerosis with Aggressive Lipid Lowering (REVERSAL) trial, 502 patients were randomized to either a moderate lipid-lowering strategy (pravastatin 40 mg daily) or an intensive lipid-lowering strategy (atorvastatin 80 mg daily) for 18 months.[3] Treatment resulted in reduction of LDL-C to 79 mg/dL with atorvastatin and 110 mg/dL with pravastatin. While atheroma volume increased by 2.7% in pravastatin-treated patients ($p < 0.001$ compared with baseline), there was no significant change as compared with baseline in atorvastatin-treated patients (−0.4%; p = NS compared with baseline). In addition to the lipid-lowering effect, C-reactive protein (CRP) was lowered 36.4% by atorvastatin and 5.2% by pravastatin and changes in CRP correlated with the rate of plaque progression and remodeling,[11,13] suggesting a central role of inflammation in plaque progression and remodeling.

The ESTABLISH trial investigated the effect of early statin treatment on plaque volume in 70 patients with acute coronary syndrome (ACS).[14] All patients underwent emergent PCI,

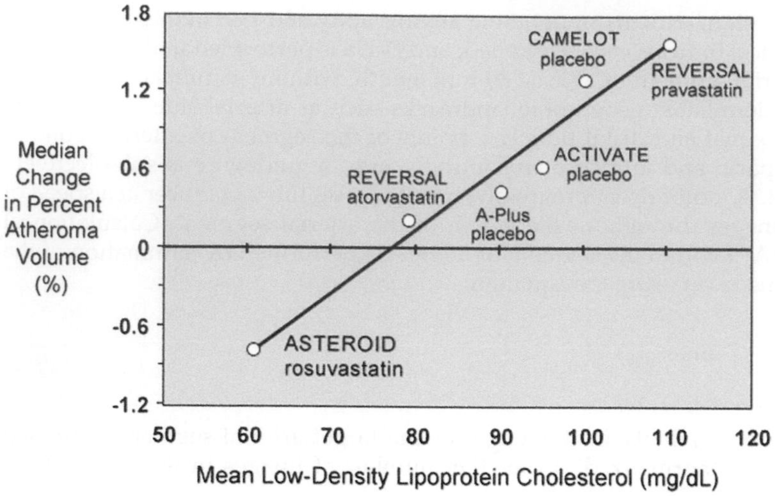

Figure 11.3 This figure shows the close correlation between mean LDL-cholesterol levels and median change in percent atheroma volume for several intravascular ultrasound trials. *Source*: Adapted form Ref. 15.

and were subsequently randomized to atorvastatin 20 mg/day or standard therapy. IVUS of nonculprit vessels was repeated after 6 months in 48 patients. LDL-C level was significantly decreased by 41.7% in the atorvastatin group compared with the control group, in which LDL-C was increased by 0.7% ($p < 0.0001$). Plaque volume was significantly decreased in the atorvastatin group ($-13.1 \pm 12.8\%$) compared with the control group ($8.7 \pm 14.9\%$; $p < 0.0001$). The percentage change in plaque volume showed a significant positive correlation with follow-up LDL-C level ($r = 0.456$, $p = 0.0011$) and percent LDL-C reduction ($r = 0.612$, $p < 0.0001$), even in patients with baseline LDL-C <125 mg/dL.

In the ASTEROID (A Study to Evaluate the Effect of Rosuvastatin On Intravascular Ultrasound–Derived Coronary Atheroma Burden) trial 507 patients had a baseline IVUS examination and received intensive statin therapy with rosuvastatin, 40 mg/day.[15] Three hundred and forty-nine patients had evaluable serial IVUS examinations after 24 months. The mean (SD) LDL-C level declined to 60.8 (20.0) mg/dL, a mean reduction of 53.2% ($p < 0.001$). Mean (SD) HDL-C level increased to 49.0 (12.6) mg/dL, an increase of 14.7% ($p < 0.001$). The mean (SD) change in PAV for the entire vessel was −0.98% (3.15%), with a median of −0.79% (97.5% CI, −1.21% to −0.53%) ($p < 0.001$ vs. baseline), consistent with regression. The results were similar for the other primary and secondary endpoint, change in nominal atheroma volume in the 10-mm subsegment with the greatest disease severity at baseline and change in normalized TAV for the entire artery, respectively.

The independent role of HDL has been further evaluated in other studies. In a small proof-of-concept study, 47 patients were randomized within 2 weeks of an ACS to receive 5 weekly infusions of either saline or reconstituted HDL particles in the form of recombinant apoA-I Milano phospholipid (ETC-216), at a dose of 15 mg/kg or 45 mg/kg.[16] Serial IVUS evaluations performed at baseline and within 2 weeks of the final infusion revealed a 4.2% reduction in atheroma volume in patients who received ETC-216. The most pronounced regression was observed in the 10-mm subsegments that contained the greatest amount of plaque at baseline.

More recently, a placebo-controlled trial examined the effect of intravenous reconstituted HDL (CSL-111) infusions.[17] One hundred and eighty-three patients had a baseline IVUS examination, and were randomly assigned to receive 4 weekly infusions of placebo (saline, $n = 60$), 40 mg/kg of reconstituted HDL (CSL-111, $n = 111$); and 80 mg/kg of CSL-111 ($n = 12$). Administration of CSL-111 40 mg/kg was associated with mild, self-limiting transaminase elevation but was clinically well tolerated. The higher-dosage CSL-111 treatment group was discontinued early because of liver-function test abnormalities. One hundred and forty-five patients had evaluable serial IVUS examinations 2 to 3 weeks after the last study infusion (after a total of 6 weeks). The percentage change in atheroma volume was −3.4% with CSL-111 and −1.6% for placebo ($p = 0.48$ between groups; $p < 0.001$ vs. baseline for CSL-111). The mean change in plaque characterization index on IVUS was significantly different between groups. Recent data from statin intervention trials demonstrate an independent relationship between change in HDL and plaque burden. In summary, HDL remains an attractive target for pharmacological intervention.[18]

Other lipid-modifying treatments with potential shown in animal and preclinical studies, including inhibition of acyl-coenzyme A:cholesterol acyltransferase (ACAT) and cholesteryl ester transfer protein (CETP) did not demonstrate benefit in clinical IVUS trials. ACAT esterifies cholesterol in a variety of tissues, and ACAT inhibition may prevent excess accumulation of cholesteryl esters in macrophages. The ACAT inhibitor avasimibe has been shown to reduce experimental atherosclerosis. In the Avasimibe and Progression of Lesions on UltraSound (A-PLUS) trial, the effects of avasimibe on human coronary atherosclerosis were investigated.[5] Six hundred and thirty-nine patients were randomized and received background lipid-lowering therapy, if necessary, to reach a target baseline LDL level <125 mg/dL. LDL cholesterol increased during the study by 1.7% with placebo, but increased by 7.8%, 9.1%, and 10.9% in the 50-, 250-, and 750-mg avasimibe groups ($p < 0.05$ in all groups). IVUS was performed at baseline and repeated after up to 24 months of treatment. The least-squares mean change at the end of treatment was 0.7 mm^3 for placebo and 7.7, 4.1, and 4.8 mm^3 for the different avasimibe groups, respectively ($p =$ NS). PAV increased by 0.4% with placebo and by 0.7%, 0.8%, and 1.0% in the respective avasimibe groups ($p =$ NS).

In the ACTIVATE (ACAT Intravascular Atherosclerosis Treatment Evaluation) study, 408 patients with angiographically documented coronary disease were randomized to receive the ACAT inhibitor pactimibe (100 mg/day) or placebo.[6] All patients received usual care for secondary prevention, including statins, if indicated. IVUS was performed at baseline and after 18 months. The change in PAV was similar in the pactimibe and placebo groups (0.69% and 0.59%, respectively; $p = 0.77$). However, secondary efficacy variables showed potentially unfavorable effects of pactimibe treatment. As compared with baseline values, the normalized TAV showed significant regression in the placebo group (-5.6 mm^3, $p = 0.001$) but not in the pactimibe group (-1.3 mm^3, $p = 0.39$; $p = 0.03$ for the comparison between groups). Similar results were found for the atheroma volume in the most diseased 10-mm subsegment. These results have cast doubt on the use of ACAT inhibitors as an effective strategy for atherosclerosis prevention.

In clinical studies, CETP inhibition has demonstrated to elevate HDL and lower LDL levels, resulting in a beneficial impact in animal models of atherosclerosis. The ILLUSTRATE (Investigation of Lipid Level management using Coronary Ultrasound To assess Reduction of Atherosclerosis by CETP Inhibition and HDL Elevation) trial tested the efficacy of CETP inhibition on the background of effective LDL lowering with atorvastatin.[7] A total of 1188 patients with coronary disease underwent intravascular ultrasonography. After treatment with atorvastatin to reduce levels of LDL-C to less than 100 mg/dL, patients were randomly assigned to receive either atorvastatin monotherapy or atorvastatin and 60 mg of torcetrapib daily. As compared with atorvastatin monotherapy, the effect of torcetrapib–atorvastatin therapy was an approximate 61% relative increase in HDL-C and a 20% relative decrease in LDL-C, reaching LDL-C-to-HDL-C ratio less than 1.0. However, torcetrapib was also associated with an increase in systolic blood pressure of 4.6 mm Hg. After 24 months, repeated intravascular ultrasonography was performed in 910 patients. The PAV increased by 0.19% in the atorvastatin-only group and by 0.12% in the torcetrapib–atorvastatin group ($p = 0.72$). A secondary measure, the change in normalized atheroma volume, showed a small favorable effect for torcetrapib ($p = 0.02$), but there was no significant difference in the change in atheroma volume for the most diseased vessel segment. The lack of effect on plaque burden, despite dramatic changes on lipid parameters, is concerning and data from clinical endpoint trials suggest potential increased clinical events. However, it is unclear if these findings are a class effect or molecule-specific adverse effects.

Extending beyond the management of lipid risk factors, the role of imaging endpoints has been demonstrated in the Comparison of Amlodipine versus Enalapril to Limit Occurrences of Thrombosis (CAMELOT) trial. The study randomized 1991 patients with coronary artery disease and a diastolic blood pressure less than 100 mm Hg to receive either amlodipine 10 mg daily, enalapril 20 mg daily, or placebo for 24 months.[19] A reduction of major adverse cardiac events was found in the amlodipine treatment group. A subgroup of 274 patients underwent serial IVUS evaluations. This group showed a trend toward less progression of atherosclerosis in the amlodipine group versus placebo ($p = 0.12$), with significantly less progression in the subgroup

Table 11.1 Selected progression and regression studies

Reference	Number of randomized patient	Duration of study	Medication	Results	Comments
Serial cross-sectional studies					
(24)	36	36 mo	Pravastatin	Less progression	
(25)	60	18 mo		Correlation between LDL, HDL, and plaque burden	Left main
(26)	40	12 mo	Simvastatin	Regression	
(27)	634		Everolimus	Less progression of intimal thickness	Transplant vasculopathy IVUS correlates with clinical outcome
Serial volumetric studies; multicenter trials					
(12)	131	12 mo	Atorvastatin	Trend in plaque volume, decreased echogenicity	Open-label
REVERSAL (3)	502	18 mo	Atorvastatin	Arrest of progression	
ESTABLISH (14)	70	6 mo	Atorvastatin	Regression	ACS
ASTEROID (15)	507	24 mo	Rosuvastatin	Regression	No control group
A-I MILANO (16)	47	5 wk	i.v. Recombinant apoA-I Milano	Regression baseline versus follow-up	Post-ACS
ERASE (17)	183	6 wk	Reconstituted HDL	Regression baseline versus follow-up, but no difference to control	
A-PLUS (5)	639	24 mo	ACAT inhibitor avasimibe	No changes	
ACTIVATE (6)	408	18 mo	ACAT inhibitor pactimibe	Worse than control in secondary endpoints	
ILLUSTRATE (7)	1188	24 mo	CETP inhibitor torcetrapib	No benefit	
CAMELOT (19)	274	24 mo	Amlodipine	Arrest of progression	Subgroup of larger clinical trial
Retrospective analysis of multicenter trials					
(21)	1515	18–24 mo	Use of β-blocker	Benefit of β-blocker	Pooled data from 4 studies
Remodeling studies					
REVERSAL (11)	210	18 mo	Atorvastatin	Constrictive remodeling with regression	Sub-study of randomized trial
(28)	39	12 mo	Simvastatin	Constrictive remodeling with regression	Single center
Ongoing studies					
PERISCOPE (29)			Pioglitazone		ClinicalTrials.gov Identifier: NCT00225277
STRADIVARIUS (30)			Rimonabant		ClinicalTrials.gov Identifier: NCT00124332

with systolic blood pressures greater than the mean ($p = 0.02$). Compared with baseline, IVUS showed progression in the placebo group ($p < 0.001$), a trend toward progression in the enalapril group ($p = 0.08$), but no progression in the amlodipine group ($p = 0.31$).

In further analysis of the IVUS subgroup, Sipahi et al. examined the effects of normal blood pressure, prehypertension, and hypertension on progression of coronary atherosclerosis.[20] In multivariable analysis, significant determinants of progression included systolic blood pressures ($r = 0.16$; $p = 0.006$) and pulse pressure ($r = 0.14$; $p = 0.02$). Patients with "hypertensive" average blood pressures had a 12.0 ± 3.6 mm^3 increase in atheroma volume, those with "pre-hypertensive" blood pressures had no major change (0.9 ± 1.8 mm^3), and those with "normal" blood pressures had a decrease of 4.6 ± 2.6 mm^3 ($p < 0.001$ by analysis of covariance; $p < 0.05$ for comparison of all pairs).

A pooled analysis of 1515 patients from four IVUS trials examined whether β-blocker therapy is associated with reduced atheroma progression in adults with known coronary artery disease.[21] The active treatment in the pooled trials included statin, calcium-channel blocker, angiotensin-converting enzyme inhibitor, and ACAT inhibitor. Changes in atheroma volume, as determined by IVUS after adjustment for possible confounders were compared in patients who did ($n = 1154$) and did not ($n = 361$) receive concomitant β-blocker treatment. The estimated annual change in atheroma volume was statistically significantly less in patients who received β-blockers. Atheroma volume statistically significantly decreased at follow-up IVUS in patients who received β-blockers ($p < 0.001$) and did not change in patients who did not receive β-blockers ($p = 0.86$). This analysis suggests that β-blockers have antiatherosclerotic effects in patient with established coronary disease.

Ongoing IVUS studies evaluate the effect of the PPAR-agonist, pioglitazone, in patients with diabetes mellitus and of the endocannibanoid receptor antagonist rimonabant on plaque progression in patients with obesity and coronary artery disease (Table 11.1).

SUMMARY AND FUTURE DIRECTIONS

The development of IVUS has extended our understanding of the natural history of atherosclerosis including progression, remodeling, and vulnerability. Atherosclerosis imaging has the potential to apply these findings into clinical endpoints. The ability to evaluate the same arterial segment at different time points provides a unique opportunity to define the impact of a wide range of antiatherosclerotic strategies on the progression of atherosclerotic plaque. Demonstrating a beneficial or detrimental impact of experimental agents on plaque progression rates has become a powerful tool in the development of new pharmacological compounds. However, proof with an intermediated endpoint has to be followed eventually by large-scale clinical event trials, in particular, as the correlation between IVUS and clinical endpoints is incompletely known.[22]

Future developments will include the development of imaging endpoints assessing morphologic characteristics of vulnerability, for example, with virtual histology,[23] and noninvasive atherosclerosis imaging.[1]

REFERENCES

1. Sankatsing RR, de Groot E, Jukema JW, et al. Surrogate markers for atherosclerotic disease. Curr Opin Lipidol 2005; 16:434–441.
2. Taylor AJ, Kent SM, Flaherty PJ, et al. ARBITER: Arterial biology for the investigation of the treatment effects of reducing cholesterol: A randomized trial comparing the effects of atorvastatin and pravastatin on carotid intima medial thickness. Circulation 2002; 106:2055–2060.
3. Nissen SE, Tuzcu EM, Schoenhagen P, et al. REVERSAL investigators. Effect of intensive compared with moderate lipid-lowering therapy on progression of coronary atherosclerosis: A randomized controlled trial. JAMA 2004; 291:1071–1080.
4. Cannon CP, Braunwald E, McCabe CH, et al. Pravastatin or Atorvastatin Evaluation and Infection Therapy-Thrombolysis in Myocardial Infarction 22 Investigators. Intensive versus moderate lipid lowering with statins after acute coronary syndromes. N Engl J Med 2004; 350:1495–1504.
5. Tardif JC, Gregoire J, L'Allier PL, et al. Avasimibe and Progression of Lesions on UltraSound (A-PLUS) Investigators. Effects of the acyl coenzyme A:cholesterol acyltransferase inhibitor avasimibe on human atherosclerotic lesions. Circulation 2004; 110:3372–3377.
6. Nissen SE, Tuzcu EM, Brewer HB, et al. ACAT Intravascular Atherosclerosis Treatment Evaluation (ACTIVATE) Investigators. Effect of ACAT inhibition on the progression of coronary atherosclerosis. N Engl J Med 2006; 354:1253–1263.

7. Nissen SE, Tardif JC, Nicholls SJ, et al. ILLUSTRATE Investigators. Effect of torcetrapib on the progression of coronary atherosclerosis. N Engl J Med 2007; 356:1304–1316.
8. Mintz GS, Nissen SE, Anderson WD, et al. American college of cardiology clinical expert consensus document on standards for acquisition, measurement and reporting of intravascular ultrasound studies (IVUS). A report of the American College of Cardiology task force on clinical expert consensus documents. J Am Coll Cardiol 2001; 37:1478–1492.
9. Glagov S, Weisenberg E, Zarins CK, et al. Compensatory enlargement of human atherosclerotic coronary arteries. N Engl J Med 1987; 316: 1353–1371.
10. Pasterkamp G, Schoneveld AH, van der Wal AC, et al. Relation of arterial geometry to luminal narrowing and histologic markers for plaque vulnerability: The remodeling paradox. J Am Coll Cardiol 1998; 32:655–662.
11. Schoenhagen P, Tuzcu EM, Apperson-Hansen C, et al. Determinants of arterial wall remodeling during lipid-lowering therapy: Serial intravascular ultrasound observations from the Reversal of Atherosclerosis with Aggressive Lipid Lowering Therapy (REVERSAL) trial. Circulation 2006; 113:2826–2834.
12. Schartl M, Bocksch W, Koschyk DH, et al. Use of intravascular ultrasound to compare effects of different strategies of lipid-lowering therapy on plaque volume and composition in patients with coronary artery disease. Circulation 2001; 104:387–392.
13. Nissen SE, Tuzcu EM, Schoenhagen P, et al. Reversal of atherosclerosis with aggressive lipid lowering (REVERSAL) Investigators. Statin therapy, LDL cholesterol, C-reactive protein, and coronary artery disease. N Engl J Med 2005; 352:29–38.
14. Okazaki S, Yokoyama T, Miyauchi K, et al. Early statin treatment in patients with acute coronary syndrome: Demonstration of the beneficial effect on atherosclerotic lesions by serial volumetric intravascular ultrasound analysis during half a year after coronary event: The ESTABLISH study. Circulation 2004; 110:1061–1068.
15. Nissen SE, Nicholls SJ, Sipahi I, et al. ASTEROID Investigators effect of very high-intensity statin therapy on regression of coronary atherosclerosis: The ASTEROID trial. JAMA 2006; 295:1556–1565.
16. Nissen SE, Tsunoda T, Tuzcu EM, et al. Effect of recombinant ApoA-I Milano on coronary atherosclerosis in patients with acute coronary syndromes: A randomized controlled trial. JAMA 2003; 290:2292–2300.
17. Tardif JC, Gregoire J, L'Allier PL, et al. Effect of rHDL on Atherosclerosis-Safety and Efficacy (ERASE) Investigators. Effects of reconstituted high-density lipoprotein infusions on coronary atherosclerosis: A randomized controlled trial. JAMA 2007; 297:1675–1682.
18. Nicholls SJ, Tuzcu EM, Sipahi I, et al. Statins, high-density lipoprotein cholesterol, and regression of coronary atherosclerosis. JAMA 2007; 297:499–508.
19. Nissen SE, Tuzcu EM, Libby P, et al. CAMELOT Investigators. Effect of antihypertensive agents on cardiovascular events in patients with coronary disease and normal blood pressure: The CAMELOT study: A randomized controlled trial. JAMA 2004; 292:2217–2225.
20. Sipahi I, Tuzcu EM, Schoenhagen P, et al. Effects of normal, pre-hypertensive, and hypertensive blood pressure levels on progression of coronary atherosclerosis. J Am Coll Cardiol 2006; 48:833–838.
21. Sipahi I, Tuzcu EM, Wolski KE, et al. Beta-blockers and progression of coronary atherosclerosis: Pooled analysis of 4 intravascular ultrasonography trials. Ann Intern Med 2007; 147:10–18.
22. Berry C, L'Allier PL, Gregoire J, et al. Comparison of intravascular ultrasound and quantitative coronary angiography for the assessment of coronary artery disease progression. Circulation 2007; 115:1851–1857.
23. Nair A, Kuban BD, Tuzcu EM, et al. Coronary plaque classification with intravascular ultrasound radiofrequency data analysis. Circulation 2002; 106:2200–2206.
24. Takagi T, Yoshida K, Akasaka T, et al. Intravascular ultrasound analysis of reduction in progression of coronary narrowing by treatment with pravastatin. Am J Cardiol 1997; 79(12):1673–1676.
25. von Birgelen C, Hartmann M, Mintz GS, et al. Relation between progression and regression of atherosclerotic left main coronary artery disease and serum cholesterol levels as assessed with serial long-term (> or = 12 months) follow-up intravascular ultrasound. Circulation 2003; 108(22):2757–2762.
26. Jensen LO, Thayssen P, Pedersen KE, et al. Regression of coronary atherosclerosis by simvastatin: A serial intravascular ultrasound study. Circulation 2004; 110(3):265–270.
27. Eisen HJ, Tuzcu EM, Dorent R, et al. RAD B253 Study Group. Everolimus for the prevention of allograft rejection and vasculopathy in cardiac-transplant recipients. N Engl J Med 2003; 349(9):847–858.
28. Jensen LO, Thayssen P, Mintz GS, et al. Effect of simvastatin on coronary lesion site remodeling: A serial intravascular ultrasound study. Cardiology 2006; 106(4):256–263.
29. Nissen SE, Nicholls SJ, Wolski K, et al. JAMA 2008; 299(13):1561–1573.
30. Nissen SE, Nicholls SJ, Wolski K, et al. JAMA 2008; 299(13):1547–1560.

12 IVUS and IVUS-derived methods for vulnerable plaque assessment

Ryan K. Kaple, Akiko Maehara, and Gary S. Mintz

INTRODUCTION

Cardiovascular disease resulting in myocardial infarction and stroke is the leading cause of mortality worldwide.[1] These events are the consequence of atherosclerotic plaque rupture or erosion complicated by thrombosis.[2] When the fibrous cap of a thin-cap fibroatheroma is disrupted, its core of thrombogenic material (necrotic tissue, macrophages, and lipids) is exposed to the luminal blood resulting in platelet aggregation and thrombus formation. Thrombosis also occurs without plaque rupture through plaque erosion, a process characterized by proliferation of smooth muscle cells in a proteogylcan matrix and less inflammation.[3,4] These events result in either acute coronary syndrome (ACS; that can be fatal) or healing and plaque progression.[5,6]

Angiography underestimates plaque burden because of vessel remodeling, an increase in arterial dimensions that compensates for and "hides" the accumulating atherosclerotic burden. Studies have shown that events leading to nonfatal ACS events most often occur at sites of moderate, nonlumen compromising disease that is angiographically silent.[7–9] These and other shortcomings of angiography led to the development of intravascular ultrasound (IVUS) followed by several second-generation intravascular imaging techniques. This chapter will review the utility of these catheter-based imaging modalities in detecting vulnerable—rupture or thrombosis-prone—plaques in coronary arteries.

GRAYSCALE IVUS

Grayscale IVUS images are derived from the amplitude of the reflected ultrasound signal; black is assigned to a low-amplitude reflection, while white is assigned to the highest amplitude reflection. The quality of an IVUS image is determined, in part, by the number of in-between shades of gray. IVUS provides real-time, in vivo, cross-sectional images allowing measurement of the arterial wall [external elastic membrane (EEM)] cross-sectional area (CSA) and lumen CSA. Atherosclerotic plaque burden and coronary artery remodeling can be calculated from these measurements.

The usefulness of grayscale IVUS has been proven through decades of validation and clinical investigation. Important grayscale IVUS uses in ACS patients include detecting or measuring plaque rupture, plaque burden, positive remodeling, and thrombus formation. Plaque ruptures are detectable at culprit lesions in approximately 50% of ACS patients, but often occur upstream or downstream from the vessel cross section with the minimum lumen area (MLA).[10,11] Secondary plaque ruptures (at sites other than the culprit lesion) have also been reported, but the exact frequency is in doubt.[12] Hong et al. reported the location of plaque ruptures in patients with ACS and stable angina.[13] One prospective grayscale IVUS study showed that the baseline characteristics of lesions that later caused acute events included more eccentric plaque, a greater plaque burden, more echolucent plaque, but no significant difference in lumen area when compared to lesions not causing acute events.[14] IVUS can detect positive vessel remodeling, a phenomenon that is more common in patients with ACS events than those with stable angina and more common at the cross-section containing plaque rupture than at the cross-section containing the MLA.[10,15–20]

However, most grayscale IVUS data on vulnerable plaque are retrospective. Traditional grayscale IVUS cannot reliably predict rupture-prone plaque. First, grayscale echolucent plaque correlates with lipid-rich material on histology in only 65% of cases.[14,21] Second, IVUS cannot detect the thin-cap overlying a rupture-prone fibroatheroma whose thickness of 65 μm is below the axial resolution of IVUS (100–150 μm).[2]

Second-generation IVUS technology has now been developed to overcome some of the shortcomings of grayscale IVUS. Virtual histology (VH) IVUS and integrated backscatter (IB)

IVUS attempt to provide real-time in vivo tissue characterization of plaque. Palpography, thermography, and vasa vasorum imaging provide "functional" data about plaque stability. However, these modalities that are based on traditional IVUS are still limited by the inherent axial resolution of IVUS of 100 to 150 μm and, potentially, the inability to image through calcium. Furthermore, clinical data on these techniques are still limited.

VIRTUAL HISTOLOGY (VH)

Radio frequency (RF) spectral analysis was designed to improve on the limitations of grayscale IVUS by providing accurate plaque characterization. This has been validated by Nair et al. who compared histology sections to the corresponding IVUS data of explanted coronary arteries.[22] Data derived from the amplitude, power, frequency, and phase of the normalized backscatter signal, allowing differentiation among tissues that have similar amplitude signals: fibrous (FI), fibrofatty (FF), dense calcium (DC), or necrotic core (NC) (Fig. 12.1B). Each tissue type is assigned a color (dark green, light green, white, and red, respectively). The most recent predictive accuracies for FI, FF, DC, and NC are 93.5%, 94.1%, 96.7%, and 96.7%, respectively, with a sensitivity and specificity ranging from 72% to 99%.[23] Thin-capped fibroatheromas (TCFAs) on VH are defined as lesions with >10% confluent necrotic core in contact with the lumen (Fig. 12.2).[24] This definition takes into consideration that the axial resolution of IVUS (150–200 μm) cannot detect thin-fibrous caps (65 μm); therefore, a necrotic core in contact with the lumen is indirect evidence of a thin fibrous cap.[2]

Current data

To date, the most consistent and convincing data on VH-IVUS are the following:

(1) VH-IVUS findings are in keeping with pathologic studies of lesion composition and morphometry. The amount of necrotic core found by VH-IVUS has been shown to be similar to that of previously reported histopathologic data (55.9% vs. 59.6% for ACS and 19% vs. 23% for stable angina).[25] VH-IVUS TCFAs are more prevalent in patients presenting with ACS than stable angina, and are most often found in the proximal sections of the vessel.[26,27] The site of plaque rupture has been shown to have a larger necrotic core than the MLA site.[28]
(2) Prior to intervention, VH-IVUS TCFAs seem to occur in the distribution of acute occlusions in patients with myocardial infarctions reported by Wang et al. and in the distribution of plaque ruptures reported by Hong et al. and are associated with positive remodeling seen in biologically active lesions.[26,29] Remodeling index has been shown to be positively correlated with the NC ($r = 0.83$, $p < 0.0001$) and inversely with FI tissue ($r = -0.45$, $p = 0.003$).[30] Positively remodeled lesions also demonstrate a more unstable profile (defined as the presence of a fibroatheroma) as compared to negatively remodeled lesions.[30]
(3) The largest NC—presumably, the most active part of the plaque—is usually not at the site of the MLA and may not be covered when stenting the most severe part of the lesion.[31]
(4) Putative distal embolization during percutaneous coronary interventional (PCI) procedures—as measured by HITS, troponin elevation, CK-MB elevation, etc.—correlate with the size of the lesion's pre-PCI NC.[32,33]

Nevertheless, it is a significant step from these important and consistent observations to using VH-IVUS as a decision-making tool in an individual patient. It is anticipated that the results of ongoing prospective studies with long-term follow-up—especially, PROSPECT (Providing Regional Observations to Study Predictors of Events in the Coronary Tree, NCT00180466) and SPECIAL (Study of Prospective Events in Coronary Intermediate Atherosclerotic Lesions, Japan)—will provide this information.

There are several limitations of VH-IVUS. All material between the lumen and EEM contour must be classified as NC, DC, FI, or FF plaque—there is no algorithm for blood or thrombus. Thrombus seen on histopathologic sections of atherectomy samples is most often classified as FI or FF on VH-IVUS depending on its age.[34] Acoustic shadowing may cause inaccuracies in plaque characterization and qualitative lesion assessment (Fig. 12.1A). Stent metal appears as white, simulating DC, accompanied by a red artifact that could be confused as an NC.

INTEGRATED BACKSCATTER IVUS

Tissue characterization by IB-IVUS uses fast Fourier transformation to extract power data from the raw IVUS signal and classify plaque into five categories: fibrous tissue, intimal hyperplasia or lipid core, calcification, thrombus, and mixed lesions (Fig. 12.1C).[35] Both IB-IVUS and VH-IVUS utilize postprocessing of IVUS power and frequency data, but use different formulas to quantitate the tissue signals. However, there is little head-to-head data comparing the two techniques.

Current data

In vivo, validation of IB-IVUS was performed by imaging explanted coronary arteries and comparing images to angioscopy and histology.[36] This study showed a significant difference between IB-IVUS signal for calcified tissue, mixed lesions, fibrous tissue, and thrombus ($p < 0.05$), but not between lipid core, intimal hyperplasia, and media. IB-IVUS has been shown to be superior to grayscale IVUS in identifying fibrous tissue and lipid pools (128 coronary artery autopsy cross sections in 42 arteries).[37] One specific limitation to this modality is that intimal hyperplasia and lipid core have similar IB-IVUS values, and differentiating between these types of tissues will require a more complex algorithm.

A recent IB-IVUS study reported the baseline and follow-up findings of 144 coronary lesions.[38] Lesions that went on to rupture (10 lesions) showed greater plaque burden, eccentricity, positive remodeling, and percentage of lipid, but less percentage of fibrous tissue. The sensitivity, specificity, and positive predictive value were 90%, 96%, and 69%, respectively, for lipid tissue and 80%, 90%, and 42%, respectively, for fibrous tissue.

PALPOGRAPHY

Palpography determines the strain on the fibrous cap overlying the plaque by analyzing the radio frequency of the reflected ultrasound signal at two pressures during the cardiac cycle (Fig. 12.1D).[39] It was originally hypothesized that measuring strain on the fibrous cap could be a surrogate measure for vulnerability.

Current data

A positive relationship has been shown between strain and the number of macrophages with an inverse relationship between strain and cap thickness and smooth muscle cell density.[40,41] Palpography has a high sensitivity (88%) and specificity (89%) for detecting lesions with a vulnerable profile on histology (thin fibrous cap, prominent macrophage content, and >40% necrotic core).[41] Highly compressible lipid-rich plaque (as compared to calcified/fibrous plaque) and shoulder regions of eccentric plaques have the highest strain.[42] High-strain lesions are more often seen in ACS than in stable angina patients and correlate with C-reactive protein levels.[43]

In a study comparing palpography and VH-IVUS, NC in contact with the lumen was an independent predictor of high strain after correcting for univariate predictors (odds ratio, 5.0; $p = 0.003$).[44] The sensitivity, specificity, positive predictive value, and negative predictive value of VH-IVUS to detect high strain on palpography was 75.0%, 44.4%, 56.3%, and 65.1%, respectively.

Palpography is limited by potential inaccuracies in strain estimates due to out of plane motion, catheter eccentricity, and tilt.[45]

THERMOGRAPHY

Activated acute inflammatory cells in atherosclerotic plaque increase the local temperature of the involved tissue primarily through the rapid metabolism of ATP by macrophages. It is known that this inflammatory process increases the likelihood of plaque rupture leading to the hypothesis that local increases in luminal temperature could help identify high-risk plaques.

Current data

Thermal heterogeneity of the vessel luminal surface, defined as having ≥ 1 measurement outside of a set background temperature range, was first identified in carotid specimens using a needle thermistor.[46] Temperature correlated directly with macrophage density and inversely correlated with smooth muscle cell density and the distance between macrophages and the lumen surface.

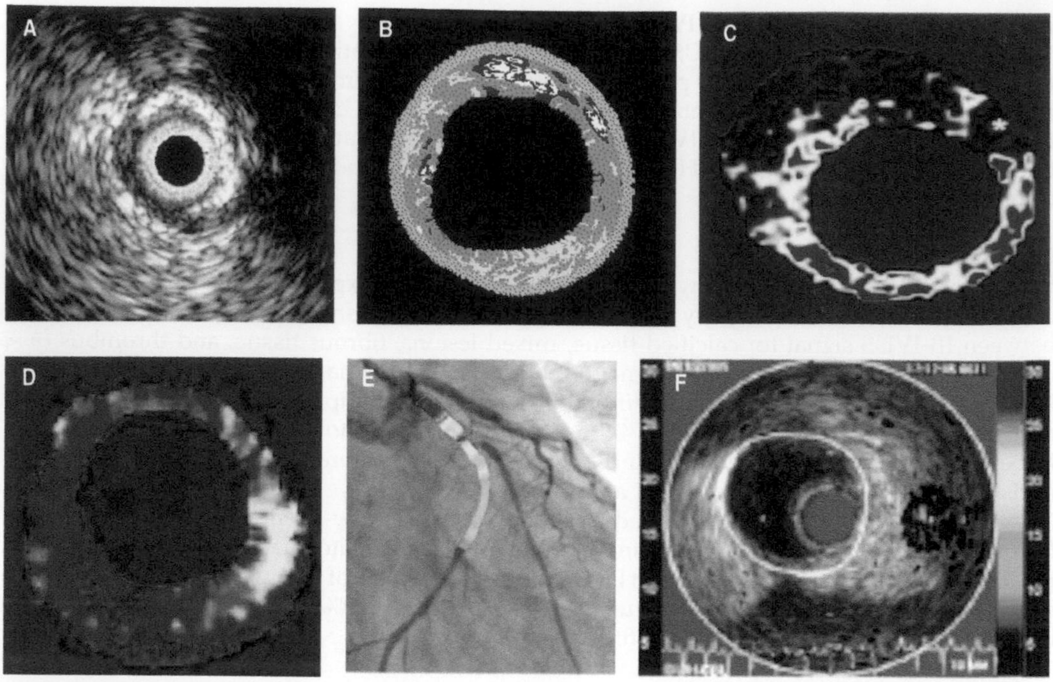

Figure 12.1 Examples of grayscale intravascular ultrasound (IVUS) and the IVUS-derived methods of vulnerable plaque detection, discussed in this chapter. (**A**) Grayscale IVUS image in cross section—this image shows an example of acoustic shadowing due to calcification. (**B**) Virtual histology IVUS—this image demonstrates a cross section that primarily comprises fibrous (*dark green*) and fibrofatty (*light green*) tissue, but contains a confluent necrotic core (*red*) with scant calcification (*white*). (**C**) Integrated backscatter IVUS—lipid material is represented in blue and fibrous material in red. *Source*: Adapted from Ref. 38. (**D**) Palpography—light colors represent high strain. *Source*: Adapted from Ref. 62. (**E**) Thermography—red and yellow represent higher temperature than the surroundings. *Source*: Adapted from Ref. 63. (**F**) Contrast vasa vasorum IVUS imaging—blue color in the area surrounding the coronary vessel represents flow in vasa vasorum. *Source*: Adapted from Ref. 60.

In vivo, studies have shown that the prevalence of temperature heterogeneity varies based on clinical presentation: 20% of stable angina, 40% of unstable angina, and 67% of ACS patients (Fig. 12.1E).[47] The greatest temperature difference between the lesion and reference segment was seen in ACS patients. One prospective study showed that temperature heterogeneity can be reversed by statin therapy.[48] Increased heterogeneity has been shown to be associated with vessel remodeling and unfavorable outcomes after PCI.[49,50]

Vasa vasorum imaging

Histopathologic studies have shown that culprit lesions in acute myocardial infarction patients have increased vasa vasorum density.[51,52] These vessels are thought to contribute to plaque instability by promoting inflammation and intraplaque hemorrhage and infiltrate.[53–55] In vivo imaging of vasa vasorum by IVUS is possible using microbubble injection (Fig. 12.1F, 12.3). There is also interest in quantization of vasa vasorum in order to provide a measure for prophylactic therapies directed at decreasing neovascularization.[56]

Current data

The feasibility of vasa vasorum imaging using microbubble contrast was first shown in atherosclerotic rabbit aortas[57] and porcine coronaries.[58] The only in vivo study to date was carried out in non–culprit lesions of 16 ACS patients.[59] A significant increase in contrast perfusion density was seen in the media/intima and adventitia ($p = 0.006$ and $p = 0.035$, respectively) after injection of microbubbles proximal to the lesions. Additional in vivo studies are necessary to understand the utility of this imaging modality.

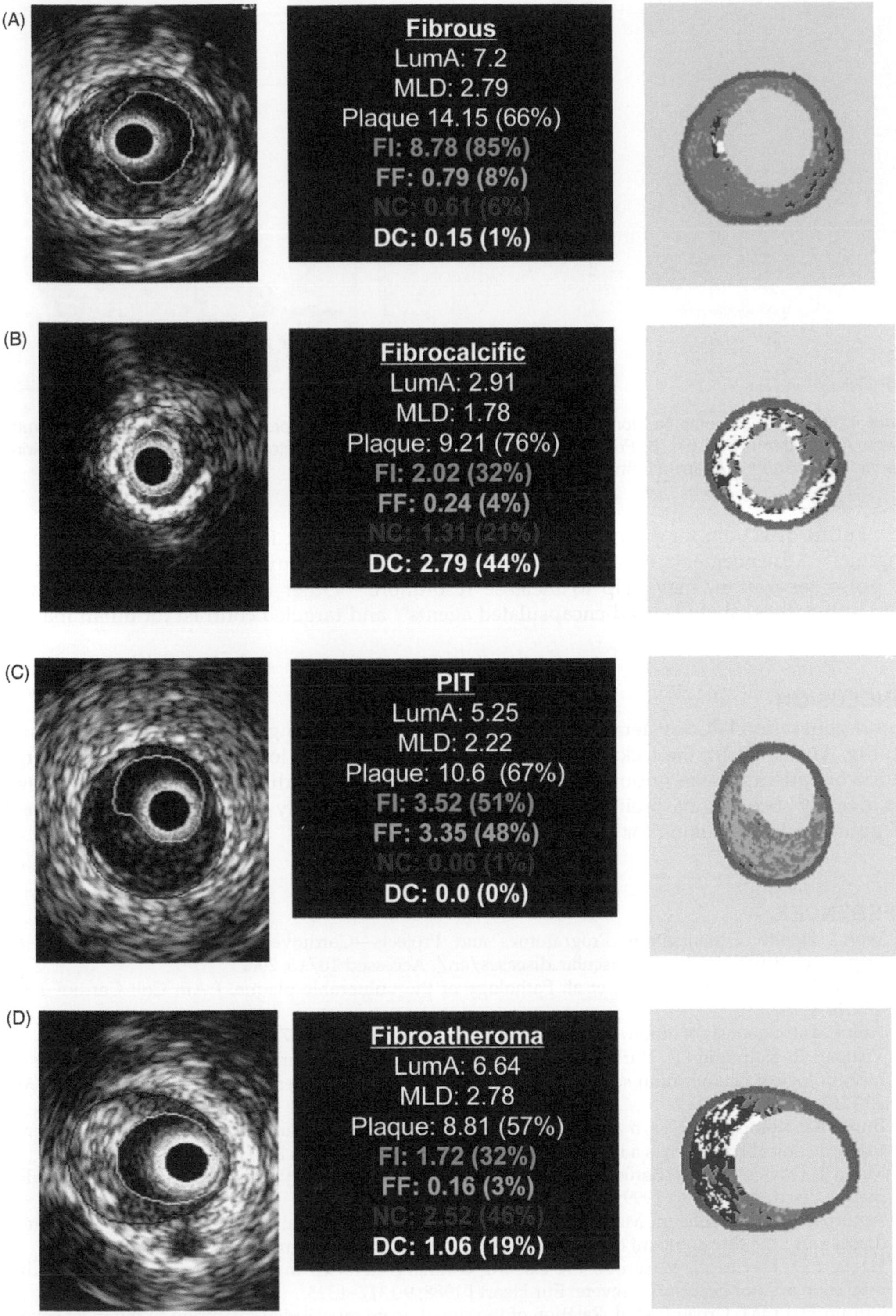

Figure 12.2 Grayscale and VH-IVUS cross-sectional images representing fibrous (**A**), fibrocalcific (**B**), pathological intimal thickening (PIT) (**C**), and fibroatheroma (**D**). Plaque component values are reported as "area (mm^2),% (of total plaque)", and plaque is reported as "area (mm^2),% (of vessel occupied by plaque)". *Abbreviation*: MLD, minimum lumen diameter.

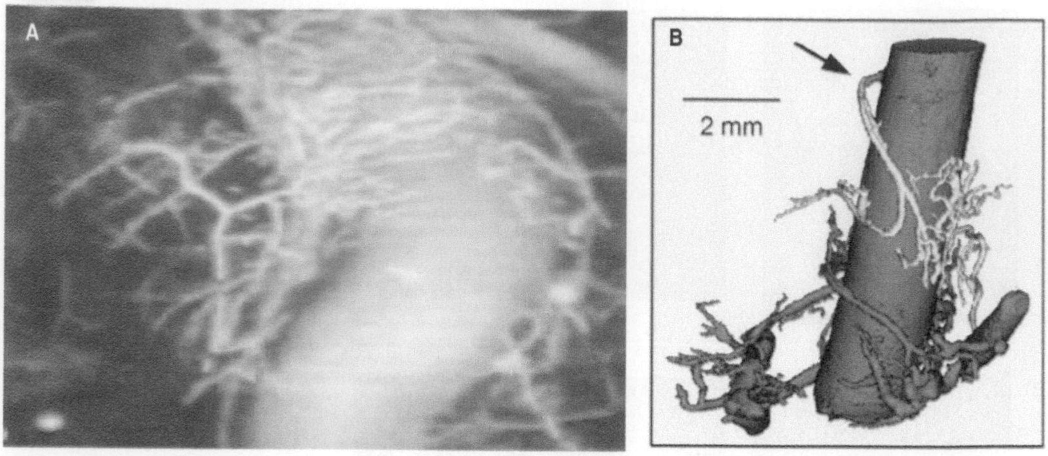

Figure 12.3 (**A**) Microcomputed tomography representation of a porcine coronary artery with vasa vasorum. *Source*: Adapted from Ref. 51. (**B**) Postmortem injection of silicone polymer into human coronary artery showing vasa vasorum. *Source*: Adapted from Ref. 64.

Future directions for this modality include contrast harmonic IVUS and three-dimensional imaging.[60] Advancements in signal acquisition, such as pulse-inversion extraction and spatial pulse separation, may help to increase resolution.[61] Other contrast materials are also being tested; these include lipid-encapsulated agents[61] and targeted contrast for inflammatory particles.

CONCLUSION

Second-generation IVUS systems have enhanced the understanding of plaque composition and stability. At this point, the lack of prospective clinical data with long-term follow-up in large cohorts of patients leaves important questions unanswered regarding the clinical utility. However, there is encouraging preliminary data regarding their ability to define patient prognosis and guide decision-making for the care of individual patients.

REFERENCES

1. World Health Organization. Programmes and Projects—Cardiovascular Disease. Available at: http://www.who.int/cardiovascular_diseases/en/. Accessed 10/15, 2007.
2. Virmani R, Burke AP, Farb A, et al. Pathology of the vulnerable plaque. J Am Coll Cardiol 2006; 47:C13–C18.
3. Falk E. Pathogenesis of atherosclerosis. J Am Coll Cardiol 2006; 47:C7–C12.
4. Virmani R, Kolodgie FD, Burke AP, et al. Lessons from sudden coronary death: A comprehensive morphological classification scheme for atherosclerotic lesions. Arterioscler Thromb Vasc Biol 2000; 20:1262–1275.
5. Burke AP, Kolodgie FD, Farb A, et al. Healed plaque ruptures and sudden coronary death: Evidence that subclinical rupture has a role in plaque progression. Circulation 2001; 103:934–940.
6. Mann J, Davies MJ. Mechanisms of progression in native coronary artery disease: Role of healed plaque disruption. Heart 1999; 82:265–268.
7. Ambrose JA, Tannenbaum MA, Alexopoulos D, et al. Angiographic progression of coronary artery disease and the development of myocardial infarction. J Am Coll Cardiol 1988; 12:56–62.
8. Hackett D, Davies G, Maseri A. Pre-existing coronary stenoses in patients with first myocardial infarction are not necessarily severe. Eur Heart J 1988; 9:1317–1323.
9. Giroud D, Li JM, Urban P, et al. Relation of the site of acute myocardial infarction to the most severe coronary arterial stenosis at prior angiography. Am J Cardiol 1992; 69:729–732.
10. Maehara A, Mintz GS, Bui AB, et al. Morphologic and angiographic features of coronary plaque rupture detected by intravascular ultrasound. J Am Coll Cardiol 2002; 40:904–910.
11. Tinana A, Mintz GS, Weissman NJ. Volumetric intravascular ultrasound quantification of the amount of atherosclerosis and calcium in nonstenotic arterial segments. Am J Cardiol 2002; 89:757–760.

12. Rioufol G, Finet G, Ginon I, et al. Multiple atherosclerotic plaque rupture in acute coronary syndrome: A three-vessel intravascular ultrasound study. Circulation 2002; 106:804–808.
13. Hong MK, Mintz GS, Lee CW, et al. The site of plaque rupture in native coronary arteries: A three-vessel intravascular ultrasound analysis. J Am Coll Cardiol 2005; 46:261–265.
14. Yamagishi M, Terashima M, Awano K, et al. Morphology of vulnerable coronary plaque: Insights from follow-up of patients examined by intravascular ultrasound before an acute coronary syndrome. J Am Coll Cardiol 2000; 35:106–111.
15. Schoenhagen P, Ziada KM, Kapadia SR, et al. Extent and direction of arterial remodeling in stable versus unstable coronary syndromes: An intravascular ultrasound study. Circulation 2000; 101: 598–603.
16. von Birgelen C, Klinkhart W, Mintz GS, et al. Plaque distribution and vascular remodeling of ruptured and nonruptured coronary plaques in the same vessel: An intravascular ultrasound study in vivo. J Am Coll Cardiol 2001; 37:1864–1870.
17. Nakamura M, Nishikawa H, Mukai S, et al. Impact of coronary artery remodeling on clinical presentation of coronary artery disease: An intravascular ultrasound study. J Am Coll Cardiol 2001; 37:63–69.
18. Schoenhagen P, Vince DG, Ziada KM, et al. Association of arterial expansion (expansive remodeling) of bifurcation lesions determined by intravascular ultrasonography with unstable clinical presentation. Am J Cardiol 2001; 88:785–787.
19. Gyongyosi M, Yang P, Hassan A, et al. Arterial remodelling of native human coronary arteries in patients with unstable angina pectoris: A prospective intravascular ultrasound study. Heart 1999; 82:68–74.
20. Smits PC, Pasterkamp G, de Jaegere PP, et al. Angioscopic complex lesions are predominantly compensatory enlarged: An angioscopy and intracoronary ultrasound study. Cardiovasc Res 1999; 41: 458–464.
21. Prati F, Arbustini E, Labellarte A, et al. Correlation between high frequency intravascular ultrasound and histomorphology in human coronary arteries. Heart 2001; 85:567–570.
22. Nair A, Kuban BD, Obuchowski N, et al. Assessing spectral algorithms to predict atherosclerotic plaque composition with normalized and raw intravascular ultrasound data. Ultrasound Med Biol 2001; 27:1319–1331.
23. Nair A, Margolis MP, Kuban BD, et al. Automated coronary plaque characterisation with intravascular ultrasound backscatter: Ex vivo validation. EuroIntervention 2007; 3:113–120.
24. Carlier SG, Mintz GS, Stone GW. Imaging of atherosclerotic plaque using radiofrequency ultrasound signal processing. J Nucl Cardiol 2006; 13:831–840.
25. Kolodgie FD, Virmani R, Burke AP, et al. Pathologic assessment of the vulnerable human coronary plaque. Heart 2004; 90:1385–1391.
26. Hong MK, Mintz GS, Lee CW, et al. Comparison of virtual histology to intravascular ultrasound of culprit coronary lesions in acute coronary syndrome and target coronary lesions in stable angina pectoris. Am J Cardiol 2007; 100:953–959.
27. Valgimigli M, Rodriguez-Granillo GA, Garcia-Garcia HM, et al. Distance from the ostium as an independent determinant of coronary plaque composition in vivo: An intravascular ultrasound study based radiofrequency data analysis in humans. Eur Heart J 2006; 27:655–663.
28. Rodriguez-Granillo GA, Garcia-Garcia HM, Valgimigli M, et al. Global characterization of coronary plaque rupture phenotype using three-vessel intravascular ultrasound radiofrequency data analysis. Eur Heart J 2006; 27:1921–1927.
29. Wang JC, Normand SL, Mauri L, et al. Coronary artery spatial distribution of acute myocardial infarction occlusions. Circulation 2004; 110:278–284.
30. Rodriguez-Granillo GA, Serruys PW, Garcia-Garcia HM, et al. Coronary artery remodeling is related to plaque composition. Heart 2006; 92:388–391.
31. Kaple RK, Carlier SG, Sano K, et al. The axial distribution of atherosclerotic plaque components: An in vivo volumetric intravascular ultrasound radiofrequency analysis of lumen stenosis, necrotic core, and vessel remodeling. Eur Heart J 2007; 28(Abstract Supplement):681.
32. Kawaguchi R, Oshima S, Jingu M, et al. Usefulness of virtual histology intravascular ultrasound to predict distal embolization for ST-segment elevation myocardial infarction. J Am Coll Cardiol 2007; 50:1641–1646.
33. Kawamoto T, Okura H, Koyama Y, et al. The relationship between coronary plaque characteristics and small embolic particles during coronary stent implantation. J Am Coll Cardiol 2007; 50: 1635–1640.
34. Nasu K, Tsuchikane E, Katoh O, et al. Impact of intramural thrombus on the accuracy of tissue characterization by virtual histology. Eur Heart J 2007; 28(Abstract Supplement): 675–676.

35. Kawasaki M, Takatsu H, Noda T, et al. Noninvasive quantitative tissue characterization and two-dimensional color-coded map of human atherosclerotic lesions using ultrasound integrated backscatter: Comparison between histology and integrated backscatter images. J Am Coll Cardiol 2001; 38: 486–492.
36. Kawasaki M, Takatsu H, Noda T, et al. In vivo quantitative tissue characterization of human coronary arterial plaques by use of integrated backscatter intravascular ultrasound and comparison with angioscopic findings. Circulation 2002; 105:2487–2492.
37. Kawasaki M, Bouma BE, Bressner J, et al. Diagnostic accuracy of optical coherence tomography and integrated backscatter intravascular ultrasound images for tissue characterization of human coronary plaques. J Am Coll Cardiol 2006; 48:81–88.
38. Sano K, Kawasaki M, Ishihara Y, et al. Assessment of vulnerable plaques causing acute coronary syndrome using integrated backscatter intravascular ultrasound. J Am Coll Cardiol 2006; 47:734–741.
39. de Korte CL, van der Steen AF, Cespedes EI, et al. Intravascular ultrasound elastography in human arteries: Initial experience in vitro. Ultrasound Med Biol 1998; 24:401–408.
40. Loree HM, Kamm RD, Stringfellow RG, et al. Effects of fibrous cap thickness on peak circumferential stress in model atherosclerotic vessels. Circ Res 1992; 71:850–858.
41. Schaar JA, De Korte CL, Mastik F, et al. Characterizing vulnerable plaque features with intravascular elastography. Circulation 2003; 108:2636–2641.
42. de Korte CL, Sierevogel MJ, Mastik F, et al. Identification of atherosclerotic plaque components with intravascular ultrasound elastography in vivo: A Yucatan pig study. Circulation 2002; 105:1627–1630.
43. Schaar JA, Regar E, Mastik F, et al. Incidence of high-strain patterns in human coronary arteries: Assessment with three-dimensional intravascular palpography and correlation with clinical presentation. Circulation 2004; 109:2716–2719.
44. Rodriguez-Granillo GA, Garcia-Garcia HM, Valgimigli M, et al. In vivo relationship between compositional and mechanical imaging of coronary arteries. Insights from intravascular ultrasound radiofrequency data analysis. Am Heart J 2006; 151:1025.e1021–e1026.
45. Konofagou E, Ophir J. A new elastographic method for estimation and imaging of lateral displacements, lateral strains, corrected axial strains and Poisson's ratios in tissues. Ultrasound Med Biol 1998; 24:1183–1199.
46. Casscells W, Hathorn B, David M, et al. Thermal detection of cellular infiltrates in living atherosclerotic plaques: Possible implications for plaque rupture and thrombosis. Lancet 1996; 347:1447–1451.
47. Stefanadis C, Diamantopoulos L, Vlachopoulos C, et al. Thermal heterogeneity within human atherosclerotic coronary arteries detected in vivo: A new method of detection by application of a special thermography catheter. Circulation 1999; 99:1965–1971.
48. Stefanadis C, Toutouzas K, Vavuranakis M, et al. Statin treatment is associated with reduced thermal heterogeneity in human atherosclerotic plaques. Eur Heart J 2002; 23:1664–1669.
49. Varnava AM, Mills PG, Davies MJ. Relationship between coronary artery remodeling and plaque vulnerability. Circulation 2002; 105:939–943.
50. Stefanadis C, Toutouzas K, Tsiamis E, et al. Increased local temperature in human coronary atherosclerotic plaques: An independent predictor of clinical outcome in patients undergoing a percutaneous coronary intervention. J Am Coll Cardiol 2001; 37:1277–1283.
51. Barger AC, Beeuwkes R III, Lainey LL, et al. Hypothesis: Vasa vasorum and neovascularization of human coronary arteries. A possible role in the pathophysiology of atherosclerosis. N Engl J Med 1984; 310:175–177.
52. Tenaglia AN, Peters KG, Sketch MH Jr, et al. Neovascularization in atherectomy specimens from patients with unstable angina: Implications for pathogenesis of unstable angina. Am Heart J 1998; 135:10–14.
53. Moulton KS, Vakili K, Zurakowski D, et al. Inhibition of plaque neovascularization reduces macrophage accumulation and progression of advanced atherosclerosis. Proc Natl Acad Sci USA 2003; 100:4736–4741.
54. Kolodgie FD, Gold HK, Burke AP, et al. Intraplaque hemorrhage and progression of coronary atheroma. N Engl J Med 2003; 349:2316–2325.
55. Milei J, Parodi JC, Alonso GF, et al. Carotid rupture and intraplaque hemorrhage: Immunophenotype and role of cells involved. Am Heart J 1998; 136:1096–1105.
56. Kolodgie FD, Narula J, Yuan C, et al. Elimination of neoangiogenesis for plaque stabilization: Is there a role for local drug therapy? J Am Coll Cardiol 2007; 49:2093–2101.
57. Goertz DE, Frijlink ME, Tempel D, et al. Contrast harmonic intravascular ultrasound: A feasibility study for vasa vasorum imaging. Invest Radiol 2006; 41:631–638.
58. Vavuranakis M, Papaioannou TG, Kakadiaris IA, et al. Detection of perivascular blood flow in vivo by contrast-enhanced intracoronary ultrasonography and image analysis: An animal study. Clin Exp Pharmacol Physiol 2007; 34:1319–1323.

59. Vavuranakis M, Kakadiaris IA, O'Malley SM, et al. A new method for assessment of plaque vulnerability based on vasa vasorum imaging, by using contrast-enhanced intravascular ultrasound and differential image analysis. Int J Cardiol 2008; 130(1):23–29.
60. Goertz DE, Frijlink ME, Tempel D, et al. Contrast harmonic intravascular ultrasound: A feasibility study for vasa vasorum imaging. Invest Radiol 2006; 41:631–638.
61. Goertz DE, Frijlink ME, de Jong N, et al. Nonlinear intravascular ultrasound contrast imaging. Ultrasound Med Biol 2006; 32:491–502.
62. Schaar JA, van der Steen AF, Mastik F, et al. Intravascular palpography for vulnerable plaque assessment. J Am Coll Cardiol 2006; 47:C86–C91.
63. Hamdan A, Assali A, Fuchs S, et al. Imaging of vulnerable coronary artery plaques. Catheter Cardiovasc Interv 2007; 70:65–74.
64. Ritman EL, Lerman A. The dynamic vasa vasorum. Cardiovasc Res 2007; 75:649–658.

13 Evaluation of acute and chronic microvascular coronary disease

Eulógio Martinez and Pedro A. Lemos

FUNCTIONAL ANATOMY OF THE CORONARY ARTERIAL SYSTEM

The coronary arterial system is divided into three functionally distinct main compartments. The first compartment comprises the large epicardial coronary arteries, which run onto the outer surface of the heart and have a diameter >500 μm. These vessels exert a capacitance function, with practically no resistance to blood flow.[1,2] An intermediate compartment comprises the prearterioles, which diameter ranges from approximately 100 to 500 μm. Measurements of intracoronary pressure indicate that vessels up to 100 μm are responsible for ~45% of total coronary vascular resistance.[3] As a result of their extramyocardial position and wall thickness, these vessels are not under direct vasomotor control by diffusible myocardial metabolites. The third, more distal, compartment is composed of the intramural arterioles (diameter <100 μm), which are responsible for most of the resistance to coronary flow. At the level of coronary arterioles, myocardial blood flow is finely regulated to match with the tissue oxygen consumption.[2]

Increase in blood flow induces vasodilatation of epicardial coronary vessels and proximal arterioles by endothelium-dependent mechanisms.[4] When aortic pressure increases, distal prearterioles undergo myogenic vasoconstriction that results in a constant pressure just proximal to the next compartment, the arterioles.[5] Arterioles are the ultimate level at which coronary blood flow is regulated to match the delivery of oxygen and nutrients to the local metabolic demand.[2]

INTRACORONARY METHODS TO ASSESS THE FUNCTION OF MYOCARDIAL MICROCIRCULATION

The direct assessment of the structure or function of the coronary microcirculation is currently not possible in humans. Instead, the measurement of coronary blood flow has commonly used to evaluate the functional status of the coronary microvasculature.

The coronary blood flow can be accurately quantified by intracoronary techniques, which includes mainly two methods that utilize dedicate 0.014 in. coronary guidewires: (*i*) ultrasound measurement of blood flow velocity according to the Doppler principle and (*ii*) total blood flow measurement by thermodilution.

Sensor-tipped Doppler flow wires for intracoronary use have been developed and are available to be utilized in clinical practice, with a very low complication rate.[6] Current Doppler wires are 0.014 in. in diameter, which makes possible their intracoronary insertion down to distal epicardial vessels without disturbing the flow pattern. A 28°-wide ultrasound beam is generated at the distal tip of the wire, which provides a large sample volume 4 mm from the tip of the wire (Fig. 13.1). When optimal wire position inside the lumen is obtained (i.e., distal tip freely in the luminal space, avoiding contact with the vessel wall), the Doppler wire ensures a reliable measurement of peak flow velocity with minimal dependence on guidewire position.

During Doppler flow velocity measurement, spectral flow velocity data [along with electrocardiogram (ECG) tracing] are displayed in real time (Fig. 13.2). The following parameters are usually computed: time-averaged peak velocity (APV) normalized to the cardiac cycle (cm/s), which is the time average of the spectral peak velocity waveform of 2 cardiac cycles; average systolic peak velocity (ASPV; cm/s); average diastolic peak velocity (ADPV; cm/s); and the ratio of average diastolic-to-average systolic velocity (Fig. 13.2; Table 13.1). It is important to emphasize that, although normal limits for Doppler-derived parameters have been described, interpretation of each of these indices must be made in the context of a broad understanding of other Doppler variables as well as angiographic and clinical characteristics. A limitation of the Doppler wire is that it measures flow velocity rather than volumetric blood flow. However,

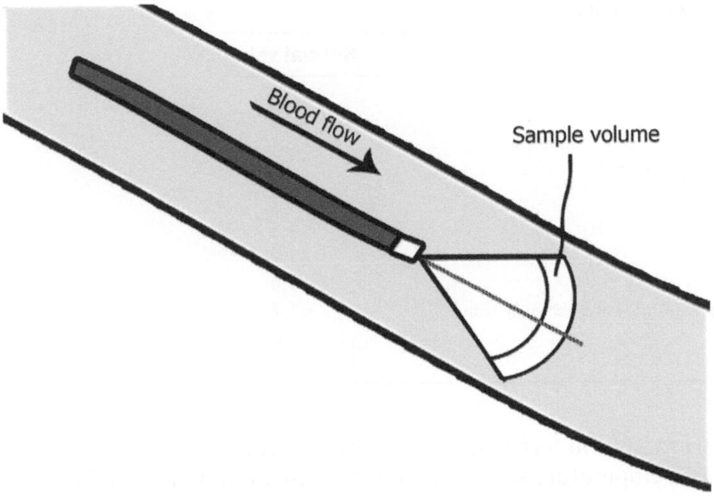

Figure 13.1 Sensor-tipped Doppler flow wire. A 28°-wide ultrasound beam is generated at the distal tip of the wire, which provides a sample volume 4 mm from the tip of the wire.

if the sectional area of target artery remains constant across the measurement conditions (e. g., between basal and hyperemic measurements), any detected change in flow velocity necessarily parallels the changes in volumetric flow. Thus, in practice, to avoid marked variations and, therefore, "freeze" the epicardial vessel size, intracoronary nitrates are usually administered to improve the reliability of multiple Doppler measurements.

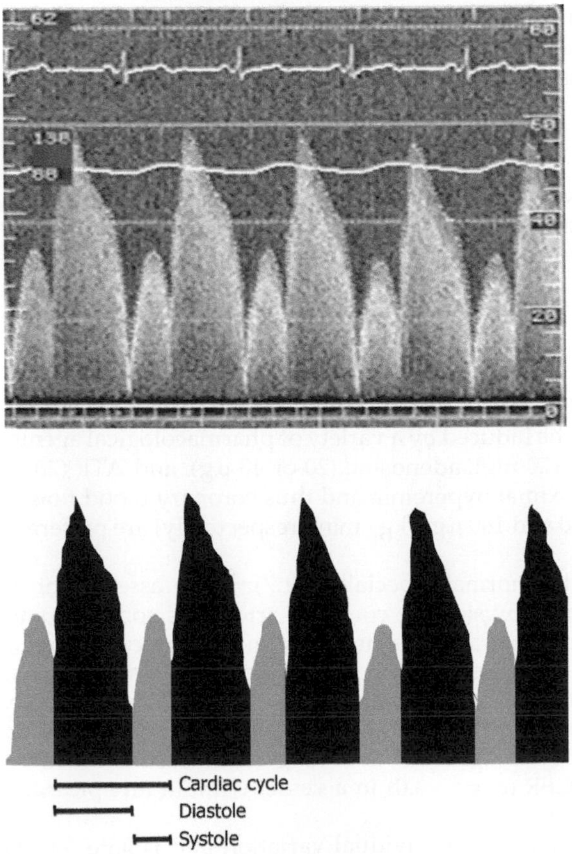

Figure 13.2 Intracoronary Doppler tracing of the left anterior descending artery. Note that the flow velocity during the systolic phase is smaller than during diastole. The time-averaged peak velocity (APV) is calculated for the whole cardiac cycle (35 cm/s in the example). The average systolic peak velocity is also calculated for the systolic and for the diastolic phases, together with the ratio of average diastolic to average systolic velocity (ratio = 2.7 in the example).

Table 13.1 Intracoronary Doppler measurements

Parameter	Normal value
Average peak velocity (APV)[39–42]	
Basal (cm/s)	≥20
Hyperemic (cm/s)	≥30
Diastolic/systolic mean velocity ratio (DSVR)[39–43]	
Left anterior descending artery	>1.7
Left circumflex artery	>1.5
Proximal right coronary artery (RCA)	>1.2
Distal RCA and posterior descending artery	>1.4
Translesional velocity gradient (or proximal/distal velocity ratio)[39–45]	<1.7
Distal coronary flow reserve[42,45,46]	≥2.0
Relative coronary flow reserve[42]	1.0

More recently, a novel thermodilution technique for measuring coronary blood flow has been developed, using a pressure/temperature sensor-tipped 0.014 in. guidewire.[7] Initial studies have shown a significant correlation between thermodilution and Doppler measurements, both experimentally[7] and in humans.[8] However, further evaluation revealed differences of 20% between the two methods in approximately one-fourth of the cases.[9,10] A latter experimental study compared both Doppler and thermodilution intracoronary measurements against a gold standard flow measurement obtained through an external flow probe.[11] That study demonstrated that both techniques significantly correlate with directly measured blood flow. However, the thermodilution-derived measurements clearly showed a closer agreement with the gold standard indices.[11] It is important to note that, apart from the possible better performance in measuring the blood flow, the thermodilution wires are potentially advantageous compared with Doppler wires, because the pressure-derived fractional flow reserve (FFR) can be measured simultaneously. As detailed in another chapter of this book, the FFR gives an epicardial-specific assessment of the coronary flow resistance. Therefore, the conjoint assessment of FFR and total coronary flow measurements helps in distinguishing epicardial and microvascular dysfunctions.

CORONARY FLOW RESERVE

Coronary flow reserve (CFR) is the ratio between the hyperemic coronary blood flow to the basal blood flow. In other words, CFR measures the magnitude of the maximal increase in coronary flow, in comparison to the blood flow measured at baseline.

$$\text{CFR} = \text{Maximal (hyperemic) coronary flow} \div \text{Baseline coronary flow}$$

Since blood flow is determined by the microvascular resistance, maximal blood flow, and therefore the CFR, are ultimately dependent on the microcirculatory coronary function.

In practice, maximal coronary flow can be induced by a variety of pharmacological agents. Intracoronary administration of papaverine (20 mg), adenosine (20 or 40 μg), and ATP (20 or 40 μg) have proven effective in inducing maximal hyperemia and thus coronary blood flow.[12] However, intravenous adenosine or ATP (140 and 180 μg/(kg · min), respectively) are preferred when steady-state hyperemia are needed.[12]

A CFR <2.0 is frequently considered abnormal (specially <1.7).[13] The assessment of microvascular dysfunction in regions irrigated by stenotic coronary arteries is complex, and the evaluation of the microvascular function in such cases depends on the clinical context.[2] Therefore, the "diagnosis" of microvascular disease is better undertaken in cases where the presence of epicardial stenoses has been ruled out, either by angiography or other methods (e. g., FFR, intravascular ultrasound). In this context, patients without epicardial obstructions who present with a flow reserve <2.0 can be reliably "diagnosed" as having microvascular coronary dysfunction. Conversely, a frankly normal CFR (e. g., >3.0) in a vessel without an epicardial stenosis reliably excludes small-vessel disease.

CFR is known to have marked intra- and inter-individual variation and isolate results must be interpreted with cautious. Furthermore, for the optimal application of intracoronary

Table 13.2 Mechanisms and conditions associated with microvascular dysfunction[2]

Mechanism	Associated conditions
Luminal obstruction	Spontaneous microembolization in acute coronary syndromes Iatrogenic embolization during percutaneous coronary intervention
Vascular wall infiltration	Infiltrative heart diseases
Vascular remodeling	Hypertrophic cardiomyopathy, systemic arterial hypertension
Vascular paucity	Aortic stenosis, systemic arterial hypertension
Perivascular fibrosis	Aortic stenosis, systemic arterial hypertension
Endothelial dysfunction	Smoking, hyperlipidemia, diabetes
Smooth muscle cell dysfunction	Hypertrophic cardiomyopathy, systemic arterial hypertension
Autonomic dysfunction	Coronary recanalization
Extramural vascular compression	Aortic stenosis, systemic arterial hypertension, hypertrophic cardiomyopathy
Reduction in diastole and perfusion time	Aortic stenosis

Doppler, it is mandatory an in-depth understanding of the limitations of the method. Most importantly, both baseline and maximal flow measurements are sensitive to changes in hemodynamic conditions.

CORONARY MICROVASCULAR DYSFUNCTION

Microvascular dysfunction occurs secondary to several pathophysiological mechanisms, which may act isolated or in association to increase myocardial microvascular resistance and/or impair the microvascular vasodilatory capacity (Table 13.2).

Recently, Camici and Crea have suggested classifying the coronary microvascular dysfunction into four types: (1) dysfunction occurring in the absence of coronary artery disease or myocardial diseases, (2) dysfunction in the presence of myocardial diseases, (3) dysfunction in the presence of obstructive epicardial disease, and (4) iatrogenic dysfunction.

Microvascular dysfunction without coronary artery disease, or myocardial diseases, has been described among smokers,[14] patients with hyperlipidemia,[15–20] diabetes,[21–24] and hypertension.[25]

Patients without evidence of obstructive epicardial, who present with angina-like chest pain are commonly referred as having Syndrome X. Reduced CFR has been consistently reported in a subset of patients with Syndrome X, suggesting that coronary microvascular dysfunction is the probable cause of the symptoms and that it would be more appropriate to diagnose these patients as having "microvascular angina."[26–28] Indeed, such diagnosis might be strongly considered for symptomatic patients who present reduced CFR and angiographically normal coronaries, or normal FFR, or normal relative CFR (ratio of CRF in two separate coronary territories) (Fig. 13.3).[29]

Microvascular dysfunction has been documented to be markedly present in patients with hypertrophic cardiomyopathy,[30,31] and to be an important predictor of long-term outcomes for this population.[32,33] Also, patients with dilated cardiomyopathy have been found to often present microvascular dysfunction.[34,35] Other cardiac diseases for which microvascular dysfunction has been shown to occur include aortic stenosis and infiltrative heart diseases (e. g., Anderson-Fabry disease). Interestingly, patients with obstructive coronary artery disease may present abnormal CFR even in regions supplied by angiographically normal coronary arteries, a fact that may have an important role in reducing the global ischemic threshould.[36]

In patients with acute coronary syndromes, coronary microvascular dysfunction is an important factor in determining the severity of myocardial ischemia in the territory of a critical lesion. Recently, it has been demonstrated that patients with unstable angina may have transient episodes of ischemia that are associated with an increase in coronary microvascular resistance, which may be improved by platelet GP IIb/IIIa blockade with abciximab.[37]

Acute impairment of microvascular coronary function may occur in the setting of reperfusion for acute myocardial infarction (AIM), either following primary percutaneous coronary intervention or fibrinolytic therapy. Also, acute microvascular dysfunction may appear as a complication during percutaneous coronary intervention, even for non-AMI patients. The so-called

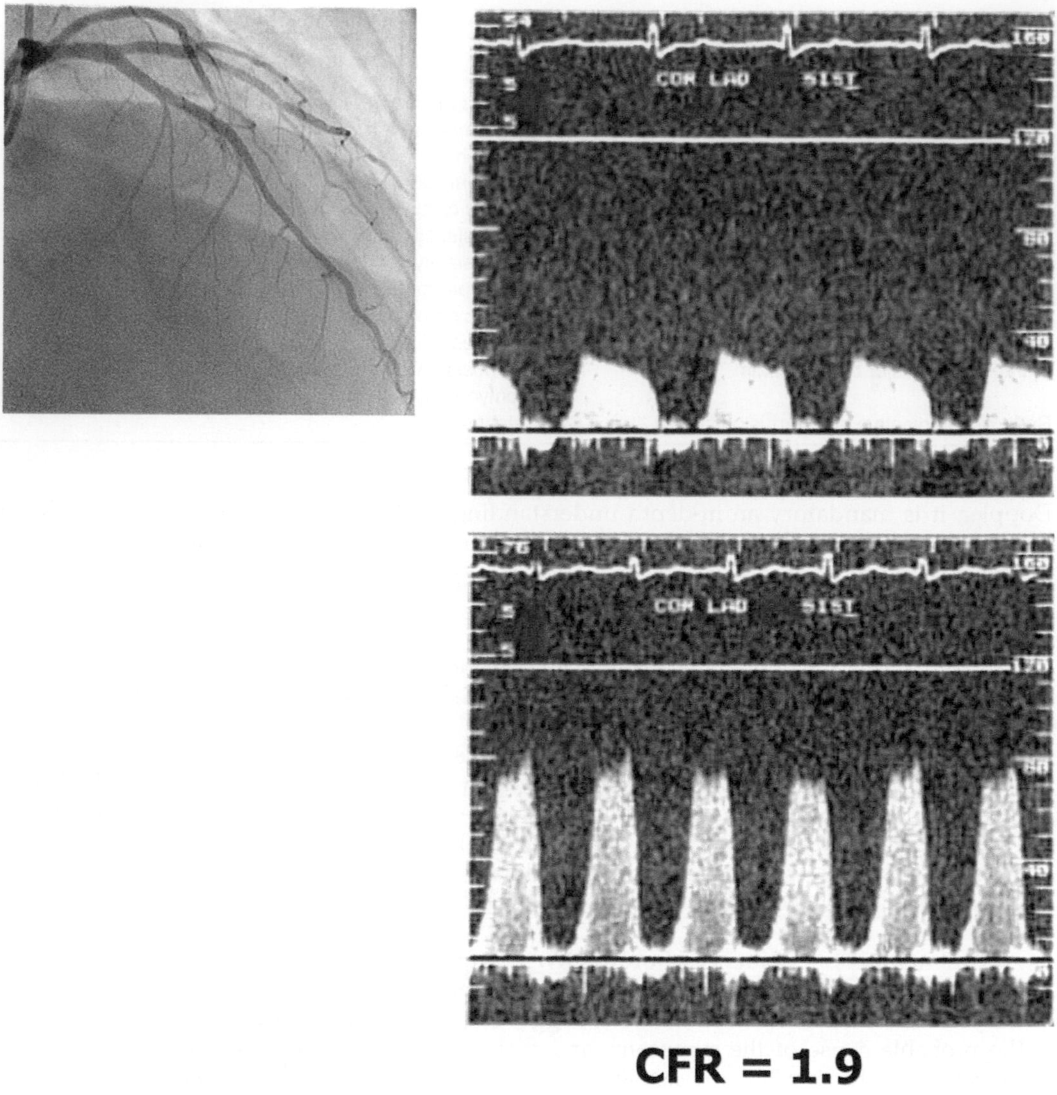

Figure 13.3 Intracoronary Doppler tracing (left anterior descending artery) at baseline (*top, right*) and during maximal hyperemia with intravenous adenosine (*bottom*). Note that there is an increase in blood flow velocity after the infusion of the vasodilator. However, the ratio baseline/hyperemia (i.e., the coronary flow reserve) is 1.9. The CRF <2.0 and the presence of angiographically normal coronaries (*top, left*) suggest the diagnosis of microvascular dysfunction.

"no-reflow" phenomenon is defined as a non–perfusion state in the presence of unobstructed epicardial vessel, which occurs as a consequence of extreme lack of microvascular integrity. It typically occurs in patients with AIM who have undergone successful recanalization of the culprit artery. However, "no-reflow" may occur in other high-risk patient populations treated with coronary angioplasty, such as those with degenerated saphenous vein grafts. No-reflow events have been reported to be associated with typical intracoronary Doppler tracing, characterized a systolic retrograde flow together with a rapid deceleration ($\leq$600 ms) of diastolic flow and a negative diastolic/systolic flow velocity ratio.[38]

CONCLUSIONS

Microvascular dysfunction is a relatively frequent condition that is rather underdiagnosed. Both isolate microvascular dysfunction and its association with other cardiac conditions have been demonstrated to have clinical and prognostic relevance. Invasive intracoronary methods, either with Doppler-derived parameters or with thermodilution techniques, may add in diagnostic information to patients with suspected or known impaired microvascular coronary function.

REFERENCES

1. De Bruyne B, Hersbach F, Pijls NH, et al. Abnormal epicardial coronary resistance in patients with diffuse atherosclerosis but "Normal" coronary angiography. Circulation 2001; 104:2401–2406.
2. Camici PG, Crea F. Coronary microvascular dysfunction. N Engl J Med 2007; 356:830–840.
3. Marcus ML, Chilian WM, Kanatsuka H, et al. Understanding the coronary circulation through studies at the microvascular level. Circulation 1990; 82:1–7.
4. Lupi A, Buffon A, Finocchiaro ML, et al. Mechanisms of adenosine-induced epicardial coronary artery dilatation. Eur Heart J 1997; 18:614–617.
5. Kuo L, Chilian WM, Davis MJ. Coronary arteriolar myogenic response is independent of endothelium. Circ Res 1990; 66:860–866.
6. Qian J, Ge J, Baumgart D, et al. Safety of intracoronary Doppler flow measurement. Am Heart J 2000; 140:502–510.
7. De Bruyne B, Pijls NH, Smith L, et al. Coronary thermodilution to assess flow reserve: Experimental validation. Circulation 2001; 104:2003–2006.
8. Pijls NH, De Bruyne B, Smith L, et al. Coronary thermodilution to assess flow reserve: Validation in humans. Circulation 2002; 105:2482–2486.
9. McGinn AL, White CW, Wilson RF. Interstudy variability of coronary flow reserve. Influence of heart rate, arterial pressure, and ventricular preload. Circulation 1990; 81:1319–1330.
10. Gaster AL, Korsholm L, Thayssen P, et al. Reproducibility of intravascular ultrasound and intracoronary Doppler measurements. Catheter Cardiovasc Interv 2001; 53:449–458.
11. Fearon WF, Farouque HM, Balsam LB, et al. Comparison of coronary thermodilution and Doppler velocity for assessing coronary flow reserve. Circulation 2003; 108:2198–2200.
12. De Bruyne B, Pijls NH, Barbato E, et al. Intracoronary and intravenous adenosine 5′-triphosphate, adenosine, papaverine, and contrast medium to assess fractional flow reserve in humans. Circulation 2003; 107:1877–1883.
13. Heller LI, Cates C, Popma J, et al. Intracoronary Doppler assessment of moderate coronary artery disease: Comparison with 201Tl imaging and coronary angiography. FACTS Study Group. Circulation 1997; 96:484–490.
14. Kaufmann PA, Gnecchi-Ruscone T, di Terlizzi M, et al. Coronary heart disease in smokers: Vitamin C restores coronary microcirculatory function. Circulation 2000; 102:1233–1238.
15. Gould KL, Martucci JP, Goldberg DI, et al. Short-term cholesterol lowering decreases size and severity of perfusion abnormalities by positron emission tomography after dipyridamole in patients with coronary artery disease. A potential noninvasive marker of healing coronary endothelium. Circulation 1994; 89:1530–1538.
16. Dayanikli F, Grambow D, Muzik O, et al. Early detection of abnormal coronary flow reserve in asymptomatic men at high risk for coronary artery disease using positron emission tomography. Circulation 1994; 90:808–817.
17. Czernin J, Barnard RJ, Sun KT, et al. Effect of short-term cardiovascular conditioning and low-fat diet on myocardial blood flow and flow reserve. Circulation 1995; 92:197–204.
18. Pitkanen OP, Raitakari OT, Niinikoski H, et al. Coronary flow reserve is impaired in young men with familial hypercholesterolemia. J Am Coll Cardiol 1996; 28:1705–1711.
19. Pitkanen OP, Nuutila P, Raitakari OT, et al. Coronary flow reserve in young men with familial combined hyperlipidemia. Circulation 1999; 99:1678–1684.
20. Kaufmann PA, Gnecchi-Ruscone T, Schafers KP, et al. Low density lipoprotein cholesterol and coronary microvascular dysfunction in hypercholesterolemia. J Am Coll Cardiol 2000; 36:103–109.
21. Nitenberg A, Valensi P, Sachs R, et al. Impairment of coronary vascular reserve and ACh-induced coronary vasodilation in diabetic patients with angiographically normal coronary arteries and normal left ventricular systolic function. Diabetes 1993; 42:1017–1025.
22. Pitkanen OP, Nuutila P, Raitakari OT, et al. Coronary flow reserve is reduced in young men with IDDM. Diabetes 1998; 47:248–254.
23. Yokoyama I, Momomura S, Ohtake T, et al. Reduced myocardial flow reserve in non-insulin-dependent diabetes mellitus. J Am Coll Cardiol 1997; 30:1472–1477.
24. Di Carli MF, Janisse J, Grunberger G, et al. Role of chronic hyperglycemia in the pathogenesis of coronary microvascular dysfunction in diabetes. J Am Coll Cardiol 2003; 41:1387–1393.
25. Laine H, Raitakari OT, Niinikoski H, et al. Early impairment of coronary flow reserve in young men with borderline hypertension. J Am Coll Cardiol 1998; 32:147–153.

26. Galiuto L, Sestito A, Barchetta S, et al. Noninvasive evaluation of flow reserve in the left anterior descending coronary artery in patients with cardiac syndrome X. Am J Cardiol 2007; 99:1378–1383.
27. Epstein SE, Cannon RO III. Site of increased resistance to coronary flow in patients with angina pectoris and normal epicardial coronary arteries. J Am Coll Cardiol 1986; 8:459–461.
28. Cemin R, Erlicher A, Fattor B, et al. Reduced coronary flow reserve and parasympathetic dysfunction in patients with cardiovascular syndrome X. Coron Artery Dis 2008; 19:1–7.
29. Cannon RO III, Camici PG, Epstein SE. Pathophysiological dilemma of syndrome X. Circulation 1992; 85:883–892.
30. Camici P, Chiriatti G, Lorenzoni R, et al. Coronary vasodilation is impaired in both hypertrophied and nonhypertrophied myocardium of patients with hypertrophic cardiomyopathy: A study with nitrogen-13 ammonia and positron emission tomography. J Am Coll Cardiol 1991; 17:879–886.
31. Gistri R, Cecchi F, Choudhury L, et al. Effect of verapamil on absolute myocardial blood flow in hypertrophic cardiomyopathy. Am J Cardiol 1994; 74:363–368.
32. Cecchi F, Olivotto I, Gistri R, et al. Coronary microvascular dysfunction and prognosis in hypertrophic cardiomyopathy. N Engl J Med 2003; 349:1027–1035.
33. Olivotto I, Cecchi F, Gistri R, et al. Relevance of coronary microvascular flow impairment to long-term remodeling and systolic dysfunction in hypertrophic cardiomyopathy. J Am Coll Cardiol 2006; 47:1043–1048.
34. Canetti M, Akhter MW, Lerman A, et al. Evaluation of myocardial blood flow reserve in patients with chronic congestive heart failure due to idiopathic dilated cardiomyopathy. Am J Cardiol 2003; 92:1246–1249.
35. Neglia D, Parodi O, Gallopin M, et al. Myocardial blood flow response to pacing tachycardia and to dipyridamole infusion in patients with dilated cardiomyopathy without overt heart failure. A quantitative assessment by positron emission tomography. Circulation 1995; 92:796–804.
36. Sambuceti G, Parodi O, Marzullo P, et al. Regional myocardial blood flow in stable angina pectoris associated with isolated significant narrowing of either the left anterior descending or left circumflex coronary artery. Am J Cardiol 1993; 72:990–994.
37. Marzilli M, Sambuceti G, Testa R, et al. Platelet glycoprotein IIb/IIIa receptor blockade and coronary resistance in unstable angina. J Am Coll Cardiol 2002; 40:2102–2109.
38. Kawamoto T, Yoshida K, Akasaka T, et al. Can coronary blood flow velocity pattern after primary percutaneous transluminal coronary angioplasty [correction of angiography] predict recovery of regional left ventricular function in patients with acute myocardial infarction? Circulation 1999; 100:339–345.
39. Segal J, Kern MJ, Scott NA, et al. Alterations of phasic coronary artery flow velocity in humans during percutaneous coronary angioplasty. J Am Coll Cardiol 1992; 20:276–286.
40. Ofili EO, Kern MJ, Labovitz AJ, et al. Analysis of coronary blood flow velocity dynamics in angiographically normal and stenosed arteries before and after endolumen enlargement by angioplasty. J Am Coll Cardiol 1993; 21:308–316.
41. Ofili EO, Labovitz AJ, Kern MJ. Coronary flow velocity dynamics in normal and diseased arteries. Am J Cardiol 1993; 71:3D–9D.
42. Kern MJ. Coronary physiology revisited: Practical insights from the cardiac catheterization laboratory. Circulation 2000; 101:1344–1351.
43. Kajiya F, Tsujioka K, Ogasawara Y, et al. Analysis of flow characteristics in poststenotic regions of the human coronary artery during bypass graft surgery. Circulation 1987; 76:1092–1100.
44. Donohue TJ, Kern MJ, Aguirre FV, et al. Assessing the hemodynamic significance of coronary artery stenoses: Analysis of translesional pressure-flow velocity relations in patients. J Am Coll Cardiol 1993; 22:449–458.
45. Kern MJ, Aguirre FV, Bach RG, et al. Translesional pressure-flow velocity assessment in patients: Part I. Cathet Cardiovasc Diagn 1994; 31:49–60.
46. Joye JD, Schulman DS, Lasorda D, et al. Intracoronary Doppler guide wire versus stress single-photon emission computed tomographic thallium-201 imaging in assessment of intermediate coronary stenoses. J Am Coll Cardiol 1994; 24:940–947.

14 Collateral function assessment

Steffen Gloekler and Bernhard Meier

INTRODUCTION

Long before the era of interventional cardiology, Heberden was the first to describe the phenomenon of angina pectoris, already including the walking-through phenomenon. This symptom was later attributed to recruitment of collateral vessels during exercise. However, the following two centuries favored the concept of coronary end-arteries rather than that of a functional human coronary collateral circulation.[1] With the advent of percutaneous coronary intervention (PCI) in 1977, antegrade revascularization of stenotic vessels became a mainstay for treatment of coronary artery disease (CAD). Because one-third to one-fifth of CAD patients are not amenable to PCI and some are not candidates for surgical revascularization either, the need for alternative methods like promotion of collateral growth has arisen. In parallel, invasive methods for the assessment of coronary collaterals have been introduced and evaluated.[2,3] Quantitative collateral assessment by invasive means has markedly advanced insight into the functional relevance of the coronary collateral circulation: In CAD, the amount of collateral flow is a pivotal protective factor with respect to infarct size[4,5] and mortality (Fig. 14.1).[6] Infarct size is determined by the duration of coronary occlusion, the anatomic area (or myocardial mass) at risk for infarction, collateral flow to the infarct-related artery, myocardial preconditioning and oxygen consumption at the time of occlusion.[7]

Apart from shortening door-to-balloon time and optimizing medical therapy, the so far untreatable determinant of infarct size, collateral flow, may be therapeutically promoted (therapeutic collateral promotion; TCP) by different approaches (e.g., with colony-stimulating factor therapy). In this context, accurate assessment of coronary collateral function will be increasingly relevant, especially in context of serial measurements within protocols for TCP.

Since collateral flow and antegrade coronary flow are competitive forces, collaterals can only be assessed during vascular occlusion of the epicardial artery—be it naturally (in case of a chronic total occlusion; CTO) or artificially (in case of a temporary balloon occlusion of the coronary artery).

CHRONIC TOTAL OCCLUSION (CTO) MODEL

In case of CTO of a coronary artery without myocardial infarction, its entire perfusion area (i.e., the area at risk) has to be supplied by collaterals. These collaterals are often sufficient to reduce the area at risk to zero, that is, preventing myocardial infarction altogether (Fig. 14.2).[8] Most likely, there is a gray zone of individuals never undergoing coronary angiography because of collateralized CTOs without angina pectoris. In case of a CTO with normal left ventricular wall motion, the supplying collaterals of the occluded region must have been "sufficient" to prevent myocardial infarction. In case of antegrade restoration of flow, collateral function regresses to approximately 60% of the initial value, but remains recruitable with the potential to reach the initial value in case of chronic reocclusion.[9,10]

ACUTE CORONARY BALLOON-OCCLUSION MODEL

In the majority of patients with CAD undergoing invasive assessment, there is no CTO, but there may be a certain degree of collateralization to the ischemic region of the stenotic artery. For assessment of collateral function, a temporary episode of balloon occlusion (Fig. 14.3) to completely block the antegrade coronary blood flow is required.

During collateral assessment in normal coronary arteries, inflation of the angioplasty balloon should be performed at slowly increasing low pressure (1–2 atm) using an adequate-size balloon (Fig. 14.4). Documenting the proof of total occlusion by stop of the contrast agent should be obtained to avoid falsely high "collateral flow." The standard time of balloon occlusion is 60 seconds. After deflation and pullback of the balloon, the integrity of the vessel has to be checked by final angiography. For prevention of vasospasm, as a consequence of occluding a normal

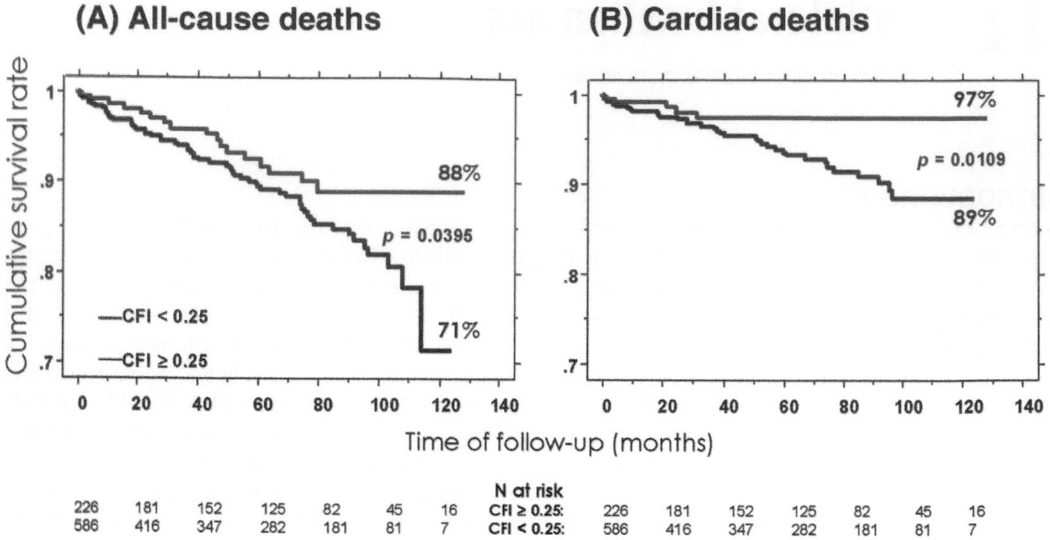

Figure 14.1 Benefit in all-cause (**A**) and cardiac mortality (**B**) in patients with sufficient collateral function (collateral flow index >25%; *red curves*) above poor collateral function (collateral flow index <25%; *black curves*).

artery, the administration of a transdermal nitrate patch for 12 hours is recommended. In our experience, briefly occluding a normal coronary artery observing the above recommendations is a safe procedure.

Principally, there are various more or less accurate methods for assessment of collateral flow to the perfusion area of a coronary artery of interest.

QUALITATIVE METHODS FOR CORONARY COLLATERAL FUNCTION ASSESSMENT

Angina pectoris during balloon occlusion

The most simple, but highly variable method to assess the clinical impact of collaterals in a situation of acute recruitment by balloon occlusion is to ask the patient about angina pectoris. This dichotomizes patients in two groups, that is, an epidemiologically larger group with

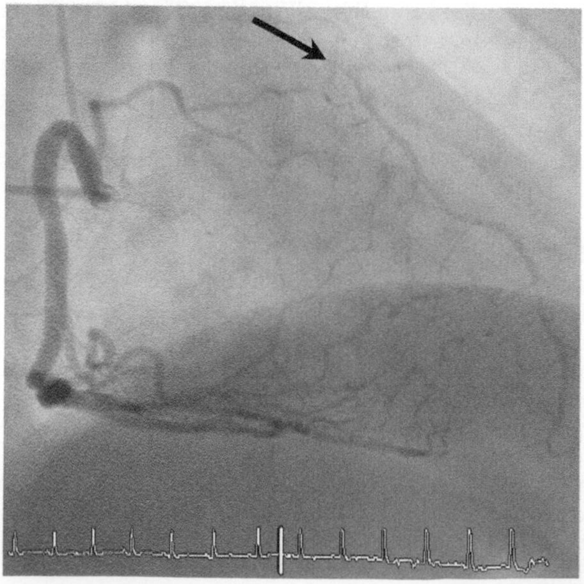

Figure 14.2 CTO (*arrow*) of the left anterior descending coronary artery (LAD), revealed by dye injection into the right coronary artery (RCA): A conus branch and septal collaterals interconnect the perfusion territories of both coronary arteries.

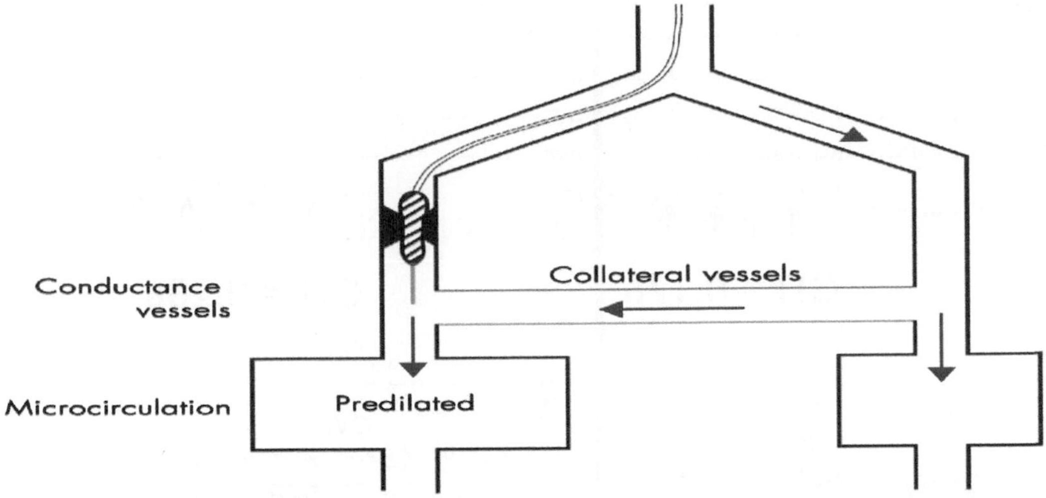

Figure 14.3 Schematic illustration of the principle of collateral assessment in the balloon-occlusion model. The transducer of a pressure or Doppler guidewire is positioned distal to the temporary occlusion. The detected pressure (P_{occl}) or flow velocity (V_{occl}) originates from collateral vessels (except for the central venous counter pressure, which has to be also recorded and subtracted from P_{occl} for calculation of CFI), which exclusively supply the vascular territory during blockage of antegrade coronary flow.

insufficient collaterals and a smaller group with sufficient collaterals (present, respectively, absent angina pectoris).

The predictive value of this method for determination of electrocardiography (ECG) signs of ischemia during occlusion or quantitative collateral flow levels is low.

In case of TCP, however, intra-individual changes of angina pectoris during brief arterial occlusion can be regarded as a valuable endpoint, indicating the clinical relevance of collaterals.

Pros: Easy and costless to perform; no technical equipment needed.
Contras: Large interindividual and likely intraindividual variability; qualitative collateral assessment.
Conclusion: Helpful for crude risk stratification.

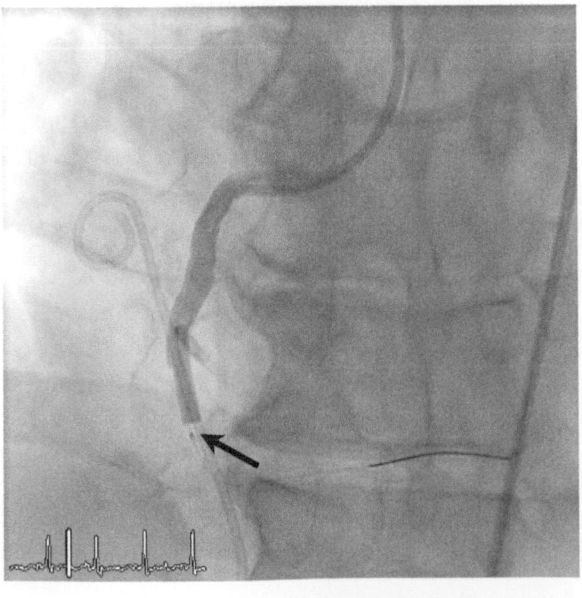

Figure 14.4 Angiographic confirmation of total balloon occlusion of the proximal right coronary artery during simultaneous collateral flow assessment with a pressure guidewire. The black arrow indicates the stop of the contrast medium proximal to the inflated balloon.

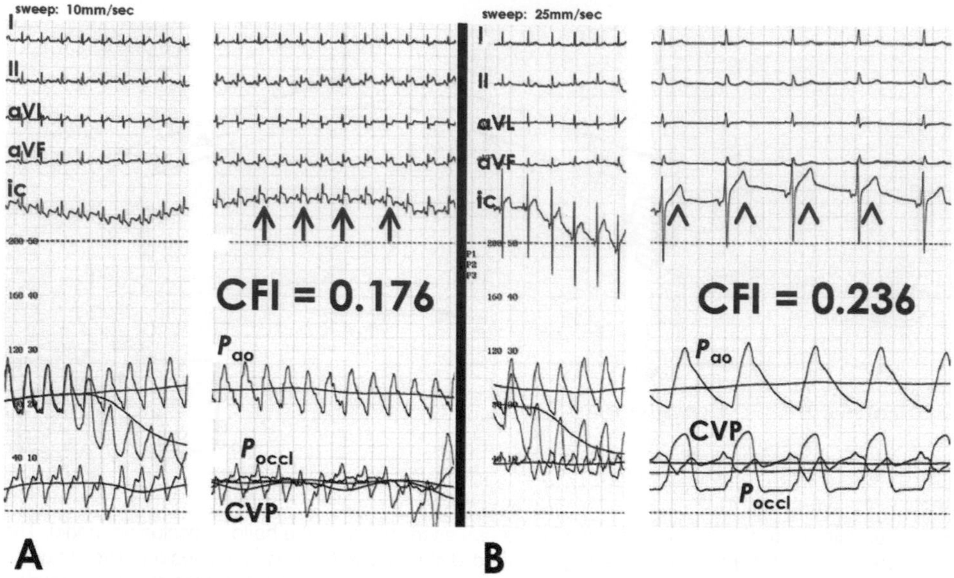

Figure 14.5 Pressure and ECG tracings of two patients with different amounts of collateral flow. The left side of Panel (**A**) and (**B**) shows the beginning of balloon inflation with subsequent pressure drop of the distal coronary pressure (P_{occl}). The right side of each panel shows pressures during balloon occlusion. In the fist patient with insufficient collateral flow and angina pectoris during vessel occlusion (**A**), both external and ic. ECG tracings (*upper part*) show marked ST-elevations (*arrows*). The second patient (**B**) has sufficient collaterals: He experienced no angina and ic. and external ECG (*arrowheads*) revealed no ischemic repolarization during vessel occlusion.

ECG during balloon occlusion

Similar to the sudden pathological occlusion of a coronary artery in case of an infarction, the artificial balloon occlusion causes acute ischemic repolarization patterns (i.e., ST-segment–elevation or –depression) on the external and on the intracoronary (ic.) ECG. The external ECG is part of the standard setting in the catheterization laboratory and an ic. ECG can be easily obtained via the angioplasty guidewire.[11] ST-segment changes >0.1 mV on the ic. or external ECG during occlusion indicate collaterals insufficient to prevent myocardial ischemia. The territory of left coronary artery (LCA) has been shown to be more susceptible signs of ischemia during a 120-second period of coronary occlusion than that of the right coronary artery (RCA).[12]

Similar to angina pectoris (AP), the ECG is also a dichotomous method for collateral function characterization (Figs. 14.5 and 14.9). In a follow up study of our group, cardiac deaths and cardiac death or myocardial infarction occurred more often in the group with pathologic ST-segment elevation than in that without pathologic ST-segment elevation.[13] The ECG threshold between sufficient and insufficient collaterals is equivalent to a relative collateral flow of approximately 25%.

Pros: Easy and costless to obtain; more accurate than angina pectoris.

Contras: Large interindividual variability; variable with the vessel examined qualitative collateral assessment.

Conclusion: Helpful for crude risk stratification.

Regional left ventricular (LV) function

In case of a CTO, the presence of normal LV-wall motion qualifies collaterals as sufficient to prevent myocardial infarction (Fig. 14.6).[8] Unfortunately, in a substantial fraction of CTOs, collateral function is not sufficient to prevent an infarction (Fig. 14.7, for comparison). In case of stenotic, but not occluded coronary arteries, ECG revealed that regional systolic and diastolic LV function is directly related to the amount of collateral flow to this territory during 60 seconds of coronary artery occlusion.[14] However, since the majority of cases are not CTOs, LV-angiography

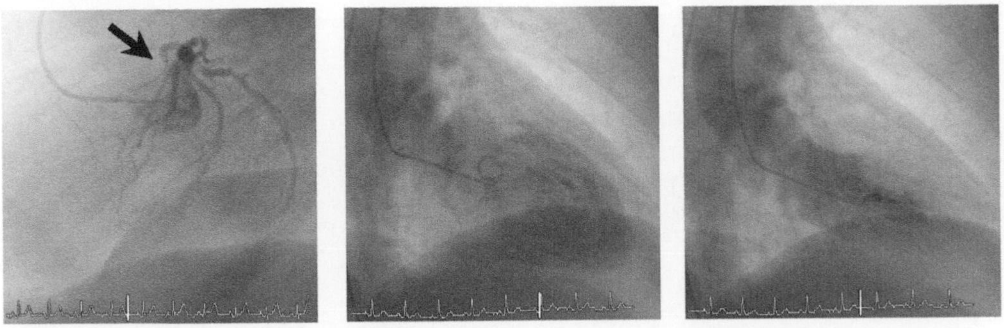

A B C

Figure 14.6 CTO with sufficient collateral function, normal LV function, and no myocardial infarction: (**A**) chronic total occlusion (*arrow*) of left anterior descending coronary artery (LAD) (**B**) end-diastolic LV angiogram, and (**C**) end-systolic LV angiogram.

simultaneously with coronary occlusion is rather impractical (since a second catheter is needed) and too imprecise for assessing collateral flow.

Pros: In case of CTOs with normal LV-function no further collateral assessment necessary to characterize collateral flow as sufficient.
Contras: Not applicable in stenotic arteries without a second catheter or simultaneous echocardiography ; qualitative collateral assessment.
Conclusion: In CTOs applicable, otherwise too elaborate for limited information.

In general, most of the above methods do not require special equipment or expenses. However, their variability is high and they allow only qualitative assessment of collateral function.

ANGIOGRAPHIC AND SENSOR-DERIVED METHODS FOR CORONARY COLLATERAL FUNCTION ASSESSMENT

Qualitative angiographic classification

The coronary angiographic assessment, first described by Rentrop et al., qualifies naturally or balloon-occluded coronary arteries according to the degree (0–3) of retrograde filling of the collateral receiving epicardial artery by collateral vessels from the collateral supplying vessel[15] as follows (Fig. 14.8): 0, no filling; 1, small side branches filled; 2, filling of part of the major branch; and 3, main vessel entirely filled.

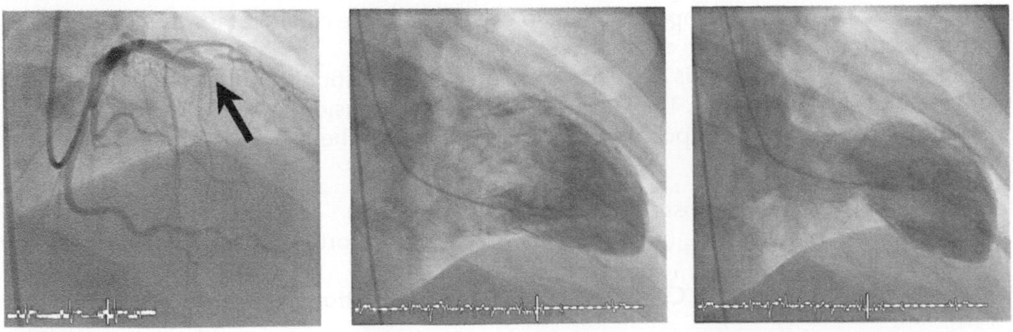

A B C

Figure 14.7 CTO with insufficient collateral function, impaired LV function, anterior wall myocardial infarction: (**A**) acute total occlusion of LAD distal to the second septal branch (*arrow*) (**B**) end-diastolic LV angiogram, (**C**) end-systolic LV angiogram.

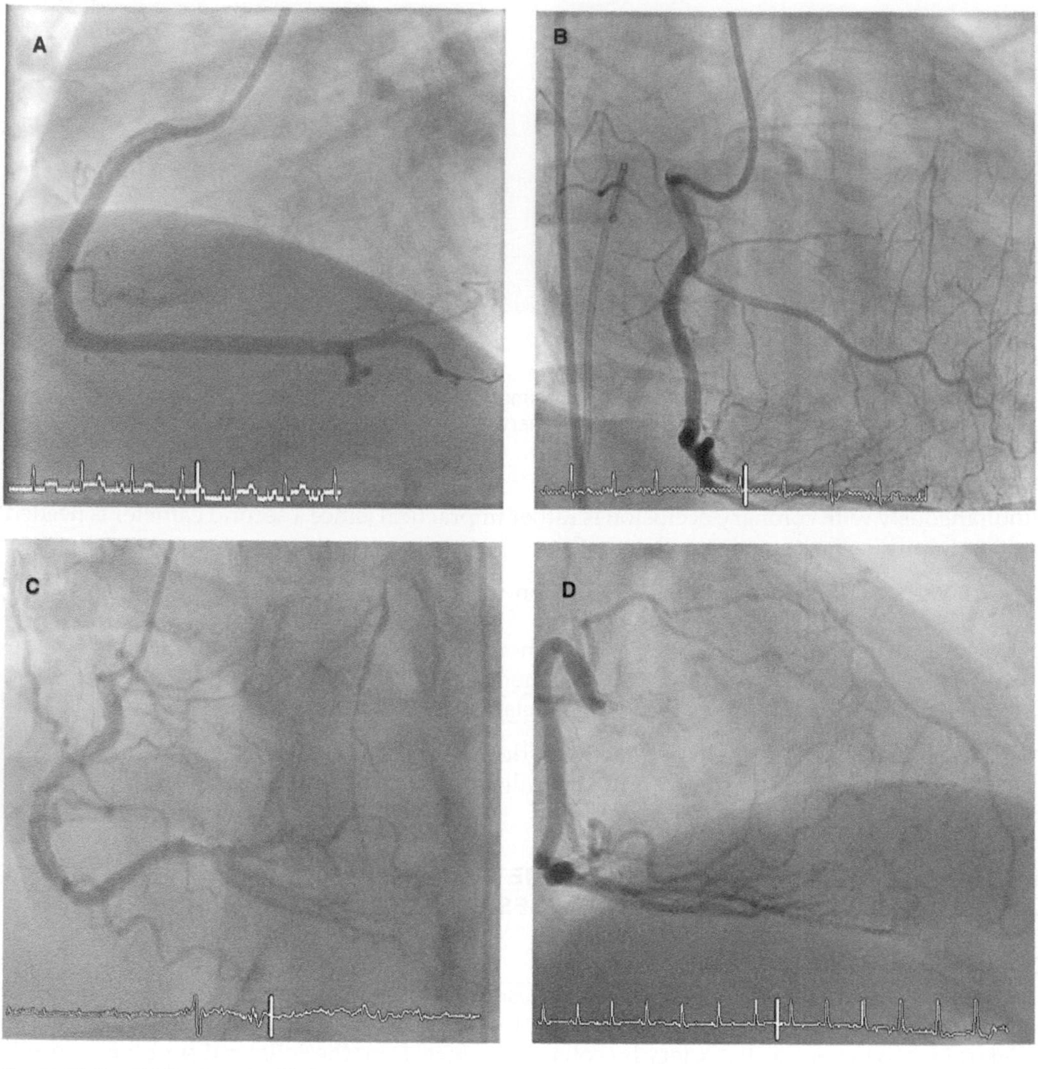

Figure 14.8 (**A**) Rentrop 0, (**B**) Rentrop 1, (**C**) Rentrop 2, and (**D**) Rentrop 3.

In the absence of CTO, the qualification of recruitable collaterals requires the insertion of two catheters, that is, one for temporary balloon occlusion of the collateral receiving artery and one for contrast injection into the collateral supplying artery.

Therefore, this procedure is applied rarely and classification of collaterals is limited to spontaneously visible collaterals. The fact of omitting total occlusion by a balloon renders maximal recruitment of collaterals impossible and partly, therefore, the sensitivity of this qualitative method is low.

Pros: In case of CTOs easy and costless to perform.
Contras: Otherwise too elaborate (2nd catheter) for limited information; qualitative collateral assessment.
Conclusion: Appropriate only for CTOs and crude risk stratification.

Semi-quantitative classification (washout collaterometry)

Another method, which avoids a second catheter access and is semi-quantitative is the so-called "washout collaterometry"[16]: A brief balloon occlusion is performed in the ipsilateral vessel promptly after antegrade contrast dye injection. The dye is then trapped distal to the site of occlusion and can be washed out only by collateral flow originating from the ipsilateral or contralateral coronary arteries. Depending on the degree of collateral flow, more or less heart cycles are required to wash out the trapped dye.

In a study of our group, we found an inverse correlation between contrast washout time and collateral flow index ($r = 0.72, p < 0.0001$). In case of washout within 11 heart beats, collateral flow is sufficient to prevent ischemia.

Pros: Easy and costless to perform. Assesses both ipsilateral and contralateral collaterals. No need for 2nd catheter.
Contras: Semi-quantitative.
Conclusion: Applicable in all coronary vessels; suitable for more accurate risk stratification.

Quantitative intracoronary pressure or Doppler measurements (CFI_p or CFI_v)

The coronary wedge pressure is defined as the mean distal coronary pressure as obtained during occlusion of the artery for at least 30 seconds.[11] In all vessels with a wedge pressure of 30 mm Hg or higher, collaterals were present in the cited study. Since the mid-1990s, pressure and Doppler-tipped angioplasty guidewires have been available and collateral flow can be quantitatively assessed by simultaneous measurement of aortic pressure, intracoronary velocity or pressure distal to the stenosis during and after a standardized balloon occlusion of 60 seconds. The simultaneously obtained pressure and the subsequently recorded velocity parameters allow calculating the collateral flow index (CFI),[3] which represents collateral flow as a fraction of antegrade flow via the nonoccluded vessel.

Based on the reasonable assumption that the occlusive pressure or flow velocity is directly and closely related to collateral flow, relative collateral-to-normal flow is calculated as shown below (Figs. 14.5 and 14.9). In case of calculation of the pressure-derived CFI (CFI_p), the central venous pressure (CVP) has to be subtracted from the aortic (P_{ao}) and distal (P_{occl}) pressures and CFI is calculated as:

$$CFI_P = \frac{P_{occl} - CVP}{P_{ao} - CVP}$$

The velocity-derived CFI is obtained by measuring coronary flow velocity distal to the occlusion (V_{occl}), and by determining coronary flow velocity during vessel patency at the same site ($V_{nonoccl}$) (Fig. 14.10); CFI_v is calculated as:

$$CFI_v = \frac{V_{occl}}{V_{nonoccl}}$$

Using a combined pressure/velocity wire, a collateral resistance index (R_{coll}; mm Hg/cm $\times$ sec^{-1}) can be calculated if the velocity time integral is taken[17]:

$$R_{coll} = \frac{P_{ao} - P_{occl}}{V_{occl}}$$

Pros: Feasible in most coronary arteries; pressure measurements robust.
Contras: Expensive. In complex coronary anatomy challenging to maneuver the sensor wire; potential for dissection or thrombotic occlusion of vessel. Flow velocity measurements more susceptible for artifacts.
Conclusion: Gold standard for collateral quantification. Applicable in most coronary arteries. Appropriate for exact risk stratification and quantitative monitoring of TCP.

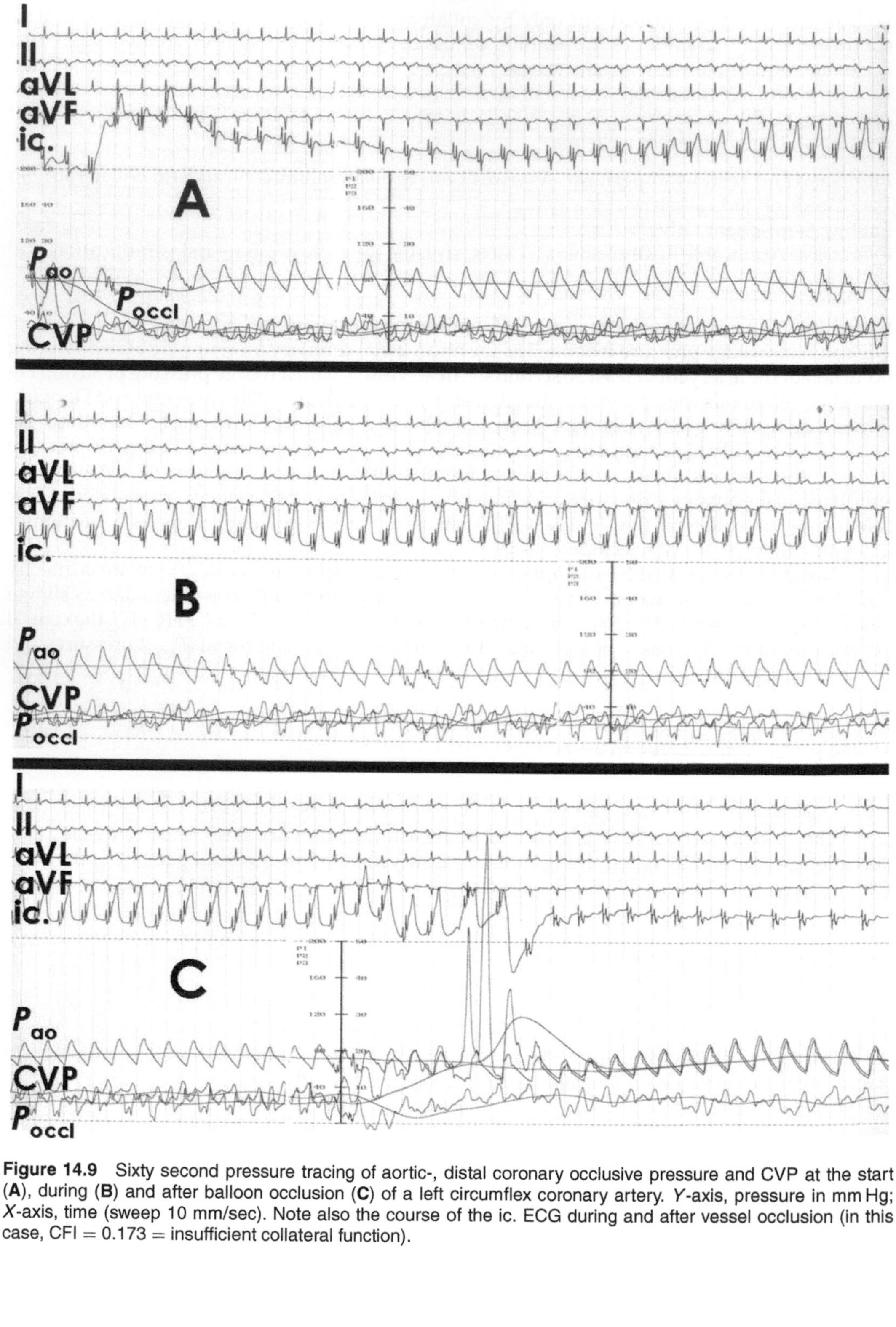

Figure 14.9 Sixty second pressure tracing of aortic-, distal coronary occlusive pressure and CVP at the start (**A**), during (**B**) and after balloon occlusion (**C**) of a left circumflex coronary artery. *Y*-axis, pressure in mm Hg; *X*-axis, time (sweep 10 mm/sec). Note also the course of the ic. ECG during and after vessel occlusion (in this case, CFI = 0.173 = insufficient collateral function).

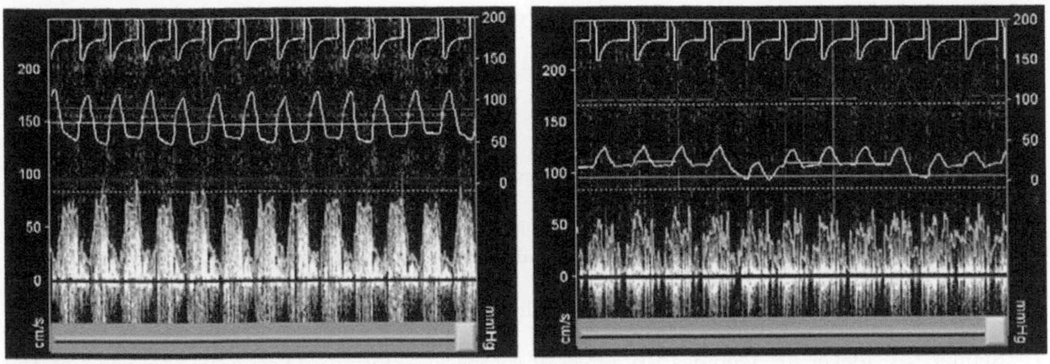

A B

Figure 14.10 Combined pressure and flow velocity tracings obtained in the left circumflex artery. In the upper part of the figures, ECG (*white*), P_{ao} (*red*), and P_{occl} (*yellow*) are depicted. The lower part of both panels shows the Doppler velocity spectra. Panel (**A**) shows pressures and flow velocity during normal antegrade coronary flow in the presence of a stenotic lesion. Panel (**B**) shows the same parameters during balloon occlusion. Left side of *X*-axis, flow velocity in cm/sec; right side, pressure in mm Hg.

Perfusion-derived collateral assessment (CPI)

Absolute myocardial blood flow (MBF; mL/min × gram myocardial mass) is the gold standard to assess myocardial perfusion. Apart from positron emission tomography (PET), myocardial contrast echocardiography (MCE) has been shown to be able to detect MBF accurately.[18] Collateral-derived MBF has also been determined during balloon occlusion and compared to simultaneously obtained CFI.[19] In this validation study, it was hypothesized that CPI accurately reflects CFI_p: $CPI = MBF_{coll}/MBF$.

CFI_p and CPI showed an excellent agreement ($r^2 = 0.92$).[19] Conversely, collateral-derived MBF measurements by MCE during balloon occlusion proved that the pressure-derived CFI exactly reflects collateral relative to normal myocardial perfusion in humans.

In case of simultaneous determination of occlusive pressure by pressure guidewire and MBF by MCE, the absolute collateral resistance can be calculated as: $R_{coll} = P_{ao} - P_{occl}/MBF_c$ (dyn·sec·cm^{-5}).

Pros: Noninvasive assessment of collateral flow in case of CTOs.
Contras: Complex procedure; needs additional operator for ultrasound scanner. Variable quality of image acquisition. Extensive postprocessing.
Conclusion: Appropriate for exact risk stratification and monitoring of TCP in case of CTOs.

CONCLUSIONS

The human coronary collateral circulation

(1) contributes to prevention of ischemia in approximately 25% to 30% of patients with CAD,
(2) contributes to reduction of the area at risk, and thus infarct size,
(3) reduces future cardiovascular events,
(4) improves overall survival,
(5) can be promoted therapeutically by several approaches, and
(6) should be assessed accurately and quantitatively.

Today, the gold standard for clinical assessment of coronary collateral function is the invasive, pressure- or Doppler sensor–derived CFI.

REFERENCES

1. Cohnheim J, von Schulthess-Rechberg A. Ueber die Folgen der Kranzarterienverschliessung für das Herz. Virch Arch Pathol 1881; 85:790–795.
2. Pijls NH, van Son JA, Kirkeeide RL, et al. Experimental basis of determining maximum coronary, myocardial, and collateral blood flow by pressure measurements for assessing functional

stenosis severity before and after percutaneous transluminal coronary angioplasty. Circulation 1993; 87:1354–1367.

3. Seiler C, Fleisch M, Garachemani A, et al. Coronary collateral quantitation in patients with coronary artery disease using intravascular flow velocity or pressure measurements. J Am Coll Cardiol 1998; 32:1272–1279.
4. Habib GB, Heibig J, Forman SA, et al. Influence of coronary collateral vessels on myocardial infarct size in humans. Results of phase I Thrombolysis in Myocardial Infarction (TIMI) trial. The TIMI Investigators. Circulation 1991; 83:739–746.
5. Elsman P, van't Hof AW, de Boer MJ, et al. Role of collateral circulation in the acute phase of ST-segment-elevation myocardial infarction treated with primary coronary intervention. Eur Heart J 2004; 25:854–858.
6. Meier P, Zbinden R, Togni M, et al. Coronary collateral function long after drug-eluting stent implantation. J Am Coll Cardiol 2007; 49:15–20.
7. Reimer KA, Ideker RE, Jennings RB. Effect of coronary occlusion site on ischaemic bed size and collateral blood flow in dogs. Cardiovasc Res 1981; 15:668–674.
8. Gloekler S, Rutz T, Seiler C. Six simultaneously employed methods to gauge the coronary collateral flow of the decade. Kardiovaskuläre Medizin 2007; 10:298–300.
9. Perera D, Kanaganayagam GS, Saha M, et al. Coronary collaterals remain recruitable after percutaneous intervention. Circulation 2007; 115(15):2015–2021.
10. Werner GS, Emig U, Mutschke O, et al. Regression of collateral function after recanalization of chronic total coronary occlusions: A serial assessment by intracoronary pressure and Doppler recordings. Circulation 2003; 108:2877–2882.
11. Meier B, Luethy P, Finci L, et al. Coronary wedge pressure in relation to spontaneously visible and recruitable collaterals. Circulation 1987; 75:906–913.
12. De Marchi SF, Meier P, Oswald P, et al. Variable ECG signs of ischemia during controlled occlusion of the left and right coronary artery in humans. Am J Physiol Heart Circ Physiol 2006; 291:H351–H356.
13. Meier P, Gloekler S, Zbinden R, et al. Beneficial effect of recruitable collaterals: A 10-year follow-up study in patients with stable coronary artery disease undergoing quantitative collateral measurements. Circulation 2007; 116:975–983.
14. Seiler C, Pohl T, Lipp E, et al. Regional left ventricular function during transient coronary occlusion: Relation with coronary collateral flow. Heart 2002; 88:35–42.
15. Rentrop KP, Cohen M, Blanke H, et al. Changes in collateral channel filling immediately after controlled coronary artery occlusion by an angioplasty balloon in human subjects. J Am Coll Cardiol 1985; 5:587–592.
16. Seiler C, Billinger M, Fleisch M, et al. Washout collaterometry: A new method of assessing collaterals using angiographic contrast clearance during coronary occlusion. Heart 2001; 86:540–546.
17. Seiler C, Fleisch M, Billinger M, et al. Simultaneous intracoronary velocity- and pressure-derived assessment of adenosine-induced collateral hemodynamics in patients with one- to two-vessel coronary artery disease. J Am Coll Cardiol 1999; 34:1985–1994.
18. Vogel R, Indermuhle A, Reinhardt J, et al. The quantification of absolute myocardial perfusion in humans by contrast echocardiography: Algorithm and validation. J Am Coll Cardiol 2005; 45:754–762.
19. Vogel R, Zbinden R, Indermuhle A, et al. Collateral-flow measurements in humans by myocardial contrast echocardiography: Validation of coronary pressure-derived collateral-flow assessment. Eur Heart J 2006; 27:157–165.

15 Merits and limitations of FFR for the evaluation of ambiguous lesions

Special attention to ostial location, bifurcation, tandem lesion, ectasic vessel, in-stent restenosis, and diffuse disease

Clarissa Cola and Manel Sabaté

INTRODUCTION

Coronary angiography remains the "gold standard" for the diagnosis of epicardial coronary artery disease. However, precise quantification of lesions severity is limited because of the complex three-dimensional geometry of epicardial plaques. Moreover, coronary physiology and physiopathological effects of lesions cannot be determined.[1–3] Accurate identification of both normal and diseased vessel segments is complicated by diffuse disease as well as by angiographic artefacts of contrast streaming, image foreshortening, and calcification. Bifurcation or ostial lesion locations may be obscured and difficult to assess by overlapping branch segments. Measurements of coronary pressure and flow provide complementary information to the anatomic characterization of coronary disease obtained by both angiographic and intravascular ultrasound examinations. In particular, fractional flow reserve (FFR) has been demonstrated to be a useful tool to easily and reliably assess lesions significance and physiopathology.[4] FFR in the catheterization laboratory can facilitate timely and more objective decision making about therapy, especially in complex and difficult settings. Table 15.1 summarizes current recommendations for the application of physiologic measurements with FFR, and shows how its use in more complex settings is still under investigation.[5] In this chapter, we describe the utility and limitations of this technique in particular complex situations, such as ostial location, bifurcation, tandem lesions, ectasic vessel, and in-stent restenosis (Table 15.1).

LEFT MAIN AND AORTO-OSTIAL LESIONS

Ostial lesions assessment and their real significance is often a problem for the interventionalist because of the technical limitations of angiography in this setting. This problem is especially critical when the left main coronary artery (LMCA) is involved. Furthermore, in patients with multivessel disease, uncertainty about the contribution of the LMCA to the clinical syndrome may confuse the issue of whether to perform percutaneous coronary intervention (PCI) or surgery. FFR is used to assess LMCA narrowings, with specific technical considerations. In general, for the evaluation of aorto-ostial lesions, the engagement of the guiding catheter must be very careful and it is necessary to use intravenous adenosine instead of intracoronary injection to achieve a stable maximal hyperemia. In particular, because of the potential for the guiding catheter to obstruct blood flow across an ostial narrowing, FFR measurements should be performed with the guiding catheter disengaged from the coronary ostium. Initially, the guiding catheter and wire pressures should be equalized before the guiding catheter is seated. Then, the guiding catheter is seated and the pressure wire is advanced into the artery. The guiding catheter is then disengaged and the intravenous adenosine infusion initiated. After 1 to 2 minutes, FFR is calculated, and thereafter the wire can be pulled back slowly to identify the exact location of the pressure drop.

In case of a distal left main narrowing, this procedure may be performed twice, first with the pressure wire in the left anterior descending artery and again with the wire in the circumflex artery.

The same technique is applied to the assessment of right coronary artery ostial lesion, with particular attention to the guiding catheter engagement and flow obstruction. In this case, as for the LMCA also, the catheter is disengaged before measuring the FFR.

Table 15.1 Recommendations for physiological assessment with FFR in the Catheter Laboratory

Applications of physiologic measurements in the catheterization laboratory			
PCI guideline recommended uses		**Applications of coronary pressure under study**	
Assessment of intermediate coronary stenoses (30–70% luminal narrowing) in patients with anginal symptoms. Coronary pressure or Doppler velocimetry may also be useful as an alternative to perform noninvasive functional testing to determine whether an intervention is warranted.	Class IIa, *level of evidence: B*	Determination of one or more culprit stenoses (either serially or in separate vessels) in patients with multivessel disease	N/D
		Evaluation of ostial or distal left main and ostial right lesions, especially when these regions cannot be well visualized by angiography.	N/D
Assessment of the success of PCI in restoring flow reserve and to predict the risk of restenosis.	Class IIb, *level of evidence: C*	Guidance for treatment of serial stenoses in a coronary artery.	N/D
		Determination of significance of focal treatable region in vessel with diffuse coronary artery disease.	N/D
Evaluation of patients with anginal symptoms without an apparent angiographic culprit lesion.	Class IIb, *level of evidence: C*	Determination of prognosis after stent deployment.	N/D
		Assessment of stenosis in patients with previous (nonacute, lasting >6 days) myocardial infarction.	N/D
Routine assessment of the severity of angiographic disease in patients with a positive, unequivocal noninvasive functional study is not recommended.	Class III, *level of evidence: C*	Assessment of lesions in patients with treated unstable angina Pectoris	N/D
		Assessment of the collateral circulation	N/D

Figure 15.1 demonstrates the influence of engagement of guiding catheter in coronary artery ostia and the obstruction of different catheter sizes. Figure 15.2 demonstrates how the pressure changes due to the engagement of the catheter can alter FFR results.

The use of FFR in isolated LMCA stenosis has been examined in 54 patients.[6] In 30 patients with an FFR <0.75, surgery was performed, while in the remaining 24 patients with an FFR ≥0.75, medical therapy was chosen to be performed. After a follow-up of 3 years, no differences in event-free survival rate or functional class were seen between the groups. None of the patients in the medical group experienced myocardial infarction or died. Although limited data has been reported so far in this scenario, the measurement of FFR in ambiguous left main is a highly practical diagnostic tool for clinical decision making.

BIFURCATION LESIONS

Angiographic evaluation of bifurcation lesions and their significance is hampered by the inherent limitations of angiography, especially the overlap of adjacent vessels, angulations, and foreshortening of the side branch origin.[7] This difficulty can be demonstrated by the need for additional angulated radiographic views, and at times, cannot be resolved despite the angiographer's best efforts. Bifurcation treatment on its turn is still technically difficult. Despite the emergence of drug-eluting stents (DES), bifurcation lesions have a higher restenosis rate, espe-

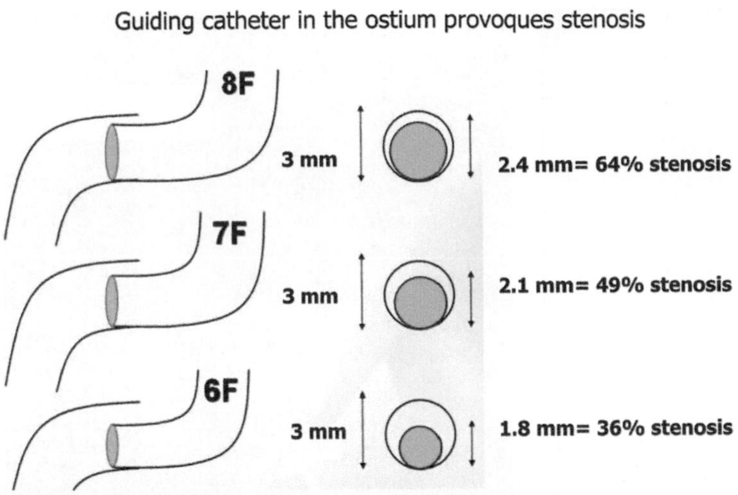

Figure 15.1 Influence of engagement of guiding catheter in coronary artery ostia and the obstruction of different catheter sizes. Every different catheter size determines a level of obstruction, according to the ostium diameter. When a plaque affects the ostium, the catheter engagement may cause an important flow obstruction, which is visualized with pressure damping. This may influence the physiologic assessment of the stenosis itself, because hyperemia may not be achieved.

cially at the ostium of the side branch in comparison with simple lesions.[7–8] Stenting of the side branch may not always be necessary and angiographic assessment of lesion morphology may not be enough to decide the best treatment option.

Physiologic determination of hemodynamic significance of bifurcation lesions can be reliably addressed with FFR. Separate FFR analysis of each branch can be performed to assess the hemodynamic significance of each stenosis and provides functional information.[7] A few studies have evaluated the role of FFR in the decision-making process to treat side branch. Koo et al.[9] evaluated the feasibility and safety of physiological assessment of jailed side branches with

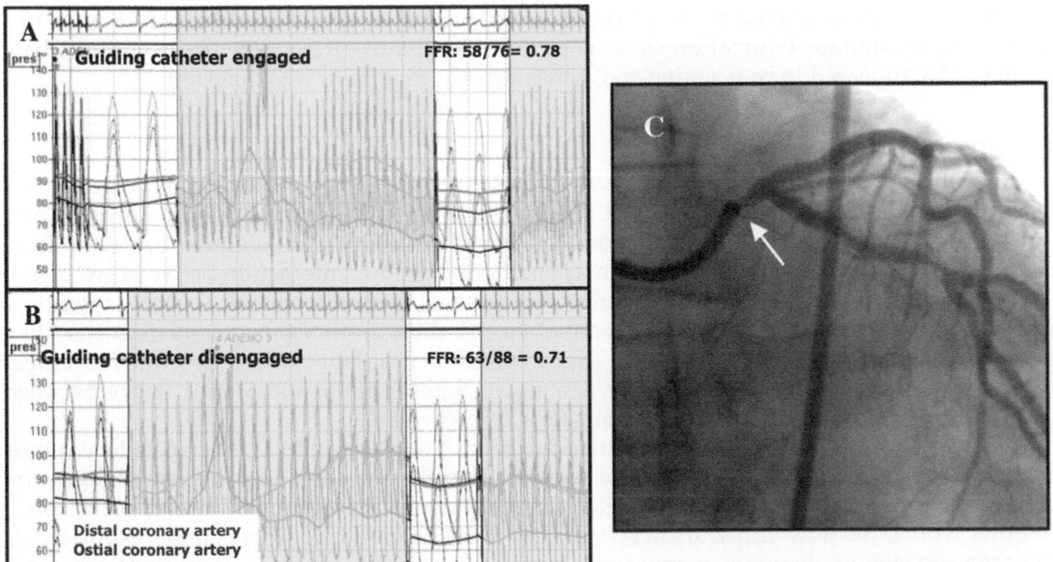

Figure 15.2 Fractional flow reserve measured in left main coronary artery (LMCA) with ostial lesion. (**A**) The measurement is performed with the guiding catheter engaged in the LMCA; FFR is 0.78. (**B**) The same assessment performed with the catheter disengaged, where the FFR gives a significant value of 0.71. (**C**) Angiography of LMCA ostial lesion.

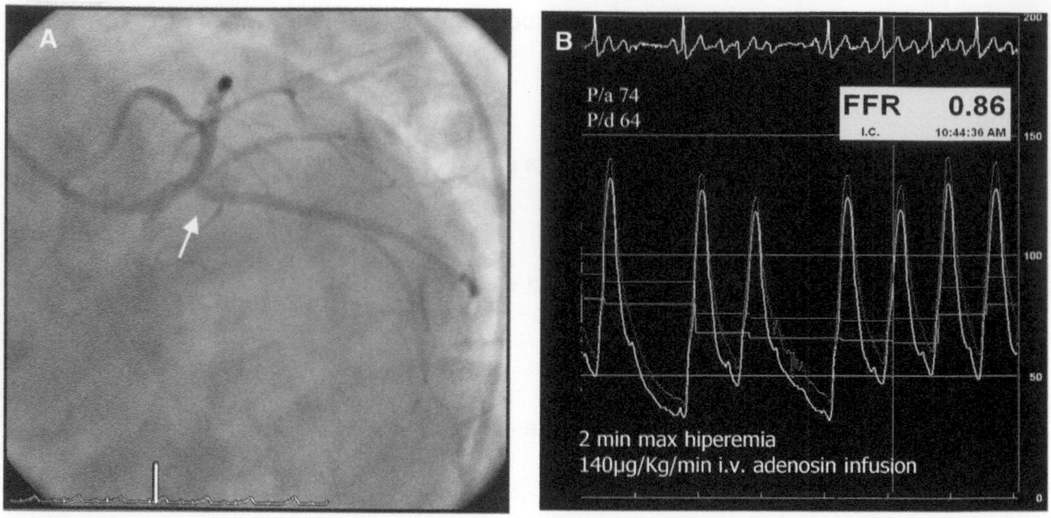

Figure 15.3 (**A**) Angiographic image showing an ambiguous bifurcation stenosis at distal left main–circumflex artery–intermediate, difficult to evaluate by means of angiography alone. (**B**) The fractional flow reserve measured on the lesion represented in panel (A); FFR value of 0.86, obtained after 2 minutes of intravenous infusion of adenosine (140 μg/kg/min). This value is not significant, so the treatment was deferred.

FFR in 97 patients. The study demonstrated that no lesion with <75% stenosis by quantitative coronary angiography (QCA) had FFR <0.75, and among 73 lesions with >75% stenosis, only 20 were functionally significant.[9] Thus, most of the lesions involving the jailed side branch might not have functional significance and do not require revascularization. Ziaee et al.[7] showed that 80% of patients with >70% stenosis of the side branch had FFR >0.75 in their cohort. In these studies, the measurement of FFR suggests that most of these lesions do not have functional significance and that intervention on these nonsignificant lesions may not be necessary. The use of FFR in the assessment of bifurcation lesions might prevent unnecessary interventions in lesions that are not functionally restrictive. The need for revascularization of the side branch in bifurcation lesions can be guided by hemodynamic parameters as determined by FFR. Figure 15.3 depicts an ambiguous bifurcation stenosis at distal left main–circumflex artery–intermediate branch. FFR appeared to be negative and, consequently, treatment was deferred.

TANDEM LESIONS

In the event where more than one stenosis is present in the same vessel, the hyperemic flow (and pressure gradient) through the first one will be influenced by the presence of the second one and vice versa. One stenosis will mask the true effect of its serial counterpart by limiting the ability to achieve maximum hyperemia. The fluid dynamic interaction between two serial stenoses depends on the sequence, severity, and distance between lesions as well as the flow rate. When the distance between two lesions is greater than six-times the vessel diameter, they generally behave independently and the overall pressure gradient is the sum of the individual pressure losses at any given flow rate. When serial stenoses are at a shorter distance between each other, they inhibit maximal hyperemic flow in that vessel.

The interpretation of FFR in the scenario of serial stenosis within a coronary artery is thus complex. Experiments document that the calculation of the apparent FFR (hyperemic pressure distal/hyperemic pressure proximal to each stenosis) overestimates the FFR of either lesion.[10] In other words, the flow impediment specific to the interrogated stenosis is underestimated as the opposite stenosis becomes more severe because maximal hyperemic flow is not achieved. For these reasons, the best way to evaluate serial stenosis is with intravenous 140 μg/kg/min adenosine induction of continuous hyperemia, which allows the pressure wire to be pulled back across the lesions. The focus of maximal gradient can be identified. Subsequent measures can be performed to evaluate the unmasked significance of other stenosis.

Branches between serial stenosis may inhibit maximal hyperemia because of "branch steal." One can imagine hyperemic flow down this branch may increase a gradient across the proximal stenosis by increasing flow, but may decrease the distal lesion gradient because of "steal" by the branch. By corollary, dilating the distal stenosis may not alter the hyperemic gradient across the proximal stenosis. Dilating the proximal stenosis may subsequently increase the gradient over the distal lesion. A similar situation exists for bifurcation lesions. A thorough understanding of the inhibition of maximal hyperemic flow caused by serial stenosis and intervening branches can allow the use of FFR in this situation. After intervention, FFR can be repeated in the remaining nontreated stenosis. From the practical point of view, one may consider first to demonstrate the presence of ischemia relative to the entire vessel and then treat the spot of the maximal drop in pressure after FFR continuous pullback under maximal hyperemia. Then reevaluate the entire segment after spot stenting and decide whether to keep treating any additional spot of relevant pressure drop. In such scenario, one would not expect to have a poststenting FFR completely normalized and an additional diagnostic tool (i.e., intravascular ultrasound) may be necessary to rule out technical problems inside the stent.

DIFFUSE DISEASE

Normal coronary arteries do not provide any relevant resistance to blood flow. This lack of resistance is identified by the absence of any pertinent decline of pressure along the epicardial coronary artery, even not at hyperemia. In diffuse disease, there is a gradual decline of coronary pressure (i.e., increasing resistance) along the coronary artery, which is best observed during hyperemia. Similarly, in patients with hemodynamically significant coronary artery disease affecting one vessel, a decline in pressure is often observed along the course of other arteries with angiographically unapparent atherosclerotic disease. De Bruyne et al.[11] demonstrated that in 37 strictly normal coronary arteries, FFR was 0.97 ± 0.02, whereas in 106 nonstenotic arteries in patients with atherosclerosis elsewhere in the coronary circulation, FFR was 0.89 ± 0.08, with frank ischemic values <0.75 in 8% of them.

As is the case in patients with serial stenosis within one coronary artery, similar considerations can be made for patients with diffuse coronary artery disease and long lesions. The pressure pullback recording at maximum hyperemia will provide the necessary information to decide if and where stenting is useful. The location of a focal pressure drops superimposed on the diffuse disease can be identified as appropriate location for stenting by the pressure pullback recording (Fig. 15.4). In the case of diffuse disease and superimposed focal lesions, it is recommended to treat only those segments with a hyperemic gradient of at least 10 mm Hg because, after placing a stent, a pressure drop of 5 to 10 mmHg is often present again after 3 to 6 months due to intimal hyperplasia. In other cases, the decline of pressure along the vessel might be so diffused that interventional treatment is not possible. In these cases, multivessel/lesion stenting can be avoided and medical treatment (or bypass surgery) is recommended. A certain amount of operator discrimination and experience is necessary for an adequate decision whether to treat these challenging vessels, but pressure measurements offer a valuable adjunct to mere angiographic guidance.[12] An additional important pitfall to consider when assessing FFR in diffuse vessel is the potential overestimation of measurements due to lack of achieving maximal hyperaemia, even after intravenous administration of adenosine. This may be specifically true in diabetic patients.[13] In this population, structural abnormalities in the coronary microcirculation, such as microaneurysm, may contribute to the impaired vasodilator response to potent coronary vasodilators. Therefore, endothelium-dependent and -independent coronary vasodilator functions may be impaired in such patients. These observations have been derived from diabetic patients with poorly controlled plasma glucose levels (HbA1 c >8.0%).[13]

MULTIVESSEL CORONARY ARTERY DISEASE

With the increasing use of coronary stents in an even more complex patient population, a frequent application of physiological assessment involves lesion selection in patients with multivessel disease. Accurate lesion selection is relevant as myocardial perfusion by means of non-invasive tests (SPECT) may fail to correctly indicate all ischemic areas in 90% of patients.[14] Often, one ischemic area may be masked by another, more severely underperfused area. Fur-

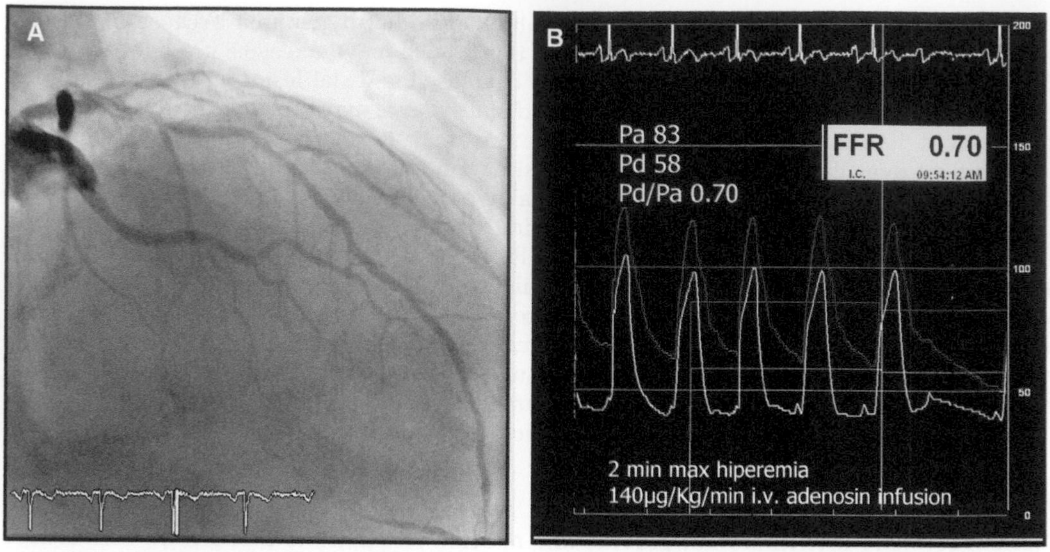

Figure 15.4 Diffuse disease in LAD coronary artery. (**A**) The angiography of a patient with diffuse stenosis in the LAD. (B) FFR results of 0.70, which lead to treatment of both the proximal and mid-segments.

thermore, when several stenoses or diffuse disease is present within one coronary artery, an abnormal myocardial hypoperfusion image cannot discriminate among the different stenosis along the length of that vessel. For clinical practice, these observations highlight those regions, which are not responsible for ischemia and may contain significant apparent narrowings, whereas other, more severe-appearing lesions may not be hemodynamically important. Coronary pressure measurements are particularly useful for localizing regions of suspected ischemia. Several small nonrandomized studies have reported the use of coronary physiology in multivessel disease.[15–18] Reiber et al. found that 4 (27%) of 15 patients with an FFR <0.75 in the territory with no perfusion abnormality had an event at 1 year, compared with 8 (9%) of 92 patients with a high FFR.[18] Data also support the safety of deferring intervention on vessels with an FFR >0.75 in patients with absent, normal, or inconclusive stress test results and multivessel coronary artery disease (CAD).[17] Moreover, in patients with multivessel disease referred for bypass surgery, patients who underwent selective PCI of hemodynamically significant stenoses had a prognosis similar to that of patients who had coronary artery bypass surgery of all angiographic diseased vessels.[14] Hence, defining the "culprit lesion" with FFR is feasible, but it is worth to notice that these studies were performed in patients with stable angina and normal ventricles: they do not validate using FFR to determine revascularization strategies in complicated scenarios involving depressed left ventricle function, diabetes mellitus, and valve disease.

IN-STENT RESTENOSIS

After stenting, about 15% to 20% of patients develop in-stent restenosis and require repeat target vessel revascularization. However, even QCA cannot reliably predict whether a stent restenosis induces ischemia. Particularly, in case of in-stent restenosis of intermediate severity (40–70%), stress perfusion myocardial scintigraphy is used for clinical decision making. FFR can be measured as a simple, reliable, and reproducible index of functional stenosis severity.[4] A FFR value <0.75 reliably identifies stenosis of native coronary arteries associated with inducible ischemia. Although FFR is reported to be a valid surrogate for myocardial scintigraphy in stenotic native coronary arteries, its utility in patients with coronary stent restenosis is unknown. Stent restenosis differs from native coronary lesions in its morphology, histology, and geometry.[19] In contrast to native coronary lesions, which may have an eccentric and complex cross-sectional geometry, stent restenosis is thought to have less-complex lesion geometry. Therefore, the lesion severity

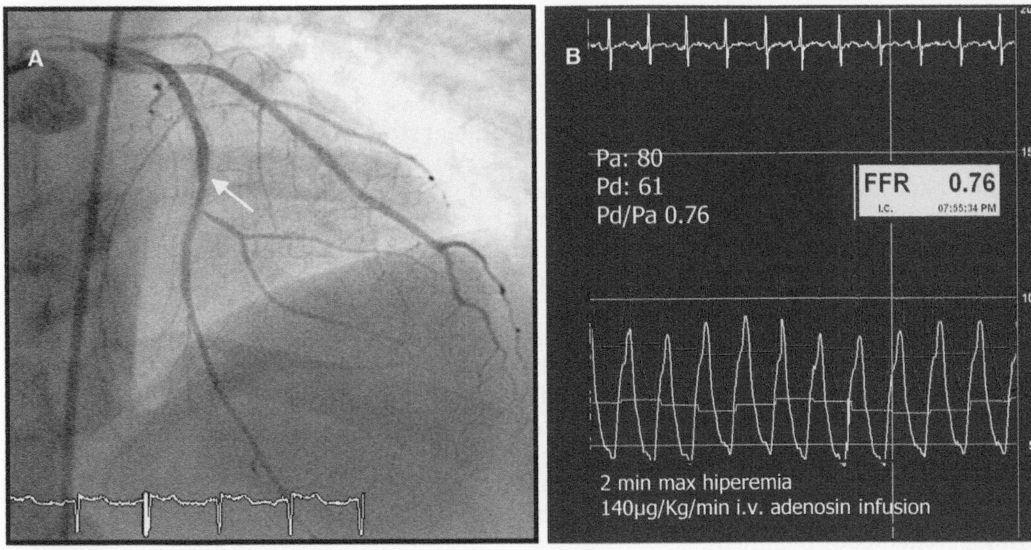

Figure 15.5 Case of in-stent restenosis. (**A**) This figure shows angiography of proximal LAD with in-stent restenosis (*white arrow*); this lesion has a borderline angiographic significance. (**B**) The physiologic assessment of the lesion shown in panel (A), with FFR 0.76—the lesion was then successfully treated with PCI.

threshold for inducing ischemia may be higher in stent restenosis than in a native lesion. Few studies addressed this issue.[20,21]

Krüger and colleagues[21] performed a small nonrandomized study and found that FFR <0.75 predicts hemodynamically significant stent restenosis, and that if FFR is >0.75, a conservative approach is justified. Moreover, the authors concluded that FFR cutoff value of 0.75 is not only valid for significant native coronary stenosis but also for stent restenosis.

The validity of this approach needs to be corroborated in a larger prospective, randomized trial, but in the clinical experience, the physiologic assessment of in-stent reestenosis significance is possible and useful for the decision making (Fig. 15.5).

ECTASIC-VESSEL

Coronary artery ectasia is characterized by disturbances in blood flow filling and washout. Angiographic signs of turbulent and stagnant flow include delayed antegrade dye filling, a segmental back flow phenomenon, and local deposition of contrast medium (stasis) in the dilated coronary segment.[22] Slow flow has been recently evaluated. In a detailed study, Akyurek et al.[23] used the Doppler wire to measure blood flow velocity and coronary flow reserve in patients with isolated coronary ectasia and in a control group. They reported a trend for lower resting blood flow velocity where coronary ectasia was present, compared with the control group. Following intracoronary administration of papaverine, a potent hyperemic stimulus, the coronary flow reserve was 1.51 in the ectasia group compared with 2.67 in the control arteries ($p = 0.001$), suggesting a combination of epicardial flow disturbances and microvascular dysfunction as the cause of myocardial ischemia. A point of interest was the estimated resting absolute volumetric flow within the ectasic vessel, found approximately three-times higher compared with control patients. Few data are available in the literature about FFR evaluation in ectasic vessel and its significance. Kim et al.,[24] with the aim to assess the mechanism of coronary dilatation on cardiac isquemia, investigated whether the slow flow and dilation causes functional stenosis and ischemia with FFR by injecting vasodilators, in a small number of subjects with unstable angina and nonsignificant stenoses at the angiogram. In this small study, the author did not find any difference in FFR evaluated with intracoronary adenosine and intracoronary nitrates. We dispose of few data in the literature, but so far FFR seems not to be the appropriate functional test to evaluate the mechanism of isquemia in the case of ectasic vessel, which could depend on the microvasculature slow flow, and not on pressure gradient.

CONCLUSIONS

In this era of expensive drug-eluting stents, a cost-effective strategy may include the determination of the hemodynamics of a stenosis in the catheterization laboratory before stenting, especially in the management of patients with multivessel disease and complex lesions. Luminography does not supply enough data to determine treatment strategy especially in complex lesions setting. Often we can end up stenting lesions, which do not need an invasive treatment; or, on the other hand, we can underestimate a severe narrowing. Some lesions that are deemed to be "hemodynamically nonsignificant" may actually be significant and should be revascularized. Hemodynamic studies can reduce the number of stents used and overall medical expenditures. The main drawback of FFR measurements occurs in the presence of microvascular disease, as this index does not take into consideration the contribution of abnormal microvasculature. Moreover, in the case of an infarction, FFR can change—it can be high for a significant lesion due to the necrotic tissue receiving blood for that given vessel.

In summary, the coronary pressure–derived FFR index is reliable for evaluating lesion-specific physiologic stenosis severity. FFR can provide us complementary information in the evaluation of ischemia beyond what can be gleaned by angiography. It is a valuable tool for clinical decision making, especially in patients with complex coronary disease, such as the above-mentioned settings, to determine the need for revascularization and the potential strategy during percutaneous treatment.

REFERENCES

1. Mintz GS, Popma JJ, Pichard AD, et al. Limitations of angiography in the assessment of plaque distribution in coronary artery disease: A systematic study of target lesion eccentricity in 1446 lesions. Circulation 1996; 93:924–931.
2. Pijls NHJ, Van Gelder B, Van der Voort P, et al. Fractional flow reserve. A useful index to evaluate the influence of an epicardial coronary stenosis on myocardial blood flow. Circulation 1995; 92:3183–3193.
3. Topol EJ, Nissen SE. Our preoccupation with coronary luminology. The dissociation between clinical and angiographic findings in ischemic heart disease. Circulation 1995; 92:2333–2342.
4. Kern MJ, Lerman A, Bech Jw, et al. Physiological assessment of coronary artery disease in the cardiac catheterization laboratory. A scientific statement from the American heart association committee on diagnostic and interventional cardiac catheterization, council on clinical cardiology. Circulation 2006; 114:1321–1341.
5. Smith SCJ, Feldman TE, Hirshfeld JWJ, et al. ACC/AHA/SCAI 2005 guideline update for percutaneous coronary intervention: A report of the American College of Cardiology/American Heart Association Task Force on Practice Guidelines (ACC/AHA/SCAI Writing Committee to Update the 2001 Guidelines for Percutaneous Coronary Intervention). percutaneous/update/index.pdf.: ACC/AHA/SCAI Writing Committee 2006.
6. Bech GJ, Droste H, Pijls NH, et al. Value of fractional flow reserve in making decisions about bypass surgery for equivocal left main coronary artery disease. Heart 2001; 86:547–552.
7. Ziaee A, Parham WA, Herrmann SC, et al. Lack of relation between imaging and physiology in ostial coronary artery narrowings. Am J Cardiol 2004; 93:1404–1407.
8. Colombo A, Moses JW, Morice MC, et al. Randomized study to evaluate sirolimus-eluting stents implanted at coronary bifurcation lesions. Circulation 2004; 109:1244–1249.
9. Koo BK, Kang HJ, Youn TJ, et al. Physiologic assessment of jailed side branch lesions using fractional flow reserve. J Am Coll Cardiol 2005; 46:633–637.
10. Pijls NHJ, De Bruyne B, Bech GJW, et al. Coronary pressure measurement to assess the hemodynamic significance of serial stenoses within one coronary artery: Validation in humans. Circulation 2000; 102:2371–2377.
11. De Bruyne B, Hersbach F, Pijls NH, et al. Abnormal epicardial coronary resistance in patients with diffuse atherosclerosis but "normal" coronary angiography. Circulation 2001; 104:2401–2406.
12. Kern MJ. Focus for the new millennium: Diffuse coronary artery disease and physiologic measurements of severity. Am Coll Cardiol Curr J Rev 2000; March/April:13–19.
13. Yanagisawa H, Chikamori T, Tanaka N, et al. Application of pressure-derived myocardial fractional flow reserve in assessing the functional severity of coronary artery stenosis in patients with diabetes mellitus. Circ J 2004; 68:993–998.
14. Botman KJ, Pijls NH, Bech JW, et al. Percutaneous coronary intervention or bypass surgery in multivessel disease? A tailored approach based on coronary pressure measurement. Catheter Cardiovasc Interv 2004; 63:184–191.

15. Chamuleau SA, Tio RA, de Cock CC, et al. Prognostic value of coronary blood flow velocity and myocardial perfusion in intermediate coronary narrowings and multivessel disease. J Am Coll Cardiol 2002; 39:852–858 [published comments in J Am Coll Cardiol 2002; 40:573 and J Am Coll Cardiol 2002; 39:859–863].
16. Chamuleau SA, Meuwissen M, van Eck-Smit BL, et al. Fractional flow reserve, absolute and relative coronary blood flow velocity reserve in relation to the results of technetium-99m sestamibi single-photon emission computed tomography in patients with two vessel coronary artery disease. J Am Coll Cardiol 2001; 37:1316–1322.
17. Chamuleau SA, Meuwissen M, Koch KT, et al. Usefulness of fractional flow reserve for risk stratification of patients with multivessel coronary artery disease and an intermediate stenosis. Am J Cardiol 2002; 89:377–380.
18. Reiber J, Schiele TM, Koeing A. Long-term safety of therapy stratification in patients with intermediate coronary lesions based on intracoronary pressure measurements. Am J Cardiol 2002; 90:1160–1164.
19. Hoffmann R, Mintz GS, Dussaillant GR, et al. Patterns and mechanisms of stent restenosis: A serial intravascular ultrasound study. Circulation 1996; 94:1247–1254.
20. Lopez-Palop R, Pinar E, Lozano I, et al. Utility of the fractional flow reserve in the evaluation of angiographically moderate in-stent restenosis. Eur Heart J 2004; 25:2040–2047.
21. Krüger S, Koch KC, Kaumanns I, et al. Use of fractional flow reserve versus stress perfusion scintigraphy in stent restenosis. Eur J Int Med 2005; 16:429–431.
22. Manginas A, Cokkinos DV. Coronary artery ectasias: Imaging, functional assessment and clinical implications. Eur Heart J 2006; 27:1026–1031.
23. Akyurek O, Berkalp B, Sayin T, et al. Altered coronary flow properties in diffuse coronary artery ectasia. Am Heart J 2003; 145:66–72.
24. Kim W, Jeong MH, Ahn YK, et al. The changes of fractional flow reserve after intracoronary nitrate and Nicorandil injection in coronary artery ectasia. Int J Cardiol 2006; 113:250–251.

16 | Clinical applications of OCT

Nobuaki Suzuki, John Coletta, Giulio Guagliumi, and Marco A. Costa

INTRODUCTION

Optical coherence tomography (OCT) is a novel optical imaging technology that provides cross-sectional tomographic imaging for biomedical structure with great spatial resolution.[1] The principle of OCT is similar to that of intravascular ultrasound (IVUS) except OCT utilizes near-infrared wavelength light instead of sound waves. The typical OCT image has a homoaxial resolution of 10 μm and a lateral resolution of 20 μm, which is 10 times higher than that of IVUS. This increased resolution, however, comes at the expense of tissue penetration. The absorption and scattering of light by biologic tissues limit OCT to a depth of ≤2 mm in endovascular tissue.[2] Yet, due to the enhanced resolution, OCT is able to detect subtle differences, which the conventional IVUS cannot depict. Endovascular images are scanned using a fiber-optic scanning catheter-endoscope. The current commercially available catheter consists of a single-mode optical fiber in a hollow rotating or translating cable that emits and scans the OCT beam radially from the catheter axis.[2] The diameter of the wire with transducer is as small as 0.014 in. Current imaging systems require proximal balloon occlusion and flush administration during image acquisition with an automated pullback speed of 1 mm/sec and creation of approximately 16 cross-sectional frames per millimeter. This level of dense longitudinal imaging coupled with incredible resolution makes OCT ideal for evaluation of vascular biology as well as the response of vascular wall to injury or device implantation. This section will focus on the clinical application of OCT and the analysis of images obtained by the most commercially available motorized pullback OCT image wire system (M2 OCT system and ImageWire, LightLab Imaging Inc., Westford, MA).

RATIONALE OF OCT IMAGING

Imaging with OCT is similar to B-mode ultrasonography, except that OCT uses low-intensity light instead of sound. The near-infrared spectrum of light is utilized because it is absorbed less by biologic tissues than visual light wavelengths. The result is improved image quality as more light can be reflected back to the transducer. Intravascular OCT utilizes a catheter terminating with a rotating single fiber-optic core, which is able to emit and receive light. The source beam is split into a signal that is sent to the sample and another that is sent to a known reference path. The micron-scale resolution of OCT is achieved through detection of very small echo delays (10–15 sec) between light reflected from the reference path and the sample. Information on the time-of-flight of the reflected light from the sample is compared to that of the reference path, which allows precise measurement of distance (low-coherence interferometry). As the wire is rotated, the beam is swept over the lumen. The data acquired is processed by a computer located within the imaging system for the creation of each cross-sectional image. Each cross-sectional is collected along the catheter pullback path and displayed in a real-time 2D array at different transverse positions (tomographic views). Imaging rates of current systems are 15 to 30 frames/sec at pullback speeds of 1 mm/sec. The complete data set is stored electronically for off-line analysis.

IMAGE ACQUISITION PROCEDURE

The creation of optimal images requires both proper vessel selection as well as strict procedural adherence. Careful analysis of the entire vessel prior to imaging includes determination of vessel caliber, and the presence of disease proximal to the target imaging segment, branch vessels, collaterals, and vessel tortuosity. Optimal vessels are between 2.5 and 3.5 mm in diameter and void of disease in the proximal segment, branch or collateral vessels as well as excessive tortuosity (<90° bend).

Key technical components include positioning of the occlusion balloon, inflation pressure, type of flush, and rate and timing of infusion. The occlusion balloon should be placed in a healthy segment of vessel to reduce risk of vessel injury. Gentle, low-pressure inflation (0.5 atm) is performed under fluoroscopic guidance. Although normal saline may be used, Lactated Ringer's solution is preferred in order to minimize arrhythmia. The automated contrast injector pump with warming cuff is used to first warm the solution to 37°C and then to infuse 0.5 cc/sec continuously through the balloon lumen. Proper timing of infusion minimizes infusion time and enables optimal timing for image acquisition. Because red blood cells absorb and scatter the OCT signal, optimal image acquisition requires removing or displacing blood from the segment of interest. To limit contamination of blood during analysis, contrast infusion should start a few seconds prior to balloon occlusion. Finally, the OCT wire should be positioned 5 to 10 mm distal to the target segment. This not only ensures that the target segment will be captured but also allows for off-line analysis adjustments of the z-offset (described below).

EVALUATION OF THE OCT IMAGES

Evaluation of coronary atherosclerosis

Previous investigation has shown that plaque rupture in acute coronary syndrome is often found at the shoulder of atheromatous plaques with a large lipid core and a thin fibrous cap, termed thin-capped fibrous atheroma (TCFA). Other seminal postmortem investigation showed that the cap thickness of TCFA associated with plaque rupture was under 65 μm.[3] Much attention has focused on plaque stabilization. Although previous research demonstrated the effect of statin therapy on regression of coronary plaque,[4] it remains unclear whether this change alters the TCFA. Until the development of OCT, no method for accurate in vivo assessment of the TCFA has been available. The ability of OCT to accurately measure fibrous-cap thickness was previously reported.[5] Not only does OCT have the required resolution to assess TCFA, it also has the potential to repeatedly assess the effect of therapies or interventions on the TCFA over multiple time points. This unique combination holds promise for future drug and device development.

Assessment of plaque characterization can also guide device selection and help predict complications in endovascular procedures, as described with IVUS.[6] Validated evaluation of plaque characteristics by OCT has already been described (Table 16.1),[7] although various factors, including distance of the plaque from the transducer or presence of residual blood in the lumen, affect the image. The limited depth of penetration with OCT may restrict assessment of the extent of the lipid pool or accurate depiction of transluminal remodeling associated with such plaques.

Further investigation for the quantitative assessment of plaque characteristics in larger caliber arteries is warranted. Plaque characterization by OCT has been validated in arteries from amputated legs[8] and cadavers,[7] however, in vivo characterization of atherosclerotic plaques has yet to be investigated.

Table 16.1 Definition of plaque characteristics in OCT images

Intimal hyperplasia	Signal-rich layer nearest lumen
Media	Signal-poor middle layer
Adventitia	Signal-rich, heterogeneous outer layer
Internal elastic lamina	Signal-rich band (~20 mm) between the intima and media
External elastic lamina	Signal-rich band (~20 mm) between the media and adventitia
Plaque	Loss of layered appearance, narrowing of lumen
Fibrous plaque	Homogeneous, signal-rich region
Macrocalcification	Large, heterogeneous, sharply delineated, signal-poor or signal-rich region or alternating signal-poor and signal-rich region
Lipid pool	Large, homogeneous, poorly delineated, signal-poor (echolucent) region
Fibrous cap	Signal-rich band overlying signal-poor region

Evaluation for percutaneous coronary intervention

Evaluation of minimal lumen diameter (MLA)

The impact of MLA on clinical outcomes in patients with contemporary percutaneous coronary intervention (PCI) has already been demonstrated.[9] However, the measurement of lumen area by means of IVUS still needs considerable manual interpolation and might be unrealistic for some clinical situations. On the other hand, coronary OCT imaging software (developed through collaboration between University Hospitals Case Medical Center Core Laboratory, Cleveland, OH, and LightLab Imaging Inc.) enables measurement of the lumen area automatically and instantaneously by utilizing the intensity differences of the lumen-wall interface (Fig. 16.1). The ability of OCT to delineate such interfaces permits less interpolation than with other clinically available imaging modalities. As such, reproducibility of measurements of MLA by OCT has been very good.[10]

Evaluation of neointimal coverage and stent apposition

The superior spatial resolution of OCT is also well suited for the evaluation of neointimal hyperplasia (NIH) and stent apposition. It has been reported that late stent thrombosis, which is a serious complication of PCI in the drug-eluting stent (DES) era, is potentially caused by delayed vascular healing.[11,12] There is also a considerable number of patients with incomplete strut

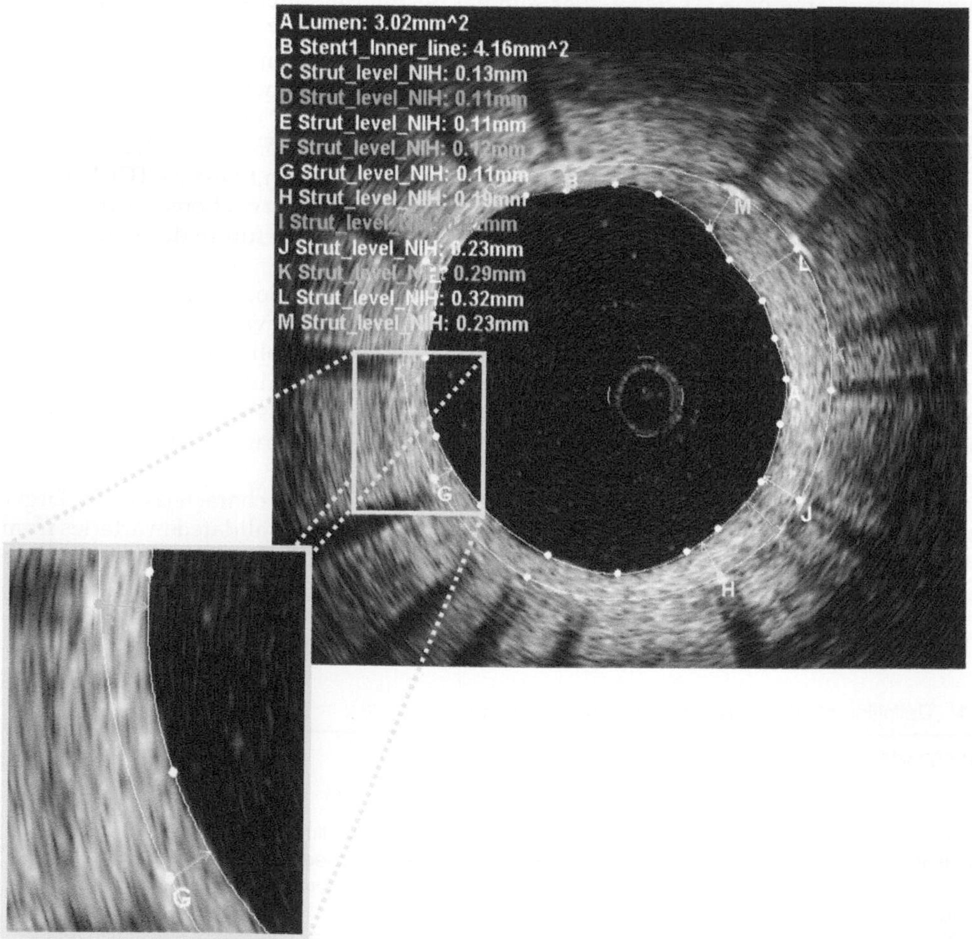

Figure 16.1 Strut-level analysis demonstrating automatic lumen contour, stent contour along the inner strut edge, and strut-level neointimal hyperplasia measurements. A portion of the image is enlarged to demonstrate the high resolution provided by optical coherence tomography (OCT).

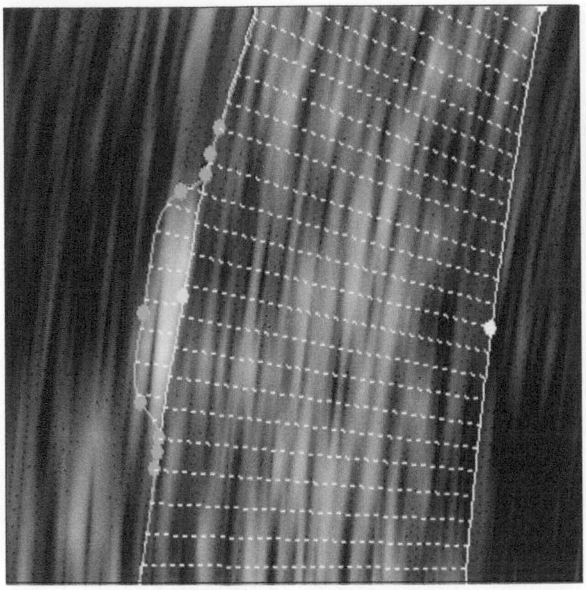

Figure 16.2 The thickness of Taxus Liberte strut reflections was measured. The mean measured thickness was 37 ± 8 μm (20–70 μm), far less than the actual strut thickness (97 μm).

coverage or malapposition even 8 months after DES implantation.[13] However, the influence of stent malapposition on clinical outcome has yet to be defined.[14,15] The superiority of OCT compared to IVUS in the detection of stent malapposition has been established.[16] Moreover, we have shown that detection of strut malapposition with OCT is accompanied with sufficient reproducibility, further bolstering this promising analysis methodology.[12] As such, OCT evaluation should be included in contemporary DES clinical trials. Consensus thresholds for optimal strut apposition and coverage with OCT must be established prior to such widespread investigation.

Evaluation of stent struts

Because the light source of OCT cannot penetrate metal, caution is advised for the interpretation of individual stent struts, as the high-intensity signal of the OCT image does not represent the morphology of the true strut. Using the previously mentioned software, the thickness of the high-intensity shadow representing a stent strut (Fig. 16.2) was determined. Thickness measurements of 2250 struts in 471 cross-sectional OCT images were obtained 6 months after Taxus Liberte stent implantation. Measurements were determined along the vector whose initial point was located at the centroid of the vessel. Interestingly, the mean measured thickness was 37 ± 8 μm (20–70 μm), which is definitely smaller than the actual strut thickness (97 μm). This inadequate strut thickness has been observed by others.[17] Therefore, the high-intensity structure cannot represent the strut thickness but is rather a reflection of the strut surface. As such, we propose that preserving a consistent selection point for the entire data set is required for accurate data reporting.

Evaluation of coronary thrombus

Recent data demonstrated the influence of thrombus burden pre-DES implantation on development of stent thrombosis.[18] Investigations with IVUS, angioscopy, and pathology have also revealed the presence of thrombus after DES implantation even at the late follow-up phase.[19,20] Seminal postmortem investigation determining the diagnostic accuracy OCT to detect coronary thrombus showed the ability of OCT to not only identify but also to differentiate red and white thrombi. Red thrombi were identified as high-backscattering protrusions inside the lumen of the artery, with signal-free shadowing in the OCT image while white thrombi were identified as low-backscattering projections in the OCT image.[21] Anecdotally, we observed a highly backscattered signal within the coronary artery of a living patient being evaluated in the follow-up phase of DES implant which appeared between consecutive sessions of OCT transducer pullback

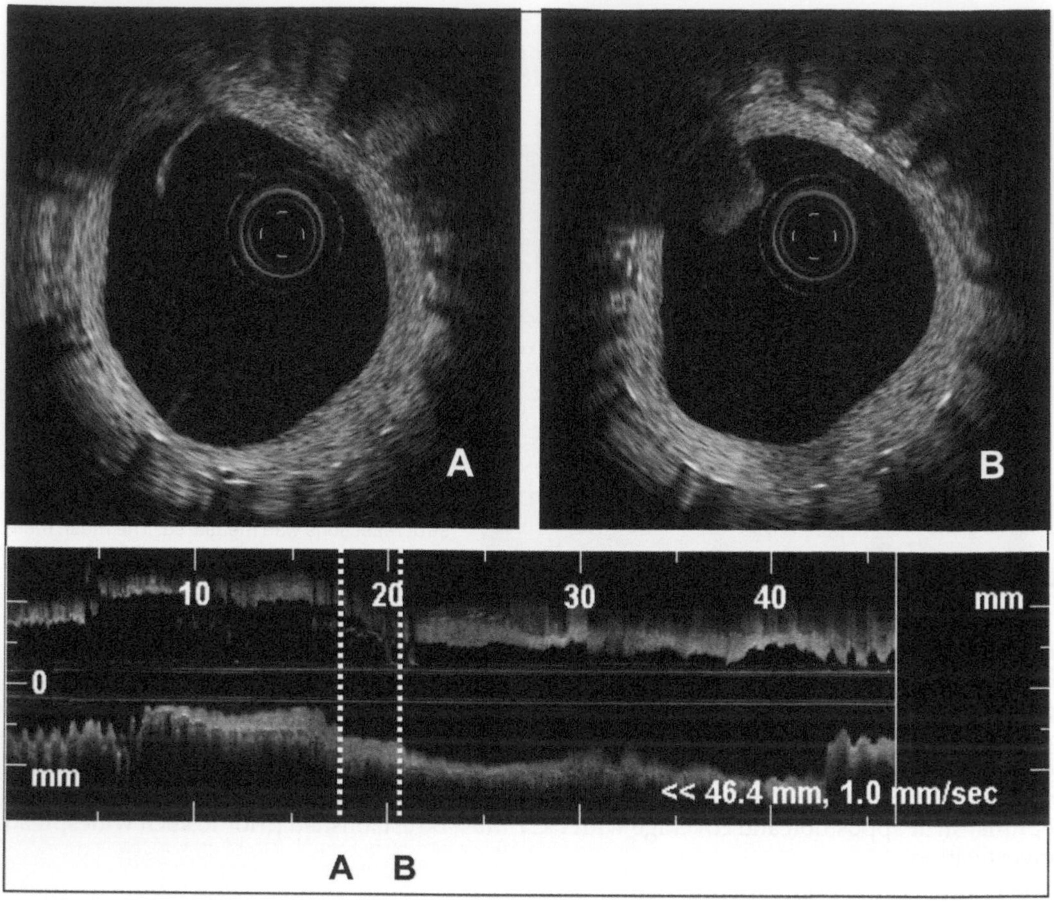

Figure 16.3 In vivo demonstration of highly backscattered intraluminal signal which appeared between consecutive OCT wire pullback procedures. This appearance is similar to the postmortem findings of thrombus.

(Fig. 16.3). With the increasing clinical use of OCT, it is apparent that similar findings need investigation beyond postmortem comparison. Careful interpretation is required to differentiate such in vivo findings.

Common image artifacts

Shadow

When the OCT signal encounters a highly reflective surface, a shadow is cast beyond this surface and away from the OCT wire. Although no meaningful data can be gathered from within this zone, some information may be inferred. An example is when a strut in close proximity to the transducer casts a large shadow on the distal lumen contour (Fig. 16.4). The resulting void may be misinterpreted as a side branch; however, careful analysis of not only the current frame but also adjacent frames will rectify similar dilemmas.

Sew-up

Rapid movement of the artery or transducer during the capture of a single frame may result in image misalignment. This appears as a sew-up artifact (Fig. 16.5). Information within the sew-up zone is uninterruptable; however, data from other areas of the frame, although not considered optimal, can be interpreted.

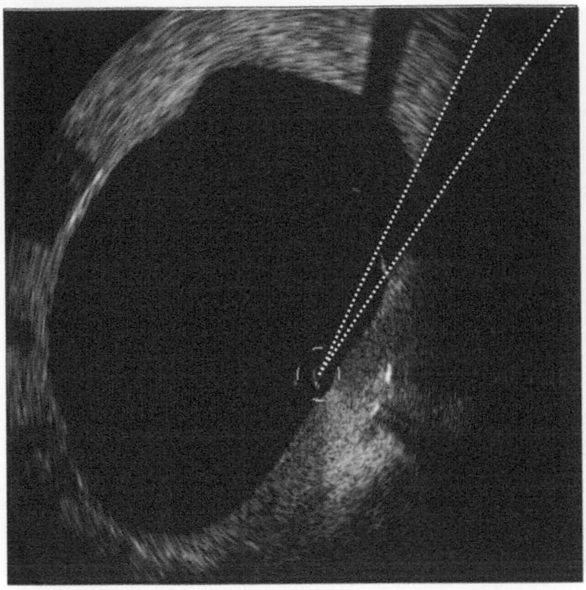

Figure 16.4 Shadow artifact created by a stent strut. The resultant loss of lumen contour maybe misinterpreted as a side branch vessel. Careful analysis of adjacent frame is warranted for such findings.

Reverberation

As with echocardiography, harmonics can create replica images occurring at fixed distances from the original object. These reverberations can occur with highly reflecting objects, such as stent struts (Fig. 16.6). This is distinguished from stent struts in overlapped stent segments by the fact that reverberation artifact occurs completely within the path of the shadow created by the original object. In stent-overlapped segments, the distal overlapped strut intensity should not exist directly behind the luminal strut signal (Fig. 16.7).

Sunflower artifact

The sunflower artifact is caused by an eccentric wire position within the vessel lumen. The slim profile of the wire allows the wire to float freely within the lumen. When it rests against the lumen wall a common strut artifact is encountered. With optimal stent expansion it is assumed that each strut resides relatively parallel to the local lumen contour. Because OCT relies on reflected

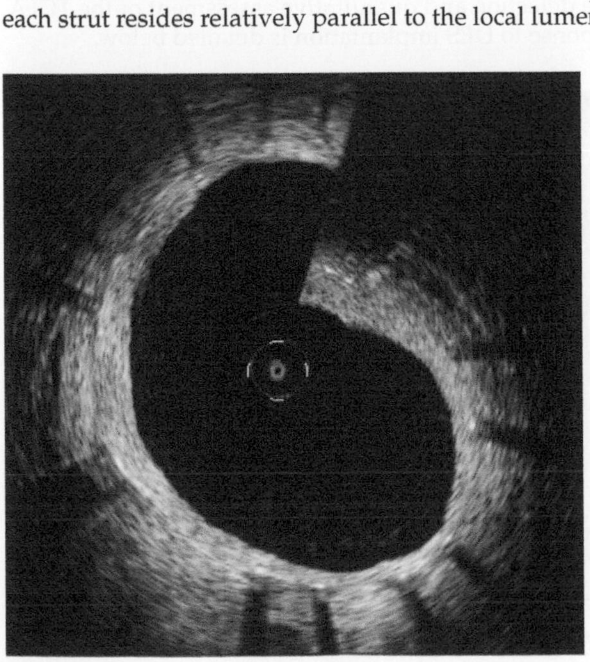

Figure 16.5 Rapid movement of the vessel or imaging wire during acquisition of a single cross-section may result in sew-up artifact.

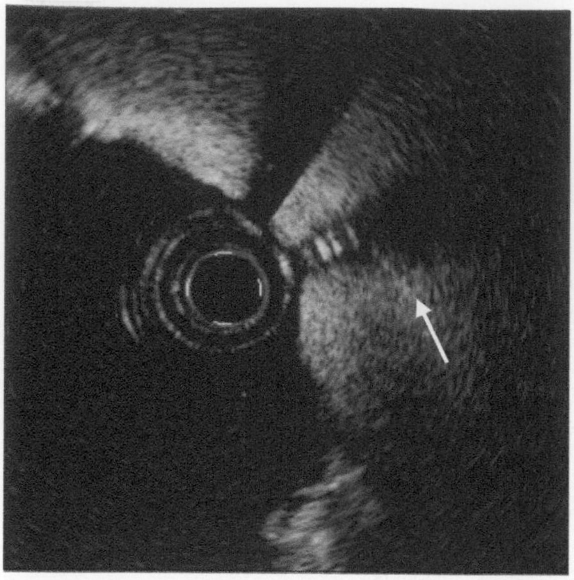

Figure 16.6 Reverberation of a highly reflective object is shown (*arrow*). The signals are maintained along the exact vector of the primary object.

light for image creation, light returns to the wire from object surfaces, which are perpendicular to the light source. Eccentric wire position may restrict the accessible surface area of stent struts to the light source. The resultant strut reflection appears to face the transducer similar to the way a sunflower "follows" the sun (Fig. 16.7). In this case, the strut is clearly not parallel to the lumen contour. An illustrated strut was inserted to further explain our hypothesis.

Development of quantitative OCT analysis

To take advantage of spatial resolution of OCT, quantitative OCT analysis is required. Although automated lumen and stent volume analysis is available with IVUS, the required automatic processes are currently in development for OCT. However, the evaluation of the vascular healing following DES implantation for individual stent strut is impossible by IVUS because of lower spatial resolution. OCT allows the establishment of quantitative "strut level" analysis. Although similar methodology can be applied to the detection and quantitative assessment of the TCFA, the process for analyzing the vascular response to DES implantation is detailed below.

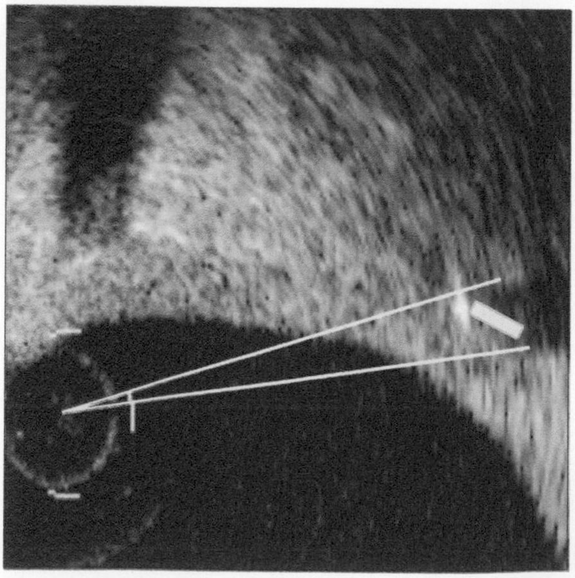

Figure 16.7 The appearance of the stent strut is always directed toward the imaging wire. This sunflower artifact is accentuated by eccentric wire position. An illustrated strut helps to demonstrate this phenomenon.

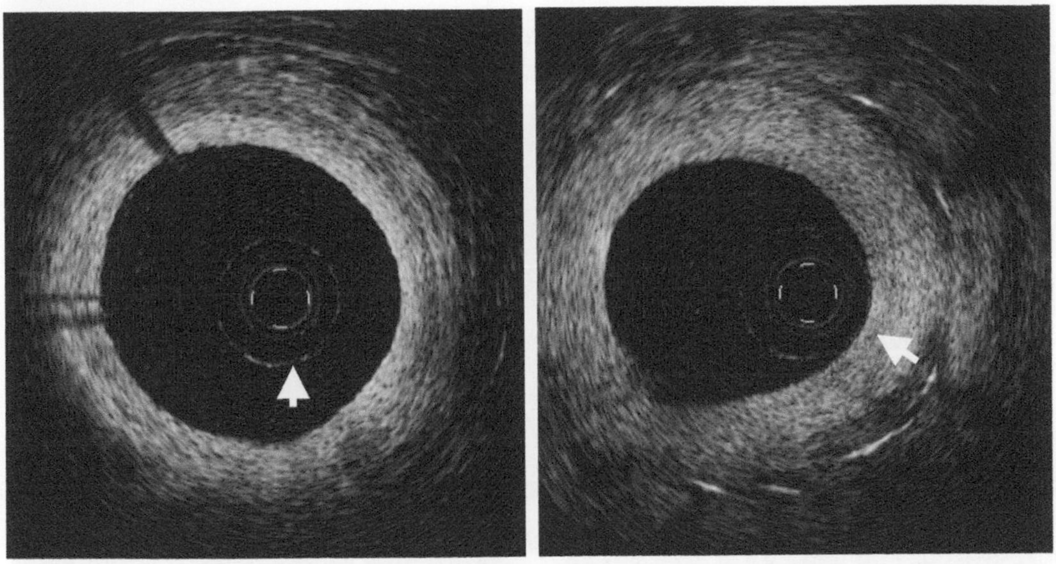

Figure 16.8 Identification of the ImageWire border for the image calibration is simplified when the wire rests upon the vessel lumen.

Calibration

Accurate calibration is mandatory to fully realize the spatial resolution of OCT. The size of the OCT image is calibrated by adjusting the z-offset. The ImageWire, which is directed in the z-axis of the image, stretches or compresses when stress, most commonly at the initiation of a pullback, is applied. The wire diameter is also affected by heat generated by the rotation of the wire throughout image acquisition. To maintain accurate measurements, the z-offset must be readjusted prior to off-line analysis. Four alignment sites corresponding to the actual outer diameter of the ImageWire are automatically superimposed upon the wire represented on each image frame. The recommended optimal z-offset occurs when the outer edge of the ImageWire sheath, delineated easily if the sheath is in contact with the lumen wall (Fig. 16.8), rests on all four alignment sites. In order to validate this method, we analyzed the known diameter of the introducing catheter with various z-offset alignments. The mean lumen diameter of the catheter was obtained when all the four alignments were on the outer edge of the ImageWire (Fig. 16.9). We investigated the optimal alignment for 13 cases. Only 2 (15.4%) cases correlated the recommended z-offset to accurate catheter measurement. The best-fit pattern was determined for each case (Fig. 16.10). In four cases, the optimal z-offset was obtained when the wire was completely contained within the fiducial marks. Thus, using a standardized z-offset showed differences of approximately ±3.9% in length and ±6.3% in area determinations, more than that of intra- or interobserver variability.[10] This may lead to significant differences in serial evaluations even within the same patient. For optimal calibration, we advocate individualized determination of z-offset for each case based upon measurement of a known reference, the guiding catheter. In cases where a known reference is not imaged, an accepted z-offset profile must be uniformly employed. For such cases, we recommend having as many marks rest upon the outer edge of the wire. This careful step will permit confident offline analysis.

Lumen area measurement

Lumen contour delineation and area measurement are performed automatically, although the minor correction is permitted and occasionally necessary (Fig. 16.1).

Stent area measurement

The stent inner line is delineated manually. A point is placed on the center of the luminal edge of each strut reflection (Fig. 16.1). The software connects these points to create a representative stent contour, which enables automatic area determination.

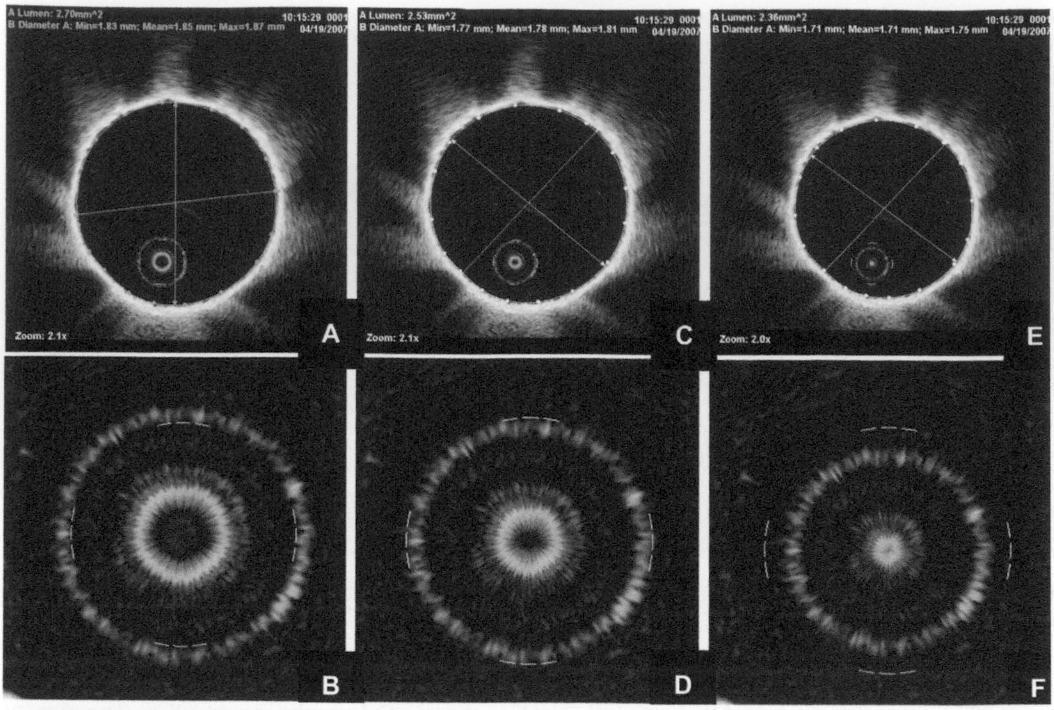

Figure 16.9 Differences in z-offset affect the accuracy of measurements. Guiding catheter (6F) lumen diameter was determined for the same cross-sectional image using three different z-offsets. The lumen measurements in (**A**), (**C**), and (**E**) were obtained from the z-offsets shown in (**B**), (**D**), and (**F**), respectively. In this case, z-offset shown in (**D**) resulted in the most accurate lumen diameter.

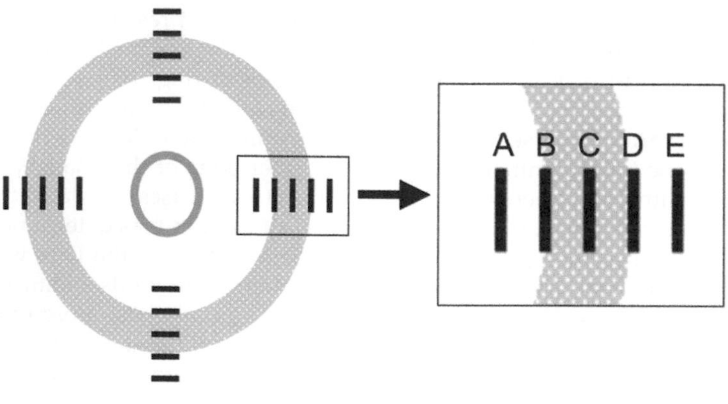

2B2C	2C2D	1C3D	4D	2D2E	3D1E	4E
1 (7.7%)	1 (7.7%)	1 (7.7%)	2 (15.4%)	3 (23.1%)	1 (7.7%)	4 (30.8%)

Figure 16.10 Optimal z-offset was determined based on the measured diameter of the guiding catheter. Actual diameter ±2.5% was defined as an acceptable measurement. The profile of the z-offset is shown by how many of the z-offset lines were classified A–E for each case, according to the illustration shown. Of the 13 cases, the z-offset with four lines on the outer edge (4D) was optimal in only two (15.4%) cases. The optimal profile of the remaining 11 cases is illustrated in the table. This data indicates that the optimal z-offset should be determined independently for each case.

Neointimal hyperplasia and malapposition measurement

An important aspect of the stent strut level analysis by OCT is the ability to evaluate the distance of each strut to the lumen in an automated fashion. The distance measured from the strut surface to the lumen along the line directed toward the lumen center will indicate NIH in the case of an embedded strut. NIH is indicated by a positive measurement along the automatically assigned vector. The area of NIH is easily extrapolated by subtracting the lumen area from the stent area (Fig. 16.1) in cross-sections demonstrating complete strut coverage. In the case of strut malapposition, the vector is directed from the strut away from the lumen center to the lumen contour. The resulting negative value indicates malapposition.

Linear extensions from stent to lumen contours

Once both stent and lumen contours are completed, the software is able to create linear extensions from the strut to the lumen for 360 lines in 1° increments. The associated measurement of NIH or strut malapposition is assigned to each ray thereby allowing regional assessment for each cross-section (Fig. 16.11).

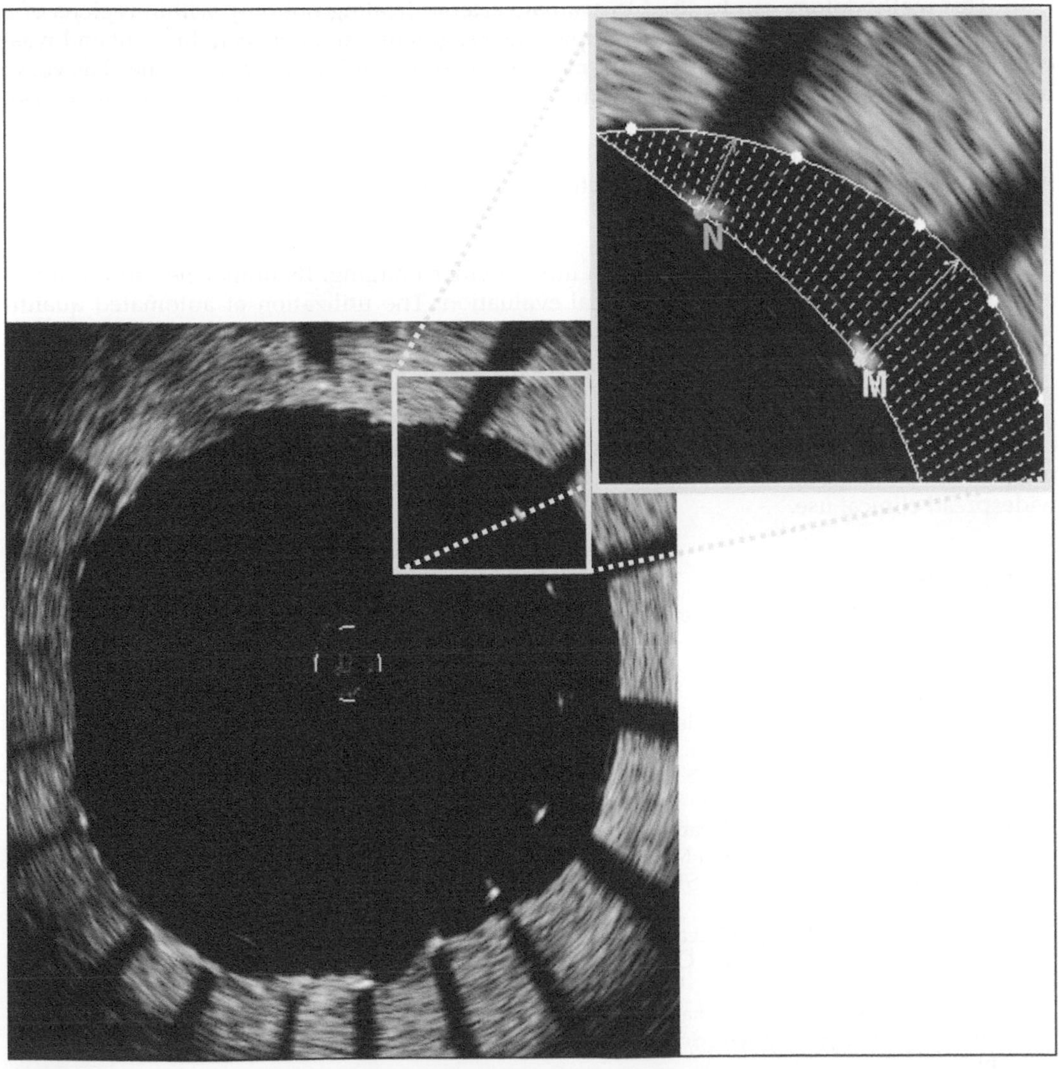

Figure 16.11 Dedicated software allows for the creation of the linear extensions between two specified contours. Using the lumen centroid as the origin of the extensions, 360 lines are provided in 1° increment. In this case, the extension can be seen between the malapposed stent struts and the underlying lumen.

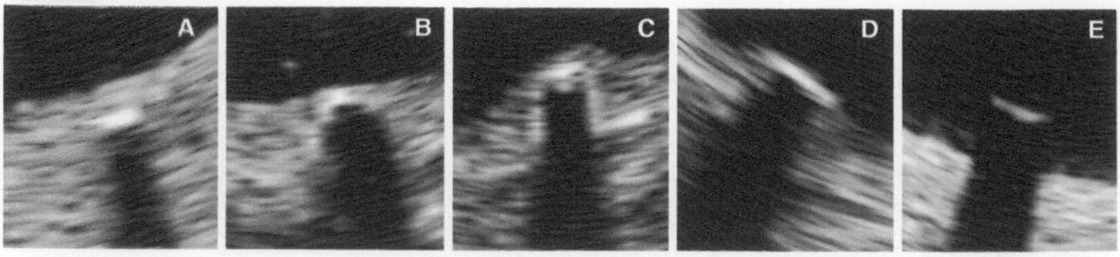

Figure 16.12 Classification of strut apposition by OCT. Frames (**A–E**) represent Types I, II, IIIa, IIIb, and IV, respectively. Type I, totally embedded strut. Type II, embedded subintimally without disruption of lumen contour. Type IIIa, completely embedded with disruption of lumen contour. Type IIIb, partially embedded with extension of strut into lumen. Type IV, complete strut malapposition (blood able to exist between strut and lumen wall).

Qualitative strut level analysis

The relationship between stent strut and vessel wall can be defined and stratified into four categories (Fig. 16.12).

This methodology can be used to evaluate arterial healing not only within regions of a single-stented segment but also in overlapped-stent segments, and between different endovascular devices. Whether this level of assessment will correlate with clinical outcomes has yet to be determined, however, this type of data may provide insight into the vascular healing process. The vascular response to stents of various strut compositions, polymer coatings or medications at varying dosages can be assessed serially. This may aide preclinical device trials and may improve current delays in device introduction for clinical use.

SUMMARY

OCT clearly represents a breakthrough in intravascular imaging. Its unmatched resolution is extremely well suited for coronary arterial evaluation. The utilization of automated quantitative systems for OCT images certainly represents a major advance for the analysis of coronary atherosclerosis and vascular response to endovascular devices in humans. As technologic advances eliminate the need for proximal balloon occlusion, increase pullback speed, and improve signal-to-noise ratio to allow better visual penetration into the vessel wall, the clinical role of intravascular OCT will inevitably be expanded. It is anticipated that software improvements enabling on-line automated quantitative analysis will further propel OCT into widespread clinical use.

REFERENCES

1. Huang D, Swanson EA, Lin CP, et al. Optical coherence tomography. Science 1991; 254:1178–1181.
2. Fujimoto JG. Optical coherence tomography for ultrahigh resolution in vivo imaging. Nat Biotechnol 2003; 21:1361–1367.
3. Burke AP, Farb A, Malcom GT, et al. Coronary risk factors and plaque morphology in men with coronary disease who died suddenly. N Engl J Med 1997; 336:1276–1282.
4. Nissen SE, Nicholls SJ, Sipahi I, et al. Effect of very high-intensity statin therapy on regression of coronary atherosclerosis: The ASTEROID trial. JAMA 2006; 295:1556–1565.
5. Kume T, Akasaka T, Kawamoto T, et al. Measurement of the thickness of the fibrous cap by optical coherence tomography. Am Heart J 2006; 152:755.e1–755.e4.
6. Kawaguchi R, Oshima S, Jingu M, et al. Usefulness of virtual histology intravascular ultrasound to predict distal embolization for ST-segment elevation myocardial infarction. J Am Coll Cardiol 2007; 50:1641–1646.
7. Jang IK, Bouma BE, Kang DH, et al. Visualization of coronary atherosclerotic plaques in patients using optical coherence tomography: Comparison with intravascular ultrasound. J Am Coll Cardiol 2002; 39:604–609.
8. Meissner OA, Rieber J, Babaryka G, et al. Intravascular optical coherence tomography: Comparison with histopathology in atherosclerotic peripheral artery specimens. J Vasc Interv Radiol 2006; 17:343–349.
9. Sonoda S, Morino Y, Ako J, et al. Impact of final stent dimensions on long-term results following sirolimus-eluting stent implantation: Serial intravascular ultrasound analysis from the sirius trial. J Am Coll Cardiol 2004; 43:1959–1963.

10. Suzuki Y, Guagliumi G, Sirbu V, et al. Validation of a novel automated optical coherence tomography analysis system for evaluation of vascular healing after DES implantation. Am J Cardiol 2007; 100:140L.
11. Virmani R, Guagliumi G, Farb A, et al. Localized hypersensitivity and late coronary thrombosis secondary to a sirolimus-eluting stent: Should we be cautious? Circulation 2004; 109:701–705.
12. Sousa JE, Costa MA, Farb A, et al. Images in cardiovascular medicine. Vascular healing 4 years after the implantation of sirolimus-eluting stent in humans: A histopathological examination. Circulation 2004; 110:e5–e6.
13. Siqueira DA, Abizaid AA, Costa Jde R, et al. Late incomplete apposition after drug-eluting stent implantation: Incidence and potential for adverse clinical outcomes. Eur Heart J 2007; 28:1304–1309.
14. Hong MK, Mintz GS, Lee CW, et al. Late stent malapposition after drug-eluting stent implantation: An intravascular ultrasound analysis with long-term follow-up. Circulation 2006; 113:414–419.
15. Tanabe K, Serruys PW, Degertekin M, et al. Incomplete stent apposition after implantation of paclitaxel-eluting stents or bare metal stents: Insights from the randomized TAXUS II trial. Circulation 2005; 111:900–905.
16. Bouma BE, Tearney GJ, Yabushita H, et al. Evaluation of intracoronary stenting by intravascular optical coherence tomography. Heart 2003; 89:317–320.
17. Tanigawa J, Barlis P, Di Mario C. Intravascular optimal coherence tomography: Optimisation of image acquisition and quantitative assessment of stent strut apposition. Eurointerv 2007; 3:128–136.
18. Sianos G, Papafaklis MI, Daemen J, et al. Angiographic stent thrombosis after routine use of drug-eluting stents in ST-segment elevation myocardial infarction: The importance of thrombus burden. J Am Coll Cardiol 2007; 50:573–583.
19. Suzuki N, Angiolillo D, Monteiro C, et al. Variable histological and ultrasonic characteristics of restenosis after drug-eluting stents. Int J Cardiol. 2008; 130:444–448.
20. Awata M, Kotani J, Uematsu M, et al. Serial angioscopic evidence of incomplete neointimal coverage after sirolimus-eluting stent implantation: Comparison with bare-metal stents. Circulation 2007; 116:910–916.
21. Kume T, Akasaka T, Kawamoto T, et al. Assessment of coronary arterial thrombus by optical coherence tomography. Am J Cardiol 2006; 97:1713–1717.

17 Viability assessment and cardiac function

Carlos Eduardo Rochitte and Tiago Senra

INTRODUCTION

Cardiac function, generally expressed as, but not restricted to, left ventricular (LV) function, is of critical importance as it relates to mortality and clinical prognosis in a broad range of cardiac pathologies.[1] Cardiovascular magnetic resonance (CMR) has the unique capability of precisely determining LV function without geometric assumptions due to its three-dimensional (3-D) nature and high temporal and spatial resolutions.[2] In coronary artery disease (CAD), myocardial viability is another important parameter, as patients with LV dysfunction but with viable myocardium undergoing revascularization can benefit from up to an 80% reduction in annual mortality.[3] Evaluation of myocardial viability by CMR using late gadolinium enhancement (LGE) protocols in these patients is now considered a gold standard.[4,5]

This chapter will discuss the technical and clinical considerations of cardiac magnetic resonance in the evaluations of patients with CAD.

CARDIAC FUNCTION ASSESSMENT—TECHNIQUES AND APPLICATIONS

Cardiac function is currently evaluated using CMR by a fast gradient–echo pulse sequence called steady-state free precession (SSFP). This technique allows the acquisition of 20 to 40 images per heart cycle synchronized to the electrocardiogram in a single expiratory breath-hold providing optimal temporal resolution and delineation of endocardial and epicardial contours. Images acquired by SSFP techniques show a dark myocardium and bright blood cavity with high signal and contrast-to-noise ratios, which in association with very short repetition and echo times allows optimal use of parallel imaging and results in excellent temporal resolution and image quality. Imaging is independent of acoustic windows and may be performed in any desired plane.

LV systolic function is analyzed from short-axis images that span the entire left ventricular chamber from base to apex, thus allowing the use of true 3-D quantification methods using Simpson's rule, which is known to be superior to 2-D methods of LV quantification (Fig. 17.1).[6] In addition, the well-defined endocardial and epicardial borders on SSFP images allow easy and reproducible manual as well as semiautomated contour detection of inner and outer LV borders, leading to accurate LV mass and function measurements (Fig. 17.2). The higher accuracy in the evaluation of LV function by CMR has led to a reduction in sample size requirements for studies of remodeling in heart failure, resulting in cost-effective implications in clinical research.

LV mass is an important predictor of morbidity and mortality, especially in patients with systemic hypertension. Here, CMR has also been considered the reference method for the evaluation of LV mass due to its high accuracy and low interobserver variability.[6] Diastolic function can be assessed by two different techniques using CMR: (1) the phase contrast evaluation of flow in the mitral valve generates velocity and volumetric curves of transmitral flow similar to Doppler imaging; and (2) the peak filling rate is a technique that relies on the detection of volumetric changes in the LV over time on cine dynamic images. Although diastolic function can be precisely evaluated by CMR, this application has been less frequently used in the clinical routine, due to its lower temporal resolution compared to echocardiography.

Regional myocardial function is best evaluated by myocardial tagging, an imaging protocol that consists of saturated lines that label the myocardium throughout the cardiac cycle and can be used to quantify any deformation or abnormality. This protocol allows precise and objective evaluation and quantification of systolic segment dysfunction in different clinical scenarios such as in CAD (at rest or during pharmacologic stress) as well as diastolic segment dysfunction such as in pericardial adherence (Fig. 17.3).

The dynamic CMR imaging techniques described above can also be used for the evaluation of right ventricle (RV) function, especially important in patients with congenital heart disease, primary pulmonary hypertension, or arrhythmogenic right ventricular dysplasia. Importantly,

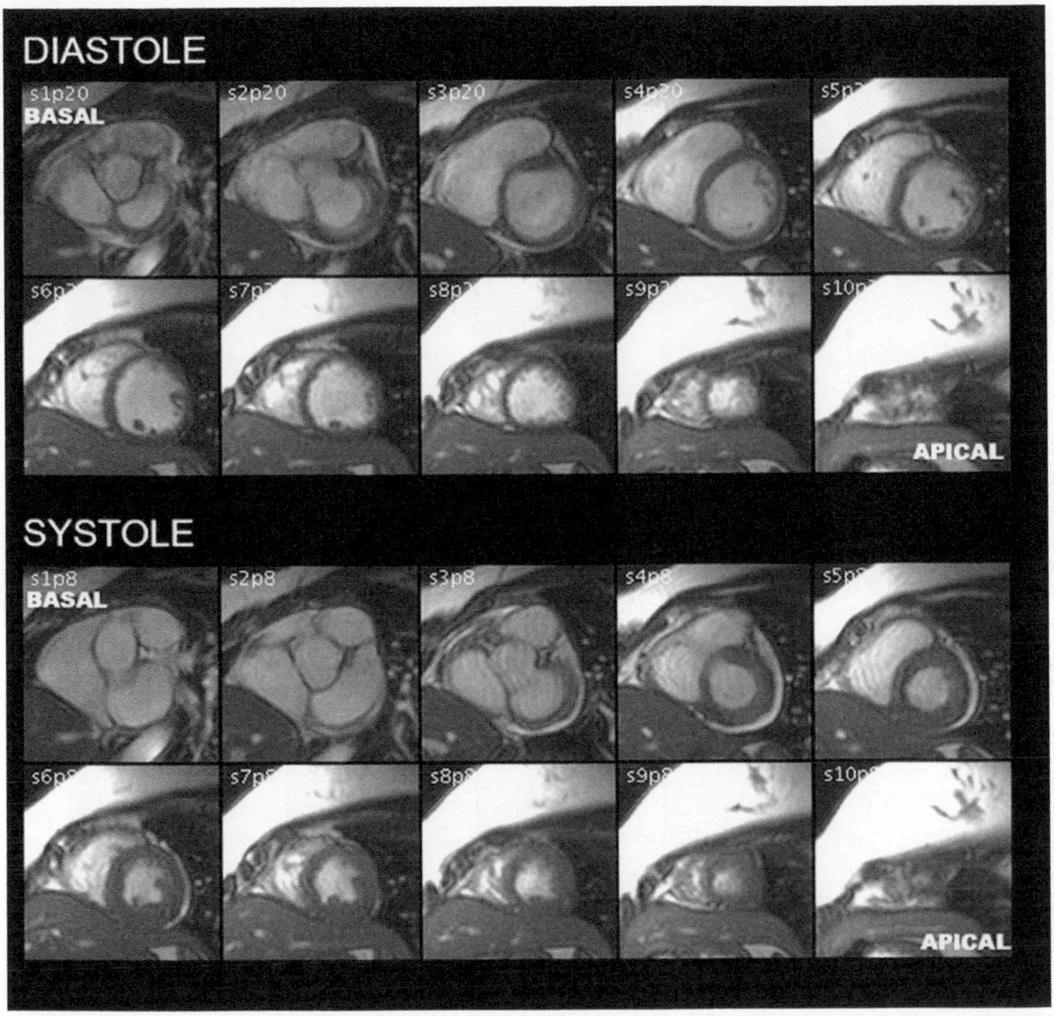

Figure 17.1 Short-axis SSFP images depicting the LV in diastole (*upper panel*) and systole (*bottom panel*) from base to apex in a patient with normal function.

normal LV and RV function parameters have been shown to be dependent on age, sex, and body surface area.[7,8]

At rest, regional wall thinning and akinesia raise the suspicion of absence of myocardial viability due to myocardial injury. However, these parameters are not definitive in myocardial viability determination,[9] as they do not directly address the presence of viable cells, which is best assessed using the LGE imaging technique.

Wall motion abnormalities can be detected using pharmacological CMR stress testing, with the use of high-dose dobutamine (up to 40 μg/kg/min plus atropine and metoprolol, in a protocol similar to stress echocardiography). New wall motion abnormalities during stress testing have been used as a surrogate for the diagnosis of myocardial ischemia (Fig. 17.4), whereas myocardial viability can be detected using low-dose dobutamine (up to 20 μg/kg/min) CMR imaging, where areas of akinesia or dyskinesia that improve contractility indicate preserved myocardial viability.[10]

MYOCARDIAL VIABILITY ASSESSMENT—TECHNIQUES AND APPLICATIONS

CMR is currently considered as one of the best available clinical tools for myocardial viability assessment. Several imaging techniques have been developed over the last years to assess myocardial viability using CMR, including segment contractility evaluation during low-dose

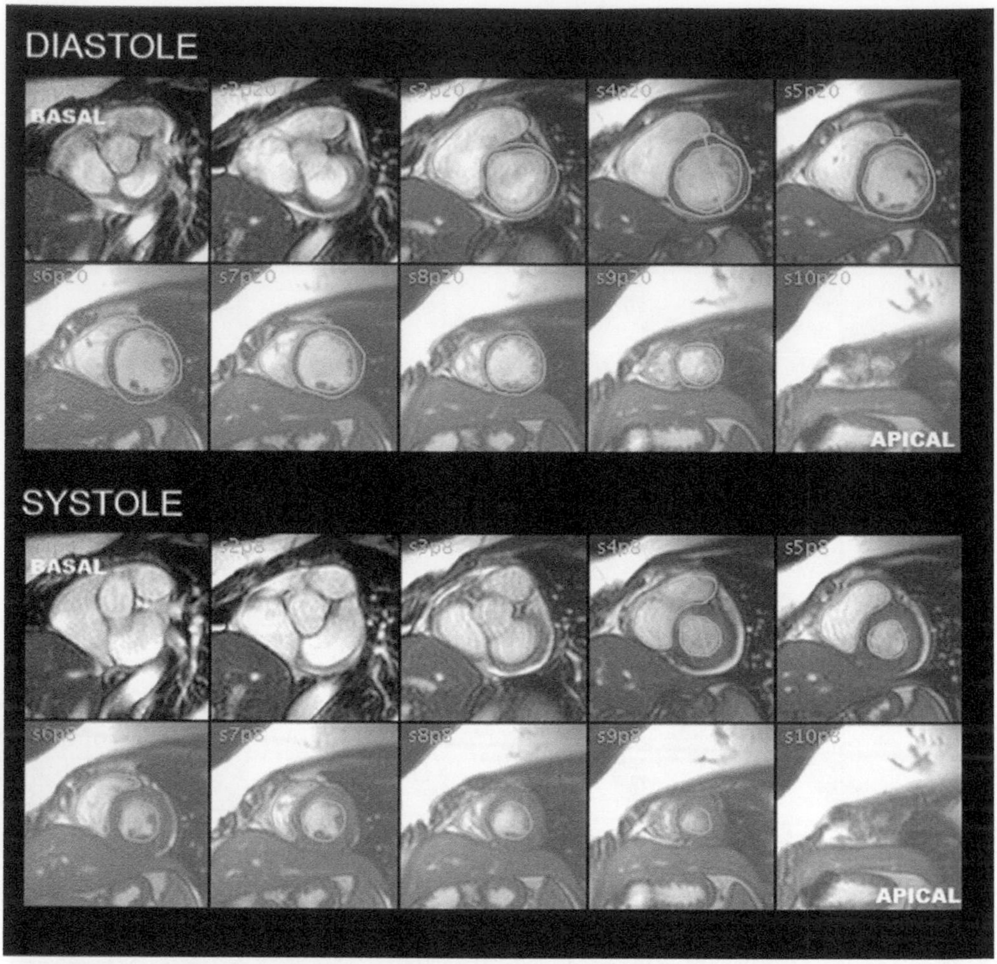

Figure 17.2 Short-axis SSFP images depicting RV and LV function measurements by the Simpson's method with manual delineation of endocardial and epicardial contours in diastole (*upper panel*) and systole (*bottom panel*) in the same patient mentioned in Figure 17.1.

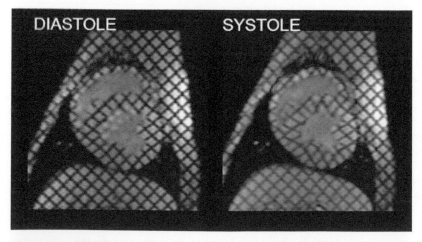

Figure 17.3 Short-axis tagging images in a canine experiment showing the gridlines in end-diastole and end-systole. Note the deformation of the myocardial tag lines during end-systole compared to the thoracic wall lines without any deformation.

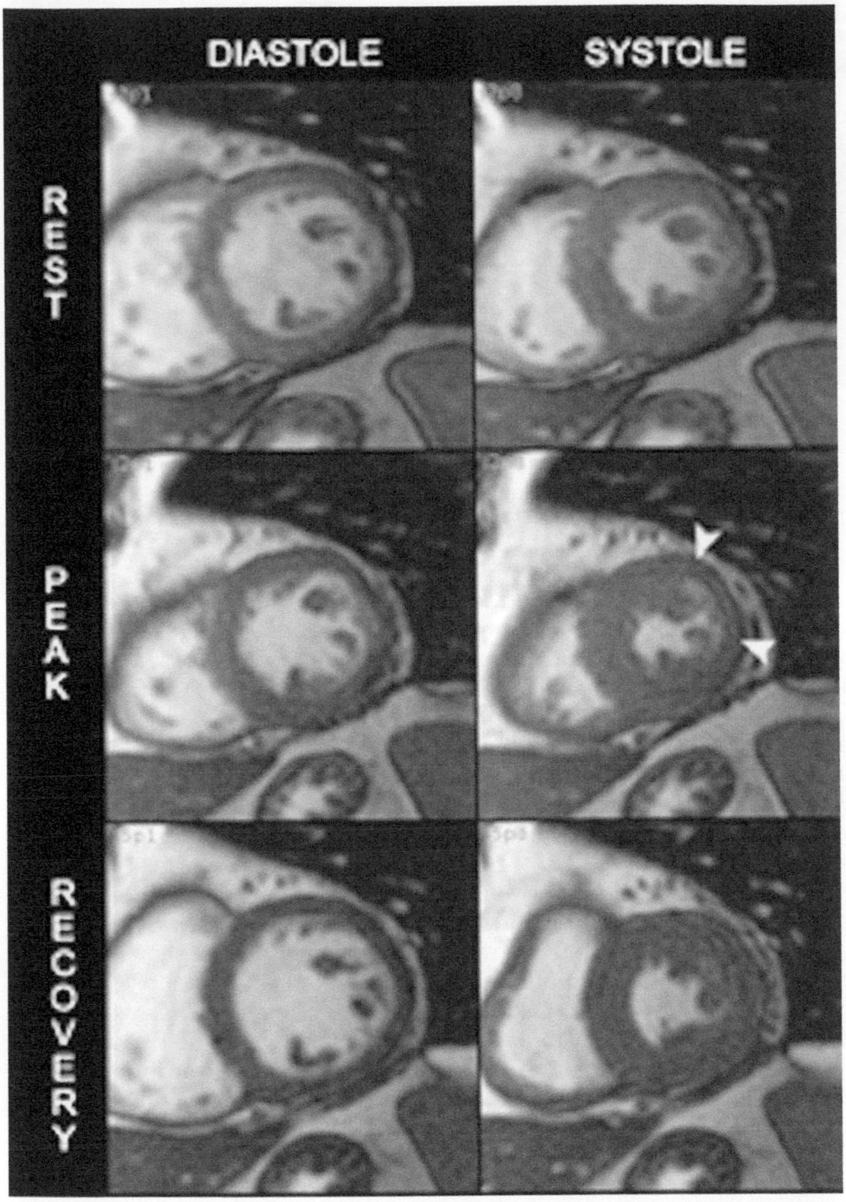

Figure 17.4 Short-axis SSFP images acquired at rest (*upper row*), peak stress with dobutamine infusion (*middle row*) and recovery with metoprolol (*bottom row*) in diastole (*left column*) and systole (*right column*). Note the new wall-motion abnormality in the anterolateral segment (segment between arrowheads) seen during systolic stress images that is absent at rest and disappeared at recovery, indicating myocardial ischemia.

dobutamine infusion, systolic myocardial thickening, sodium imaging,[11] and analysis of the energetic/metabolic profile through spectroscopy.

However, LGE is the most commonly used imaging technique in clinical practice due to its close correlation to clinical and pathological data, ease of use, and lack of any pharmacological stress. LGE has also been shown to have prognostic value in ischemic and nonischemic cardiac pathologies.[12,13]

The principles for LGE detection in myocardial infarct imaging using gadolinium-based contrast CMR were initially proposed by Lima and colleagues.[14] Later, several authors validated LGE quantifications of myocardial infarction in different clinical scenarios and established its prognostic value.[15]

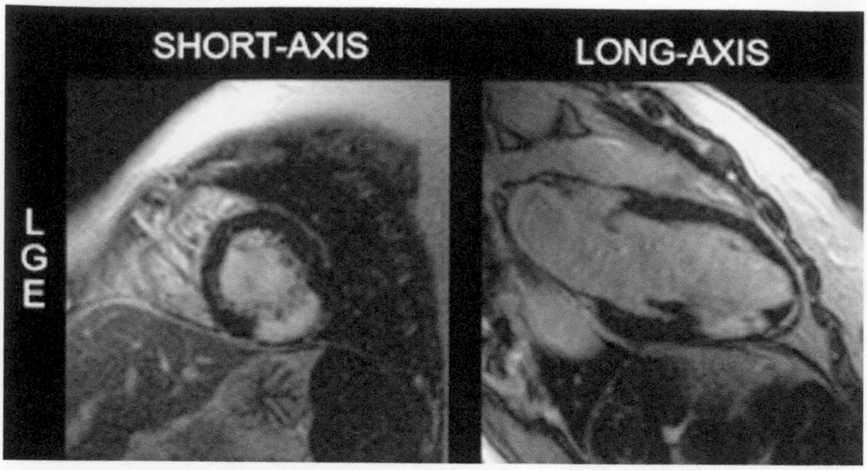

Figure 17.5 Late gadolinium enhancement images of a patient post–acute myocardial infarction showing an inferolateral midventricle transmural infarct.

LGE technique relies on the kinetics of intravenous gadolinium-based contrast media, which does not penetrate the intact cellular membrane, and thus the intracellular space. Normal myocardial tissue is comprised mostly of intracellular volume, represented by the myocytes. The remaining volume is occupied by interstitial and vascular space. In areas of myocardial infarction, necrosis and myocyte cell membrane rupture lead to an increased extracellular space and altered contrast kinetics. Areas of chronic myocardial fibrosis and scarring have large extracellular space as well, as these areas are primarily comprised of sparse collagen fibers and few fibroblasts. Within theses areas of increased extracellular space, contrast washout is delayed compared to the normal myocardium, reaching a peak difference in concentration around 10 to 20 minutes after contrast injection.

LGE imaging protocols are based on T1-weigthed fast gradient–echo pulse sequences, with an inversion-recovery preparatory pulse and an inversion time adjusted to null normal myocardium signal, which appears black in these images. Optimizing visualization of myocardial infarct zones relies on the use of gadolinium and T1-weighted images and the nulling of surrounding normal myocardium signal, obtained by adjusting inversion recovery times, typically from 200 to 300 ms. This leads to an enhanced contrast between the two areas and generates differences in signal intensity between normal and injured myocardium of up to 1080% (Fig. 17.5). Recently, technical developments have become available that allow fast and 3-D image acquisition of LGE. Such pulse sequences allow single breath-hold, navigator 3-D acquisition, and real-time acquisition.[16]

High contrast-to-noise ratios and superior spatial resolution allow precise visualization and quantification not only of necrosis or fibrosis in CAD, but also detection of other causes of increased extracellular space, such as myocitolisis, inflammation, and myocardial infiltration found in other cardiomyopathies such as hypertrophic cardiomyopathy (Fig. 17.6), Chagas disease (Fig. 17.7), myocarditis and infiltrative diseases among others. The reproducible and accurate delineation of infarcted and injured myocardium by manual tracing or by the use of automated software analysis provide measurements of infarct size or myocardial fibrosis mass with undisputable precision.

Importantly, infarct size measurements correlate well with histology in acute myocardial infarction ($R = 0.99$; $p < 0.001$), subacute myocardial infarction ($R = 0.99$; $p < 0.001$) as well as in chronic myocardial infarction settings ($R = 0.97$; $p < 0.001$).[17] Recently, myocardial infarction detection by CMR has been validated in a prospective, double-blinded multicenter international trial.[18] In a direct comparison, CMR was superior to single-photon emission computed tomography (SPECT) in the detection of subendocardial infarcts and in the reproducibility of infarcted mass quantification.[19] Even focal, percutaneous intervention–related infarcts, causing small increases of myocardial necrosis markers, such as troponin and CKMB releases, can be

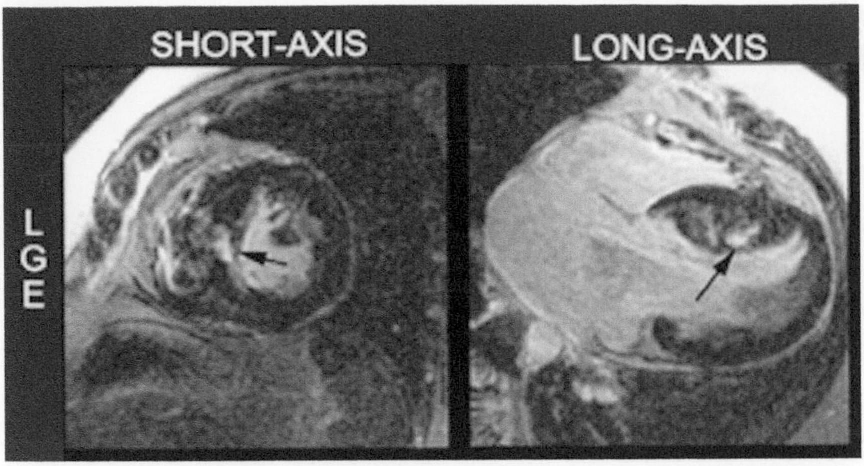

Figure 17.6 Late gadolinium enhancement images of a patient with hypertrophic cardiomyopathy showing myocardial fibrosis in the septum (*arrows*).

identified by CMR. It is now well recognized that although small, these microinfarcts have prognostic significance.

Importantly, infarct size determined by CMR has prognostic value in the acute myocardial infarct patient.[20] Even though a direct correlation between myocardial fibrosis and malignant ventricular arrhythmias has not been demonstrated, LGE volume correlates with inducible ventricular tachycardia/fibrillation during electrophysiology studies in these patients. In this regard, LGE technique, with its high spatial resolution and contrast-to-noise ratio, has provided the opportunity to analyze interface areas between normal myocardium and infarct, the so-called "gray zone" or "border zone." The extent of the "gray zone" has also been associated with inducible ventricular arrhythmias. Currently, this area has been the focus of clinical investigation in an attempt to identify better criteria for the indication of implantable cardiac defibrillators.

In addition, CMR is capable of identifying areas of microvascular obstruction or no-reflow phenomenon, another marker of severe myocardial injury with prognostic value in the context of acute myocardial infarct.[21] These areas are generally subendocardial and appear black within the infarct area during the first minutes after contrast injection, due to slow wash in of contrast media.[22] Capillary obstruction with neutrophils, red cells and endothelial cell debris, interstitial

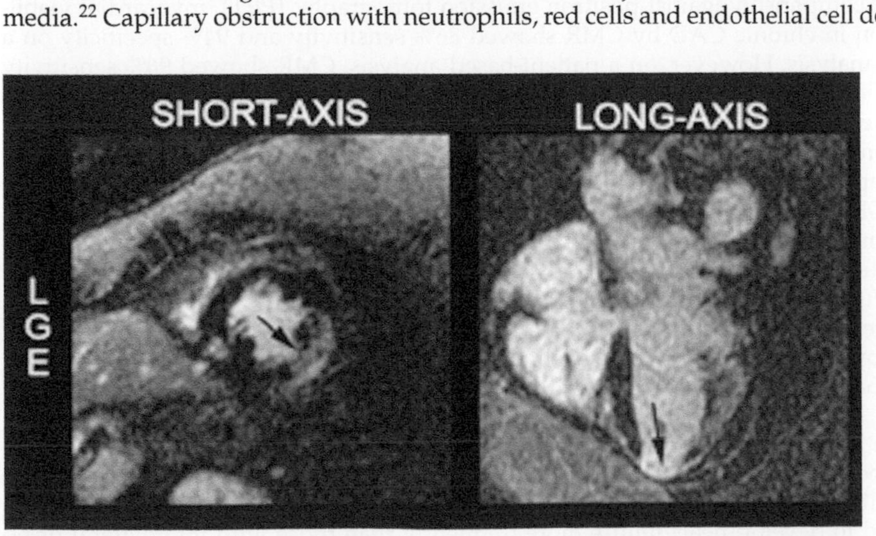

Figure 17.7 Late gadolinium enhancement images of a patient with Chagas disease showing epicardial myocardial fibrosis in the apical lateral segment (short axis, *arrow*) and transmural myocardial fibrosis in the apex (long axis, *arrow*).

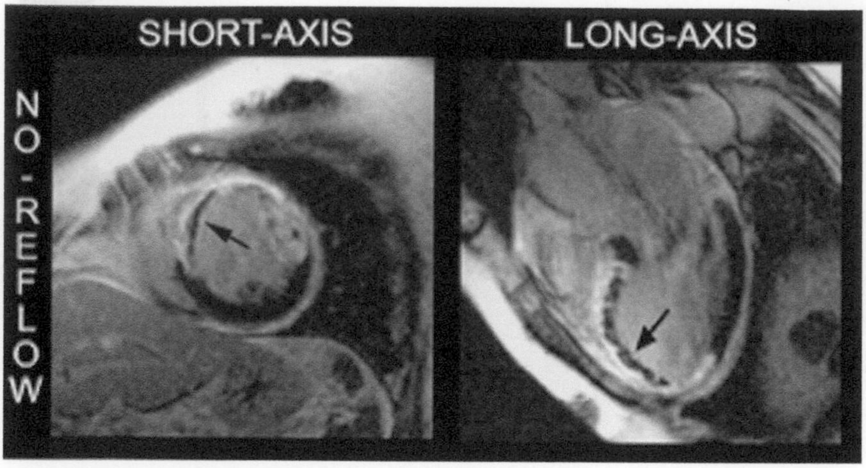

Figure 17.8 Late gadolinium enhancement images of a patient post–acute myocardial infarction showing anteroseptal microvascular obstruction or "no-reflow" (*arrows*).

edema, and swollen myocytes are among the proposed mechanisms of this phenomenon that result in the slow wash in of gadolinium (Fig. 17.8).

In patients with CAD, LV dysfunction is an important prognostic marker. However, segment or global LV dysfunction may not only reflect irreversible injury such as myocardial necrosis and fibrosis, but also reversibility with myocardial stunning and hibernation. Determination of viable segments is important in selecting patients for revascularization and predicting ventricular remodeling postinfarct.[23] Determining myocardial viability by CMR relies on the transmural extent of LGE areas. Previous studies have shown that most segments with LGE representing less than 50% of myocardial segmental area recover to normal contractility after revascularization, being therefore viable; however, segments with LGE representing more than 50% of myocardial segmental area have much poorer rates of contractile recovery after revascularization, and are therefore not considered viable (Fig. 17.9).[24] The relationship between contractile function and the transmural extent of infarct is complex and depends on LV cavity characteristics and the viability status of the neighboring segments.

In a direct comparison against positron emission tomography (PET), myocardial viability determination in chronic CAD by CMR showed 86% sensitivity and 94% specificity on a segment-based analysis. However, on a patient-based analysis, CMR showed 96% sensitivity and 100% specificity. Disagreement between imaging methods occurred more frequently in the detection of subendocardial infarcts, which is particularly challenging to PET due to its lower spatial resolution.[25]

A recent approach called multimodality CMR refers to CMR visualization algorithms that combine LGE analysis with myocardial perfusion and regional contractility; multimodality CMR has proven to be more effective in the detection of myocardial ischemia and viability.[26] In the immediate post–myocardial infarction setting, the transmural extent of LGE inversely correlates with functional recovery after 8 to 12 weeks.[27]

Beyond the diagnostic utility in CAD, LGE CMR is useful in a broad range of cardiomyopathies and provides prognostic value as well. In hypertrophic cardiomyopathy, LGE is found in up to 80% of patients and may correlate with the prevalence of classic risk factors for sudden cardiac death.[28] LGE has been proven to represent fibrosis rather than myocardial disarray in patients with hypertrophic cardiomyopathy. Patients with myocarditis often present with distinctive mesocardial patterns of LGE which may be correlated to specific viral etiologies underlying the disease and provide prognostic insight.[29] Specifically, patients with septal mesocardial LGE tend to develop heart failure more frequently than those with inferolateral or no LGE.[30] Interestingly, 30% of patients with idiopathic heart failure have similar LGE pattern, suggesting myocarditis as a possible etiology for the syndrome in this patient population.[31] In Chagas disease, LGE can present in several different patterns, but correlates well with disease

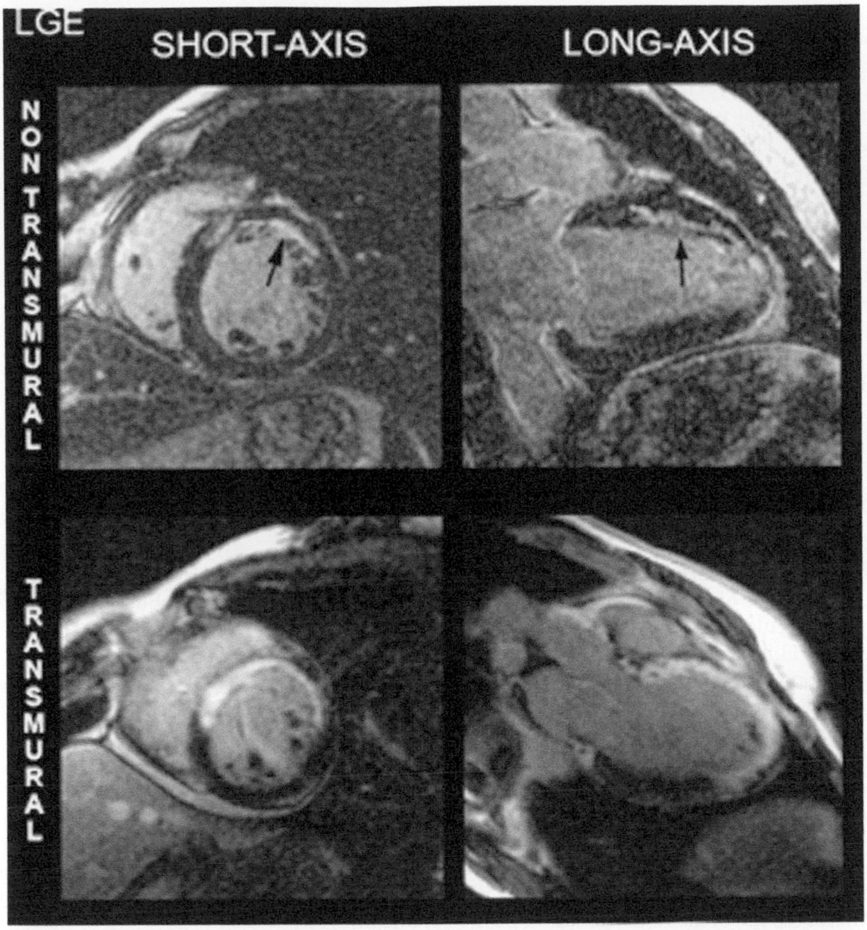

Figure 17.9 Late gadolinium enhancement images of two patients post–acute myocardial infarction showing an anterior nontransmural infarct (*upper panel, arrows*) and an anteroseptal transmural infarct (*lower panel*).

progression, LV function, and heart failure symptoms.[32] Recently, our group demonstrated that the amount of myocardial fibrosis correlated to a validated clinical score of prognosis (Rochitte CE).[33]

Moreover, the combined use of cardiac function assessment protocols and LGE is an extremely valuable tool in the evaluation of several cardiomyopathies, such as endomyocardiofibrosis, Löffler disease, infiltrative diseases (e.g. amyloidosis, sarcoidosis, Fabry's disease, mitochondrial diseases, etc.), ARVD, muscular dystrophy,[34] valvular disease, peripartum cardiomyopathy, and hypertensive cardiomyopathy, as it might have different patterns in each of the different pathologies.

CONCLUSION

Cardiovascular magnetic resonance has become an important first-line noninvasive diagnostic study in a broad range of clinical settings including precise evaluation of cardiac function and myocardial viability in coronary artery disease, as well as in the diagnostic evaluation of nonischemic cardiomyopathies.

Late gadolinium enhancement and cardiac function imaging protocols by CMR add clinically important diagnostic and prognostic information, providing invaluable insight into clinical decision making. The unique characteristics of CMR, its high image resolution and the growing evidence supporting this technology in clinical cardiology have positioned CMR as an indispensable diagnostic modality in modern cardiology.

REFERENCES

1. White HD, Norris RM, Brown MA, et al. Left ventricular end-systolic volume as the major determinant of survival after recovery from myocardial infarction. Circulation 1987; 76:44–51.
2. Longmore DB, Klipstein RH, Underwood SR, et al. Dimensional accuracy of magnetic resonance in studies of the heart. Lancet 1985; 1:1360–1362.
3. Allman KC, Shaw LJ, Hachamovitch R, et al. Myocardial viability testing and impact of revascularization on prognosis in patients with coronary artery disease and left ventricular dysfunction: A meta-analysis. J Am Coll Cardiol 2002; 39:1151–1158.
4. Pennell DJ, Sechtem UP, Higgins CB, et al. Clinical indications for cardiovascular magnetic resonance (CMR): Consensus panel report. J Cardiovasc Magn Reson 2004; 6:727–765.
5. Rochitte CE, Pinto IM, Fernandes JL, et al. Cardiovascular magnetic resonance and computed tomography imaging guidelines of the Brazilian Society of Cardiology. Arq Bras Cardiol 2006; 87:e60–e100.
6. Myerson SG, Bellenger NG, Pennell DJ. Assessment of left ventricular mass by cardiovascular magnetic resonance. Hypertension 2002; 39:750–755.
7. Maceira AM, Prasad SK, Khan M, et al. Normalized left ventricular systolic and diastolic function by steady state free precession cardiovascular magnetic resonance. J Cardiovasc Magn Reson 2006; 8:417–426.
8. Tandri H, Daya SK, Nasir K, et al. Normal reference values for the adult right ventricle by magnetic resonance imaging. Am J Cardiol 2006; 98:1660–1664.
9. Kim RJ, Shah DJ. Fundamental concepts in myocardial viability assessment revisited: When knowing how much is "alive" is not enough. Heart 2004; 90:137–140.
10. Nagel E, Lehmkuhl HB, Bocksch W, et al. Noninvasive diagnosis of ischemia-induced wall motion abnormalities with the use of high-dose dobutamine stress MRI: Comparison with dobutamine stress echocardiography. Circulation 1999; 99:763–770.
11. Rochitte CE, Kim RJ, Hillenbrand HB, et al. Microvascular integrity and the time course of myocardial sodium accumulation after acute infarction. Circ Res 2000; 87:648–655.
12. Kwong RY, Chan AK, Brown KA, et al. Impact of unrecognized myocardial scar detected by cardiac magnetic resonance imaging on event-free survival in patients presenting with signs or symptoms of coronary artery disease. Circulation 2006; 113;2733–2743.
13. McCrohon JA, Moon JC, Prasad SK, et al. Differentiation of heart failure related to dilated cardiomyopathy and coronary artery disease using gadolinium-enhanced cardiovascular magnetic resonance. Circulation 2003; 108:54–59.
14. Lima JA, Judd RM, Bazille A, et al. Regional heterogeneity of human myocardial infarcts demonstrated by contrast-enhanced MRI. Potential mechanisms. Circulation 1995; 92:1117–1125.
15. Wu E, Judd RM, Vargas JD, et al. Visualisation of presence, location, and transmural extent of healed Q-wave and non-Q-wave myocardial infarction. Lancet 2001; 357:21–28.
16. Saranathan M, Rochitte CE, Foo TK. Fast, three-dimensional free-breathing MR imaging of myocardial infarction: A feasibility study. Magn Reson Med 2004; 51:1055–1060.
17. Kim RJ, Fieno DS, Parrish TB, et al. Relationship of MRI delayed contrast enhancement to irreversible injury, infarct age, and contractile function. Circulation 1999; 100:1992–2002.
18. Kim RJ, Albert TS, Wible JH, et al. Performance of delayed-enhancement magnetic resonance imaging with gadoversetamide contrast for the detection and assessment of myocardial infarction: An international, multicenter, double-blinded, randomized trial. Circulation 2008; 117:629–637.
19. Wagner A, Mahrholdt H, Holly TA, et al. Contrast-enhanced MRI and routine single photon emission computed tomography (SPECT) perfusion imaging for detection of subendocardial myocardial infarctus: An imaging study. Lancet 2003; 361:374–379.
20. Wu KC, Zerhouni EA, Judd RM, et al. Prognostic significance of microvascular obstruction by magnetic resonance imaging in patients with acute myocardial infarction. Circulation 1998; 97: 765–772.
21. Wu KC, Zerhouni EA, Judd RM, et al. Prognostic significance of microvascular obstruction by magnetic resonance imaging in patients with acute myocardial infarction. Circulation 1998; 97:765–772.
22. Rochitte CE, Lima JA, Bluemke DA, et al. Magnitude and time course of microvascular obstruction and tissue injury after acute myocardial infarction. Circulation 1998; 98:1006–1014.
23. Silva JC, Rochitte CE, Júnior JS, et al. Late coronary artery recanalization effects on left ventricular remodelling and contractility by magnetic resonance imaging. Eur Heart J 2005; 26:36–43.
24. Kim RJ, Wu E, Rafael A, et al. The use of contrast-enhanced magnetic resonance imaging to identify reversible myocardial dysfunction. N Engl J Med 2000; 343:1445–1453.
25. Klein C, Nekolla SG, Bengel FM, et al. Assessment of myocardial viability with contrast-enhanced magnetic resonance imaging: Comparison with positron emission tomography. Circulation 2002; 105:162–167.

26. Klem I, Heitner JF, Shah DJ, et al. Improved detection of coronary artery disease by stress perfusion cardiovascular magnetic resonance with the use of delayed enhancement infarction imaging. J Am Coll Cardiol 2006; 47:1630–1638.
27. Choi KM, Kim RJ, Gubernikoff G, et al. Transmural extent of acute myocardial infarction predicts long-term improvement in contractile function. Circulation 2001; 104:1101–1107.
28. Moon JC, McKenna WJ, McCrohon JA, et al. Toward clinical risk assessment in hypertrophic cardiomyopathy with gadolinium cardiovascular magnetic resonance. J Am Coll Cardiol 2003; 41:1561–1567.
29. Mahrholdt H, Goedecke C, Wagner A, et al. Cardiovascular magnetic resonance assessment of human myocarditis: A comparison to histology and molecular pathology. Circulation 2004; 109:1250–1258.
30. Mahrholdt H, Wagner A, Deluigi CC, et al. Presentation, patterns of myocardial damage, and clinical course of viral myocarditis. Circulation 2006; 114:1581–1590.
31. McCrohon JA, Moon JC, Prasad SK, et al. Differentiation of heart failure related to dilated cardiomyopathy and coronary artery disease using gadolinium-enhanced cardiovascular magnetic resonance. Circulation 2003; 108:54–59.
32. Rochitte CE, Oliveira PF, Andrade JM, et al. Myocardial delayed enhancement by magnetic resonance imaging in patients with Chagas' disease: A marker of disease severity. J Am Coll Cardiol 2005; 46:1553–1558.
33. Uellendahl, MM. Detecção de fibrose miocárdica pela ressonância magnética cardiovascular em portadores de doença de Chagas: correlação com as formas clínicas e prognóstico. [tese], São Paulo: Faculdade de Medicina, Universidade de São Paulo; 2007. http://www.teses.usp.br/teses/disponiveis/5/5131/tde-20022009-133403/.
34. Silva MC, Meira ZM, Gurgel Giannetti J, et al. Myocardial delayed enhancement by magnetic resonance imaging in patients with muscular dystrophy. J Am Coll Cardiol 2007; 49:1874–1879.

18 Cardiovascular interventional MR imaging

Frank Wacker and Michael Bock

INTRODUCTION

Image-guided, minimally invasive procedures have steadily grown in importance for the treatment of cardiovascular diseases. Increasingly complex interventional procedures are challenging many treatments that used to be within the realm of both, cardiac and thoracic surgery. During these procedures, instruments such as needles, catheters, stents, and stent grafts are inserted into the human body under image guidance. Not only the procedures but also the imaging modalities, which are used to control and monitor these procedures have become technically more complex. In the past, X-ray image guidance was the stronghold for cardiovascular image guidance. The main advantage of X-ray fluoroscopy is real-time imaging with image acquisition and display rates of 10 or more frames per second. However, X-ray–based imaging techniques do utilize ionizing radiation and the lack of soft-tissue contrast limits their applicability in complex anatomical sites. Therefore, methods such as intravascular ultrasound (IVUS) and fusion of preacquired computed tomography (CT) and magnetic resonance (MR) images with fluoroscopy have been increasingly applied during cardiovascular interventions to add information that is essential to perform challenging interventional procedures.

Since the mid-1980s, when MRI has been introduced widely as a clinical tool, MRI has become a highly acclaimed imaging modality for vascular and cardiac imaging. At the same time increasing interest in interventional procedures under MR guidance was expressed and first papers on MR-guided biopsies were published. At the beginning, long image acquisition times made cardiovascular imaging time-consuming and limited access to the patient placed in a large magnet structure prohibited a widespread use of MRI during interventional procedures. However, MRI has several advantages over other imaging modalities: MR images have an excellent soft-tissue contrast, the imaging slices can be oriented in all the three dimensions without restrictions, and MRI is not using any ionizing radiation. Additionally, MRI can provide both morphologic and functional information about blood flow, diffusion, perfusion, tissue oxygenation, and changes in tissue temperature. Currently, no other imaging modality alone offers such wealth information. This makes MRI an attractive imaging method for both diagnostic and therapeutic procedures.

With the improvements in MR hardware, fast data acquisition and image reconstruction have become possible over the recent years. New magnet types have been designed that facilitate access to the patient in the center of a magnet. Modern commercial MR systems have the ability for real-time MRI sequences using fast pulse sequences and parallel imaging techniques. This allows for image acquisition at frame rates of up to 10 images/sec, so that the motion of interventional instruments can be visualized even in challenging anatomical regions such as the rapidly moving heart or pulsating vessels like the aorta. With these technical advances, MR-guided interventions have evolved from a pure research application to a clinical method over the last decade. Main applications for MR-guided procedures are biopsies in the breast, the brain, the prostate, and other organs, as well as percutaneous MR-guided thermal ablation procedures. Clinical trials have shown that MRI is an excellent tool for target localization, interactive puncture guidance, thermal monitoring, and therapy control.

MR imaging–guided cardiovascular interventions are still a research topic with a large number of preclinical applications and some that have already entered the clinical arena over the last decade. The challenges are temporal and spatial resolution of MR sequences which are already sufficient for certain application such as vena cava filter placement or aortic stent graft implantation. For others such as intracerebral coiling or coronary stent placement, the methods need to be further improved before they can be applied in a clinical setting. Another challenge is that clinically approved and certified catheters, guidewires, and other interventional materials for the MR environment are not commercially available, and many applications rely on device prototypes.

In the following overview, the technical aspects such as the system design of the MR scanner, rapid image acquisition techniques, and fast image reconstruction algorithms, as well as dedicated catheters and instruments will be discussed that are required for MR-guided cardiovascular interventions. The safety of the current procedures will be discussed and experimental and clinical applications will be presented.

INTERVENTIONAL MR SYSTEMS

A cardiovascular interventional MR system should offer the clinician good access to the patient without any compromise in image quality, rapid image acquisition, as well as fast image reconstruction and display. For this purpose several MR system designs have been proposed.

Vertical magnets

Vertical C-arm–shaped magnets create a magnetic field between two magnet pole shoes. Historically, these open-configuration magnets were used in the first interventional MR systems. Access to the patient from at least three directions similar to conventional C-arm fluoroscopy units facilitated percutaneous biopsies and drainage procedures. Unfortunately, the magnet pole shoes are significantly larger than the image detectors in X-ray fluoroscopy; thus patient access can still be challenging. Initially, C-arm magnets were often built using permanent or resistive magnets at lower field strengths below 1 T, which compromised the achievable signal-to-noise ratio (SNR) compared to current diagnostic MR unit operating at $B_0 \geq 1.5$ T. In addition, C-arm magnets are often equipped with gradient systems with maximum amplitudes of G_{max} <25 mT/m, whereas modern diagnostic MR systems offer gradient systems with G_{max} up to 45 mT/m, so that C-arm systems are limited in their achievable image frame rate. Recently, superconducting magnets with a C-arm design have been realized that operate at higher field strengths up to 1 T (Philips Panorama) that provide images with a quality similar to conventional high-field MR units. Unfortunately, the increasing field strength also reduces the patient access, because the diameter of the pole shoes increases.

Solenoid magnets

Today, most diagnostic MR systems use superconducting closed-bore solenoid magnets for field generation. Since these MR systems are widely available and offer a high SNR in combination with fast image acquisition techniques, at present an increasing number of interventions are performed in closed-bore superconducting MR magnets. In closed-bore solenoid magnets direct access to the patient is challenging, but during endovascular procedures the access port for the catheter is typically separated by a distance of 40 to 80 cm from the interventional target, such as the heart, which allows the clinician to operate on the target area at magnet iso-center while standing close to the magnet opening. Superconducting solenoid magnet MR systems are equipped with very strong whole body gradient systems [typical G_{max} of up to 45 mT/m, slew rates of up to 170 T/(m · s)], so that image update rates of 5 to 10 images per second can be realized technically.

New magnet designs further reduced the magnet length from 2 m and more to about 160 cm for a 1.5-T magnet, and recently, even a 120-cm-long 1.5-T magnet (Siemens Magnetom Espree) has been introduced. This ultra-short magnet additionally offers a 70-cm bore diameter, which further improves patient access. With decreasing magnet length, the B_0 field homogeneity is reduced, and only a limited field of view (FOV) of 35 cm can be effectively used for imaging. For vascular interventions, the limited FOV can be challenging, however, in cardiac applications this size of the FOV is sufficient to cover both the heart and the adjacent blood vessels.

Combined X-ray and MR-systems

Rarely is MRI the only imaging modality used to guide an intervention. During a procedure performed under MRI guidance, an additional X-ray control might be needed, as MR-compatible instruments such as guidewires are rarely available, and the use of MRI with these devices might compromise patient safety. To facilitate the transport between MRI and X-ray imaging units, so-called XMR systems have been developed that combine an MRI system with an angiography unit. With a dedicated MR system (GE Signa SP, "double donut") even simultaneous MR and X-ray imaging has been experimentally demonstrated,[1] however, the commercially available XMR systems connect the MRI to the angiography unit with a specially designed patient transport device.[2] The use of two separate imaging modalities assures that both conventional angiography and MRI are performed with optimal image quality. Furthermore, the modalities can be used independently when a combined procedure is not scheduled.

To combine the excellent soft-tissue contrast of MRI with the good device contrast of X-ray imaging during an XMR procedure, MR images need to be merged with the X-ray data. The merging procedure requires images that are carefully corrected for image distortion of the individual modality.[3] Data merging is particularly indicated during cardiac interventions, when the X-ray images delineate the metal components of catheter and guidewire, and the MR images show the anatomy of the heart.

MR-compatible instrumentation

Interventional procedures require hardware installations in the MR environment that differ from those of diagnostic MR suites.

Dedicated display devices are required to rapidly present the real-time image data to the radiologist and the support personnel with a latency of below a few 100 ms. Monitors (often of TFT type) can be used for this application which are largely resistant to influences by the static magnetic field, and that are additionally equipped with a radio-frequency (RF) shield to avoid RF interference with the MR data acquisition. The monitors are often mounted to the ceiling or can be moved in the room using a dedicated trolley. For larger image displays that can be seen by all persons in the magnet room, video projectors and back projection screens are used.

Patient monitoring is mandatory during any interventional procedure. In the magnet room, commercially available RF-shielded echocardiography (ECG) leads are used, and they are often combined with dedicated ECG systems that are largely immune to interferences from gradient-induced voltages, which facilitate heart rhythm detection. However, even with these systems, distorted ECG signals are seen, which is a consequence of the so-called magneto-hydrodynamic effect. Artifactual ECG distortions might be misinterpreted as arrhythmia or ST-segment changes, which makes close monitoring during cardiac procedures more challenging than with X-ray.

ECG and other metallic leads and cables are also prone to heating due to coupling to the electric RF fields. This heating is particularly pronounced when the length of the electrically conducting structures approaches the B_0-dependent resonance length. At field strength of 1.5 T, temperature differences of up to 44 K have been observed.[4] To reduce the risk of skin burns, loop configurations of metallic cables should be avoided and such cables should not have contact with the patients skin. Furthermore, all objects such as infusion pumps, anesthesia trays, ventilators, etc. in the RF cabin need to be carefully screened for ferromagnetic components, as these could become lethal missiles in the vicinity of the magnet. To avoid these risks, the use of ferromagnetic instruments needs to be prohibited or the personnel must be trained to keep these instruments at a safe distance from the magnet (e.g., the 0.5 mT line) at any time during the intervention.

In the course of an MR-guided intervention, the high gradient amplitudes and the rapid gradient switching required for real-time imaging can lead to excessive noise at sound pressure levels of up to 120 dB. Gradient noise makes ear protection mandatory for both the patient and the personnel, and communication within the RF cabin and with the outside control room becomes challenging. Passive noise suppression has been proposed by encasing the gradient tube into a vacuum chamber and direct mounting of the gradient to the ground (e.g., Pianissimo gradients, Toshiba), which can reduce gradient noise by 20 to 30 dB. For an improved communication, dedicated headphones that are immune to RF interference have been developed.

DEVICE LOCALIZATION

An essential element of cardiovascular interventional MRI is the tracking of the interventional devices. Many device-tracking techniques have been proposed for both percutaneous and intravascular interventions,[5,6] which were initially categorized as either active and passive. These terms have been abandoned over the recent years, as a clear definition of the term active is hardly possible. In the following passive methods as well as techniques that involve electrically active elements such as direct currents, inductively coupled coils, RF coils, or direct field measurements are described.

MR-visible markers

Instruments are often either MR-invisible (e.g., plastic catheters), or they cause artifacts (e.g., ferromagnetic implants), which can be so large that they obscure the instrument's location. For device localization therefore markers are attached to the instruments that either amplify (positive) or reduce (negative) the MR signal.

Reduced signals can be achieved with paramagnetic substances such as dysprosium oxide, which can be attached to the surface of the instruments as a coating.[7,8] For markers with a negative contrast a separation is easily achieved between the signal void and the surrounding tissue if the marker is placed in a homogeneous signal-carrying tissue. In tissues with low-signal intensities (e.g., the lung), however, the susceptibility artifact can hardly be detected.

Positive signals have been created with T1-shortening contrast agents that are filled into the interior of the instrument (e.g., a catheter) or that are mixed into the coating material.[9,10] If enough space is available, small marker reservoirs filled with a contrast agent solution can be attached to the instrument, which are then imaged with heavily T1-weighted imaging techniques such as short-TR spoiled gradient echo pulse sequences (FLASH).

A new image needs to be acquired for each update of the device coordinates in image based localization, which can be challenging under real-time conditions even if parallel imaging and temporal interpolation techniques are used. Longer acquisition times might be tolerated in stereotactic applications where intruments need to be localized to compare their current position with the planned trajectory. To overcome the temporal limitations, projection imaging has been used for device tracking. Here, thick 2D slabs are used to rapidly detect the markers in the imaging volume. When combined with incomplete refocusing of the transverse magnetization, negative contrast markers can also be localized with projection imaging. Here the signal void is converted into a positive signal by refocusing only the signal in the strong static field gradients around the markers (white marker phenomenon).[11]

Image-based passive tracking has the advantage that no additional hardware is required, since the device location can be calculated from the images using postprocessing algorithms such as cross-correlation. The precision of the position calculation is dependent on the material constants of the instruments, the field strength, the presence of partial volume effects, the pulse sequence type, and the imaging parameters used. Passive tracking methods can only determine the instrument position if the device is contained in the current imaging slice which makes them especially suitable for tracking of rigid instruments. Flexible instruments such as intravascular catheters in tortuous vessels can be difficult to localize with these techniques.

Direct currents

A signal void close to the instrument can not only be created by MR-visible markers but also by a direct current that is flowing through an integrated wire.[2] The current generates a local inhomogeneous magnetic field, which creates a local signal void in the MR image. Typically in intravascular catheters, currents of several 10 mA are applied in coils of 1 mm diameter, and the size of the signal void is controlled by the current amplitude. Two images are acquired with and without current, that is, without and with signal void, and the device is then automatically localized in the difference image.

Direct currents can also be used to actively steer the catheters. When the magnetic field of the integrated coil is not parallel to the main magnetic field of the MR, the integrated coil experienes a torque, which can be exploited to steer the catheter around edges in the vessels.[12] Unfortunately, active steering requires significantly higher currents which can cause Ohmic heating of the steering coils and which may be dangerous in case of device failure.

Inductively coupled resonance circuits

Besides the static magnetic field B_0, the interaction of the devices with the MR system's B_1 radiofrequency fields can also be used for localization. Therefore small resonance circuits consisting of a coil (i.e., an inductor) and a capacitance can be attached to the devices. The resonance frequency of the circuit is matched with the proton resonance frequency of the MR system. During RF excitation the resonance circuit locally amplifies the B_1 field in the inductor via inductive coupling, and a substantially higher flip angle is observed within the tracking coil. To detect only signal from the tracking coil, very low flip angles are applied outside the coil, so that only the interior of the small inductor is experiencing an RF excitation. For rapid device tracking, this signal can be acquired with a projection technique (i.e., without time-consuming phase encoding) in all the three spatial directions, which provides the x, y, and z coordinates of the coil in less than 20 ms.[13]

A major advantage of inductive coupling is that the resonance circuit is not directly connected to the receiver of the MRI system, and, thus, does not require additional cables or premplifiers in the devices. Furthermore, existing imaging coils can be used for signal reception. Inductively coupled coils can only be used at a single field strength as they are tuned to the resonance frequency of the MR system. Inductively coupled coils can not only applied for instrument tracking, but can also be used for high-resolution imaging. Therefore, the metallic structures of stents or vena cava filters are converted into inductively coupled coils by the addition of suitable capacitors.[14,15] The resonant implants can then be used to image re-stenosis or thrombus formation at their interior.

Radio frequency coils for tracking and profiling

Tracking and profiling of devices can also be realized with small radio frequency coils that are attached to the instruments.[16,17] As opposed to inductively coupled coils, which have no direct connection with the MR system, these coils are directly connected to the MR receiver, and the MR signal is read out together with that of the surrounding imaging coils. Again, projection data are rapidly acquired in x, y, and z direction using a nonselective RF excitation. Thus, the instrument position can be interrogated with 50 updates per second and more, and the position can be superimposed onto a previously acquired image data set (roadmap).

Only the position information is updated with a roadmap technique, which limits its use to static anatomical situations, for example, intracranial interventions. In the abdomen, breathing and heart motion constantly change the local anatomy, and the acquisition of new MR images is frequently required. Therefore, a fast imaging pulse sequence (e.g., balanced SSFP, true FISP) is applied after the instrument position is measured. If the position information is used to automatically realign the imaging slice, this automatic tracking technology allows the operator to control the imaging process through the motion of the catheter.[18,19] At matrix sizes of 128 to 256, image update rates of 3 to 6 Hz have been achieved with fast imaging pulse sequences, which was further doubled with real-time parallel imaging.[20,21]

With a single tracking coil at the catheter tip, the visualization of the catheter shaft can be difficult during an intravascular interention and catheter looping can be hard to detect. The total length of the catheter can be delineated (profiling) with an additional guidewire antenna in the catheter lumen. Here, so-called extended inner conductor antennas have been proposed where the guidewire consists of a coaxial cable where the outer braiding is removed over a certain section near the tip.[22,23] Instrument tracking and profiling can be combined when a twisted pair profiling coil and a solenoid tracking coil are integrated into the device. Small coils at the catheter tip have not only been used for instrument tracking in endovascular interventions, but also for high-resolution imaging of the vessel wall.[24,25]

Profiling and tracking coils require a direct connection to the receiver of the MR system, which is realized with long electrically conducting cables. The electric fields of the transmitting RF coil (typically, the body coil) can couple with these structures, which can result in severe RF heating, and, thus, compromises patient safety. The risk of RF heating can be reduced by the integration of electronic elements such as cable traps, baluns, or even transformer which shorten the effective electronic length of the cable segments below the field strength–dependent resonance length.[26–28]

Gradient fields

The instrument position can also be determined in the MR system when the spatially varying gradient fields are measured. The gradient fields can be assessed with three orthogonal Hall probes, and the sensor position is determined through a comparison with known gradient control signals.[29] Field measurements have also commercially been implemented with orthogonal coils that detect the voltages induced during gradient ramping. The coils can be integrated into devices such as endoscopes, needle holders, and even into an electrophysiology catheter. Alternatively field measurements can also be realized with an optical sensor made of an optically active crystal (e.g., Terbium—Gallium–Garnet) that utilizes the Faraday effect to avoid any electrically conducting structure.[30] An advantage of gradient field measurements is that device position and MR image information can be acquired simultaneously, because gradient activity is present during MR image acquisition on all the three spatial axes.

INTERVENTIONAL MRI PULSE SEQUENCES

In any MR imaging sequence, spatial resolution, temporal resolution, contrast-to-noise ratio, and SNR must be balanced to meet the demands encountered in the clinical setting. For interventional procedures, a high temporal resolution of the image updates is required. This is realized with short image acquisition times in combination with short image reconstruction times that must not exceed its acquisition time to avoid an increasing time lag between data acquisition and image display. The following pulse sequences have shown to be advantageous for many interventional applications.

Fast low-angle shot (FLASH)

The spoiled gradient echo pulse sequence, also known as fast low-angle shot (FLASH), is historically one of the earliest pulse sequences used for real-time imaging. Compared to spin echo pulse sequences, very low flip angles (€ = 5°–30°) are used for RF excitation, and only a fraction of the longitudinal magnetization is utilized. Between two RF excitations, the transverse magnetization is completely spoiled so that the image contrast is determined by T1 only. The strong T1 weighting is advantageous for interventional MRI, if, for example, the distribution volume of therapeutic agents mixed with a T1-shortening contrast agent needs to be visualized.

One of the most important applications of T1-weighted FLASH pulse sequences is contrast-enhanced MR angiography (cMRA). With fast, time-resolved 3D FLASH MRA pulse sequences, the transit of a contrast bolus after intra-arterial injection can be visualized, and the perfusion of an organ can be assessed at least semi-quantitatively. Contrary to procedures under X-ray guidance, however, contrast agents are not imperatively necessary to verify the catheter position and the vessels distal to the catheter, as the morphology of both vessels and adjacent organs is directly visible in the MR image.

For intravascular contrast agents, a 3D FLASH pulse sequence with better spatial resolution can be used to image the whole vascular anatomy after steady-state distribution has been achieved, since such agents significantly shorten the long intrinsic T1 time of blood over an extended period of time, so that the interior of the blood vessel becomes visible in the FLASH images. Thus, with a single injection of contrast agent both vascular anatomy and organ perfusion can be assessed. Finally, the increased MR signal in the blood vessels is also advantageous for tracking of devices with RF coils (cf. sections, radio frequency coils for tracking and profiling and gradient fields), since a higher MR signal is detected.

Steady-state free precession

A second important real-time imaging pulse sequence is the balanced steady-state free precession pulse sequence (bSSFP, trueFISP, FIESTA). The bSSFP sequence timing is similar to that of a FLASH pulse sequence; however, all gradient moments are balanced, so that between two RF excitations no gradient-induced phases accumulate. Thus, the transverse magnetization is not spoiled but completely refocused within one TR, and the image contrast depends on the ratio of T1 and T2. The T2/T1 ratio is high for liquids, and thus bSSFP sequences provide a significantly higher SNR for liquid-filled spaces and blood vessels than FLASH pulse sequences. bSSFP sequences are susceptible to artifacts from off-resonances, which are visible as dark bands in the images.

Other sequences for real-time imaging

Echo planar imaging (EPI), spiral imaging, or even rapid spin echo pulse sequences have also been proposed for interventional MRI. Often, these sequences require modifications over their conventional diagnostic counterparts to make them suitable for interventional procedure guidance. Single-shot EPI pulse sequences often suffer from artifacts such as off-resonance shifts, N/2-ghosts, or image distortion. If, however, not all, but only a certain fraction (e.g., 3–7 lines) of the k-space lines are acquired per RF excitation, these segmented EPI sequences combine very short acquisition times with high-quality MR images.

Spin echo pulse sequences are advantageous for interventional MRI because susceptibility artifacts from metallic instruments are highly reduced. The long spin echo acquisition times can be significantly reduced, when multiple refocusing of the spin echo with different phase encoding steps (RARE) is performed in combination with half-Fourier data acquisition (HASTE) and Local-Look excitation (inner volume excitation). Nevertheless, for cardiovascular interventions, spin echo sequences with image update rates of one image/s or less are usually too slow.

APPLICATIONS

Cardiovascular procedures utilize devices such as catheters and guidewires to access a target organ that is often separated from the skin entry point by several decimeters. This distance is advantageous for interventional MRI, as the interventionalist can be standing next to the magnet opening, whereas the target organ is located at magnet isocenter of a short bore magnet.

Historically, MR-guided cardiovascular interventions were first tested in animal models with instrument prototypes to evaluate the feasibility of uncomplicated interventional procedures. At present, more complex interventions have been performed under MR-guidance. Outside the heart, several groups have reported angioplasty, recanalization of chronic total occlusions, and endovascular stenting and stent-graft placements in the aorta and carotid, iliac, and renal arteries.[31–38] Different embolization techniques have also been utilized under MRI guidance.[11,39,40]

In the cardiac realm, myocardial ablations, septum occlusions, atrial septal punctures, as well as labeled cell deliveries have been performed under the guidance of MRI.[41–45] For aortic valve replacement,[46,47] MR imaging guidance provides important information on the location of the aortic root as well as the origin of the coronary arteries. However, the susceptibility artifact-based device visualization of aortic valves makes exact placement challenging. Cardiac electrophysiology and myocardial ablation under MR guidance could be an alternative to current functional guidance techniques which use electrograms and electromagnetic mapping in combination with image guidance using X-ray fluoroscopy or ultrasound. Electroanatomic mapping with pre-acquired MR images has recently been reported, and electrophysiology catheter prototypes for real-time MR imaging guidance have also been established.[48] With MRI guidance for myocardial injections, targeting of myocardial tissue can be performed in real time, coil- and antenna-based catheters facilitate exact delivery, and successful delivery can be reliably tracked with MRI. In contrast to X-ray fluoroscopy, MR guidance allows differentiation of infarcted and viable myocardium.[49] However, it remains unclear if precise cell delivery is advantageous in a clinical setting and the devices used for both, myocardial ablation as well as myocardial injections are not yet available for clinical trials. Transarterial coronary artery catheterizations, angioplasties, and stent placements under MRI guidance are continuously being presented from many groups, mainly in healthy animals. When treating a delicate structure such as a stenosed coronary artery, however, current real-time MRI guidance techniques meet their limits. Although one can work around a high temporal resolution by using gating techniques, the spatial resolution that comes with real-time MR imaging techniques is well beyond the requirements for most coronary interventions.

MRI-guided cardiovascular procedures in patients have so far only been applied at a limited number of centers. The main limitation is the lack of clinically approved instruments. In the cardiac area, the London group at Guys Hospital has conducted cardiac catheter maneuvers in children using an XMR suite.[3] According to the "as-low-as-reasonably-achievable" (ALARA) principle in radiation protection, the use of MR-guided interventions is particularly favorable in children and younger adults, since no radiation is applied with MRI. For young patients even low-radiation doses need to be avoided, as these patients have a higher sensibility and a higher probability to experience the negative consequences of the radiation in their remaining life span. Therefore, MR-guided interventions might soonest replace endovascular interventions under X-ray guidance in young patients suffering from congenital heart disease and arrhythmia.

To overcome limitations due to MR-incompatible instruments, the London group performed the cardiovascular interventions in these patients in an X-MR system, where the instruments are placed in the heart under X-ray guidance and the patient is then transferred to the MR system.

In Regensburg, Germany, MRI-guided stent placements were performed after positioning of the stent under fluoroscopy in patients with limb claudication.[50] In Basel, Switzerland and Regensburg, selective intra-arterial MR angiography of the legs was performed.[51,52] The Stanford group has done TIPS procedures using an MR system with an integrated flat panel X-ray unit. In this study, the authors found that the use of MRI guidance lead to a reduced number of puncture attempts compared to a historical control group.[53] In most of the clinical pilot studies, however, the workflow was often copied from established procedures under fluoroscopy or DSA. Such proof of concept studies are important in the process of establishing MRI-guided cardiovascular procedures to show general feasibility of MR-guided endovascular interventions. However, for many of these procedures, practicability, cost, procedure time, and spatial, as well as temporal resolution are currently in favor of conventional X-ray angiography and fluoroscopy. Applications that clearly profit from MR-guidance, that demonstrate the inherent strength of MRI, and that are currently difficult to perform or even impossible under X-ray fluoroscopy guidance alone still need to be developed to broaden the range of use for interventional MR imaging–guided procedure.

REFERENCES

1. Fahrig R, Butts K, Rowlands JA, et al. A truly hybrid interventional MR/X-ray system: Feasibility demonstration. J Magn Reson Imaging 2001; 13(2):294–300.
2. Adam G, Glowinski A, Neuerburg J, et al. Catheter visualization in MR-tomography: Initial experimental results with field-inhomogeneity catheters. Rofo FortschrGebRontgenstrNeuen BildgebVerfahr 1997; 166(4):324–328.
3. Razavi R, Hill DL, Keevil SF, et al. Cardiac catheterisation guided by MRI in children and adults with congenital heart disease. Lancet 2003; 362(9399):1877–1882.
4. Nitz WR, Oppelt A, Renz W, et al. On the heating of linear conductive structures as guide wires and catheters in interventional MRI. J Magn Reson Imaging 2001; 13(1):105–114.
5. Wacker FK, Hillenbrand CM, Duerk JL, et al. MR-guided endovascular interventions: Device visualization, tracking, navigation, clinical applications, and safety aspects. Magn Reson Imaging Clin N Am 2005; 13(3):431–439.
6. Bock M, Wacker FK. MR-guided intravascular interventions: Techniques and applications. J Magn Reson Imaging 2008; 27(2):326–338.
7. Wacker FK, Reither K, Branding G, et al. Magnetic resonance-guided vascular catheterization: Feasibility using a passive tracking technique at 0.2 Telsa in a pig model. J Magn Reson Imaging J Magn Reson Imaging 1999; 10(5):841–844.
8. Bakker CJ, Smits HF, Bos C, et al. MR-guided balloon angioplasty: In vitro demonstration of the potential of MRI for guiding, monitoring, and evaluating endovascular interventions. J Magn Reson Imaging 1998; 8(1):245–250.
9. Unal O, Li J, Cheng W, et al. MR-visible coatings for endovascular device visualization. J Magn Reson Imaging 2006; 23(5):763–769.
10. Omary RA, Frayne R, Unal O, et al. MR-guided angioplasty of renal artery stenosis in a pig model: A feasibility study. J Vasc Interv Radiol 2000; 11(3):373–381.
11. Bakker CJ, Seppenwoolde JH, Bartels LW, et al. Adaptive subtraction as an aid in MR-guided placement of catheters and guidewires. J Magn Reson Imaging 2004; 20(3):470–474.
12. Settecase F, Sussman MS, Wilson MW, et al. Magnetically-assisted remote control (MARC) steering of endovascular catheters for interventional MRI: A model for deflection and design implications. Med Phys 2007; 34(8):3135–3142.
13. Quick HH, Zenge MO, Kuehl H, et al. Interventional magnetic resonance angiography with no strings attached: Wireless active catheter visualization. Magn Reson Med 2005; 53(2):446–455.
14. Quick HH, Kuehl H, Kaiser G, et al. Inductively coupled stent antennas in MRI. Magn Reson Med 2002; 48(5):781–790.
15. Kivelitz D, Wagner S, Schnorr J, et al. A vascular stent as an active component for locally enhanced magnetic resonance imaging: Initial in vivo imaging results after catheter-guided placement in rabbits. Invest Radiol 2003; 38(3):147–152.
16. Leung DA, Debatin JF, Wildermuth S, et al. Real-time biplanar needle tracking for interventional MR imaging procedures. Radiology 1995; 197(2):485–488.

17. Dumoulin CL, Souza SP, Darrow RD. Real-time position monitoring of invasive devices using magnetic resonance. Magn Reson Med 1993; 29(3):411–415.
18. Wacker FK, Elgort D, Hillenbrand CM, et al. The catheter-driven MRI scanner: A new approach to intravascular catheter tracking and imaging-parameter adjustment for interventional MRI. Am J Roentgenol 2004; 183(2):391–395.
19. Bock M, Volz S, Zuhlsdorff S, et al. MR-guided intravascular procedures: Real-time parameter control and automated slice positioning with active tracking coils. J Magn Reson Imaging 2004; 19(5):580–589.
20. Bock M, Muller S, Zuehlsdorff S, et al. Active catheter tracking using parallel MRI and real-time image reconstruction. Magn Reson Med 2006; 55(6):1454–1459.
21. Muller S, Umathum R, Speier P, et al. Dynamic coil selection for real-time imaging in interventional MRI. Magn Reson Med 2006; 56(5):1156–1162.
22. Ocali O, Atalar E. Intravascular magnetic resonance imaging using a loopless catheter antenna. Magn Reson Med 1997; 37(1):112–118.
23. Quick HH, Kuehl H, Kaiser G, et al. Interventional MRA using actively visualized catheters, TrueFISP, and real-time image fusion. Magn Reson Med 2003; 49(1):129–137.
24. Hofmann LV, Liddell RP, Arepally A, et al. In vivo intravascular MR imaging: Transvenous technique for arterial wall imaging. J Vasc Interv Radiol 2003; 14(10):1317–1327.
25. Hillenbrand CM, Jesberger JA, Wong EY, et al. Toward rapid high resolution in vivo intravascular MRI: Evaluation of vessel wall conspicuity in a porcine model using multiple imaging protocols. J Magn Reson Imaging 2006; 23(2):135–144.
26. Ladd ME, Quick HH. Reduction of resonant RF heating in intravascular catheters using coaxial chokes. Magn Reson Med 2000; 43(4):615–619.
27. Weiss S, Vernickel P, Schaeffter T, et al. Transmission line for improved RF safety of interventional devices. Magn Reson Med 2005; 54(1):182–189.
28. Krafft A, Muller S, Umathum R, et al. B1 field-insensitive transformers for RF-safe transmission lines. Magma 2006; 19(5):257–266.
29. Scheffler K, Korvink JG. Navigation with Hall sensor device for interventional MRI. Proceedings of the 11th ISMRM Meeting and Exhibition, 2004:950.
30. Bock M, Umathum R, Sikora J, et al. A Faraday effect position sensor for interventional magnetic resonance imaging. Phys Med Biol 2006; 51(4):999–1009.
31. Raman VK, Karmarkar PV, Guttman MA, et al. Real-time magnetic resonance-guided endovascular repair of experimental abdominal aortic aneurysm in swine. J Am Coll Cardiol 2005; 45(12):2069–2077.
32. Eggebrecht H, Kuhl H, Kaiser GM, et al. Feasibility of real-time magnetic resonance-guided stent-graft placement in a swine model of descending aortic dissection. Eur Heart J 2006; 27(5):613–620.
33. Wacker FK, Reither K, Ebert W, et al. MR image-guided endovascular procedures with the ultrasmall superparamagnetic iron oxide SH U 555 C as an intravascular contrast agent: Study in pigs. Radiology 2003; 226(2):459–464.
34. Feng L, Dumoulin CL, Dashnaw S, et al. Feasibility of stent placement in carotid arteries with real-time MR imaging guidance in pigs. Radiology 2005; 234(2):558–562.
35. Omary RA, Gehl JA, Schirf BE, et al. MR imaging versus conventional X-ray fluoroscopy-guided renal angioplasty in swine: Prospective randomized comparison. Radiology 2006; 238(2):489–496.
36. Elgort DR, Hillenbrand CM, Zhang S, et al. Image-guided and -monitored renal artery stenting using only MRI. J Magn Reson Imaging 2006; 23(5):619–627.
37. Buecker A, Neuerburg JM, Adam GB, et al. Real-time MR fluoroscopy for MR-guided iliac artery stent placement. J Magn Reson Imaging 2000; 12(4):616–622.
38. Raval AN, Karmarkar PV, Guttman MA, et al. Real-time magnetic resonance imaging-guided endovascular recanalization of chronic total arterial occlusion in a swine model. Circulation 2006; 113(8):1101–1107.
39. Fink C, Bock M, Umathum R, et al. Renal embolization: Feasibility of magnetic resonance-guidance using active catheter tracking and intraarterial magnetic resonance angiography. Invest Radiol 2004; 39(2):111–119.
40. Larson AC, Wang D, Atassi B, et al. Transcatheter intraarterial perfusion: MR monitoring of chemoembolization for hepatocellular carcinoma–feasibility of initial clinical translation. Radiology 2008; 246(3):964–971.
41. Bücker A, Spüntrup E, Grabitz R, et al. Magnetic resonance-guided placement of atrial septal closure device in animal model of patent foramen ovale. Circulation 2002; 106(4):511–515.
42. Yang X, Atalar E. MRI-guided gene therapy. FEBS Lett 2006; 580(12):2958–2961.
43. Lederman RJ, Guttman MA, Peters DC, et al. Catheter-based endomyocardial injection with real-time magnetic resonance imaging. Circulation 2002; 105(11):1282–1284.
44. Rickers C, Jerosch-Herold M, Hu X, et al. Magnetic resonance image-guided transcatheter closure of atrial septal defects. Circulation 2003; 107(1):132–138.

45. Kraitchman DL, Tatsumi M, Gilson WD, et al. Dynamic imaging of allogeneic mesenchymal stem cells trafficking to myocardial infarction. Circulation 2005; 112(10):1451–1461.
46. Kuehne T, Yilmaz S, Meinus C, et al. Magnetic resonance imaging-guided transcatheter implantation of a prosthetic valve in aortic valve position: Feasibility study in swine. J Am Coll Cardiol 2004; 44(11):2247–2249.
47. Saeed M, Henk CB, Weber O, et al. Delivery and assessment of endovascular stents to repair aortic coarctation using MR and X-ray imaging. J Magn Reson Imaging 2006; 24(2):371–378.
48. Susil RC, Yeung CJ, Halperin HR, et al. Multifunctional interventional devices for MRI: A combined electrophysiology/MRI catheter. Magn Reson Med 2002; 47(3):594–600.
49. Saeed M, Martin AJ, Lee RJ, et al. MR guidance of targeted injections into border and core of scarred myocardium in pigs. Radiology 2006; 240(2):419–426.
50. Manke C, Nitz WR, Lenhart M, et al. Stentangioplastie von Beckenarterienstenosen unter MRT-Kontrolle: Erste klinische Ergebnisse. Fortschr Röntgenstr 2000; 172(1):92–97.
51. Paetzel C, Zorger N, Bachthaler M, et al. Feasibility of MR-guided angioplasty of femoral artery stenoses using real-time imaging and intraarterial contrast-enhanced MR angiography. Fortschr Röntgenstr 2004; 176(9):1232–1236.
52. Huegli RW, Thalhammer C, Jacob AL, et al. Intra-arterial MR-angiography on an open-bore MR-scanner compared to digital-subtraction angiography of the infra-popliteal runoff in patients with peripheral arterial occlusive disease. Eur J Radiol 2007.
53. Kee ST, Ganguly A, Daniel BL, et al. MR-guided transjugular intrahepatic portosystemic shunt creation with use of a hybrid radiography/MR system. J Vasc Interv Radiol 2005; 16(2 Pt 1):227–234.

19 Role of MDCT for the diagnosis of coronary anomalies and fistulae

Stephan Achenbach and Dieter Ropers

NORMAL CORONARY ANATOMY AND CORONARY ANOMALIES

Normal coronary artery anatomy is characterized by two ostia centrally located in the right and left sinus of Valsalva of the aortic root, slightly cranial to the aortic valve. The main left coronary artery originates from the left ostium, branching into the left anterior descending coronary artery and circumflex coronary artery. The latter follows a course in the left atrioventricular groove, while the former travels in the anterior interventricular sulcus toward the apex of the heart. The right coronary artery arises from the right coronary ostium. The vessel then follows the right atrioventricular groove and usually ends as a posterior descending artery in the posterior interventricular sulcus (Fig. 19.1).

Congenital anomalies of the coronary arteries are rare conditions. They may occur isolated or in association with congenital heart disease. Their incidence is estimated to be approximately between 0.3% and 1.5%.[1–4] In patients with congenital heart disease, the incidence is higher. For example, up to 12% of patients with Tetralogy of Fallot have an anomalous coronary artery distribution.[5] Even though the majority of coronary anomalies lack hemodynamic significance, possible consequences include myocardial infarction and sudden death. In young athletes, coronary artery anomalies are the second most common cause of sudden death due to structural heart disease.[2] The coronary artery anomalies most likely to cause ischemia, or ventricular tachycardia are anomalous origin of the left coronary artery from the pulmonary artery (Bland–White–Garland syndrome), large coronary arteriovenous fistulas, and those anomalies associated with a coronary artery coursing between the great vessels. Other coronary artery anomalies are rarely associated with symptoms or sudden death. Exact anatomic definition of coronary artery anomalies and their course is therefore vital to initiate appropriate management. Invasive coronary angiography, due to its projectional nature, can have difficulties regarding the exact definition of the course of anomalous coronary vessels.[3] Furthermore, selective cannulation of abnormal coronary ostia can be challenging and sometimes impossible, which further complicates analysis by invasive angiography. Noninvasive imaging tools are therefore of high diagnostic importance and especially computed tomography, which renders an isotropic, three-dimensional (3-D), high-resolution data set, is well suited for the analysis of anomalous coronary anatomy.

NONINVASIVE IMAGING FOR THE DETECTION OF CORONARY ARTERY ANOMALIES

Echocardiography and Magnetic Resonance Imaging

Echocardiography (ECG) is usually limited to the detection of the origin of coronary artery anomalies and their very first proximal path.[5] A possible exception are coronary artery fistula, which may be visualized when they have a large lumen, especially in pediatric patients.[6,7]

Magnetic resonance imaging theoretically constitutes an ideal tool for noninvasive cardiac imaging. It does not involve exposure to radiation and, in most cases, neither requires injection of contrast agent. Numerous studies have shown that magnetic resonance angiography has the potential to visualize the coronary arteries and it has also repeatedly been shown to permit the detection of the origin and course of anomalous coronary arteries with high accuracy.[8,9] In fact, the use of magnetic resonance imaging is considered an "appropriate" indication in a recent multisocietal consensus statement on the appropriateness of cardiac magnetic resonance and computed tomography imaging.[10] However, patients with implanted pacemakers or defibrillators cannot be studied by magnetic resonance imaging and the method requires substantial experience in performing the investigation and interpretation of the results. Furthermore, long

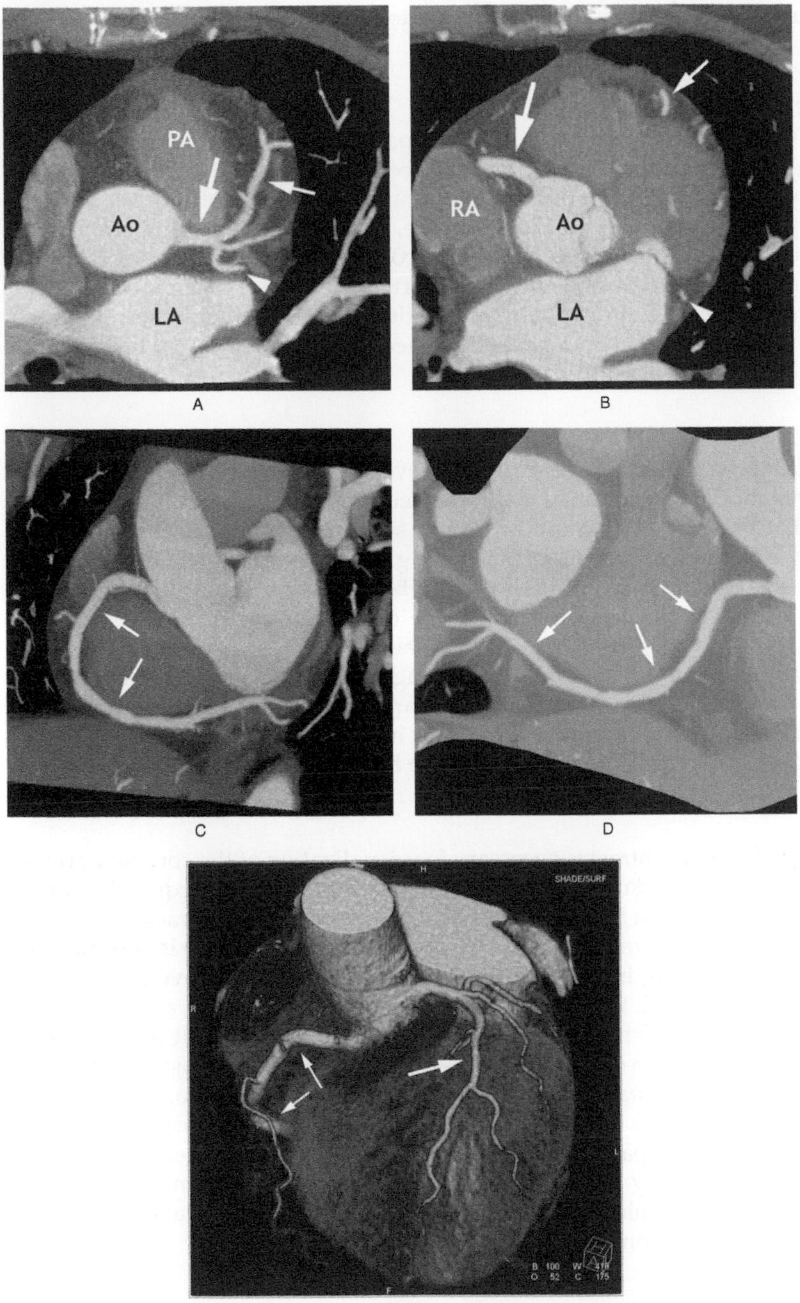

Figure 19.1 Normal coronary anatomy in contrast-enhanced multidetector CT (here: 64-slice CT). (**A**) Origin of the left main coronary artery (*large arrow*) from the aortic root. The left main coronary artery trifurcates into the left anterior descending coronary artery (*small arrow*), ramus intermedius, and left circumflex coronary artery (*arrowhead*). (**B**) Origin of the right coronary artery (*large arrow*) from the aortic root, just above the right coronary cusp of the aortic valve. Cross-section of the mid-left anterior descending coronary artery (*small arrow*) and left circumflex coronary artery (*arrowhead*). (**C**) So-called "maximum intensity projections" can be rendered in oblique planes and allow visualization of long vessel segments. Here, the right coronary artery (*arrows*) is visualized using a 5-mm-thick maximum intensity projection. (**D**) "Curved multiplanar reconstructions" are used to display an entire coronary artery in a single two-dimensional image by creating an image plane that follows the vessel course (here: right coronary artery, *arrows*). However, all structures surrounding the coronary vessel are distorted so that this type of visualization is of limited utility for the analysis of coronary anomalies. (**E**) Three-dimensional reconstruction showing the left and right coronary artery. *Abbreviations:* Ao, aorta; PA, pulmonary artery; LA, left atrium; RA, right atrium.

scan times can be required to fully depict all coronary arteries and the data set is not always fully isotropic.

Multidetector computed tomography (MDCT)

Due to the rapid evolution of CT technology during the past years, it has become possible to achieve reliable imaging of the coronary arteries. Both CT technology and scan protocols have to be chosen appropriately to achieve sufficiently high temporal and spatial resolution for coronary artery imaging. Usually, CT systems with 16 slices or more, as well as a slice collimation of less than 1.0 mm will be considered appropriate to analyze coronary artery anomalies. The scan protocol will be the same as for the detection of coronary artery stenoses, but some adjustments can be made to lower the amount of contrast agent or radiation exposure, since image quality for the detection of coronary anomalies does not necessarily need to be as high as for visualization of coronary artery stenoses.

Patient preparation

A certain degree of patient preparation is necessary to achieve optimal image quality in coronary CT angiography. Patients should be instructed about the necessary breathhold commands (and it should be verified that they are able to follow them), since all imaging needs to be done in a reliable inspiratory breathhold. Nitrates are usually given to patients when imaging for coronary artery stenoses is attempted, but this may not be necessary if only the analysis of coronary anomalies is planned. Lowering the heart rate of the patient is important for 16- and 64-slice CT, since it substantially improves image quality.[11] In most cases, short-acting β-blockers, either orally (approximately 1 hour before CT imaging) or intravenously (immediately before CT data acquisition) are applied, with a target heart rate of <65/min, optimally even <60/min. With newer Dual Source CT systems, diagnostic image quality can in almost all cases be also achieved for higher heart rates and lowering of the heart rate is not required.[12,13]

Contrast injection

Intravenous injection of iodinated contrast is necessary for visualization of the coronary arteries by CT. In order to assure correct timing of contrast injection relative to CT data acquisition, either a "bolus tracking" technique or a "test bolus" protocol can be used. In "bolus tracking," the CT density in a predefined region of interest (for example, in the ascending aorta) is continuously monitored as contrast agent is being injected, and once the density rises above a predefined threshold, data acquisition is initiated. When the "test bolus" technique is used, a small amount of contrast agent is injected (e. g., 10 mL), and the time to peak enhancement in the aorta is measured. This time interval is used to determine the delay between contrast injection and data acquisition for the CT angiography data set. For the CT angiography acquisition, contrast agent (300 mg iodine/mL or more) is usually injected at a rate of 4 to 5 mL/sec, but it can be increased to 6 or even 7 mL/sec in very heavy patients, and it can be lowered to 3 mL/sec or less if only visualization of the course of coronary anomalies is desired and contrast volume is of concern. The duration of contrast injection should approximately be the same as that of data acquisitions, but should not be shorter than 10 seconds.

Data acquisition

For data acquisition in coronary CT angiography, the scanner settings are chosen to provide maximum spatial and temporal resolution. Gantry rotation is chosen at maximum speed and slice collimation is chosen as thin as the detectors provide. Pitch values (speed of table movement relative to gantry rotation) depend on the heart rate. While tube voltage is typically fixed at 120 kV, tube current can be modified depending on the patient's size. The patient's ECG is recorded along with the CTA data and this information is used for retrospectively ECG-gated image reconstruction. Reconstructed data sets typically consist of 200 to 300 thin transaxial images with a thickness of 0.5 to 0.75 mm and a slice increment of 0.3 to 0.5 mm (to allow some overlap of slices). Image data sets are typically reconstructed in diastole, just before onset of atrial contraction, but especially in higher heart rates reconstruction during late systole may provide better image quality.

Strategies to lower radiation exposure

Patients who are investigated for the presence of anomalous coronary arteries are often young. It is therefore necessary to avoid excessive radiation dose and strategies to lower dose during CT data acquisition should be applied whenever possible. Three concepts are available to lower dose: First, the patient's ECG can be used as a signal to modulate X-ray tube output during data acquisition. Since image reconstruction will most likely only be performed in diastole (especially if heart rate is low), tube output during systole can be reduced substantially (most frequently by about 80%). This can lead to a reduction in radiation exposure of about 50%.[14,15] In patents with high heart rates and in patients with irregular heart rates, it may not be possible to use ECG-gated tube current modulation. Second, choice of tube voltage has a substantial influence on radiation exposure. While most coronary CT angiography examinations are performed using 120 kV tube voltage; the use of 100 kV tube voltage leads to a reduction of radiation exposure by approximately 40%. The downside is higher image noise. In our experience, however, image noise will not be problematic unless body weight is high and we routinely use 100 kV in all patients with a body weight below 90 kg. A third strategy is to use prospective ECG triggering instead of retrospective ECG gating. In this mode, also called "step-and-shoot" mode, images are only acquired during one predefined time instant (usually in diastole), and in the remaining interval, the X-ray tube is switched off completely while the patient table is advanced to the next scan level. Radiation doses as low as 1 to 3 mSv have been reported.[16] However, the ability to reconstruct during more than one time instant in the coronary cycle is lost when prospective ECG triggering is used.

Image postprocessing

Coronary CT angiography provides a nearly isotropic data set consisting of approximately 200 to 300 transaxial images. Several image postprocessing methods are available to review the data set and analyze the coronary arteries as to their origin and course as well as to the presence of coronary artery stenoses. Cross-sectional, two-dimensional (2-D) imaging is the best method for reviewing the exact spatial relationship of the coronary vessels and neighboring structures. Three-dimensional rendering can help to create a better visual impression of anatomy.

Transaxial slices

Careful review of thin cross-sectional slices in transaxial orientation is the basis and mainstay of analysis for coronary CT angiography. Transaxial slices are reviewed in an interactive fashion using postprocessing workstations and the evaluator should always personally review and manipulate the data set and not rely on prerendered reconstructions (Fig. 19.2).

Maximum intensity projection

In maximum intensity projection ("MIP"), thicker slices are rendered to display longer segments of the coronary arteries in a single image, thus facilitating analysis of the course and continuity of coronary arteries. Typical thickness is approximately 5 mm, but varies according to the individual situation. MIP is especially useful for the analysis of tortuous vessel segments and bifurcations. The major drawback of MIP rendering is the fact that adjacent structures can overlap, which renders the respective segment impossible (Fig. 19.2).

Multiplanar reconstruction

Multiplanar reconstruction makes use of the near-isotropic nature of most cardiac CT data sets and allows to create new imaging planes in any desired orientation to facilitate visualization of coronary segments and analysis of their spatial relationship with neighboring vessels. Multiplanar reconstruction can be combined with MIP imaging to display longer vessel segments in the same image and to compensate for slight tortuosity. "Curved multiplanar reconstruction" uses curved planes that are fitted to the vessel centerline and allows to display the entire course of a coronary artery in one single image. This is mainly used to display coronary artery patency versus stenosis. Because of the curved reference plane, curved multiplanar reconstructions do not allow to reliably assess the relationship of coronary arteries to adjacent structures such as the great vessels and cardiac chambers. For the analysis of anomalous coronary anatomy, curved multiplanar reconstruction is therefore of limited utility (Fig. 19.2).

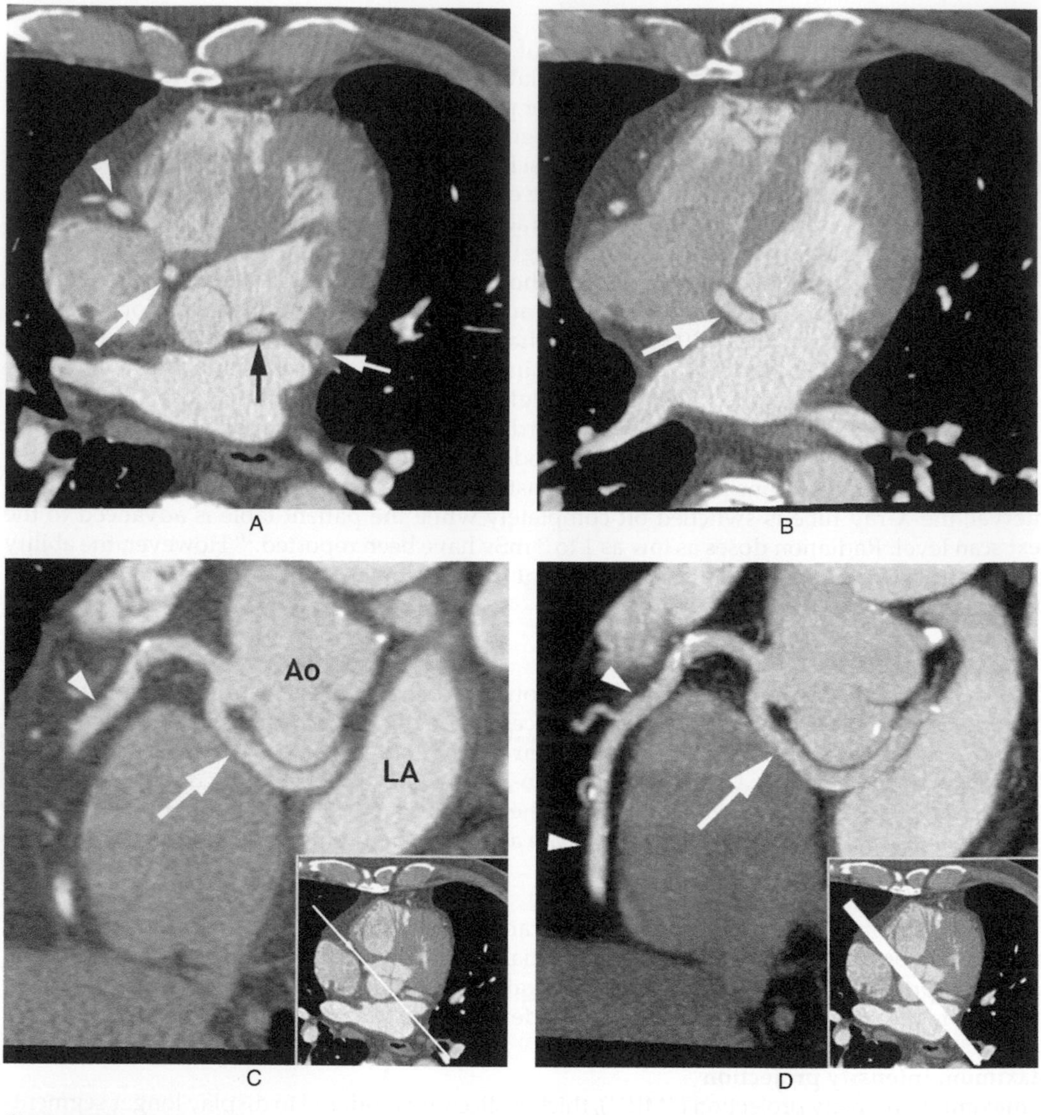

Figure 19.2 Image postprocessing methods used to visualize coronary artery anomalies by CT. The patient in this example has an anomalous left circumflex coronary artery arising from the right sinus of Valsalva and following a path behind and below the aortic root. (**A**) Transaxial slice showing cross-sections of the left circumflex coronary artery just distal to its origin from the right sinus of Valsalva (*large arrow*), the ascending segment of the anomalous left circumflex coronary artery after it has passed below the aortic root (*small black arrow*), and the distal segment of the left circumflex coronary artery in the coronary sulcus (*small white arrow*). The arrowhead points at a cross-section of the right coronary artery. (**B**) Transaxial slice showing the segment of the anomalous left circumflex coronary artery that passes just below the aortic root (*arrow*). This is the typical image for this anomaly, which is the most frequent variant of anomalous coronary arteries. (**C**) Multiplanar reconstruction in an oblique plane that shows the very proximal segment of the anomalous left circumflex coronary artery (*large arrow*), as the vessel arises from the right sinus of Valsalva (with a common ostium with the right coronary artery) and then takes a course behind and below the aortic root. Right coronary artery (*arrowhead*). The image inset shows the orientation of the oblique plane. (**D**) "Maximum intensity projection" (5 mm thickness), using the exact same orientation as the image in part (C). The thicker image allows to visualize longer segments of the coronary arteries (*large arrow*, anomalous left circumflex coronary artery; *arrowheads*, right coronary artery). The image inset shows the orientation of the oblique plane. (**E**) "Curved multiplanar reconstruction." This form of reconstruction allows to display the entire course of the anomalous left circumflex coronary artery (*arrows*). However, the anatomy of all surrounding structures is distorted which makes assessment of the vessel course impossible. (**F**) Three-dimensional reconstruction, seen from an anterior view (*large arrows*, anomalous left circumflex artery; *arrowhead*, left anterior descending coronary artery). (**G**) Three-dimensional reconstruction, seen from a posterior view (*large arrows*, anomalous left circumflex artery; *small arrows*, right coronary artery). *Abbreviations*: Ao, aorta; LA, left atrium.

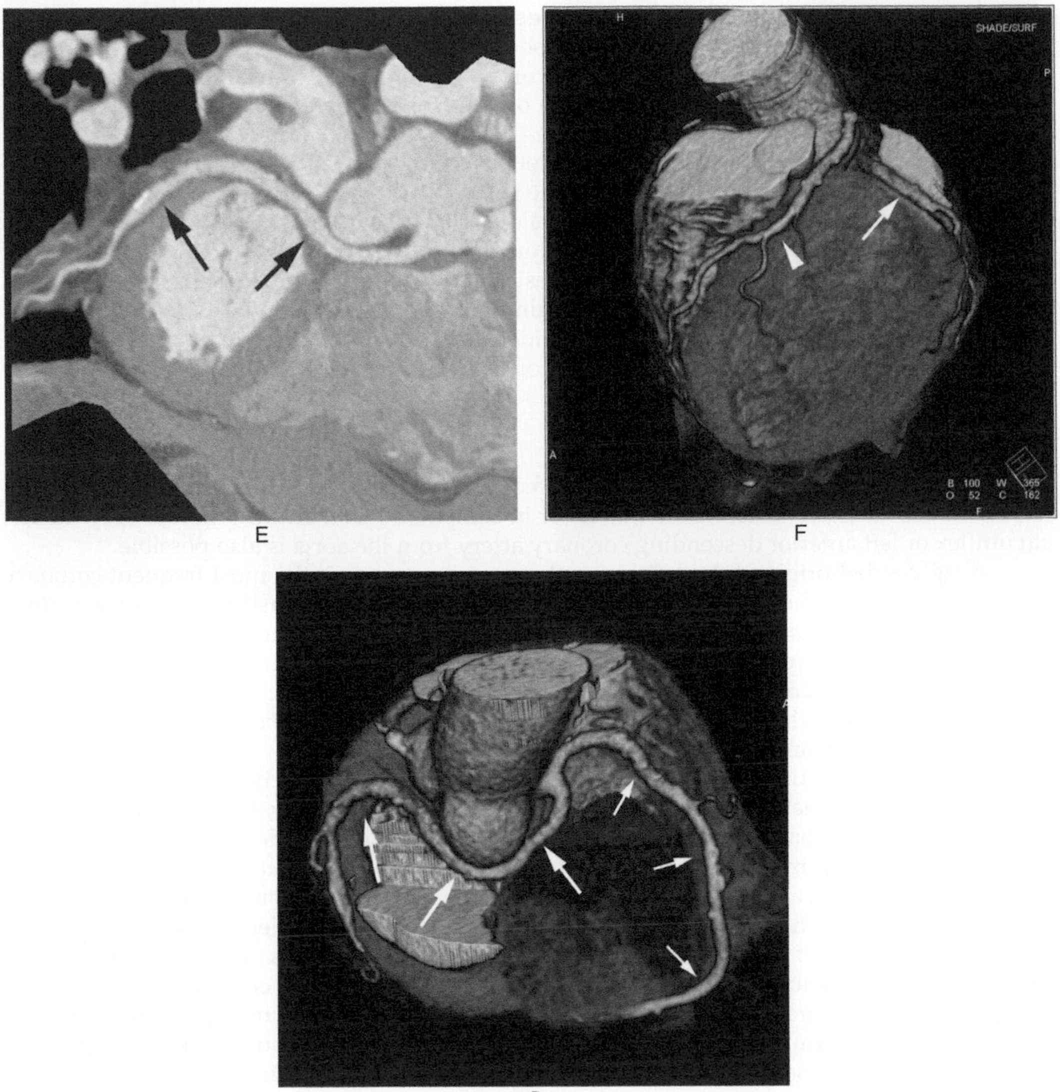

E F

G

Figure 19.2 *(Continued)*

Three-dimensional reconstruction

Three-dimensional images permit impressive visualization of cardiac and coronary anatomy. However, their use for diagnostic purposes has several drawbacks. First, segmentation is required (with usually at least some and often a great extent of manual input) (Fig. 19.1) in order to remove overlapping structures and display the coronary arteries. Secondly, the course of anomalous arteries that pass between the great arteries or deep within the heart can often only be partly visualized in 3-D reconstructions, since overlapping structures will prevent visualization of the entire vessel. Third, 3-D imaging always uses at least some degree of thresholding, which results in a loss of information and, for example, may make it impossible to discern between coronary arteries and veins, or to separate coronary calcification from contrast-enhanced lumen. 3-D reconstruction should therefore only be sparingly used for the analysis of anomalous coronary vessels, never without analyzing the 2-D, original data set. For displaying and demonstrating coronary anatomy to patients and referring physicians, 3-D images may in some (but not all) cases be useful (Fig. 19.2).

Visualization of anomalous coronary arteries by computed tomography

Because of its high spatial resolution and the isotropic nature of the obtained data set, coronary CT angiography is ideally suited for assessing coronary anomalies. The examination is rapid and straightforward to perform, and the available options for postprocessing allow exact analysis of the anomalous coronary anatomy.

Numerous scientific studies[17–23] as well as countless case reports have been published that highlight the potential and unique clinical utility of contrast-enhanced CT imaging for the detection and analysis of anomalous coronary vessels. Some of the most frequent and typical findings are outlined below. Clinically, coronary CT angiography may not only be applied as a first-line imaging test when coronary anomalies are suspected, for example, in young individuals with chest pain and/or syncope, but it is also often applied after anomalous coronary anatomy has accidentally been identified in invasive coronary angiography, and exact clarification of the origin and course of the anomalous vessel is required.

Anomalies of the left coronary artery

Anomalies of the left coronary artery can affect the left main, left anterior descending, and left circumflex coronary artery, either alone or in combination. Aberrant origin of only the left circumflex or left anterior descending coronary artery from the aorta is also possible.

A right-sided origin of the left circumflex coronary artery is the most frequent coronary anomaly and is of no hemodynamic relevance. In cardiac CT, it can easily be recognized since the left circumflex coronary artery can be traced from its origin (either at the right coronary ostium, from the aorta, or the very proximal right coronary artery), below and behind the aortic root, and into the left coronary sulcus (Fig. 19.2).

Characteristic is the short, horizontal passage of the left circumflex coronary artery immediately below and posterior to the aortic root (Fig. 19.2B).

When the left main or left anterior descending coronary artery arises from the right sinus of Valsalva, the anomalous artery can either follow a prepulmonary, inter-arterial (between the aorta and pulmonary artery) or retroaortic course to the left side (Fig. 19.3). While the prepulmonary and retroaortic courses are considered harmless, a left coronary artery passing between the aorta and pulmonary artery may potentially be compressed between the two great arteries, which have been associated with ischemia and sudden cardiac death.[2] One of the most important roles of CT imaging in assessing anomalous coronary arteries is to differentiate an intra-arterial course of an aberrant, right-sided left coronary artery from a "subpulmonary" or "transseptal" course. While the first is considered malignant, the "subpulmonary" course is assumed to be harmless. The high spatial resolution and the isotropic, 3-D nature of the CT data set make this modality ideally suited to determine such fine differences (Fig. 19.4).

Anomalies of the right coronary artery

The most frequent anomaly of the right coronary artery is its ectopic origin from the left sinus of Valsalva, with subsequent passage between the aorta and pulmonary artery. As opposed to an ectopic left coronary artery following this path, and inter-arterial course of the right coronary artery is considered to be of no clinical consequence if incidentally discovered in asymptomatic individuals.[24] Transaxial slices in CT imaging will allow immediate detection of this anomaly. Next to this typical variant, the right coronary artery may arise from many other locations. Figure 19.5 shows an unusual example of a right coronary artery arising from the mid-left anterior descending coronary artery.

Bland–White–Garland syndrome

In "Bland–White–Garland syndrome" (anomalous left coronary artery from the pulmonary artery, "ALCAPA"), the left main coronary artery originates from the pulmonary artery instead of the aorta. Usually, this disease is diagnosed in childhood but can sometimes remain undetected until adult life. Through collaterals from the right coronary artery, oxygenized blood will usually be transported to left coronary system and a left-to-right shunt ensues (blood flow from the aorta, through the normal right coronary artery and via collaterals retrogradely into the

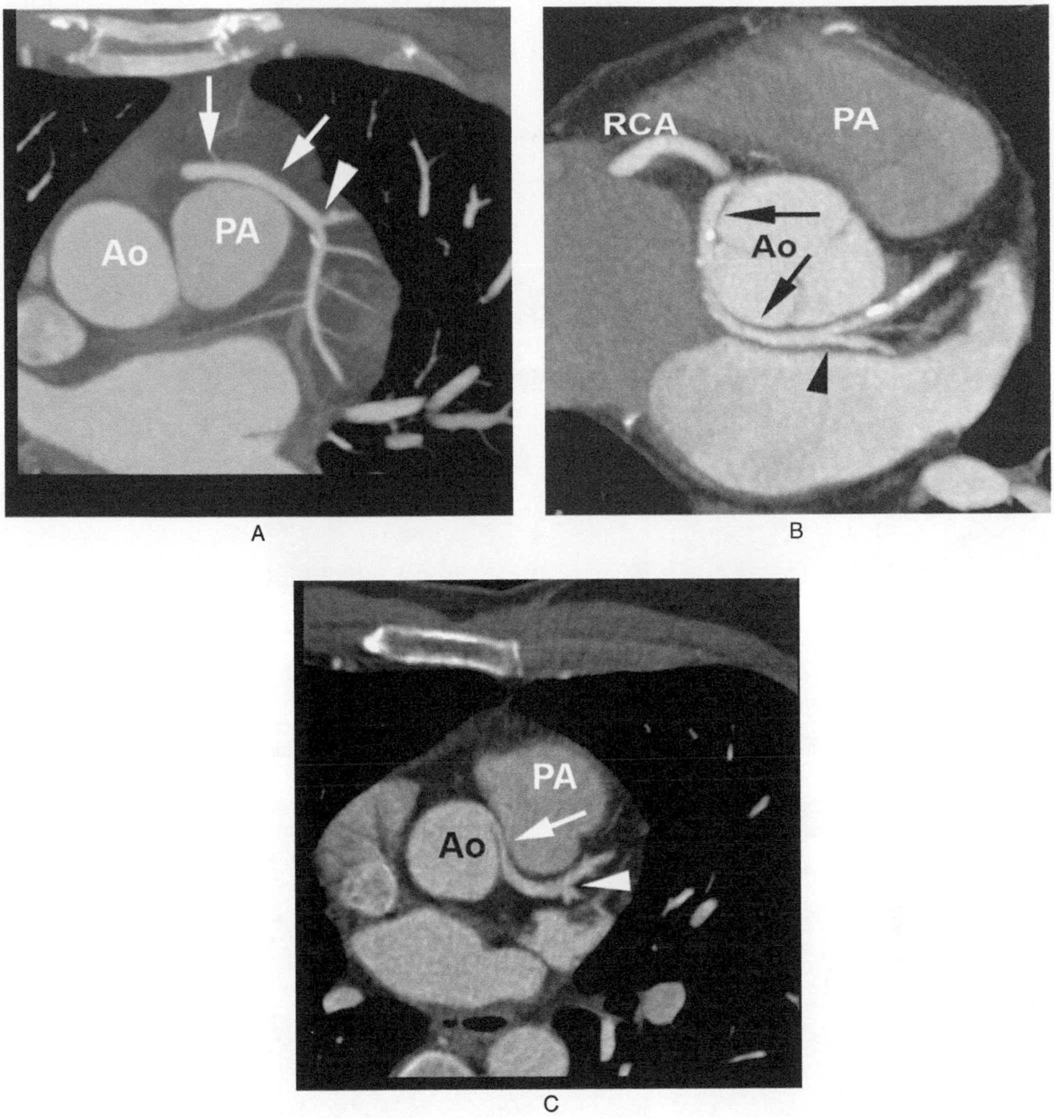

Figure 19.3 Three different variants of a right-sided left coronary artery as demonstrated by CT ("maximum intensity projections"). (**A**) Right-sided left main coronary artery with a prepulmonary or anterior course. "Maximum intensity projection" (5 mm thickness; MDCT 64) visualizing the left main coronary artery (*arrows*) taking a path anterior to the PA. The arrowhead indicates the bifurcation of the left main stem in the left anterior descending coronary artery (LAD) and the left circumflex coronary artery (CX). (**B**) Right-sided left main coronary artery with a retroaortic or posterior course. "Maximum intensity projection" (5 mm thickness; MDCT 64) demonstrates the left main coronary artery (*arrows*) with a path posterior to the aortic root. The arrowhead indicates the bifurcation of the left main stem into the left anterior descending coronary artery (LAD) and the left circumflex coronary artery (CX). (**C**) Right-sided left main coronary artery with an interarterial or preaortic course. "Maximum intensity projection" (5 mm thickness; MDCT 64) demonstrates the left main coronary artery (*arrow*) with a path between the Ao and the PA. The arrowhead indicates the bifurcation of the left main stem into the left anterior descending coronary artery and the left circumflex coronary artery. *Abbreviations*: Ao, ascending aorta; PA, pulmonary artery; RCA, right coronary artery.

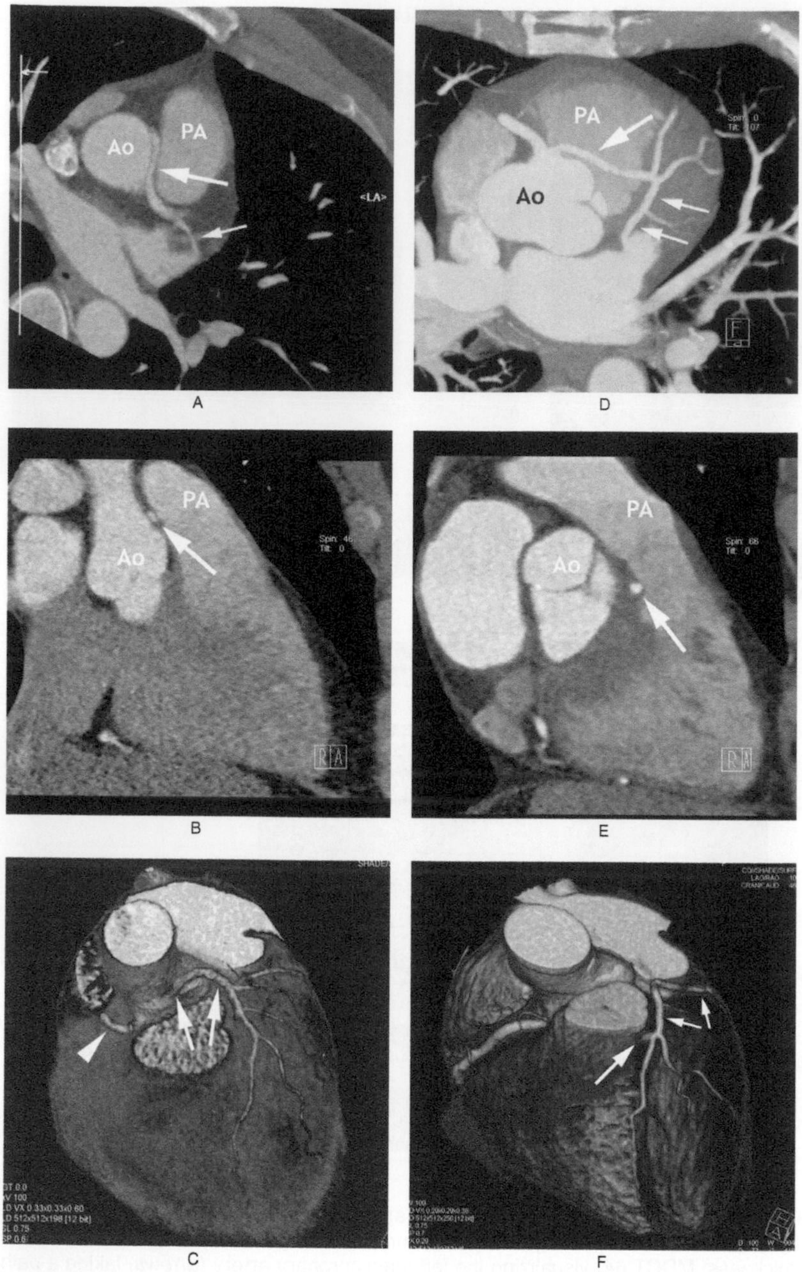

Figure 19.4 Differentiation between a right-sided left coronary artery with an inter-arterial path from a right-sided left coronary artery with a transseptal (subpulmonary) course using coronary CT angiography. (**A**) Right-sided left main coronary artery with an inter-arterial (or preaortic) course. A "maximum intensity projection" (5 mm thickness) demonstrates the left main coronary artery (*arrow*) with a path between the Ao and the PA. The small arrow points at the left circumflex coronary artery. (**B**) In an oblique multiplanar reconstruction (slightly angulated sagittal plane), it can be appreciated that the left main coronary artery (*arrow*) passes between the Ao and PA. (**C**) Three-dimensional reconstruction. After manual segmentation to remove the PA, the interarterial course of the left main coronary artery (*arrows*) between the Ao and PA is clearly visualized. The arrowhead indicates the right coronary artery. (**D**) Right-sided left main coronary artery with a transseptal (also called "subpulmonary") course. A "maximum intensity projection" (5 mm thickness) demonstrates the left main coronary artery (*large arrow*) with a path caudal to the PA within the interventricular septum. The small arrows indicate the left circumflex coronary artery. (**E**) In an oblique multiplanar reconstruction (slightly angulated sagittal plane), it can be appreciated that the left main coronary artery (*arrow*) does not have a position immediately between the Ao and the PA. Instead, it is embedded in the septal myocardium and passes somewhat below the PA. (**F**) Three-dimensional reconstruction demonstrating the left main coronary artery surfacing from the septum in the mid-part of the anterior interventricular groove (*arrow*). The small arrows indicate the left circumflex coronary artery. *Abbreviations:* Ao, ascending aorta; PA, pulmonary artery.

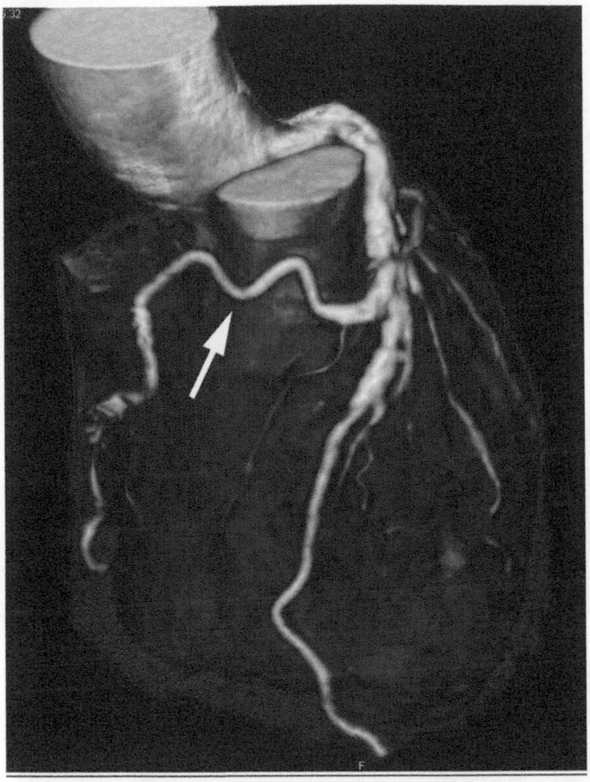

Figure 19.5 Three-dimensional CT reconstruction demonstrating a right coronary artery (*arrow*) originating from the mid-segment of the left anterior descending coronary artery. In this very unusual variant, the anomalous right coronary artery crosses the right ventricular outflow tract as it courses towards the right interventricular groove.

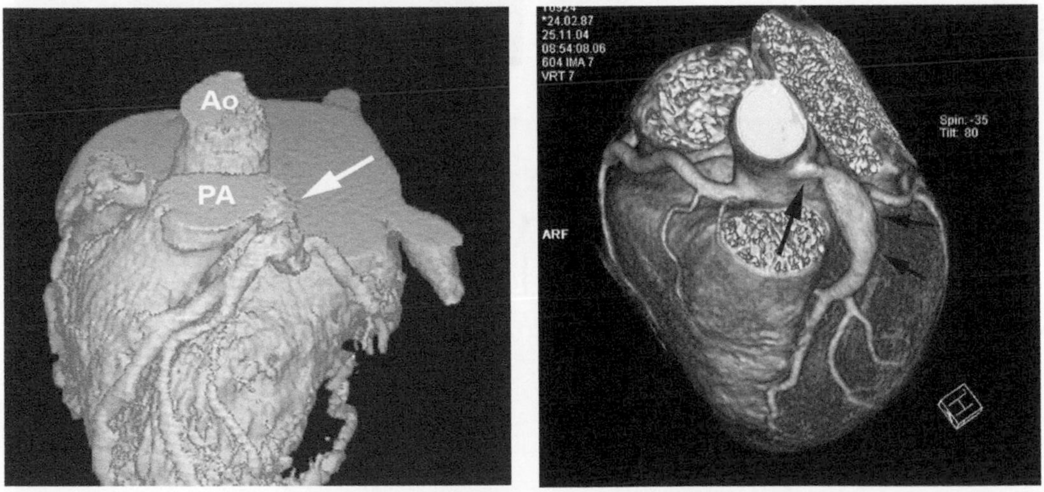

A B

Figure 19.6 Three-dimensional CT reconstructions of a patient with a left coronary artery originating from the pulmonary artery ("Bland–White–Garland syndrome" or ALCAPA) before surgical correction and several follow-ups after the operation. (**A**) Three-dimensional reconstruction obtained by contrast-enhanced electron beam CT in a 12-year-old girl. The left coronary artery originating from the PA can clearly be seen (*arrow*). Some artifacts are caused by lack of sufficient breathhold. The coronary arteries are of large caliber since collaterals from the right coronary artery to the left coronary artery form a left-to-right shunt. (**B**) Three-dimensional CT reconstruction (64-slice MDCT) 5 years after surgical repair with reimplantation of the left main coronary artery (*arrow*) into the Ao. CT demonstrates a mild stenosis of the left main stem with some poststenotic dilatation of the left anterior descending coronary artery (*small arrows*) *Abbreviations*: Ao, ascending aorta; PA, pulmonary artery.

abnormal left coronary artery, from where it flows into the pulmonary artery). As a result of the high flow, the coronary arteries are enlarged. The anatomy is easily displayed by computed tomography. When surgical correction is attempted, CT imaging may be able to provide information to the surgeon as to whether the abnormal ostium can be reimplanted into the aortic root or whether placement of a bypass graft is necessary (Fig. 19.6).

Coronary fistulae

A large variety of coronary fistulae are possible. They connect the coronary arteries to a lower-pressure system. Small coronary fistulae (e.g., from a coronary artery—most frequently the left anterior descending coronary artery—to the pulmonary artery) can be difficult to identify in CT imaging because of the often very tortuous course and the small caliber. However, these vessels lack hemodynamic relevance (Fig. 19.7). Very infrequently, coronary arteries can drain

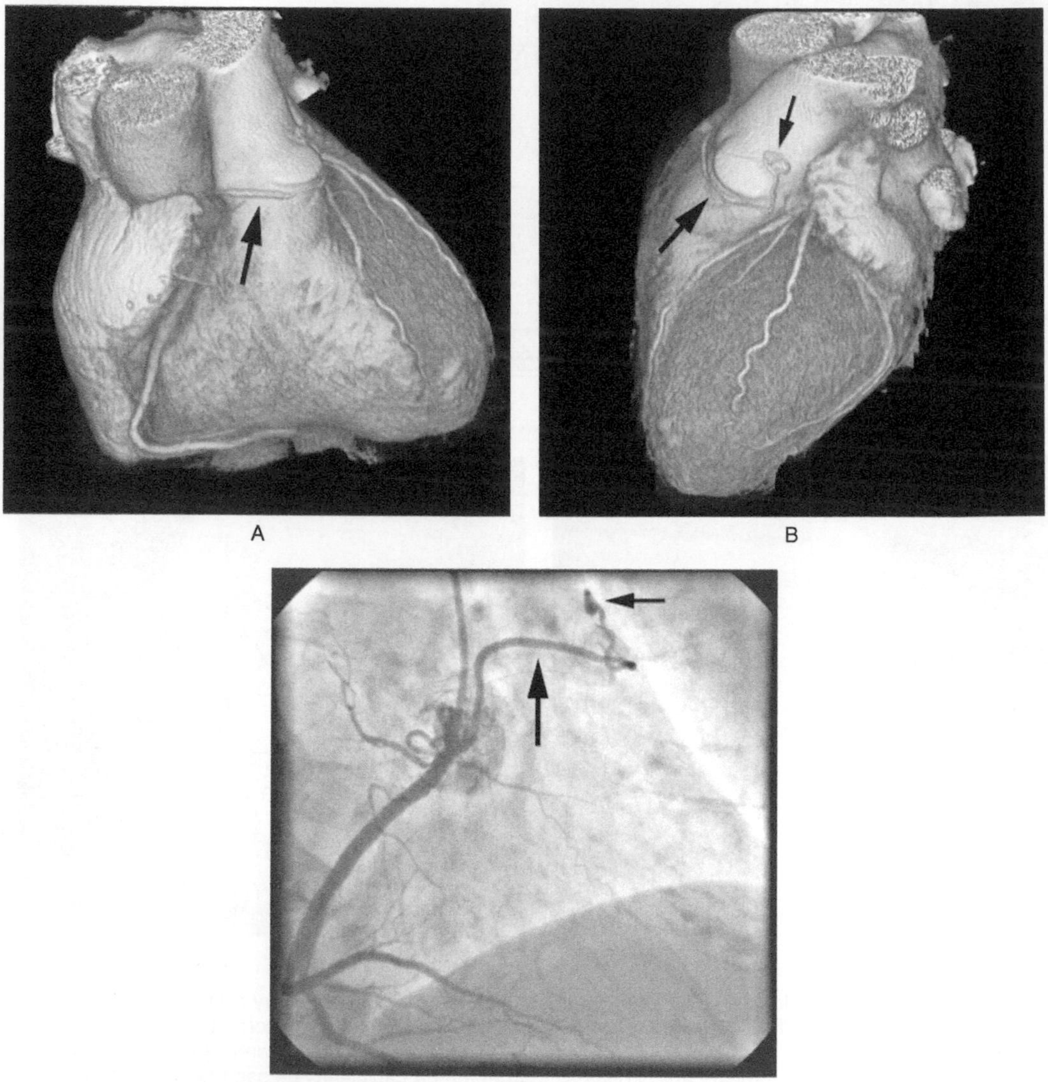

Figure 19.7 Coronary artery to pulmonary artery fistula. These fistulae are usually small and can potentially be missed in contrast-enhanced CT. (**A,B**) Three-dimensional reconstructions obtained by contrast-enhanced 16-slice CT in a patient with a very small fistula from the proximal right coronary artery (*black arrows*) to the pulmonary artery. The large arrows indicate the course of the fistula, the small arrow points at the connection to the pulmonary artery. (**C**) Corresponding invasive angiogram in RAO projection.

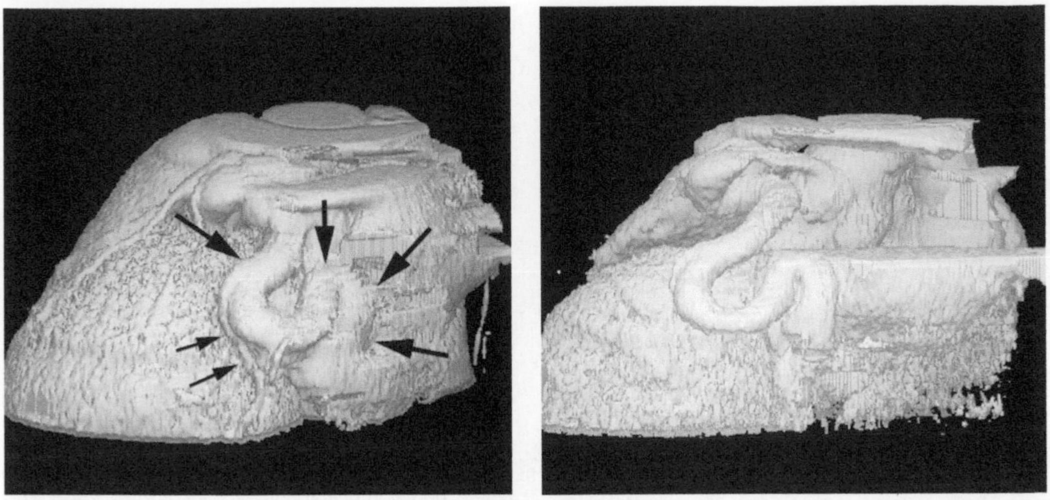

Figure 19.8 Large fistula from the left circumflex coronary artery to the coronary sinus in a 48-year-old woman with a cardiac murmur. (**A**) A three-dimensional reconstruction obtained by contrast-enhanced electron beam CT shows a very large, tortuous vessel from the left main to the coronary sinus (*large arrows*). This vessel represents the left circumflex artery. It gives rise to an obtuse marginal branch of normal diameter (*small arrows*). (**B**). Three-dimensional reconstruction with higher thresholding allows better appreciation of the tortuous course of the coronary fistula.

into one of the atria, the coronary sinus, or the right ventricle. In these cases, the high flow often leads to a very large diameter and substantial tortuosity of the fistulous vessel. The tortuosity can cause difficulties in tracing the course of such fistula in CT imaging, but careful analysis of the transaxial images will usually reveal the exact anatomy. If 3-D reconstruction is used to display the large, tortuous fistula, the rendering threshold must often be set very high in order to correctly delineate the anomalous artery (Fig. 19.8).

Pediatric patients

Coronary artery anomalies can be a relevant clinical question in pediatric patients, especially in the context of congenital heart disease.[3] For example, up to 12% of all patients with Fallot's Tetralogy have anomalous coronary arteries.[25] Exact delineation of these vessels can be of importance for surgical correction of the congenital heart defect. CT is ideally suited to visualize coronary anomalies in pediatric patients. Even in patients unable to cooperate with breathholding, sufficiently precise data sets can often be obtained in free breathing, thus obviating the need for sedation or anaesthesia (Fig. 19.9). Care has to be taken to avoid unnecessarily high-radiation exposure in these pediatric patients. Along with selecting low mAs values, tube current should be lowered to 80 kV, which substantially lowers the effective dose.

SUMMARY

Although the majority of coronary artery anomalies lack hemodynamic significance, possible consequences include myocardial infarction and sudden death. The exact anatomic definition of a coronary artery anomaly is therefore extremely important. Contrast-enhanced multidetector row spiral CT (MDCT) with retrospective ECG gating allows the noninvasive detection and definition of anomalous coronary arteries. In the often young patients, imaging parameters should be adjusted in order to keep radiation dose as low as reasonably achievable. Simple postprocessing tools such as review of the axial slices, multiplanar reconstruction, and maximum intensity projection are often most useful for analysis of the data sets; 3-D rendering can facilitate demonstration of the results. Numerous studies have demonstrated that CT imaging allows both the detection and also the exact delineation of anomalous coronary anatomy with high

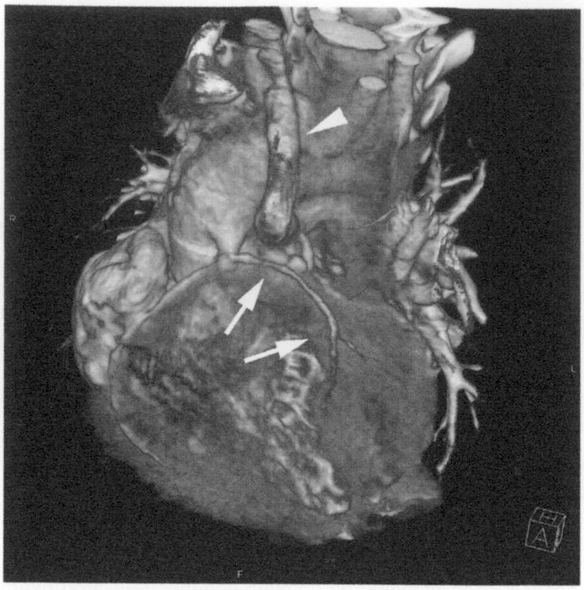

Figure 19.9 Coronary anomaly in a pediatric patient. In this 3-year old with Tetralogy of Fallot (a cavo-pulmonary shunt had been placed in a postpartal surgical procedure), an anomalous left anterior descending coronary artery arises from the right coronary ostium and crosses the right ventricular outflow tract (*large arrows*). This data set was obtained by contrast-enhanced dual source CT in free breathing, without anaesthesia or sedation.

accuracy. In fact, CT imaging constitutes a "de facto" gold standard for the delineation of anomalous coronary vessels.

REFERENCES

1. Roberts WC. Major anomalies of coronary arterial origin seen in adulthood. Am Heart J 1986; 111: 941–963.
2. Angelini P, Velasco JA, Flamm S. Coronary anomalies: Incidence, pathophysiology, and clinical relevance. Circulation 2002; 105:2449–2454.
3. Lipsett J, Cohle SD, Perry PJ, et al. Anomalous coronary arteries: A multicenter paediatric autopsy study. Pediatr Pathol 1994; 14:287–300.
4. Click RL, Holmes DR, Vlietstra RE, et al. and the Participants of the Coronary Artery Surgery Study (CASS). Anomalous coronary arteries: Location, degree of atherosclerosis and effect on survival—A report from the Coronary Artery Surgery Study. J Am Coll Cardiol 1989; 13:531–537.
5. Jureidini SB, Marino CJ, Singh GK, et al. Abberant coronary arteries: A reliable echocardiographic screening method. J Am Soc Echocardiogr 2003; 16:756–763.
6. Liang CD, Ko SF, Huang CF, et al. Echocardiographic evaluation of coronary artery fistula in pediatric patients. Pediatr Cardiol 2005; 26:745–750.
7. Arat N, Gurel OM, Biyikoglu FS, et al. Coronary artery to left ventricular fistula demonstrated by transthoracic echocardiography. Eur J Echocardiogr 2008; 9:121–122.
8. Bunce NH, Lorenz CH, Keegan J, et al. Coronary artery anomalies: Assessment with free-breathing three-dimensional coronary MR angiography. Radiology 2003; 227:201–208.
9. Casolo G, Del Meglio J, Rega L, et al. Detection and assessment of coronary artery anomalies by three-dimensional magnetic resonance coronary angiography. Int J Cardiol 2005; 103;317–322.
10. ACCF/ACR/SCCT/SCMR/ASNC/NASCI/SCAI/SIR 2006 appropriateness criteria for cardiac computed tomography and cardiac magnetic resonance imaging: A report of the American College of Cardiology Foundation Quality Strategic Directions Committee Appropriateness Criteria Working Group, American College of Radiology, Society of Cardiovascular Computed Tomography, Society for Cardiovascular Magnetic Resonance, American Society of Nuclear Cardiology, North American Society for Cardiac Imaging, Society for Cardiovascular Angiography and Interventions, and Society of Interventional Radiology. J Am Coll Cardiol 2006; 48:1475–1497.
11. Achenbach S. Cardiac CT: State of the art for the detection of coronary arterial stenosis. J Cardiovasc Comput Tomogr 2007; 1:3–20.
12. Accuracy of dual-source CT coronary angiography: First experience in a high pre-test probability population without heart rate control. Eur Radiol 2006; 16:2739–2747.
13. Achenbach A, Anders K, Kalender WA. Dual-source cardiac computed tomography: Image quality and dose considerations. Eur Radiol Feb 26, 2008 [Epub ahead of print].

14. Einstein AJ, Henzlova MJ, Rajagopalan S. Estimating risk of cancer associated with radiation exposure from 64-slice computed tomography coronary angiography. JAMA 2007; 298:317–323.
15. Hausleiter J, Meyer T, Hadamitzky M, et al. Radiation dose estimates from cardiac multislice computed tomography in daily practice. Circulation 2006; 113:1305–1310.
16. Hsieh J, Londt J, Vass M, et al. Step-and-shoot data acquisition and reconstruction for cardiac x-ray computed tomography. Med Phys 2006; 33(11):4236–4248.
17. Ropers D, Moshage W, Daniel WG, et al. Visualisation of coronary artery anomalies and their anatomic course by contrast-enhanced electron beam tomography and three-dimensional reconstruction. Am J Cardiol 2001; 87:193–197.
18. Memisoglu E, Hobikoglu G, Tepe MS, et al. Congenital coronary anomalies in adults: Comparison of anatomic course visualization by catheterangiography and electron beam CT. Catheter Cardiovasc Interv 2005; 66:34–42.
19. van Ooijen PM, Dorgelo J, Zijlstra F, et al. Detection, visualization and evaluation of anomalous coronary anatomy on 16-slice multidetector-row CT. Eur Radiol 2004; 14:2163–2171.
20. Shi H, Aschoff AJ, Brambs HJ, et al. Multislice CT imaging of anomalous coronary arteries. Eur Radiol 2004; 14:2172–2181.
21. Datta J, White CS, Gilkeson RC, et al. Anomalous coronary arteries in adults: Depiction at multidetetctor row CT angiography. Radiology 2005; 235:812–818.
22. Schmitt R, Froehner S, Brunn J, et al. Congenital anomalies of the coronary arteries: Imaging with contrast-enhanced, multidetector computed tomography. Eur Radiol 2005; 15;1110–1121.
23. Schmid M, Achenbach S, Ludwig J, et al. Visualization of coronary artery anomalies by contrast-enhanced multi-detector row spiral computed tomography. Int J Cardiol 2006; 111;430–435.
24. Gersony WM. Management of anomalous coronary artery from the contralateral sinus. J Am Coll Cardiol 2007; 50:2083–2084.
25. Burch GH, Sahn DJ. Congenital coronary artery anomalies: The pediatric perspective. Coronary Artery Disease 2001; 12:605–616.

20 Coronary stenosis evaluation with CT angiography

Koen Nieman

COMPUTED TOMOGRAPHY

Computed tomography (CT) is a cross-sectional X-ray imaging technique. Differentiation of structures is based on the varying roentgen attenuation of different tissues. Generated roentgen rays are emitted in the shape of a fan or cone from one side of the gantry. After passing through an object, the remaining photons are collected and measured by roentgen detectors on the opposite side. By measuring the (attenuation of the) roentgen a so-called projection is created. During rotation of the tube and detectors around the object, a large number of these projections are acquired. From these combined angular projections the variation of attenuation can be calculated throughout a cross-sectional plane using sophisticated image reconstruction algorithms.

Original CT scanners, which are now referred to as single-slice sequential scanners, acquired one cross-sectional (axial) image at a time. Mechanical restrictions required that after each slice acquisition, the system would unwind the cables that connect the rotating elements (roentgen tube and detectors) to the stationary base. Slip-ring technology removed this physical connection, allowing continuous tube-detector rotation and the development of spiral CT. In spiral CT, continuous tube-detector rotation is combined with continuous table advancement. From the table's perspective, the trajectory of the tube-detectors unit resembles a spiral or helix, hence the name (Fig. 20.1). The obvious advantage of spiral CT is faster imaging which accelerated the development of CT angiography.

Instead of a single row of detector elements, current CT scanners are equipped with multiple rows of very small detectors, improving both the scan speed as well as the ability to image small structures, such as the coronary arteries.

Over the years, the rotation speed of mechanical CT has gradually improved. An important innovation to improve temporal resolution has been the combined application of two tube-detector units within one CT system. Dual-source CT significantly improves temporal resolution, which is very important for motion-free imaging of the coronary arteries (Fig. 20.2).

CARDIAC CT IMAGING

For the current 64-slice CT scanners, the total width of the detectors is approximately 2 to 4 cm, which means that a minimum of 5 to 10 acquisitions are required to cover the entire heart (12–15 cm). Consecutive data segments can only be combined in a sensible manner when they have been acquired during the same phase of cardiac contraction. This can be achieved by synchronizing either the data acquisition and/or the image reconstruction to the cardiac cycle (Fig. 20.3). In spiral CT, ECG synchronization is generally accomplished by retrospective ECG-gating: the recorded patient's ECG trace during the scan serves to select "iso-cardiophasic" data, from which images are then reconstructed. Alternatively, sequential cardiac imaging protocols (available on sequential CT scanners, including electron-beam CT, as well as spiral CT scanners) operate a prospective ECG-triggered data acquisition; each consecutive acquisition (of one or more slices) is triggered on-line by the patient's ECG. Because ECG-gated spiral CT acquisition is faster, less sensitive to arrhythmia, allows overlapping image reconstruction, as well as reconstruction of many different cardiac phases, this is currently the preferred method. However, concerns regarding the inherently high radiation dose of spiral CT protocols have led to renewed interest in ECG-triggered sequential CT protocols for angiographic applications.

To image a fast-moving structure such as the heart, sufficient temporal resolution is needed to avoid motion artifacts such as blurring. The temporal resolution of CT is limited by the rotation velocity. In cardiac CT, the minimum number of projections needed for image reconstruction can be acquired during a 180° rotation. Therefore, the temporal resolution (comparable to the

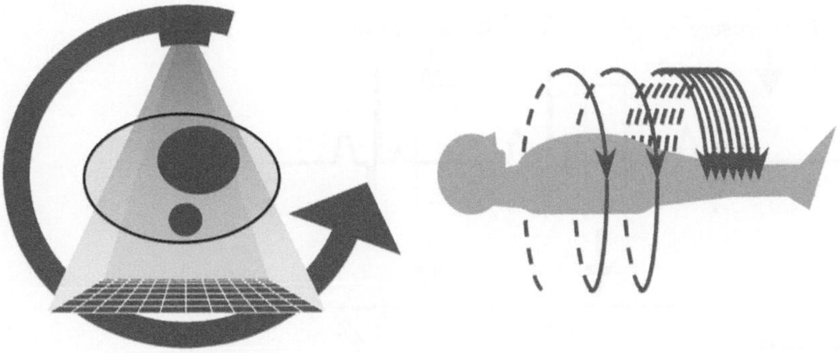

Figure 20.1 A roentgen source emits a cone-shaped roentgen beam across the gantry. On the opposite side, the detectors collect the attenuated roentgen. The X-ray source and the detectors spiral around the patient approximately 2–3 times/sec.

shutter time on a camera), equals the time needed to complete a 180° rotation, which depends on the rotation velocity of the scanner. If the rotation velocity of a CT system is 400 ms, then the temporal resolution is 200 ms. Technically impressive, but still fairly long considering the fast and continuous motion of the heart and the coronary arteries. Although the rotation velocity of CT has gradually increased over the years, further acceleration is challenged by

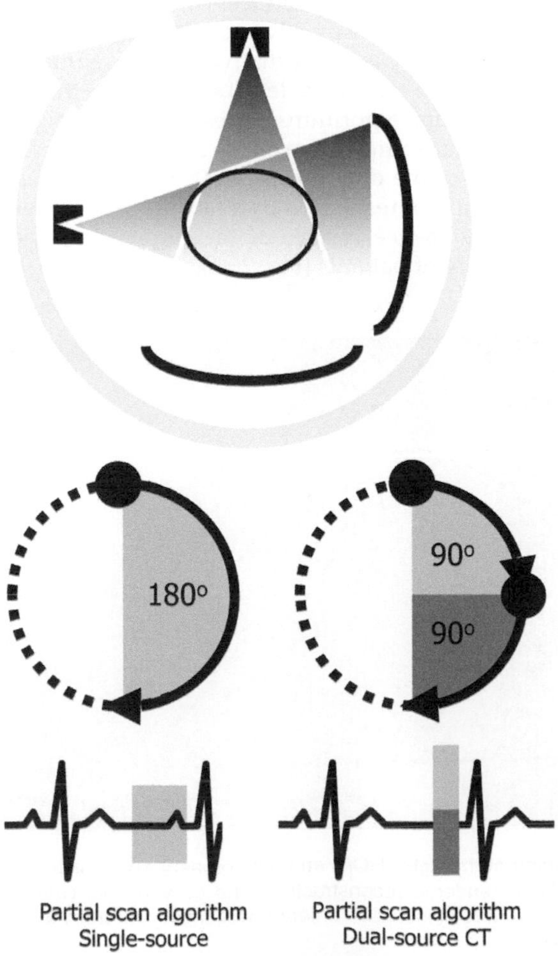

Figure 20.2 Dual-source CT scanners are equipped with two tube-detector units mounted at an angular offset of 90°. While single-source CT requires a 180° rotation, dual-source CT requires a 90° rotation to acquire the minimal amount of projections to reconstruct an image.

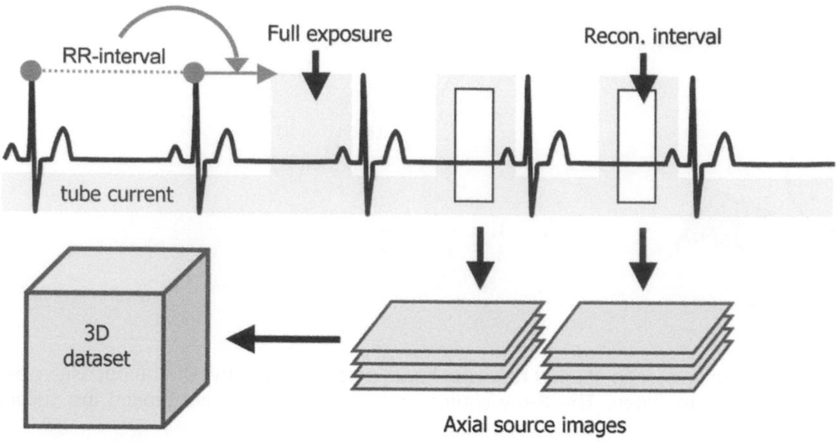

Figure 20.3 Retrospective ECG-gated image reconstruction: data acquired during the same phase of consecutive heart cycles are selected to reconstruct phase-consistent slices, which are combined to form a 3D CT angiogram. Prospective ECG-triggered tube modulation, based on the previous heart cycles full output of the tube is restricted to the desired imaging phase, which minimizes the total radiation exposure.

the immense centrifugal forces resulting from spinning the heavy tube-detector unit at high speed. Therefore, alternative solutions to improve the temporal resolution of cardiac CT are (becoming) available. Pharmacological modulation of the heart rate reduces cardiac motion and prolongs the duration of the end-diastolic phase. β-Blockers are mostly used, although calcium antagonists as well as anxiolytics may serve similar purposes. Alternatively, multisegmental reconstruction algorithms combine data from consecutive cardiac cycles to shorten the effective temporal resolution. The efficiency of these reconstruction algorithms varies depending on the heart rate and rhythm regularity during the scan. Dual-source CT systems are equipped with two tube-detector units, each of which acquires half of the data during a 90° rotation instead of the usual 180° rotation, thereby improving the temporal resolution by a factor 2. The current temporal resolution of cardiac CT can provide motion-free images of the coronary arteries during late-diastole and/or end-systole in the majority of patients (Fig. 20.4).

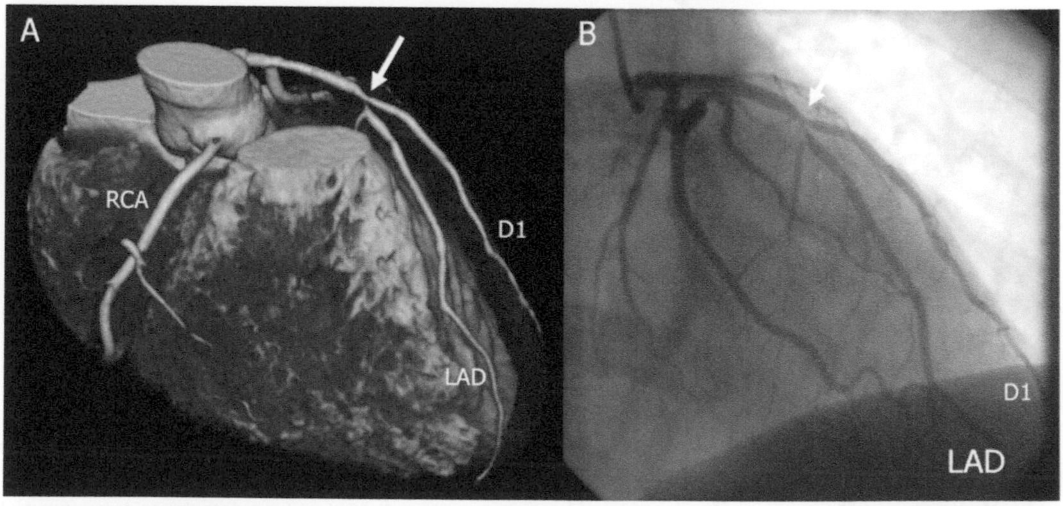

Figure 20.4 LAD bifurcation lesion motion-free imaging of the right (RCA) and left coronary artery, including modest-sized side branches, presented as a 3D volume–rendered reconstruction. The conventional catheter angiogram has been provided for comparison of the lesion (*arrow*) in the left anterior descending coronary artery (LAD) at the bifurcation of the first diagonal branch (D1).

Table 20.1 Meta-analysis of the accuracy of 16- and 64-slice CT to detect significant coronary obstruction per coronary segment, per main vessel, and per patient

Analysis	Sensitivity (%)	Specificity (%)	PPV (%)	NPV (%)	LR+	LR−	DOR
Segments	81	93	68	97	21.54	0.11	189.32
Vessels	82	91	81	92	11.80	0.08	146.45
Patients	96	74	83	94	5.36	0.05	133.05

Abbreviations: LR+, positive likelihood ration; LR−, negative likelihood ration; DOR, diagnostic odds ration.
Source: Adapted from Ref. 8.

CT CORONARY ANGIOGRAPHY

Coronary imaging challenges the performance capacity of CT in several ways. Imaging the continuously moving coronary arteries requires high temporal resolution. Imaging disease in these small branches requires sufficient spatial resolution. The scan needs to be fast to acquire all data within the time of a single breath hold (despite a relatively low table speed). Finally, one will need sufficient contrast between the coronary lumen and surrounding tissues (by intravenous contrast medium injection) and sufficient contrast-to-noise ratio.

In 2001, the ability of mechanical CT to detect obstructive coronary disease was demonstrated with promising diagnostic accuracy using 4-slice CT systems.[1,2] However, the scan required a long breath-hold (35–40 seconds). Additionally, a substantial percentage of examinations were not interpretable, often due to motion artifacts in patients with a faster heart rate.[3] Current technologies, 64-slice CT (with β-blocker premedication) or dual-source CT, show more reliable diagnostic accuracy for the detection of coronary stenosis in comparative studies with invasive angiography.[4–8] Varying per study the exclusion rate has dropped to 0% to 12%. Apart from motion artifacts, which may persist particularly in patients with a higher heart rate, extensive calcification is a remaining cause of non-interpretability. A meta-analysis of 16- and 64-slice CT studies reported an 81% sensitivity and 93% specificity to detect (segmental) coronary artery stenosis (Table 20.1).[8] The positive predictive value was somewhat lower—68%, largely because of the overestimation of disease severity in calcified vessel segments. Because CT can well exclude disease in normal vessels, the negative predictive value of CT is 97%. Partially because of the high disease prevalence in most studies, the sensitivity increases to 96% on a per-patient level, while the specificity decreases to 74%. Even on a per-patient level the negative predictive value remains high—94%. Most 64-slice studies were performed with β-blocker premedication to minimize motion artifacts. The first published results with dual-source CT show comparable diagnostic performance with 64-slice CT, but without the use of β-blockers (Figs. 20.5

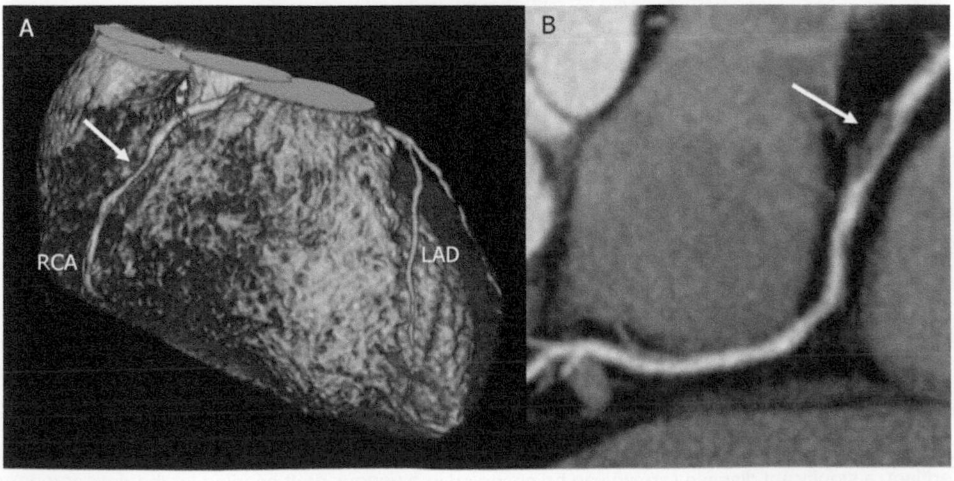

Figure 20.5 Noncalcified, stenotic lesion (*arrow*) in the right coronary artery (RCA) by CTA, presented as a 3D volume–rendered reconstruction (**A**) and a curved maximum-intensity projection (**B**).

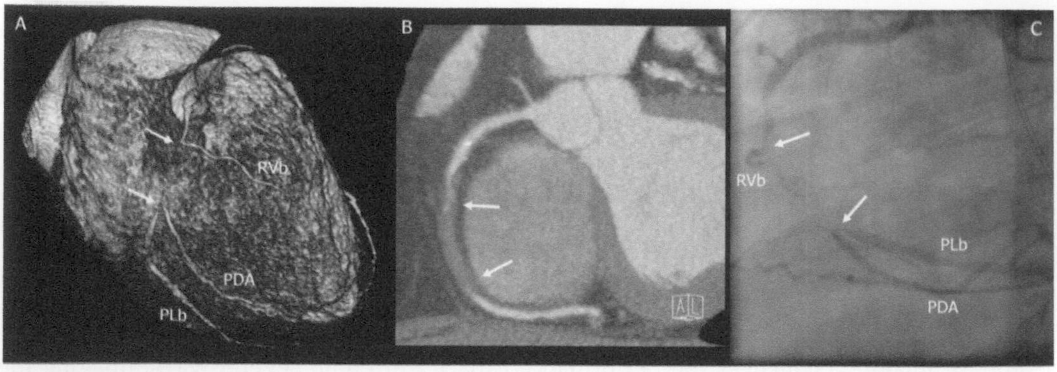

Figure 20.6 Complete occlusion (*between arrows*) of the mid-segment of the right coronary artery (RCA) between the right ventricular branch (RVb) and the (early) bifurcation of the posterior descending branch (PDA) and a posterolateral branch (PLb). In this case, the occluded segment contains only minimal amounts of calcification. Simultaneous injection of contrast into the left and right system allows visualization of the proximal and distal RCA by catheter angiography.

and 20.6).[9] The limited spatial resolution of CT, as well as artifacts from motion or calcium, limits the ability of CT to accurately quantify coronary stenoses, which showed modest correlation with quantitative invasive angiography.[5,6]

CT AFTER CORONARY REVASCULARIZATION

Patients who underwent percutaneous or surgical coronary revascularization are more likely to develop complaints in the future due to (long-term) failure of the procedure (in-stent restenosis or graft disease) or progressive coronary artery disease elsewhere. CT imaging after stenting or bypass graft surgery poses different challenges.

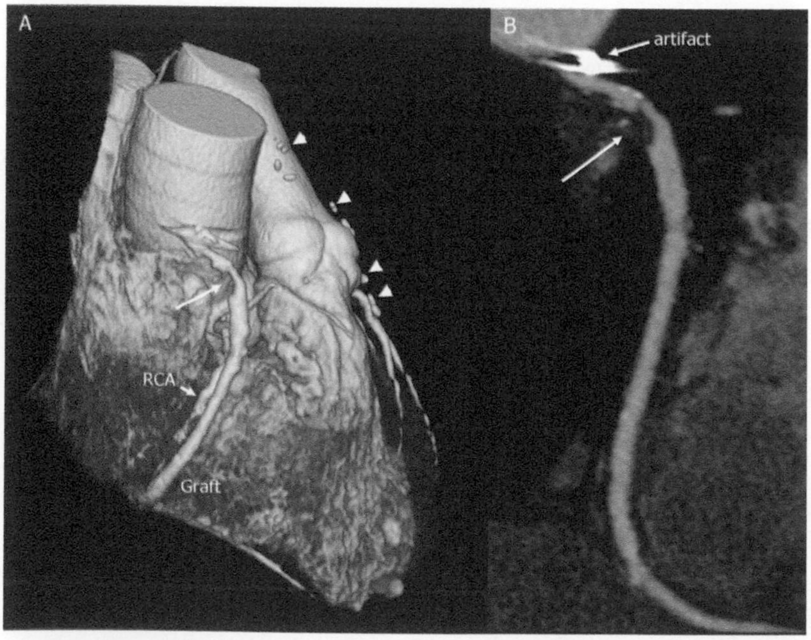

Figure 20.7 Graft disease by CTA. Despite the unevaluable proximal anastomosis to the ascending aorta due to a metal artifact, a significant disease (*arrow*) can be observed in a venous graft heading for the right coronary artery (RCA). Metal clips in the anterior mediastinum (*arrowheads*) remain visible after occlusion of a left internal mammary graft.

Table 20.2 Selected CT imaging studies after bypass graft surgery

			Graft occlusion (100%)		Graft stenosis (50–99%)		Coronary stenosis (>50%)	
References	CT	*N*	Excl (%)	Acc (%)	Excl (%)	Acc (%)	Excl (%)	Acc (%)
(10)	4	24	3	98	7	90	33	80
(11)	16	96	13	100	0	98	NR	NR
(12)	16	51	6	100	26	95	NR	NR
(13)	64	50	0	100	0	95	9	90
(14)	64	52	0	99	0	95	0	81

Generation of CT scanner (CT), study population size (*N*), excluded segments/patients (excl), accuracy as the number of true (positive/negative) observations divided by the total (acc); not reported (NR).

Coronary artery bypass grafts are generally larger and move less compared to the coronary arteries, which makes them easier to image by noninvasive imaging techniques (Fig 20.7). Additionally, grafts rarely show calcified disease and tend to occlude, rather than narrow, which is easier to detect. Occasionally, interpretation of the lumen is complicated by artifacts caused by metal within the vicinity of the graft (indicators near the graft ostium of the graft, vascular clips, sternal sutures). Nevertheless, comparative studies using 4-, 16- and 64-slice CT have demonstrated excellent accuracy to detect or exclude graft disease (Table 20.2).[10–14] More challenging is the assessment of the coronary arteries in patients who underwent bypass graft surgery. Even with state-of-the–art technology, diffuse, calcified coronary artery disease prevents accurate assessment of these vessels.[10,13,14] Therefore, CT is most useful when the condition of the grafts is the primary indication (Fig. 20.8). In symptomatic patients who return many years after surgery, when progressive coronary disease is more likely than graft failure to cause complaints, CT (or any other angiographic technique for that matter) may be unable to identify the culprit lesion.

Metal stents cause artifacts that affect interpretability of the lumen within the stent. To what degree the lumen is obscured depends on the stent material, the thickness of the struts, and the diameter of the device.[15,16] Regardless of the stent design, high-image quality is generally needed to confidently assess coronary stents. Comparative studies with conventional angiography report varying results.[17–19] When the stent is completely occluded CT will often be able to detect this (Fig. 20.9). However, in case of noncomplete in-stent restenosis CT is less

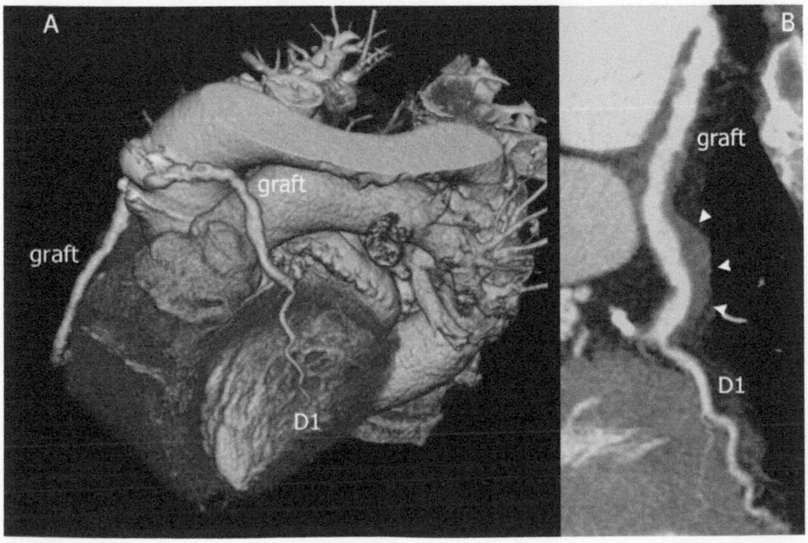

Figure 20.8 Diffuse, aneurysmatic disease (*arrowheads*) can be visualized by CTA in an otherwise patent venous graft to a diagonal branch (D1).

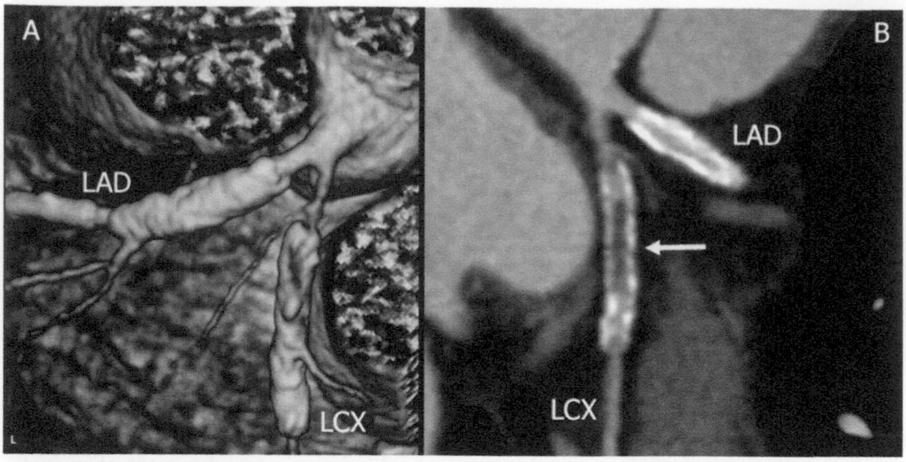

Figure 20.9 CT coronary angiogram of an occluded stent (*arrow*) in the left circumflex coronary artery (LCx). The stent in the left anterior descending coronary artery (LAD) is patent. The metal in the stent causes bright blooming effects, which make the struts appear thinker. Because of the high attenuation of the stent, the in-stent lumen cannot be assessed well on 3D volume–rendered images (**A**), as compared to cross-sectional (curved MPR) images (**B**).

reliable (Fig. 20.10).[19] Particularly for smaller stents there is a tendency to overestimate disease severity. Assessment of larger stents, for instance in the left main coronary artery or grafts, is more reliable.[14,20]

HOW TO EVALUATE A CORONARY CT SCAN

As mentioned previously, noninvasive coronary imaging challenges the capabilities of current CT technology. Unfortunately, the minimal required image quality cannot be achieved in all patients. Even when optimal image quality is available, interpretation of findings can be difficult and requires experience. The amount of raw data created during a scan is enormous, and several postprocessing tools are available to aid in the evaluation of the cardiac CT imaging data.

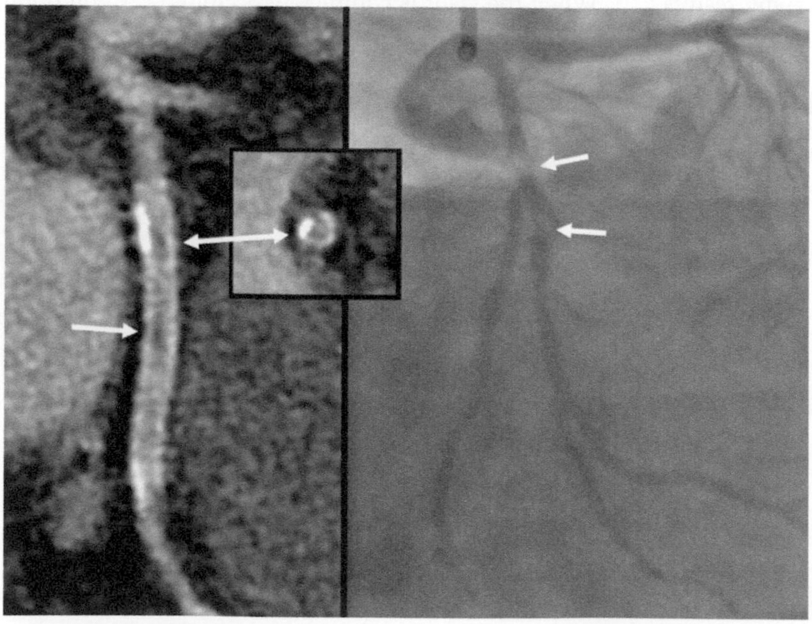

Figure 20.10 The stented left circumflex branch contains two stenotic lesions (*arrows*) which can be identified on CT (**A**), although not as clearly as compared to the conventional coronary angiogram (**B**).

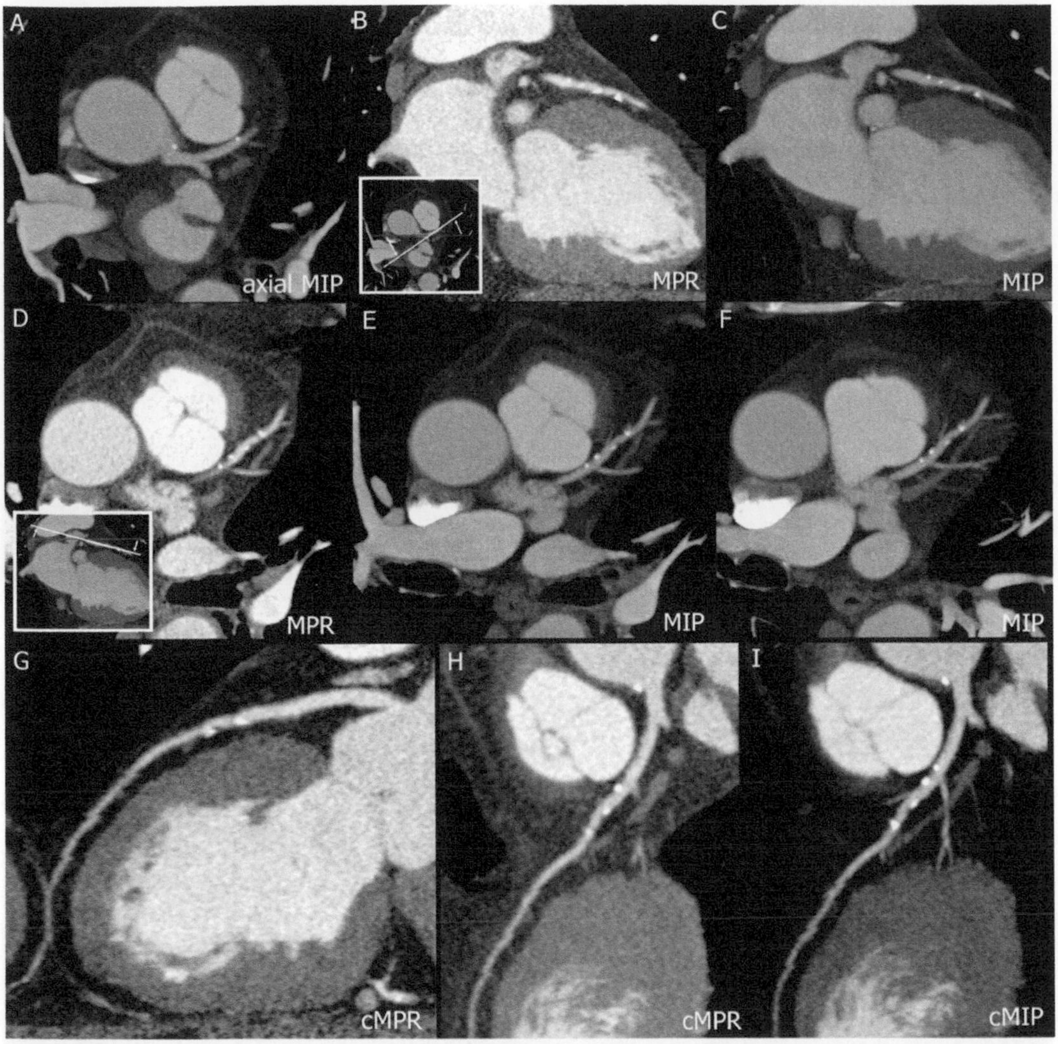

Figure 20.11 CT postprocessing techniques. Axial planes, regular, or as maximum-intensity projections (MIP) (**A**). Multiplanar reformations (MPRs) are (double-oblique) cross-sections that can show a longer section of the vessel within a single view. The inset shows how a plane, orthogonal to the plane in the inset, is positioned and rotated to visualize the proximal part of the left anterior descending coronary artery (**B,D**). By creating an MIP, which displays the highest densities within a thin slab, the contrast between the vessel and the surroundings increases (**C,E**). By increasing the slab thickness more (of the) branches come in plane (**F**). Curved MPRs (**G,H**) and curved MIPs (**I**) are curved cross-sections (or thin slabs) positioned along the course of the vessel to show the entire vessel in a single view.

Merely flipping through the axial source images will often suffice to exclude stenosis in the absence of excessive atherosclerotic disease (calcifications) and good image quality. In the remaining (majority of) cases, additional postprocessing tools will be required (Fig. 20.11). Multiplanar reformations (MPR) are cross-sectional planes through the 3D data set, which can be positioned and angulated to view a vessel of interest longitudinally or in short-axis (Fig. 20.11). Smaller branches are more easily interpreted using thin-slab maximum-intensity projections (MIP). Instead of a true MPR cross-section, MIP images display the highest attenuation values within a thin slab (3–7 mm), allowing visualization of longer segments of tortuous branches. Instead of a flat cross-section, curved MPRs or MIPs are created along the course of a vessel through the 3D data set. The folded-out result shows the vessel in cross-section along its entire

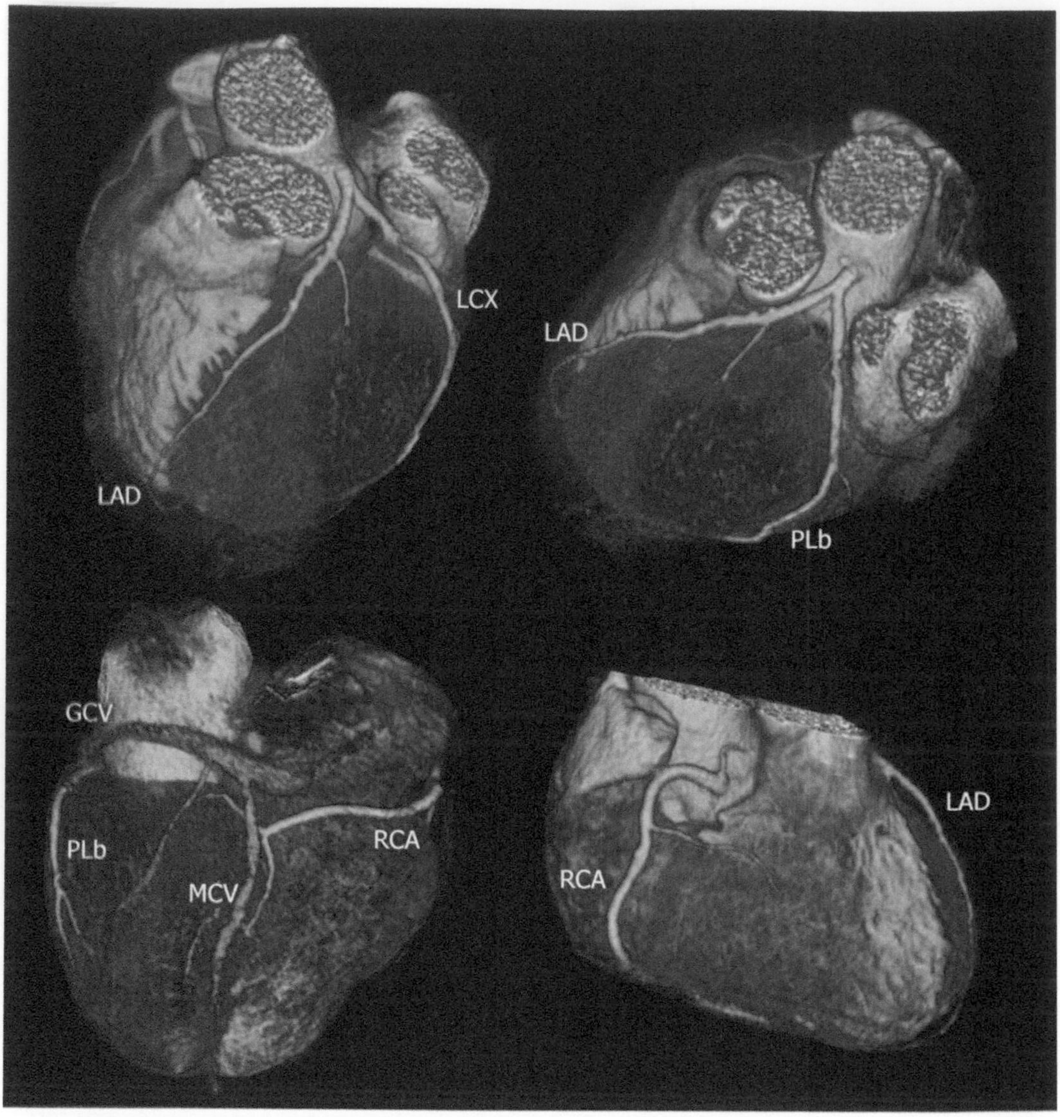

Figure 20.12 Volume-rendered images depict a 3D image of the CT angiogram. Color and opacity of the voxels are determined by the attenuation value of these image elements and their position within the volume relative to the point of view. 3D reconstructions are attractive and instructive means to correspond findings. *Abbreviations*: LAD, left anterior descending coronary artery; RCA, right coronary artery; LCx, left circumflex branch; PLb, posterolateral branch, GCV, great cardiac vein; MCV, medial cardiac vein.

course. Finally, 3D volume rendered images can be created by attributing color and transparency to the voxels within the 3D volume, depending on the attenuation value of the image elements (Fig. 20.12). The result is a 3D recreation of the CT angiogram that can be viewed from any angle. These appealing images can be useful to present and communicate findings. They are, however, less reliable in the initial assessment of the data. Over the recent years applications have been automated, allowing automated vessel tracking and 3D volume segmentation.

Considering the limited spatial resolution of CT, the presence of subtle motion blurring and calcifications, coronary lesions are often semi-quantified as nonsignificant (<50%), moderate (50–70%), severe (>70%), and occluded. Manual and (semi-)automated stenosis quantification tools are less reader-dependent and provide more reproducible results.

Table 20.3 AHA recommendations for the clinical use of coronary CT angiography[22]

Indication	Class	Evidence
Assessment of obstructive CAD in symptomatic individuals, particularly in low-intermediate probability	IIa	B
Screening of asymptomatic individuals	III	C
Follow-up after percutaneous intervention	III	C
Follow-up after CABG	IIb	C
Anomalous coronary arteries	IIa	C
Non-calcified plaque	III	C

Class I, evidence or general agreement that the procedure is useful and effective; Class II, conflicting evidence or divergence of opinion about the usefulness/efficacy of the procedure; Class IIa, weight of evidence/opinion is in favor of usefulness/efficacy; Class IIb, usefulness/efficacy is less well established by evidence/opinion; Class III, evidence and/or general agreement that the procedure is not useful/effective and in some cases may be harmful. Weight of evidence: high (A), intermediate (B), and low (C).

CLINICAL USE OF CT CORONARY ANGIOGRAPHY

The clinical role of noninvasive coronary angiography is still under development. *Expert Documents* and *Appropriateness Criteria* have been published to guide clinicians while various indications are further developed (Table 20.3).[21,22] Despite the good diagnostic performance of CT compared to invasive coronary angiography, the clinical role of CT coronary imaging is not yet fully established. CT does not equal the accuracy and versatility of invasive coronary investigations, and large-scale replacement of catheter angiography is unlikely in the near future. Because of the high negative predictive value, many feel that CT angiography will be particularly useful to exclude coronary artery disease in symptomatic patients with a low-to-intermediate probability of disease (Fig. 20.13).[23] Whether CT should be a first-line test in patients with stable complaints, or a secondary test after (nonconclusive) functional imaging remains a subject of debate.

In patients who present with acute chest symptoms, CT has been used successfully in a number of clinical trials.[24] When the ECG is nonconclusive and initial biomarkers are negative, CT can exclude coronary artery disease quickly and safely. Further studies are needed to assess the cost-effectiveness of this approach.

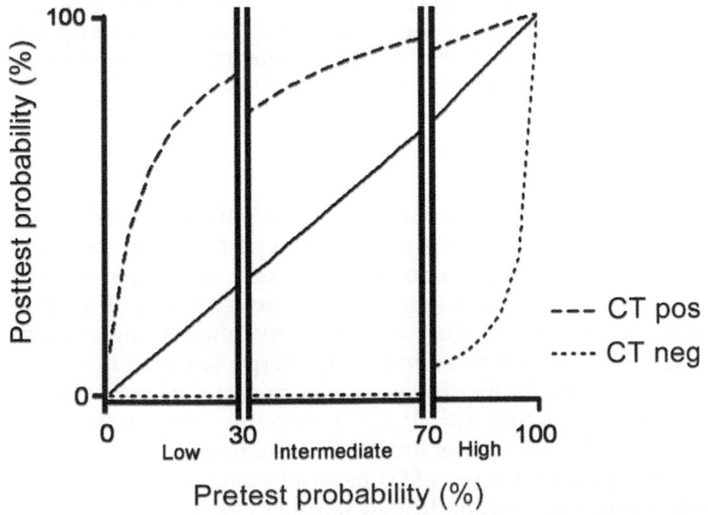

Figure 20.13 Pretest probability (Duke clinical score) and posttest probability (64-slice CT coronary angiography) of (at least one) coronary stenosis in a population of 264 individuals with stable chest pain symptoms. The results indicate that CT can be valuable to exclude significant coronary disease in individuals with a low to intermediate, rather than a high likelihood of disease. *Source*: Adapted from Ref. 23.

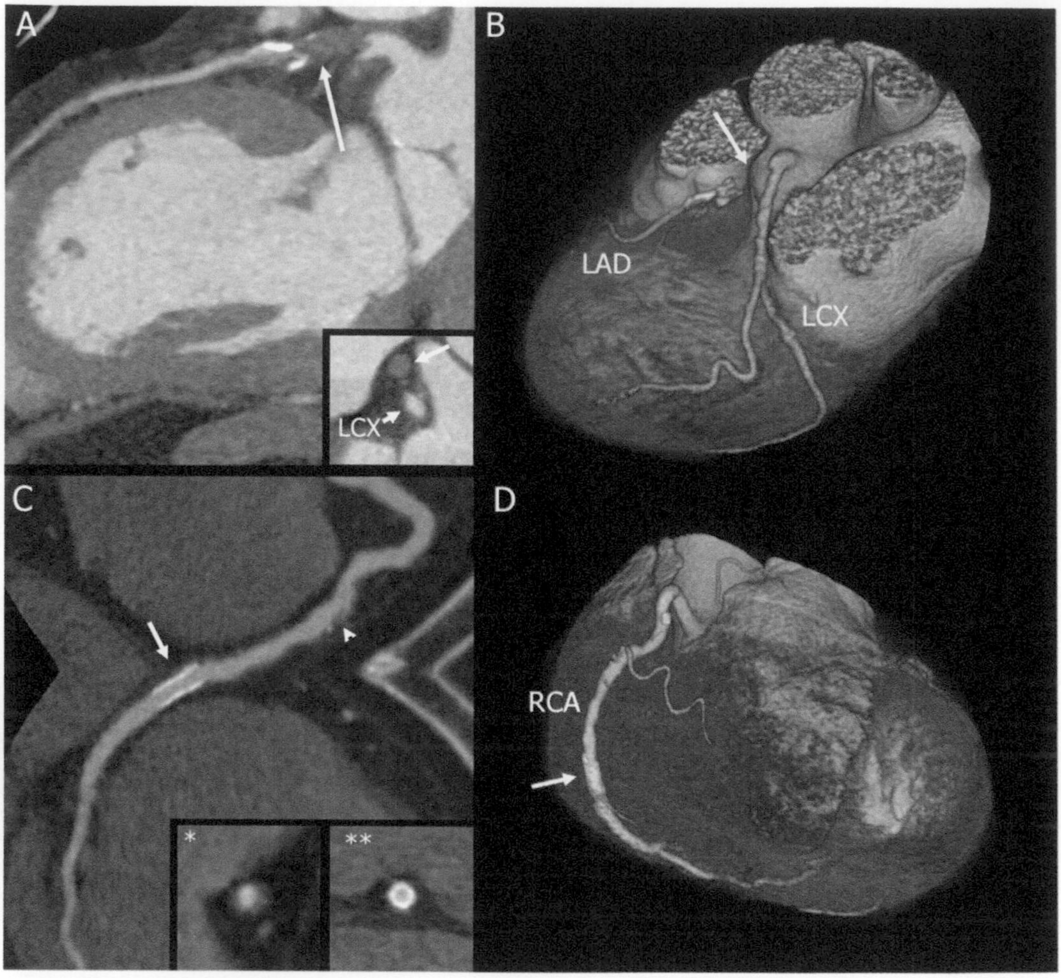

Figure 20.14 CT angiogram of a patient who previously underwent PCI of the right coronary artery (RCA), and returned with anginal symptoms. The large stent in the right coronary artery is patent (**C****,**D**). Nonstenotic plaque (*arrowhead*) containing calcified (*bright*) and noncalcified components (*dark*) was detected more proximally in the RCA (**C***). The proximal LAD is completely occluded (**A,B**). The inset (**A**) shows the low attenuation (*dark*) of the occlusion in cross-section.

Because of the unpredictable interpretability of coronary stents and inconclusive data, CT is at this point not recommended in patients that previously underwent percutaneous coronary stenting. Emerging data suggests that in selected populations with larger stents (particularly in the left main coronary artery or bypass grafts), contemporary stent designs with thin struts, or nonmetalic stents, CT can be considered as an alternative to conventional angiography (Fig. 20.14).[14,20] Although bypass grafts are well assessable by CT, interpretation of the native coronary vessels suffers from diffuse atherosclerotic disease in the majority of patients that return with symptoms late after bypass graft surgery.[13,14] CT is therefore most useful short after surgery, or when the indication for the CT scan is limited to visualization of the grafts. Other indications that are generally accepted are the use of CT as an alternative to conventional angiography when catheterization is refused, contraindicated (aortic dissection, aortic valve endocarditis) or unsuccessful (aberrant coronary arteries, proximal occlusion, coronary stents protruding into the aorta). In patients with new onset heart failure without evident coronary artery disease, CT could be useful to exclude ischemic etiology.

Because of the use of radiation, contrast media, and potential overdiagnosis of coronary artery disease, use of contrast-enhanced CT coronary imaging is discouraged as a screening tool with a low-to-intermediate probability of disease.

REFERENCES

1. Nieman K, Oudkerk M, Rensing BJ, et al. Coronary angiography with multi-slice computed tomography. Lancet 2001; 357:599–603.
2. Achenbach S, Giesler T, Ropers D, et al. Detection of coronary artery stenoses by contrast-enhanced, retrospectively electrocardiographically-gated, multislice spiral computed tomography. Circulation 2001; 103:2535–2538.
3. Giesler T, Baum U, Ropers D, et al. Noninvasive visualization of coronary arteries using contrast-enhanced multidetector CT: Influence of heart rate on image quality and stenosis detection. AJR Am J Roentgenol 2002; 179:911–916.
4. Leschka S, Alkadhi H, Plass A, et al. Accuracy of MSCT coronary angiography with 64-slice technology: First experience. Eur Heart J 2005; 26:1482–1487.
5. Raff GL, Gallagher MJ, O'Neill WW, et al. Diagnostic accuracy of noninvasive coronary angiography using 64-slice spiral computed tomography. J Am Coll Cardiol 2005; 46:552–557.
6. Leber AW, Knez A, von Ziegler F, et al. Quantification of obstructive and nonobstructive coronary lesions by 64-slice computed tomography: A comparative study with quantitative coronary angiography and intravascular ultrasound. J Am Coll Cardiol 2005; 46:147–154.
7. Mollet NR, Cademartiri F, van Mieghem CA, et al. High-resolution spiral computed tomography coronary angiography in patients referred for diagnostic conventional coronary angiography. Circulation 2005; 112:2318–2323.
8. Hamon M, Biondi-Zoccai GG, Malagutti P, et al. Diagnostic performance of multislice spiral computed tomography of coronary arteries as compared with conventional invasive coronary angiography: A meta-analysis. J Am Coll Cardiol 2006; 48:1896–1910.
9. Weustink AC, Meijboom WB, Mollet NR, et al. Reliable high-speed coronary computed tomography in symptomatic patients. J Am Coll Cardiol 2007; 50:786–794.
10. Nieman K, Pattynama PM, Rensing BJ, et al. Evaluation of patients after coronary artery bypass surgery: CT angiographic assessment of grafts and coronary arteries. Radiology 2003; 229:749–756.
11. Martuscelli E, Romagnoli A, D'Eliseo A, et al. Evaluation of venous and arterial conduit patency by 16-slice spiral computed tomography. Circulation 2004; 110:3234–3238.
12. Schlosser T, Konorza T, Hunold P, et al. Noninvasive visualization of coronary artery bypass grafts using 16-detector row computed tomography. J Am Coll Cardiol 2004; 44:1224–1229.
13. Ropers D, Pohle FK, Kuettner A, et al. Diagnostic accuracy of noninvasive coronary angiography in patients after bypass surgery using 64-slice spiral computed tomography with 330-ms gantry rotation. Circulation 2006; 114:2334–2341.
14. Malagutti P, Nieman K, Meijboom WB, et al. Use of 64-slice CT in symptomatic patients after coronary bypass surgery: Evaluation of grafts and coronary arteries. Eur Heart J 2007; 28:1879–1885.
15. Nieman K, Cademartiri F, Raaijmakers R, et al. Noninvasive angiographic evaluation of coronary stents with multi-slice spiral computed tomography. Herz 2003; 28:136–142.
16. Maintz D, Seifarth H, Raupach R, et al. 64-slice multidetector coronary CT angiography: In vitro evaluation of 68 different stents. Eur Radiol 2006; 16:818–826.
17. Gilard M, Cornily JC, Pennec PY, et al. Assessment of coronary artery stents by 16 slice computed tomography. Heart 2006; 92:58–61.
18. Cademartiri F, Schuijf JD, Pugliese F, et al. Usefulness of 64-slice multislice computed tomography coronary angiography to assess in-stent restenosis. J Am Coll Cardiol 2007; 49:2204–2210.
19. Pugliese F, Weustink AC, Van Mieghem C, et al. Dual-source coronary computed tomography angiography for detecting in-stent restenosis. Heart 2008; 94:848–854.
20. Van Mieghem CA, Cademartiri F, Mollet NR, et al. Multislice spiral computed tomography for the evaluation of stent patency after left main coronary artery stenting: A comparison with conventional coronary angiography and intravascular ultrasound. Circulation 2006; 114:645–653.
21. Budoff MJ, Achenbach S, Blumenthal RS, et al. Assessment of coronary artery disease by cardiac computed tomography: A scientific statement from the American Heart Association Committee on Cardiovascular Imaging and Intervention, Council on Cardiovascular Radiology and Intervention, and Committee on Cardiac Imaging, Council on Clinical Cardiology. Circulation 2006; 114:1761–1791.
22. Hendel RC, Patel MR, Kramer CM, et al. ACCF/ACR/SCCT/SCMR/ASNC/NASCI/SCAI/SIR 2006 appropriateness criteria for cardiac computed tomography and cardiac magnetic resonance imaging.

A report of the American College of Cardiology Foundation Quality Strategic Directions Committee Appropriateness Criteria Working Group. J Am Coll Cardiol 2006; 48:1475–1497.
23. Meijboom WB, van Mieghem CA, Mollet NR, et al. 64-Slice computed tomography coronary angiography in patients with high, intermediate, or low pretest probability of significant coronary artery disease. J Am Coll Cardiol 2007; 50:1469–1475.
24. Hoffmann U, Nagurney JT, Moselewski F, et al. Coronary multidetector computed tomography in the assessment of patients with acute chest pain. Circulation 2006; 114:2251–2260.

21 Multidetector computed tomography imaging for myocardial perfusion, viability, and cardiac function

Karl H. Schuleri, Kakuya Kitagawa, Richard T. George, and Albert C. Lardo

INTRODUCTION

Ischemic myocardium that is dysfunctional but viable has the potential to recover contractile function after revascularization. Therefore, noninvasive detection of viable myocardium in patients with chronic left ventricular (LV) dysfunction associated with coronary artery disease has important clinical implications for treatment.[1] The discrimination between viable but dysfunctional myocardium and scar tissue permits selection of patients who are most likely to benefit significantly from revascularization procedures, allowing others to avoid the risks associated with revascularization procedures when there is no clear benefit.

After myocardial infarction, the extent and degree of irreversible myocardial tissue injury are strong predictors of clinical outcomes, allowing risk stratification and evaluation of myocardial salvage.[2–5] In recent years, the success of myocardial protection after myocardial infarction has led to an ever-increasing number of patients with advanced heart disease and chronic heart failure.[6] Questions of viability and the need for repeated revascularization are also of crucial importance to this group of patients. Clinical assessment of myocardial viability is performed by single-photon emission computed tomography (SPECT), positron emission tomography (PET), stress echocardiography, or magnetic resonance imaging (MRI).[7–10] Recently, multidetector computed tomography (MDCT) has been explored beyond the capabilities of coronary artery disease assessment. The combination of fast rotation time and multislice acquisition with a high spatial resolution enables MDCT to provide additional information on myocardial perfusion, viability, and cardiac function.

MDCT PERFUSION IMAGING

First attempts to measure myocardial perfusion by CT appear as early as the late 1980s with the invention of electron beam tomography (EBT).[11,12] Early works applied indicator-dilution theory to the analysis of CT-derived time attenuation curves and reported a good correlation with microsphere myocardial blood flow (MBF) in canine models[11–14] and volunteers.[15,16] These studies, by analyzing the LV input and myocardial output functions, provided some important insights in perfusion assessment by CT. For example, studies using the dynamic spatial reconstructor demonstrated that the underestimation of MBF by CT at higher flows (above 2.5–3.5 mL/g/min) was secondary to increases in myocardial blood volume (MBV) and the relationship between MBF and MBV was then elucidated.[14] In addition, significant percentage of iodine contrast agent has been shown to retain in the myocardium after the first-pass, which is important because it affects estimates of myocardial perfusion based on transit time and MBV.[17] However, the EBT studies on myocardial perfusion was focusing on the accurate quantification of MBF and only a limited number of studies are available showing the efficacy of this modality for detecting myocardial ischemia in clinical patients. Nonetheless, a study performed in patients with coronary arterial involvement of Kawasaki disease using EBT with dipyridamole stress has demonstrated the ability of CT to potentially detect ischemic myocardium as the area of first-pass contrast deficit.[18]

Today, as the result of rapid advancement of MDCT in the coronary artery imaging, there is a growing interest to expand its application beyond coronary angiography. One of the most attractive applications is myocardial perfusion—especially simultaneous evaluation of morphology of coronary artery stenosis and its functional significance. However, this concept can become feasible on an exquisite balance of relevant factors including (A) *radiation dose*: comparison of stress and rest may be necessary for accurate diagnosis of ischemia, while this may

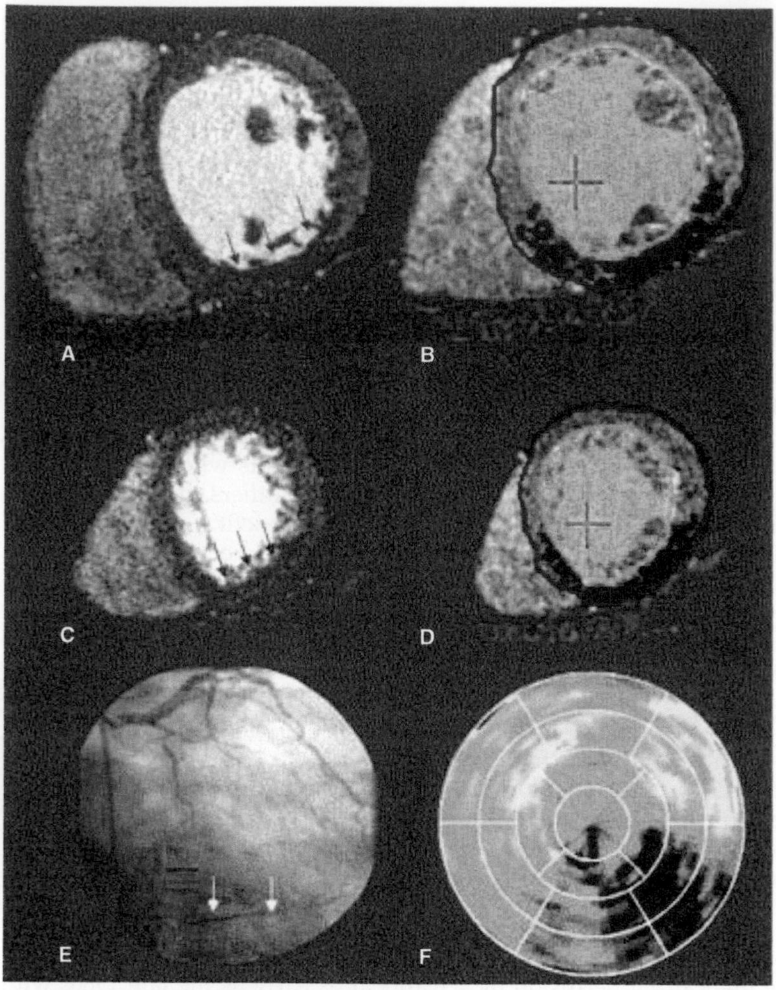

Figure 21.1 First-pass, adenosine-augmented multidetector computed tomography (MDCT) myocardial perfusion imaging in a patient referred for invasive angiography after single-photon emission computed tomography showed a fixed perfusion deficit in the inferior and inferolateral territories. Panels (**A**) and (**C**) demonstrate an inferior and inferolateral subendocardial perfusion deficit in the mid- and distal left ventricle, respectively (*arrows*). Using semiautomated function/perfusion software, myocardium meeting the perfusion deficit signal density threshold of 1 standard deviation below the remote myocardial signal density is designated in blue in panels (**B**) and (**D**). Invasive angiography shows a chronically occluded distal right coronary artery with left to right collaterals filling the posterior descending (*arrows*) and posterolateral branches (**E**). (**F**) 17-Segment polar plot of MDCT-derived myocardial signal densities. Note the hypoperfused inferior and inferolateral regions displayed in blue.

double the radiation dose; (B) *contrast dose/injection protocol*: higher contrast dose can improve the quality of coronary CTA and contrast between ischemic and normal myocardium, while increasing the nephrotoxicity and possible beam hardening artifacts; and (C) *heart rate control under pharmacologic stress*: vasodilator stress increases heart rate which can degrade image quality of coronary CTA and perfusion CT. Recent preclinical studies by George et al. have demonstrated that dynamic MDCT can also be used to quantify myocardial perfusion in a similar way to EBT[19] and ischemic myocardium can potentially be identified in a canine model of LAD stenosis by helical CT acquisition, opening the possibility of stress perfusion MDCT[20] (Fig. 21.1).

MDCT VIABILITY IMAGING

The potential role of computed tomography for the assessment of myocardial viability and the detection of myocardial infarction was first described by Gray et al. in the late 1970s studying explanted dog hearts.[21,22] In a series of elegant ex vivo work, Higgins et al. were able to show the preferential uptake of contrast media in myocardial areas damaged by acute ischemia.[23,24] Although these initial results were encouraging, and experimental data accumulated demonstrating that acute infarcts were detectable by computed tomography as regions of reduced attenuation values (hypoenhancement) compared with normal myocardium and hyperenhanced areas after contrast delivery,[25–28] the practical use of computed tomography technology was hampered by insufficient image quality. Modern MDCT systems with high temporal and spatial resolution are well suited to evaluate myocardial viability in combination with intravenous contrast. Iodinated contrast agents are biologically inert and passively diffuse in the myocardium throughout the extracellular space, with a distribution half-life of approximately 20 minutes.

There are two possible techniques to visualize injured myocardial tissue by MDCT. Iodinated intravenous contrast agents primarily remain intravascular during the early phase of first-pass circulation and thereafter they diffuse into extravascular space.[29–31] This provides the opportunity to detect (A) hypoenhanced areas early after contrast delivery which reflects areas of reduced MBF and (B) hyperenhanced areas later after the contrast agents have diffused and accumulated in the extracellular space which signifies damaged myocardium. Human and animals studies exploring MDCT viability imaging are summarized in Table 21.1.

First-pass MDCT myocardial imaging

Myocardial imaging during the first-pass circulation of an iodinated contrast agent is performed during coronary CTA acquisition. It has the ability to show the presence of an early perfusion defect characterized as an area of hypoenhanced myocardium. Nikolaou et al. were the first to demonstrate in a systematic way the significance of early hypoenhanced defects using 4-detector computed tomography in patients.[32] In this retrospective study of 106 patients, first-pass myocardial MDCT imaging could identify 23 patients with acute or chronic myocardial infarction with a diagnostic accuracy of 90% and shows a fair correlation of infarct size

Table 21.1 Human and animals studies published exploring MDCT viability imaging

References	Study population	(*N*)	Comparison modality
Animal studies			
(33)	Acute myocardial infarct[b]	5 Yorkshire pigs	Postmortem pathology Microsphere blood flow measurements
(36)	Acute myocardial infarct[a] Chronic myocardial infarct[a]	10 Monogrel dogs 7 Yorkshire pigs	Postmortem pathology Microsphere blood flow measurements
(37)	Acute myocardial infarct[a]	10 Yorkshire pigs	Delayed contrast-enhanced MRI Postmortem pathology
(34)	Acute myocardial infarct[b]	5 Yorkshire pigs	First-pass MRI
Human studies			
(32)	Acute myocardial infarct	27 patients	
(35)	Chronic myocardial infarct	16 patients	Delayed contrast-enhanced MRI
(39)	Acute Myocardial Infarct	28 patients	Delayed contrast-enhanced MRI
(38)	Acute myocardial infarct	16 patients	Delayed contrast-enhanced MRI
	Chronic myocardial infarct	21 patients	
(40)	Acute myocardial infarct	36 patients	Dobutamine stress echocardiography
(41)	Acute myocardial infarct	52 patients	Thallium-201 SPECT

[a] Intermittent coronary occlusion. Infarct areas were reperfused.
[b] Permanent coronary occlusion.

and LVEF assessed by biplane ventriculography. Experiments in porcine models of chronic coronary occlusion confirmed these initial clinical findings as a valuable approach to assess myocardial tissue composition.[33,34] The size of a first-pass perfusion defect correlated well with the extend of acute infarcts evaluated by pathology specimen and microsphere-determined MBF measurements.[33] Nikolaou et al. also assessed the diagnostic accuracy of 16-detector computed tomography in a prospective study of 30 patients. First-pass stress perfusion magnetic resonance imaging (MRI) and delayed contrast enhanced (de) MRI were compared to first-pass MDCT viability imaging at rest. MDCT detected 10/11 infarcts noted on de-MRI yielding a sensitivity, specificity, and accuracy of 91%, 79%, and 83%, respectively. Three out of six patients with hypoperfusion could be identified by MDCT. However, it should be noted that only severe ischemic perfusion defects can be detected under resting conditions. First-pass MDCT viability imaging underestimated infarct volumes on average by 18.6% compared to de-MRI.[35] At a first glance, this finding conflict with the results from the porcine model. However, the patient population was studied 3 months or longer after myocardial infarction, which reflects a completely different tissue substrate compared to the hyperacute infarct in the animal model. Moreover, in contrast to the acute total occlusion animal model, this patient population presented with reperfused infarcts.

Early clinical experience supports the approach using first-pass MDCT myocardial imaging for the diagnostic evaluation of myocardium but accurate infarct sizing seems to be limited. It is favorable that first-pass MDCT assessment has the ability to provide information without administering additional radiation or contrast dose to patients undergoing coronary CTA. However, perfusion defects are not specific for myocardial infarction. Decreased myocardial attenuation values can be detected in cases of severe local ischemia or other cardiac diseases causing perfusion inhomogeneties like hypertrophic cardiomyopathy.

Delayed contrast-enhanced MDCT imaging

Minutes following intravenous contrast, late hyperenhancement of infarcts becomes apparent (Fig. 21.2). Our laboratory was the first to report a systematic study on delayed contrast-enhanced MDCT.[36] In acute and chronic preclinic animal models of reperfused myocardial infarction injured-myocardium reached peak attenuation values 5 minutes after contrast delivery. The infarct areas were well delineated. Acute and chronic infarcts by MDCT were characterized by hyperenhancement. Infarct morphology and the transmural extent of the myocardial injury could be clearly appreciated by de-MDCT (Fig. 21.3). In addition, regions of microvascular obstruction could be detected in acute infarct areas. Microvascular obstructions are characterized by hypoenhancement. These regions of low-signal attenuation are surrounded by a region of high-signal density early after contrast injection. Over time, attenuation values slowly increases and eventually reaches the level of surrounding high HU of the infarct myocardium (Fig. 21.4).

Overall, there is an excellent agreement of infarct size with gross pathology in the setting of acute infarction, and chronic myocardial scars in preclinical animal models with a qualitative trend towards underestimation by MDCT (mean of mean −0.7 and −0.76 for acute and chronic, respectively).[36] In accordance with these results, Baks et al.[37] showed a good correlation of infarct size in an acute porcine model determined by de-MDCT and de-MRI assessed with TTC pathology infarct size ($r^2 = 0.96$ and $r^2 = 0.93$, respectively). The correlation between de-MDCT and de-MRI was excellent as well ($r^2 = 0.96$) with a slight underestimation of infarct size by de-MDCT compared to de-MRI. Similar results were demonstrated by Gerber et al.,[38] comparing de-MDCT contrast patterns to de-MRI in patients with acute and chronic infarction, respectively. The size of hypoenhanced areas during first-pass and delayed hyperenhanced areas was similar on de-MDCT and de-MRI acquisitions and showed excellent correlation. Mahnken et al.[39] studied 28 patients in the setting of reperfused infarcts and demonstrated that compared with MRI, first-pass MDCT viability imaging tends to underestimate infarct size in MDCT, whereas late enhancement images correlated well. In a multimodality approach, Habis et al.[40] took advantage of the readily delivered iodine during coronary angiography in 36 patients with acute coronary syndrome, and demonstrated that 64-MDCT without iodine re-injection immediately after an invasive catheter procedure is a promising method for early viability assessment. Dobutamine stress echocardiography was performed 2 to 4 weeks following the procedure. There was an excellent agreement between MDCT hyperenhancemet and low-dose

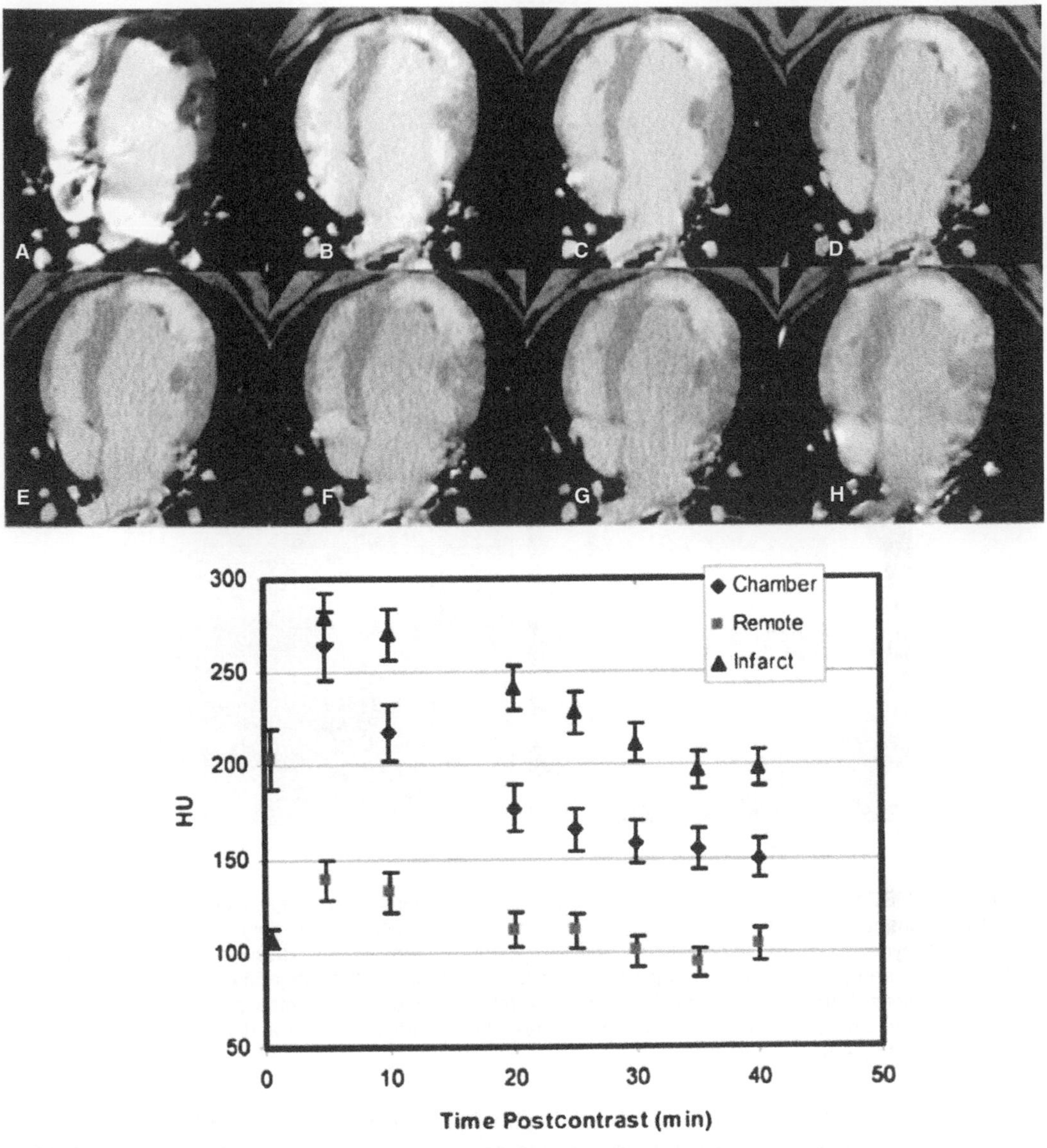

Figure 21.2 (**A–H**) Axial temporal image series demonstrating postreperfusion contrast agent kinetics after 150-mL injection of contrast. The first image (**A**) represents the first-pass image during contrast agent injection. Note that the signal density of the infarct in the first-pass is substantially lower than that of the remote myocardium and indicates a subendocardial microvascular obstruction. Five minutes after injection (**B**), the signal density of the damaged myocardial region is significantly greater than that of the remote myocardium and washes out over time. The plot represents quantitative contrast kinetics for the LV chamber, remote myocardium, and infarct after contrast injection. As can be appreciated from part (**B**), the infarct becomes well delineated and reaches peak enhancement at 5 minutes after injection and then washes out in proportion to the chamber (blood pool) and remote myocardial. *Source*: Adapted from Ref. 36.

dobutamine stress echocardiography results using a 16-segment model in 560 (97%) out of 576 segments evaluated. This study confirmed the preclinical data that the anatomical extent of myocardial infarction assessed by MDCT reflects myocardial viability. In a similar way, Sato et al.[41] studied 52 patients presenting with initial myocardial infarct. Using 64-MDCT technology without iodine re-injection 18 patients showed transmural contrast-delayed enhancement on MDCT images, 20 patients showed subendocardial contrast-delayed enhancement, and 14 patients had no contrast-delayed enhancement (Fig. 21.5). During the 6-month follow-up

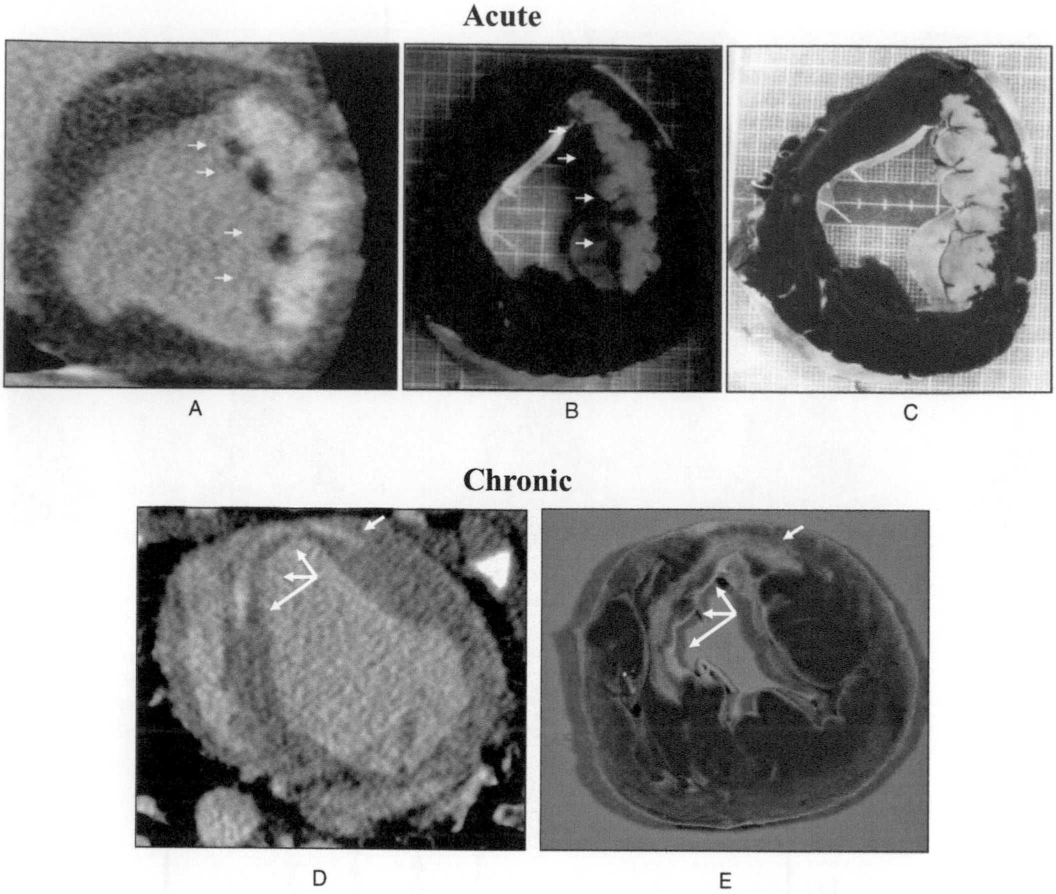

Figure 21.3 MDCT and histopathologic staining comparison of infarct morphology. **Acute myocardial infarction: (A)** Reconstructed short-axis MDCT slice 5 minutes after contrast injection demonstrating a large anterolateral infarct (hyperenhanced region) with discrete endocardial regions of microvascular obstruction (4 arrows). (B) Thioflavin S and (C) TTC staining of the same slice, which confirms the size and location of microvascular obstruction regions. **Chronic myocardial infarction**: (**D**) MDCT image reconstructed in short-axis of an 8-week-old infarct (white arrows) in a porcine model 5 minutes after contrast injection and (E) corresponding gross examination photograph.

period, LV remodeling and the number of rehospitalization for heart failure were significantly more observed in patients transmural contrast-delayed enhancement on MDCT images. Myocardial contrast-delayed enhancement patterns provide promising information regarding myocardial viability, LV remodeling, and prognosis after myocardial infarction. These studies show the feasibility of MDCT viability imaging in the next minutes after coronary angiography. All technical parameters of the studies discussed evaluating MDCT viability imaging are summarized in Table 21.2.

Mechanisms of delayed contrast enhancement in MDCT

Delayed contrast enhancement imaging is feasible with MDCT because iodinated contrast agents first passively diffuse into the increased extracellular matrix of infarcted myocardium. In the setting of acute MI, delayed enhancement is explained by myocyte necrosis, sarcomere membrane rupture, and passive diffusion of contrast into the intracellular space.[42] The mechanism of delayed hyperenhancement in chronic collagenous myocardial scar tissue is thought to be related purely to an accumulation of contrast media in the interstitial space between collagen fibers and thus an increased volume of contrast distribution in the scar tissue is compared with that of tightly packed myocytes. Therefore, accumulation of contrast material in the collagenous

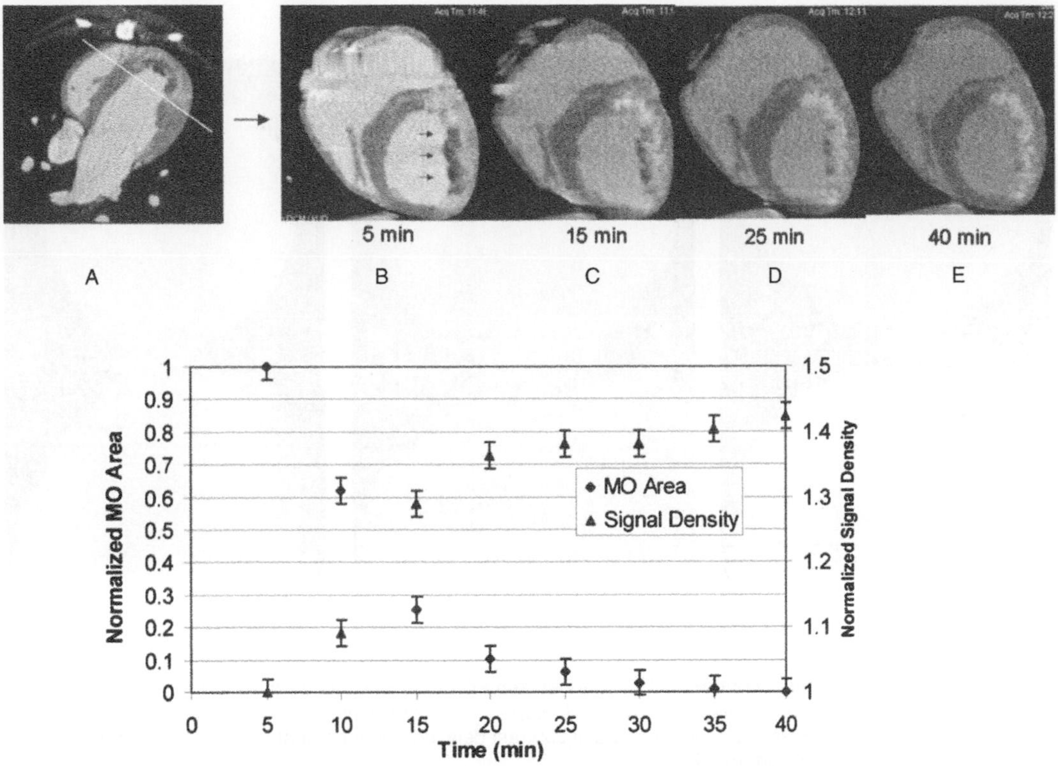

Figure 21.4 **(A)** Axial cardiac MDCT image 2 hours after LAD occlusion/reperfusion showing an orthogonal slice prescription. The large anterior region of low signal density represents a region of microvascular obstruction at the endocardial portion of the infarct. **(B–E)** Short-axis reconstruction of the same slice over time to characterize changes in the region of microvascular obstruction (arrows). As can be appreciated, the region of low signal density is surrounded by a region of high signal density early after contrast injection and then slowly increases over time and eventually reaches the level of surrounding high signal density myocardium. **(F)** Plot of both normalized size and signal density of the microvascular obstruction (MO) region over time.

scar is a passive process, and the timing between administration of contrast agents and imaging is crucial to accurately assess chronic infarct size in MDCT imaging. With respect to detailed tissue characterization for myocardial viability imaging, an important feature of MDCT is that signal density values are somewhat unique and determined by the physical properties of individual constituents of the heart including blood, viable, and nonviable myocardium that result from direct attenuation of the X-ray beam by iodine molecules.

ASSESSMENT OF CARDIAC FUNCTION WITH MDCT

The evaluation of global and regional LV function is an important part of the clinical assessment of patient with suspected coronary artery disease, ischemic, and nonischemic cardiomyopathy. Although MDCT is accurate, highly reproducible and safe, radiation exposure and use of intravenous iodinated contrast media limits its widespread use for functional assessment in the daily clinical routine. However, parameters of global and regional LV function can be regarded as additional information in patients undergoing MDCT coronary angiography to improve diagnosis and risk stratification.

Global LV function

Functional parameters such as left and right ventricular end-diastolic and end-systolic volumes, stroke volume, ejection fraction, and myocardial mass can be calculated from retrospective acquired MDCT angiography data sets. These isotropic voxel data sets allow reconstruction in arbitrary plane. For functional analysis, the slice thickness of retrospective-acquired

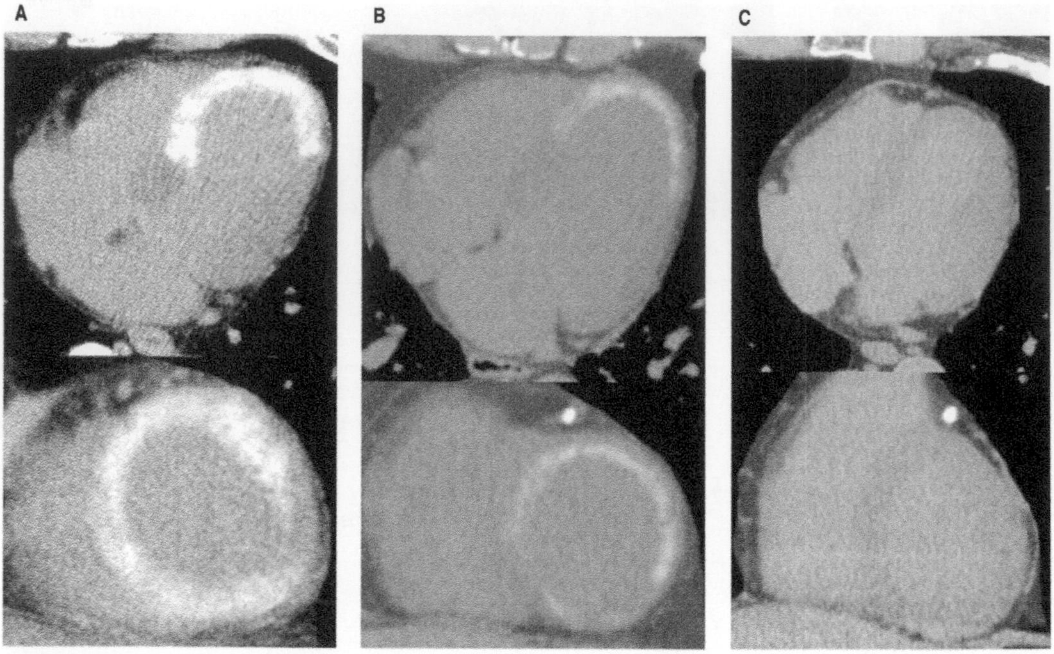

Figure 21.5 The myocardial contrast-delayed enhancement patterns were divided into three groups. Multidetector computed tomography images show axial (*upper*) and short-axis (*lower*) slices with (**A**) transmural contrast-delayed enhancement, (**B**) subendocardial contrast delayed enhancement, and (**C**) no contrast-delayed enhancement. *Source*: Adapted from Ref. 41.

Table 21.2 Technical parameters of published studies evaluating the use of MDCT viability imaging

References	Time point for viability assessment	Scanner generation (slices)	Detector collimation (mm)	Contrast dose (mL)	Tube voltage (kV)	Tube current (mA)	Gantry rotation (ms)
Animal studies							
(33)	First-pass	4	4×1.0	140	140	270	500
(36)	5 min after contrast bolus	32	32×0.5	150	135	420	400
(37)	15 min after contrast bolus	64	$32 \times 2 \times 0.6$	200	120	900	330
(34)	First-pass	16	12×1.5	40	120	30	420
Human studies							
(32)	First-pass	4	4×1.0	120	120	400	500
(35)	First-pass	16	12×0.75	100	120	500	420
(39)	First-pass	16	16×0.75	120	120	500	420
	15 min after contrast bolus		16×0.75		120	500	420
(38)	First-pass	16	16×0.75	140	140	400	420
	10 min after contrast bolus		16×1.5		90	400	420
(40)	24 ± 11 min (7–51 min)[a]	64	32×0.6	176 ± 78[b]	80/100[c]	700	330
(41)	13 ± 3 min (8–18 min)[a]	64	64×0.5	198 ± 22[b]	120	400	400

[a] After last contrast injection in the cath lab.

[b] MDCT scan were performed immediately after cath lab procedure and no additional contrast was injected for the imaging acquisition.

[c] Tube voltage was adjusted to the patients' body weight (BW). Low-voltage setting (80 kV) was applied in patients with BW below 70 kg, and high voltage (100 kV) was chosen for patient having 70-kg BW.

MDCT data sets is increased to reduce the amount of raw data, which needs to be processed for reconstruction in short-axis orientation or volumetric data sets. Usually, 10% intervals of RR-cycle are used to define the end-diastolic and end-systolic phase, resulting in 10 phases to cover the mechanical cycle of the left and right ventricle. Some investigators suggest dividing the cardiac cycle in 5% intervals for a better definition of the end-systolic or end-diastolic time instants. Global LVEF is calculated by volume threshold methods or Simpson's rule is applied by analyzing short-axis images in a semiquantitative manner.

Temporal resolution in MDCT imaging is dependent on the patient's heart rate and reconstruction method is used.[43] In technical terms, temporal resolution in MDCT imaging is defined by (A) the rotation of the X-ray tube (gantry rotation) and (B) the number of reconstructed phases. As reconstruction is usually limited to 20 phases, temporal resolution in MDCT imaging is mainly determined by the gantry rotation.

Since the introduction of multidetector rows in cardiac CT imaging, assessment of LV function has been evaluated in patient populations with suspected or manifested coronary artery disease. Early studies evaluating LV volumes and function with 4-, 8-, and 16-detector rows systems already showed a good agreement with invasive ventriculography,[44–47] 2D echocardiography,[48–54] SPECT,[54] and cardiac MRI.[54–61] However, comparison with cardiac MRI as the reference standard showed an underestimation of LVEF up to $8.5 \pm 4.7\%$.[62] Following two explanations have been proposed:

(A) The use of intravenous contrast injection, which results in a volume load during imaging that could potentially lead to this significant overestimation of LV endiastolic volume (EDV) when compared with MRI.[62–64]
(B) Most likely the limited temporal resolution caused by slow gantry rotation, which cannot be compensated with the reconstruction of additional phases seems to explain the underestimation of LVEF.

MDCT scanners with 4-, 8-, 16-, and 64-detector rows have rotation times of 500 or 420 ms resulting in a temporal resolutions of approximately 250 ms with half-segment reconstruction. However, a temporal resolution of 30 to 50 ms is required to capture maximum systolic contraction.[65] Current scanners with 64 detector rows offer rotation times as low as 330 ms, which can be further improved by multisegment reconstruction. Studies evaluating 64-MDCT technology report good agreement with 2D echocardiography[66–68] and gated SPECT[66] for functional assessment. A recent study by Annuar et al. compared 64-MDCT and cardiac MRI in 32 patients with suspected coronary artery disease. The authors report an excellent correlation between both imaging modalities for LVEF and a minor underestimation of 2.3% by MDT.[68]

The recently introduced 320-MDCT scanner system has the ability to capture a single heart beat with a gantry rotation 350 ms resulting in high temporal resolution ranging from 35 to 175 ms depending on the number of heart beat acquired. Another approach is dual-source MDCT imaging, which also enhances temporal resolution, and therefore one can expect improvement in accuracy of LV function assessment. Early reports suggest that a temporal resolution between 42 and 83 ms can be achieved with dual-source MDCT.[69,70]

As discussed, functional data are usually extracted from the coronary acquisition. Current coronary imaging protocols are designed to reduce the radiation exposure for the patient as low as possible. If so-called "ECG pulsing" protocols are applied, which reduce the radiation exposure in systole by lowering the kilovolt when the coronaries acquisition is not recommended because of intense cardiac motion, the data set can still be used for LV-function evaluation. Although, the systolic images have reduced the imaging quality, qualitative and quantitative assessment of function is possible. However, with the introduction of prospective gated imaging protocols, so called "step and shoot" acquisitions in 64-MDCT systems, functional data cannot be extracted because images are only acquired during a small window of the diastolic phase.

Regional LV function

The evaluation of coronary artery disease is not confined only to the anatomy but also to flow limiting obstruction of the coronary arteries. Information regarding regional wall motion abnormalities is crucial in terms of prognosis, timing, and choice of treatment options.

Currently, information about regional wall motion is limited to reports of visual assessment comparing MDCT to 2D echocardiography or cardiac MRI. Studies with 4- and 16-MDCT technologies showed an overall agreement for regional wall motion ranging from 82% to 98% and 88% to 91% for cardiac MRI[54,61,71] and 2D echocardiography,[48,49,52] respectively. Recently, Henneman et al.[67] reported regional wall motion in 49 patients, and showed excellent 96% overall agreement for 16- and 64-MDCT and 2D echocardiography applying the commonly used 17-segment model. It is important to be aware that high agreement was achieved in particular for the assessment of normal regional function (98%). Lower agreement was found in segments showing hypokinesia (71%) or akinesia (62%). Using exclusive 64-MDCT in a sicker population, Annuar et al. found an overall accuracy of 94.3% for 2D echocardiography and an accuracy of 82.4% for cardiac MRI. Although, 64-MDCT showed very good correlation with cardiac MRI for regional function ($r = 0.90$), only 69% segments had an identical regional wall motion score for MDCT and MRI.

Although these initial results are promising, further studies are needed to evaluate patients with reduced global function and dysfunctional segments in a quantitative way to determine the accuracy of MDCT for regional function and wall motion.

CONCLUSIONS

Assessment of myocardial viability at acceptable levels of radiation is a crucial step in making this MDCT application a clinical reality. Initial results with 64-MDCT scanners show that the tube voltage can be lowered significantly and adequate imaging quality can be achieved.[72] The advent of 320 wide-range MDCT imaging systems combined with the ability to perform segmented reconstruction and prospective gating opens new avenues for single examination of coronary pathology, perfusion, and viability assessment with relatively low-radiation doses.[73,74] Another approach is dual energy imaging with equally superior temporal resolution, which allows cardiac imaging independent of heart rate.[75,76] Dual-energy imaging has the promise to give better tissue characterization which would be an interesting addition in de-MDCT imaging. Though MDCT imaging allows accurate assessment of global LV function, other diagnostic tests without radiation exposure or the need for contrast injection are still more appealing. However, the use of MDCT to assess myocardial perfusion, viability, and scar imaging is very promising, this is still an ongoing investigation with need for improvement. Currently, expert working groups see that human data are too limited to allow clinical recommendations on the use of MDCT for the assessment of perfusion and viability.[77]

REFERENCES

1. Klocke FJ, Baird MG, Lorell BH, et al. ACC/AHA/ASNC guidelines for the clinical use of cardiac radionuclide imaging—executive summary: A report of the American College of Cardiology/American Heart Association Task Force on Practice Guidelines (ACC/AHA/ASNC Committee to Revise the 1995 Guidelines for the Clinical Use of Cardiac Radionuclide Imaging). J Am Coll Cardiol 2003; 42(7):1318–1333.
2. Schomig A, Kastrati A, Dirschinger J, et al. Coronary stenting plus platelet glycoprotein IIb/IIIa blockade compared with tissue plasminogen activator in acute myocardial infarction. Stent versus thrombolysis for occluded coronary arteries in patients with acute myocardial infarction study investigators. N Engl J Med 2000; 343(6):385–391.
3. Kastrati A, Mehilli J, Dirschinger J, et al. Myocardial salvage after coronary stenting plus abciximab versus fibrinolysis plus abciximab in patients with acute myocardial infarction: A randomised trial. Lancet 2002; 359(9310):920–925.
4. Miller TD, Christian TF, Hopfenspirger MR, et al. Infarct size after acute myocardial infarction measured by quantitative tomographic 99mTc sestamibi imaging predicts subsequent mortality. Circulation 1995; 92(3):334–341.
5. Gibbons RJ, Valeti US, Araoz PA, et al. The quantification of infarct size. J Am Coll Cardiol 2004; 44(8):1533–1542.
6. American Heart Association. Heart and Stroke Statistics—2005 Update.
7. Burt RW, Perkins OW, Oppenheim BE, et al. Direct comparison of fluorine-18-FDG SPECT, fluorine-18-FDG PET and rest thallium-201 SPECT for detection of myocardial viability. J Nucl Med 1995; 36(2):176–179.

8. Mahrholdt H, Wagner A, Judd RM, et al. Assessment of myocardial viability by cardiovascular magnetic resonance imaging. Eur Heart J 2002; 23(8):602–619.
9. Sicari R, Pasanisi E, Venneri L, et al. Stress echo results predict mortality: A large-scale multicenter prospective international study. J Am Coll Cardiol 2003; 41(4):589–595.
10. Iskandrian AS, Heo J, Schelbert HR. Myocardial viability: Methods of assessment and clinical relevance. Am Heart J 1996; 132(6):1226–1235.
11. Rumberger JA, Feiring AJ, Lipton MJ, et al. Use of ultrafast computed tomography to quantitate regional myocardial perfusion: A preliminary report. J Am Coll Cardiol 1987; 9(1):59–69.
12. Wolfkiel CJ, Ferguson JL, Chomka EV, et al. Measurement of myocardial blood flow by ultrafast computed tomography. Circulation 1987; 76(6):1262–1273.
13. Gould RG, Lipton MJ, McNamara MT, et al. Measurement of regional myocardial blood flow in dogs by ultrafast CT. Invest Radiol 1988; 23(5):348–353.
14. Wang T, Wu X, Chung N, et al. Myocardial blood flow estimated by synchronous, multislice, high-speed computed tomography. IEEE Trans Med Imaging 1989; 8(1):70–77.
15. Ludman PF, Coats AJ, Burger P, et al. Validation of measurement of regional myocardial perfusion in humans by ultrafast x-ray computed tomography. Am J Card Imaging 1993; 7(4): 267–279.
16. Bell MR, Lerman LO, Rumberger JA. Validation of minimally invasive measurement of myocardial perfusion using electron beam computed tomography and application in human volunteers. Heart 1999; 81(6):628–635.
17. Canty JM Jr, Judd RM, Brody AS, et al. First-pass entry of nonionic contrast agent into the myocardial extravascular space. Effects on radiographic estimates of transit time and blood volume. Circulation 1991; 84(5):2071–2078.
18. Naito H, Hamada S, Takamiya M, et al. Significance of dipyridamole loading in ultrafast x-ray computed tomography for detection of myocardial ischemia. A study in patients with Kawasaki disease. Invest Radiol 1995; 30(7):389–395.
19. George RT, Jerosch-Herold M, Silva C, et al. Quantification of myocardial perfusion using dynamic 64-detector computed tomography. Invest Radiol 2007; 42(12):815–822.
20. George RT, Silva C, Cordeiro MA, et al. Multidetector computed tomography myocardial perfusion imaging during adenosine stress. J Am Coll Cardiol 2006; 48(1):153–160.
21. Gray WR, Buja LM, Hagler HK, et al. Computed tomography for localization and sizing of experimental acute myocardial infarcts. Circulation 1978; 58(3 Pt 1):497–504.
22. Gray WR Jr, Parkey RW, Buja LM, et al. Computed tomography: In vitro evaluation of myocardial infarction. Radiology 1977; 122(2):511–513.
23. Higgins CB, Sovak M, Schmidt W, et al. Differential accumulation of radiopaque contrast material in acute myocardial infarction. Am J Cardiol 1979; 43(1):47–51.
24. Higgins CB, Sovak M, Schmidt W, et al. Uptake of contrast materials by experimental acute myocardial infarctions: A preliminary report. Invest Radiol 1978; 13(4):337–339.
25. Doherty PW, Lipton MJ, Berninger WH, et al. Detection and quantitation of myocardial infarction in vivo using transmission computed tomography. Circulation 1981; 63(3):597–606.
26. Higgins CB, Siemers PT, Schmidt W, et al. Evaluation of myocardial ischemic damage of various ages by computerized transmission tomography. Time-dependent effects of contrast material. Circulation 1979; 60(2):284–291.
27. Higgins CB, Siemers PT, Newell JD, et al. Role of iodinated contrast material in the evaluation of myocardial infarction by computerized transmission tomography. Invest Radiol 1980; 15(6 Suppl.):S176–S182.
28. Huber DJ, Lapray JF, Hessel SJ. In vivo evaluation of experimental myocardial infarcts by ungated computed tomography. AJR Am J Roentgenol 1981; 136(3):469–473.
29. Newhouse JH. Fluid compartment distribution of intravenous iothalamate in the dog. Invest Radiol 1977; 12(4):364–367.
30. Newhouse JH, Murphy RX Jr. Tissue distribution of soluble contrast: Effect of dose variation and changes with time. AJR Am J Roentgenol 1981; 136(3):463–467.
31. Canty JM Jr, Judd RM, Brody AS, et al. First-pass entry of nonionic contrast agent into the myocardial extravascular space. Effects on radiographic estimates of transit time and blood volume. Circulation 1991; 84(5):2071–2078.
32. Nikolaou K, Knez A, Sagmeister S, et al. Assessment of myocardial infarctions using multidetector-row computed tomography. J Comput Assist Tomogr 2004; 28(2):286–292.
33. Hoffmann U, Millea R, Enzweiler C, et al. Acute myocardial infarction: Contrast-enhanced multi-detector row CT in a porcine model. Radiology 2004; 231(3):697–701.
34. Mahnken AH, Bruners P, Katoh M, et al. Dynamic multi-section CT imaging in acute myocardial infarction: Preliminary animal experience. Eur Radiol 2006; 16(3):746–752.

35. Nikolaou K, Sanz J, Poon M, et al. Assessment of myocardial perfusion and viability from routine contrast-enhanced 16-detector-row computed tomography of the heart: Preliminary results. Eur Radiol 2005; 15(5):864–871.
36. Lardo AC, Cordeiro MA, Silva C, et al. Contrast-enhanced multidetector computed tomography viability imaging after myocardial infarction: Characterization of myocyte death, microvascular obstruction, and chronic scar. Circulation 2006; 113(3):394–404.
37. Baks T, Cademartiri F, Moelker AD, et al. Multislice computed tomography and magnetic resonance imaging for the assessment of reperfused acute myocardial infarction. J Am Coll Cardiol 2006; 48(1):144–152.
38. Gerber BL, Belge B, Legros GJ, et al. Characterization of acute and chronic myocardial infarcts by multidetector computed tomography: Comparison with contrast-enhanced magnetic resonance. Circulation 2006; 113(6):823–833.
39. Mahnken AH, Koos R, Katoh M, et al. Assessment of myocardial viability in reperfused acute myocardial infarction using 16-slice computed tomography in comparison to magnetic resonance imaging. J Am Coll Cardiol 2005; 45(12):2042–2047.
40. Habis M, Capderou A, Ghostine S, et al. Acute myocardial infarction early viability assessment by 64-slice computed tomography immediately after coronary angiography: Comparison with low-dose dobutamine echocardiography. J Am Coll Cardiol 2007; 49(11):1178–1185.
41. Sato A, Hiroe M, Nozato T, et al. Early validation study of 64-slice multidetector computed tomography for the assessment of myocardial viability and the prediction of left ventricular remodelling after acute myocardial infarction. Eur Heart J 2008; 29(4):490–498.
42. Wu KC, Lima JA. Noninvasive imaging of myocardial viability: Current techniques and future developments. Circ Res 2003; 93(12):1146–1158.
43. Dewey M, Muller M, Teige F, et al. Multisegment and halfscan reconstruction of 16-slice computed tomography for assessment of regional and global left ventricular myocardial function. Invest Radiol 2006; 41(4):400–409.
44. Juergens KU, Grude M, Fallenberg EM, et al. Using ECG-gated multidetector CT to evaluate global left ventricular myocardial function in patients with coronary artery disease. AJR Am J Roentgenol 2002; 179(6):1545–1550.
45. Heuschmid M, Kuttner A, Schroder S, et al. Left ventricular functional parameters using ECG-gated multidetector spiral CT in comparison with invasive ventriculography. Rofo 2003; 175(10): 1349–1354.
46. Hosoi S, Mochizuki T, Miyagawa M, et al. Assessment of left ventricular volumes using multi-detector row computed tomography (MDCT): Phantom and human studies. Radiat Med 2003; 21(2):62–67.
47. Boehm T, Alkadhi H, Roffi M, et al. Time-effectiveness, observer-dependence, and accuracy of measurements of left ventricular ejection fraction using 4-channel MDCT. Rofo 2004; 176(4):529–537.
48. Dirksen MS, Bax JJ, de RA,et al. Usefulness of dynamic multislice computed tomography of left ventricular function in unstable angina pectoris and comparison with echocardiography. Am J Cardiol 2002; 90(10):1157–1160.
49. Dirksen MS, Jukema JW, Bax JJ, et al. Cardiac multidetector-row computed tomography in patients with unstable angina. Am J Cardiol 2005; 95(4):457–461.
50. Schuijf JD, Bax JJ, Jukema JW, et al. Assessment of left ventricular volumes and ejection fraction with 16-slice multi-slice computed tomography; comparison with 2D-echocardiography. Int J Cardiol 2007; 116(2):201–205.
51. Schuijf JD, Bax JJ, Salm LP, et al. Noninvasive coronary imaging and assessment of left ventricular function using 16-slice computed tomography. Am J Cardiol 2005; 95(5):571–574.
52. Schuijf JD, Bax JJ, Jukema JW, et al. Noninvasive evaluation of the coronary arteries with multislice computed tomography in hypertensive patients. Hypertension 2005; 45(2):227–232.
53. Schuijf JD, Bax JJ, Jukema JW, et al. Noninvasive angiography and assessment of left ventricular function using multislice computed tomography in patients with type 2 diabetes. Diabetes Care 2004; 27(12):2905–2910.
54. Yamamuro M, Tadamura E, Kubo S, et al. Cardiac functional analysis with multi-detector row CT and segmental reconstruction algorithm: Comparison with echocardiography, SPECT, and MR imaging. Radiology 2005; 234(2):381–390.
55. Juergens KU, Grude M, Maintz D, et al. Multi-detector row CT of left ventricular function with dedicated analysis software versus MR imaging: Initial experience. Radiology 2004; 230(2):403–410.
56. Juergens KU, Maintz D, Grude M, et al. Multi-detector row computed tomography of the heart: Does a multi-segment reconstruction algorithm improve left ventricular volume measurements? Eur Radiol 2005; 15(1):111–117.
57. Juergens KU, Fischbach R. Left ventricular function studied with MDCT. Eur Radiol 2006; 16(2): 342–357.

58. Koch K, Oellig F, Kunz P, et al. Assessment of global and regional left ventricular function with a 16-slice spiral-CT using two different software tools for quantitative functional analysis and qualitative evaluation of wall motion changes in comparison with magnetic resonance imaging. Rofo 2004; 176(12):1786–1793.
59. Belge B, Coche E, Pasquet A, et al. Accurate estimation of global and regional cardiac function by retrospectively gated multidetector row computed tomography: Comparison with cine magnetic resonance imaging. Eur Radiol 2006; 16(7):1424–1433.
60. Schlosser T, Pagonidis K, Herborn CU, et al. Assessment of left ventricular parameters using 16-MDCT and new software for endocardial and epicardial border delineation. AJR Am J Roentgenol 2005; 184(3):765–773.
61. Mahnken AH, Koos R, Katoh M, et al. Sixteen-slice spiral CT versus MR imaging for the assessment of left ventricular function in acute myocardial infarction. Eur Radiol 2005; 15(4):714–720.
62. Grude M, Juergens KU, Wichter T, et al. Evaluation of global left ventricular myocardial function with electrocardiogram-gated multidetector computed tomography: Comparison with magnetic resonance imaging. Invest Radiol 2003; 38(10):653–661.
63. Heuschmid M, Rothfuss JK, Schroeder S, et al. Assessment of left ventricular myocardial function using 16-slice multidetector-row computed tomography: Comparison with magnetic resonance imaging and echocardiography. Eur Radiol 2006; 16(3):551–559.
64. Schlosser T, Pagonidis K, Herborn CU, et al. Assessment of left ventricular parameters using 16-MDCT and new software for endocardial and epicardial border delineation. AJR Am J Roentgenol 2005; 184(3):765–773.
65. Setser RM, Fischer SE, Lorenz CH. Quantification of left ventricular function with magnetic resonance images acquired in real time. J Magn Reson Imaging 2000; 12(3):430–438.
66. Henneman MM, Bax JJ, Schuijf JD, et al. Global and regional left ventricular function: A comparison between gated SPECT, 2D echocardiography and multi-slice computed tomography. Eur J Nucl Med Mol Imaging 2006; 33(12):1452–1460.
67. Henneman MM, Schuijf JD, Jukema JW, et al. Assessment of global and regional left ventricular function and volumes with 64-slice MSCT: A comparison with 2D echocardiography. J Nucl Cardiol 2006; 13(4):480–487.
68. Annuar BR, Liew CK, Chin SP, et al. Assessment of global and regional left ventricular function using 64-slice multislice computed tomography and 2D echocardiography: A comparison with cardiac magnetic resonance. Eur J Radiol 2008; 65(1):112–119.
69. Brodoefel H, Kramer U, Reimann A, et al. Dual-source CT with improved temporal resolution in assessment of left ventricular function: A pilot study. AJR Am J Roentgenol 2007; 189(5):1064–1070.
70. Mahnken AH, Bruder H, Suess C, et al. Dual-source computed tomography for assessing cardiac function: A phantom study. Invest Radiol 2007; 42(7):491–498.
71. Koch K, Oellig F, Kunz P, et al. Assessment of global and regional left ventricular function with a 16-slice spiral-CT using two different software tools for quantitative functional analysis and qualitative evaluation of wall motion changes in comparison with magnetic resonance imaging. Rofo 2004; 176(12):1786–1793.
72. Brodoefel H, Reimann A, Klumpp B, et al. Assessment of myocardial viability in a reperfused porcine model: Evaluation of different MSCT contrast protocols in acute and subacute infarct stages in comparison with MRI. J Comput Assist Tomogr 2007; 31(2):290–298.
73. Kido T, Kurata A, Higashino H, et al. Cardiac imaging using 256-detector row four-dimensional CT: Preliminary clinical report. Radiat Med 2007; 25(1):38–44.
74. Mori S, Nishizawa K, Kondo C, et al. Effective doses in subjects undergoing computed tomography cardiac imaging with the 256-multislice CT scanner. Eur J Radiol 2008; 65(3):442–448.
75. Johnson TR, Nikolaou K, Wintersperger BJ, et al. Dual-source CT cardiac imaging: Initial experience. Eur Radiol 2006; 16(7):1409–1415.
76. Matt D, Scheffel H, Leschka S, et al. Dual-source CT coronary angiography: Image quality, mean heart rate, and heart rate variability. AJR Am J Roentgen 2007; 189(3):567–573.
77. Schroeder S, Achenbach S, Bengel F, et al. Cardiac computed tomography: Indications, applications, limitations, and training requirements: Report of a Writing Group deployed by the Working Group Nuclear Cardiology and Cardiac CT of the European Society of Cardiology and the European Council of Nuclear Cardiology. Eur Heart J 2008; 29(4):531–556.

22 Evaluation of LV function in cases of global and segmental disease

Henrique Barbosa Ribeiro and Expedito E. Ribeiro

INTRODUCTION

Cardiac ventriculography is a method used in the catheterization laboratory to characterize the anatomy and function of the ventricles in patients presenting with a broad range of heart disorders including valvular, coronary artery, and congenital diseases, as well as cardiomyopathies.[1] Moreover, the left ventriculography is a major diagnostic tool to address several features (Table 22.1), including the evaluation of left ventricular (LV) function in cases of global and segmental disease. Because of all these important aspects gathered by this method it is included in the routine diagnostic catheterization protocol of the patients, except in cases where the contrast volume might be a concern, and other alternatives to contrast ventriculography are available.

TECHNIQUE

Injection catheters

In order to deliver a relatively large amount of contrast, in a short period of time, it should be used with special catheters for injection mounted into automated injection devices. This is best performed using 7F and 6F catheters that have various side holes, permitting a rapid infusion of contrast material while maintaining the catheter in a mid-ventricle position, avoiding the possible arrhythmias that can ensue. Another important issue is that catheters with an end hole only should be avoided to minimize the risk of catheter recoil during high-pressure contrast injection, which may potentially cause inadequate opacification, premature ventricle beats, or even chamber perforation.

The pigtail catheter was developed by Judkins and reaches the ventricle from any arterial access. Its end hole permits the placing of a guidewire that makes the procedure easy to perform. Its multiple side holes allow the delivery of large amounts of contrast media at a high flow rate into the ventricle. Also, the side holes help in stabilizing the catheter in a mid-ventricle position during the injection due to the counterbalanced effect of the catheter jets. Moreover, the loop shape of the catheter end precludes its direct contact with the endocardium, reducing the occurrence of ventricle premature beats.

The pigtail usually crosses easily a normal aortic valve, and even porcine aortic valve prosthesis. However, in stenotic aortic valve the use of a straight leading guidewire may be warranted. Bartsch et al.[2] reported complications of catheterization of the left ventricle in aortic stenosis in 457 patients evaluated from 1984 to 1995. The success rate was 95.2%, and higher complications rates were related to age >70 years, aortic valve areas <0.7 cm^2, and peak gradient at Doppler examination >70 mm Hg. Corroborating data from Omran et al.[3] show that 22 (22%) out of 101 patients, who underwent retrograde catheterization of the aortic valve, had focal diffusion abnormalities in the MRI cranial imaging, consistent with acute cerebral embolic event. From those patients, 3% had clinically apparent neurologic deficits. Thus, patients with aortic valve stenosis submitted to retrograde catheterization of the aortic valve have an increased risk of clinically apparent cerebral embolism, and often have silent ischemic brain lesions. They should be informed of these risks, and this procedure should be performed only in patients with less-clear noninvasive data, such as poor acoustic window, coexistent mitral valve disease, and poor LV function.

The original Judkins pigtail, with its straight shaft, has been replaced, in the routine diagnostic catheterization, by an angled pigtail that has a 145° to 155° angle at its distal end, proximal to the side holes. These catheters more frequently localize in the central as opposed to the inferoposterior region of the LV cavity. In a randomized study, 125 patients were prospectively assigned to undergo ventriculography using either of the two pigtail catheters, one

Table 22.1 Parameters assessed by left ventriculography

Ventricular morphology, volume, and thickness
Global and regional ventricular wall motion
Mitral valve morphology and integrity
Aortic valve morphology and motion
The presence, location, and size of a ventricular septal defect
Masses or calcifications in or around the heart detected by other techniques

with a straight shaft throughout its length (straight) and the other with a 145° bend placed 6.5 cm from the distal end (angled). Compared with the straight catheter, the angled catheter was easier to insert ($p = 0.038$), and it took less time to localize its correct position ($p = 0.012$).[4] Moreover, the angled catheter was less frequently accompanied by artifactual mitral regurgitation ($p = 0.038$), but was equally likely to provoke ventricular arrhythmias during injection. Nonetheless, others have shown that the opacification and overall quality of the left ventriculograms were distributed similarly between the two types of catheters.[5] Thus, adequate ventriculography can be achieved with either shape.

Other left ventriculography catheters can also be used. Among them the Sones catheter (that has an end hole and four side holes at its distal tip) is commonly used when the brachial approach is utilized. The end hole allows the insertion of the Sones catheter over a 0.035-in. straight guidewire, which makes it possible to cross even severe calcific aortic valve. In order to have a good-quality ventriculography the catheter should be placed in an axial orientation (parallel to the ventricular long axis) with the central of the tip between the LV apex and the aortic valve. Despite the fact that low injection rates may lessen the catheter recoil, this still occurs causing extrasystoles and possible harm to endocardial staining.

Injection technique

After the best catheter position in the ventricle is achieved, normally in the mid-cavity, a large amount of contrast must be delivered in a short period of time so that opacification is accomplished. This is best done using contrast material power injectors. There are many types of injectors that allow the control of both amount and rate of delivery of contrast material. At the discretion of the operator, many catheters and injection parameters may be used for LV opacification. However, we recommend in most cases the use of pigtail catheters, with a 3-second–long injection at 10 to 12 mL/second rate (total volume of ~36 mL).[1] Higher volumes can be used if an end-hole catheter is utilized, not exceeding 10 mL/sec, to avoid recoil and staining.

Filming projection

The main projection used during cardiac catheterization is 30° right anterior oblique (RAO) in order to eliminate the overlapping of the column with the LV (Fig. 22.1). This projection allows the study of the anterior, apical, and inferior segmental walls. To better assess the septal, lateral, and posterior segmental functions, normally the 60° left anterior oblique (LAO) is the best view (Fig. 22.1). The ventriculography can reliably be done with 15 frames/sec technique. If available, the biplane ventriculography is preferable since a double-projection ventriculography can be obtained with the same amount of contrast administered.

ANALYSIS OF THE VENTRICULOGRAM

The ventriculograms can be evaluated both quantitatively and qualitatively in relation to the global and regional wall function. This is frequently determined by visual estimation, however, it has been demonstrated highly variable and tends to overestimate wall motion in some segments (anterolateral) and underestimate in others (inferior). Thus, the accuracy and reproducibility of ventricular wall motion is greatly enhanced by the utilization of quantitative techniques.

The area-length technique first described in 1956 by Dodge et al.[6] is the most widely used method to quantify the LV diastolic and systolic volumes, and from them the actual left ventricular ejection fraction (LVEF; the percent of blood volume present at end-diastole that is ejected by end-systole) (Figs. 22.2 and 22.3). Currently, using computer-assisted analysis this

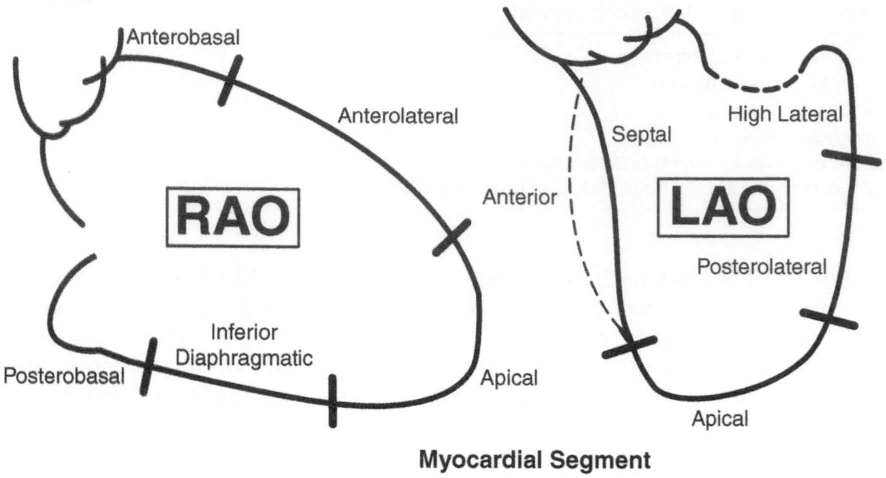

Figure 22.1 Left ventriculograms showing the 30° right anterior oblique (RAO) and the 60° left anterior oblique (LAO).

can be easily achieved. LVEF can be described as hyperdynamic (LVEF >70%), normal (LVEF 50–69%), mildly hypokinetic (LVEF 35–49%), or severely hypokinetic (LVEF <35%).[1]

Cineventriculography was the first method introduced in the routine practice to determine the LVEF. Several techniques have been developed so far, albeit cineventriculography for long time has been considered the practicable standard, in several randomized clinical trials.[7–9] Moreover, some of these trials have documented the value of its determination even in the acute phase. The PAMI-II trial included patients presenting with acute myocardial infarction (AMI) who underwent primary percutaneous coronary angioplasty (PCI).[8] Clinical and catheterization data were used to prospectively identify low risk AMI patients, who could safely be treated without intensive care, without noninvasive testing during the hospitalization, and who could be discharged on day 3. In the PAMI-II, a low-risk profile was characterized by an LVEF greater than 45% at the cineventriculography performed during the index procedure (together with age ≤70 years, one or two-vessel disease, successful PCI, and no persistent arrhythmias).

In this scenario of AMI, it has also been shown that LV function, determined at the index procedure, assessed as global or regional wall motion within the distribution of the culprit vessel, is a strong determinant of survival after primary PCI. Furthermore, an acutely depressed LVEF was found to be a powerful discriminator of death in the first few months after AMI, albeit successful primary PCI.[7]

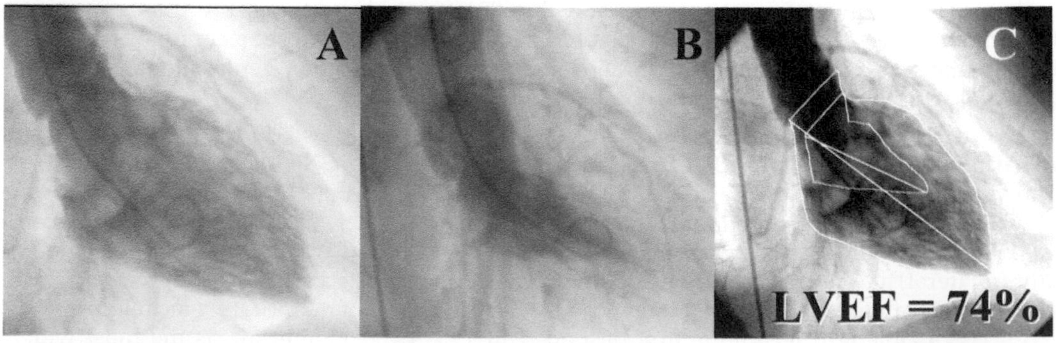

Figure 22.2 The area-length technique is the most widely used method to quantify the left ventricular diastolic (**A**) and systolic (**B**) volumes. Here is shown a hyperdynamic ventricle, with increased left ventricular ejection fraction (LVEF) (**C**).

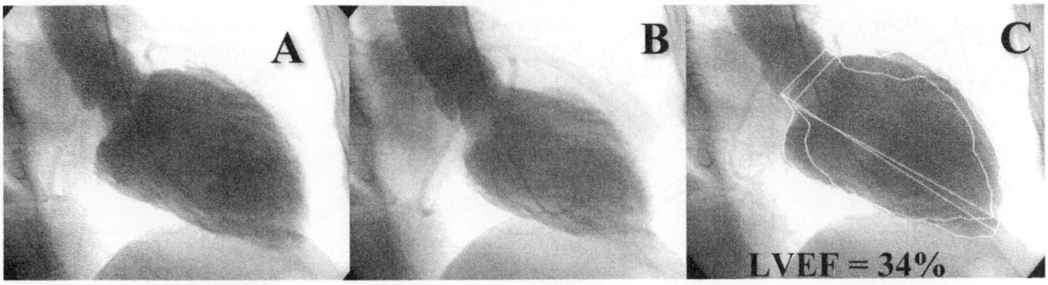

Figure 22.3 Left ventriculogram is shown in the diastole (**A**) and systole (**B**), with reduced left ventricular ejection fraction (LVEF) (**C**).

With the technological advances of other methods, the so-called noninvasive modalities have been developed, such as magnetic resonance imaging (MRI), echocardiogram, and radionuclide methods. Various studies have examined the correlation and agreement between noninvasive measurement of ejection fraction and that obtained with LV angiography.[10–12] Some reports have demonstrated good correlation between noninvasive methods and cineventriculography, what has not been confirmed by others.[12,13] For example, LVEF obtained by SPECT was significantly lower than that obtained by echocardiography.[13,14] MRI was thought to provide superior imaging quality and more accurate assessment of ejection fraction.[12,15,16] However, MRI is still relatively expensive and not routinely available. On the other hand, unenhanced echocardiography, despite readily available in most centers, resulted in an only moderate agreement with cineventriculography to determine LVEF.[12] Nonetheless, contrast-enhanced echocardiography increased its correlation with other methods, such as MRI and cineventriculography.

In the daily practice, measurement of LVEF is now performed almost uniformly by noninvasive methods. An AHA/ACC Task Force on Practice Guidelines has published recommendations on the measurement of LV function in patients with coronary disease.[17] Although each of the five techniques described above can provide accurate information, each test has certain limitations that may be important in selected patients. Moreover, it has been considered a Class I indication of echocardiography or radionuclide angiography in patients with a history of prior myocardial infarction, pathologic Q waves or symptoms or signs suggestive of heart failure to assess LV function.

In conclusion, the important practical issue may not be which technique is best, but rather, which technique is available at a particular institution and possess reasonable accuracy and reproducibility. It should be also highlighted that ventriculography is part of the coronariography exam in the catheterization laboratory, and except if contraindicated it should be performed routinely.

REGIONAL LV WALL MOTION

Regional wall motion can be graded qualitatively as normal, hypokinetic, akinetic, dyskinetic, or hyperkinetic (Fig. 22.4). The analyses of the RAO and LAO projections of the left ventricle may yield the evaluation of the following segments: anterobasal, anterolateral, anterior, apical, inferior diaphragmatic, and posterobasal (RAO projection); high lateral, posterolateral, apical, and septal (LAO projection) (Fig. 22.1).

Regional LV wall motion has been determined as a surrogate marker for coronary artery disease, with better sensitive value than global function depression. The ventricle may be evaluated by mainly two methods. First, by the construction of lines drawn from the midpoint of the major axis into the ventricular outline at intervals of a fixed number of degrees.[18] Second, by the construction of lines perpendicular to the major axis that divide the major axis into equal segments.[18,19] Currently, with the support of digital computer techniques, regional wall motion may be measured, providing quantitative evaluation of the extent of inward and/or outward movement, thus leading to the measurement of dyskinesis, hypokinesis, and akinesis of the various segments.

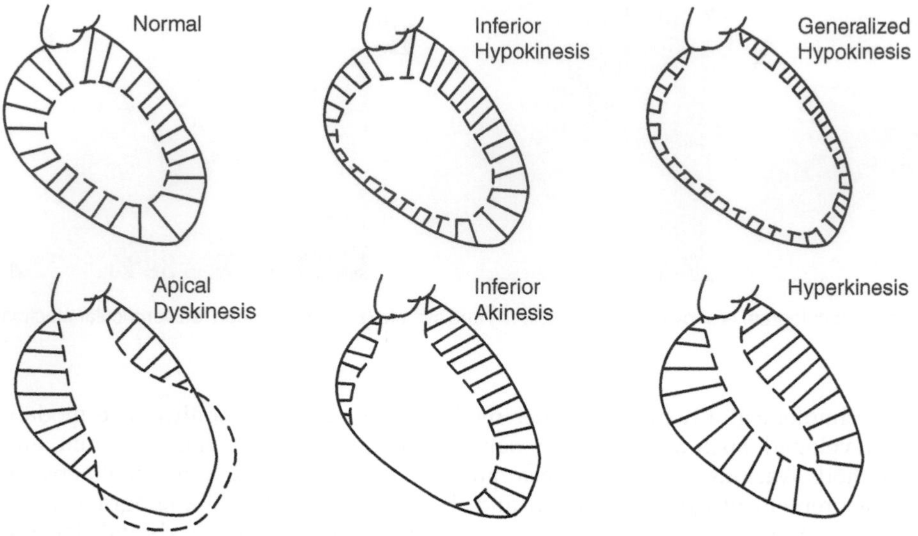

Figure 22.4 Regional wall motion can be graded qualitatively as normal, hypokinetic, akinetic, dyskinetic, or hyperkinetic.

In addition to grading the regional wall motion, it is important to distinguish reversible from irreversible contractile deficits. Chronic but potentially reversible ischemic dysfunction due to a stenotic coronary artery is so-called "hibernating" myocardium. It has been estimated that 20% to more than 50% of patients with chronic ischemic LV dysfunction have a significant amount of viable hibernating myocardium and therefore the potential for clinically important improvement in LV function after revascularization.

A variety of tests can assist in the evaluation of myocardial viability. These include myocardial perfusion imaging, positron emission tomography scanning, and dobutamine echocardiography. None of them are the objective of the present chapter. Furthermore, although rarely used clinically today, left ventriculography with an increase in segmental contraction with pharmacologic or nonpharmacologic stimulation (postextrasystolic potentiation) can be used. Assessment of regional wall motion by ventriculography, and its improvement with nitroglycerin or positive inotropic stimulation has at least two limitations: (1) subjective evaluation may not be accurate and (2) the technique used to superimpose the end-systolic silhouette on the end-diastolic silhouette may affect the assessment of regional wall motion function.

Thus, some assessments that regional wall motion function has improved or deteriorated could be erroneous. The finding of improved wall motion function would be accepted more confidently if it were reflected in improved global LV systolic function or LVEF. However, for LVEF to improve, it appears that wall motion function must improve in at least two to three myocardial regions.

Moreover, other simple clues may suggest in the ventriculograms that the hypokinesis and/or akinesis are permanent. The demonstration of calcium in the ventricle wall, obvious thinning of the wall, and the presence of mural thrombus may show irreversible damage.

COMPLICATIONS

Arrhythmias

During catheterization a variety of arrhythmias and conduction disturbances may occur. The most common ventricular premature beats may be induced by catheter introduction into the right or left ventricle or by a jet of contrast, and are generally without clinical importance or impact. Nevertheless, this can be lessened by catheter repositioning.

Ventricular tachycardia and/or fibrillation are rare complications of catheterization, with an estimated incidence reaching 0.4% of cases.

Few patients may persist with ventricular tachycardia, despite catheter removal during ventriculography. In such cases, lidocaine and amiodarone bolus, as well as cardioversion, may be necessary.

Intramyocardial injection (endocardial staining)

When unseemly ventriculography catheter positioning occurs, the contrast material can be injected within the endocardium or myocardium, especially if the catheter is placed under the papillary muscles. Thus, if a large stain occurs, medically mediated refractory ventricular arrhythmias may take place.

Fascicular block

During retrograde left cardiac catheterization, patients with preexisting right bundle branch and/or left posterior fascicular block may develop transitory complete heart block or asystole. This occurs because of the proximity of the anterior fascicle of the left bundle to the ventricle outflow. Atropine is rarely helpful in patients who develop complete heart block, but its administration is still recommended. Moreover, coughing may help support the circulation. Although temporary pacing is normally required, within 12 to 24 hours, prophylactic placement of a temporary pacemaker is not necessary, even in patients with bundle branch block or intervention in the right coronary artery.[20]

Embolism

The greatest risk related to ventriculography is the injection of thrombus or air in the ventricle. The thrombus injection can be avoided by frequent flushing of the catheter with a solution containing heparin. Besides that, if there is evidence, normally from noninvasive methods, of a thrombus in the ventricle, a lot of care should be taken with the positioning of the catheter, avoiding the apical portion (normally where the thrombus is placed). However, in our opinion if a good noninvasive image is available, this part of the examination must not be done. Another important aspect is related to air embolization, that is simply avoided by filling the injector adequately and confirming that the lines are bubbles free.

Complications of contrast material

Contrast material can yield transient complications such as hot flashes, from its vasodilatatory effect, nausea, and vomiting, in as much as 30% of patients. Moreover, radiocontrast media can lead to a usually reversible form of acute renal failure that begins within the first 12 to 24 hours after the contrast is administered, and resolves within 7 days. Less than 1% of the patients will require hemodialysis, mostly in patients with baseline plasma creatinine greater than 4 mg/dL (352 μmol/L). The major risk factors associated with contrast-induced nephropathies are (a) diabetes nephropathy, especially with renal insufficiency; (b) underlying renal insufficiency, with the plasma creatinine exceeding 1.5 mg/dL (132 μmol/L) or, estimated glomerular filtration rate less than 60 mL/min per 1.73 m^2; (c) heart failure; (d) hypovolemia; (e) percutaneous coronary intervention; (f) high total dose of contrast agent and high osmolality contrast agent; and (g) multiple myeloma.

Among the various available iodinated radiocontrast agents the lowest risk of toxicity is associated with low- or iso-osmolal agents. This new agents also reduced the incidence of hot flashes, nausea, and vomiting.

REFERENCES

1. Baim DS. Grossman's Cardiac Catheterization, Angiography, and Intervention. Philadelphia: Lippincott Williams & Wilkins, 2005:992.
2. Bartsch B, Hasse K, Voelker W, et al. Risk of invasive diagnosis with retrograde catheterization of left ventricle in patients with acquired aortic valve stenosis. Z Kardiol 1999; 88:255–260.
3. Omran H, Schmidt H, Hackenbroch M, et al. Silent and apparent cerebral embolism after retrograde catheterisation of the aortic valve in valvular stenosis: A prospective, randomised study. Lancet 2003; 361:1241–1246.
4. Lehmann KG, Yang JC, Doria RJ, et al. Catheter optimization during contrast ventriculography: A prospective randomized trial. Am Heart J 1992; 123:1273–1278.

5. Deligonul U, Jones S, Shurmur S, et al. Contrast cine left ventriculography: Comparison of two pigtail catheter shapes and analysis of factors determining the final quality. Cathet Cardiovasc Diagn 1996; 37:428–433.
6. Dodge HT, Sandler H, Ballew DW, et al. The use of biplane angiocardigraphy for the measurement of left ventricular volume in man. Am Heart J 1960; 60:762–776.
7. Halkin A, Stone GW, Dixon SR, et al. Impact and determinants of left ventricular function in patients undergoing primary percutaneous coronary intervention in acute myocardial infarction. Am J Cardiol 2005; 96:325–331.
8. Grines CL, Marsalese DL, Brodie B, et al. Safety and cost-effectiveness of early discharge after primary angioplasty in low risk patients with acute myocardial infarction. PAMI-II Investigators. Primary angioplasty in myocardial infarction. J Am Coll Cardiol 1998; 31:967–972.
9. The effects of tissue plasminogen activator, streptokinase, or both on coronary-artery patency, ventricular function, and survival after acute myocardial infarction. The GUSTO Angiographic Investigators. N Engl J Med 1993; 329:1615–1622.
10. van Royen N, Jaffe CC, Krumholz HM, et al. Comparison and reproducibility of visual echocardiographic and quantitative radionuclide left ventricular ejection fractions. Am J Cardiol 1996; 77:843–850.
11. Albrechtsson U, Eskilsson J, Lomsky M, et al. Comparison of left ventricular ejection fraction assessed by radionuclide angiocardiography, echocardiography and contrast angiocardiography. Acta Med Scand 1982; 211:147–152.
12. Hoffmann R, von Bardeleben S, ten Cate F, et al. Assessment of systolic left ventricular function: A multi-centre comparison of cineventriculography, cardiac magnetic resonance imaging, unenhanced and contrast-enhanced echocardiography. Eur Heart J 2005; 26:607–616.
13. Williams KA, Taillon LA. Left ventricular function in patients with coronary artery disease assessed by gated tomographic myocardial perfusion images. Comparison with assessment by contrast ventriculography and first-pass radionuclide angiography. J Am Coll Cardiol 1996; 27:173–181.
14. Habash-Bseiso DE, Rokey R, Berger CJ, et al. Accuracy of noninvasive ejection fraction measurement in a large community-based clinic. Clin Med Res 2005; 3:75–82.
15. Van Rossum AC, Visser FC, Sprenger M, et al. Evaluation of magnetic resonance imaging for determination of left ventricular ejection fraction and comparison with angiography. Am J Cardiol 1988; 62:628–633.
16. Cranney GB, Lotan CS, Dean L, et al. Left ventricular volume measurement using cardiac axis nuclear magnetic resonance imaging. Validation by calibrated ventricular angiography. Circulation 1990; 82:154–163.
17. Gibbons RJ, Abrams J, Chatterjee K, et al. ACC/AHA 2002 guideline update for the management of patients with chronic stable angina—summary article: A report of the American College of Cardiology/American Heart Association Task Force on practice guidelines (Committee on the Management of Patients With Chronic Stable Angina). J Am Coll Cardiol 2003; 41:159–168.
18. Herman MV, Heinle RA, Klein MD, et al. Localized disorders in myocardial contraction. Asynergy and its role in congestive heart failure. N Engl J Med 1967; 277:222–232.
19. Sniderman AD, Marpole D, Fallen EL. Regional contraction patterns in the normal and ischemic left ventricle in man. Am J Cardiol 1973; 31:484–489.
20. Harvey JR, Wyman RM, McKay RG, et al. Use of balloon flotation pacing catheters for prophylactic temporary pacing during diagnostic and therapeutic catheterization procedures. Am J Cardiol 1988; 62:941–944.

23 Current noninvasive and invasive diagnostic approach to hypertrophic cardiomyopathy

Milind Y. Desai and Samir Kapadia

INTRODUCTION

Hypertrophic cardiomyopathy (HCM) is a complex cardiovascular condition, with a potential for broad phenotypic expression such that clinical symptoms can develop during any phase of life, from infancy to more than 90 years of age.[1–7] HCM is inherited in an autosomal dominant fashion with over 12 genes identified as being involved in the phenotypic manifestation.[1,7–10] The prevalence of this genetic disorder is of the order of 1:500 in the general adult population and is one of the most common cardiac genetic disorders known.[1,7–10] Traditionally, the diagnosis of HCM has been primarily clinical, involving the use of echocardiography to evaluate for certain characteristic features such as left ventricular hypertrophy (LVH), asymmetric septal hypertrophy, systolic anterior motion of the mitral valve (SAM) with left ventricular outflow tract (LVOT) obstruction. Although there have been tremendous advances in the understanding of the genetic predisposition for this disease state, the utility of genetic study for the absolute diagnosis remains preliminary at this point of time.

CLINICAL PRESENTATION

Although the phenotypic expression in HCM is large, most patients are actually asymptomatic and diagnosed as the result of a murmur on examination, abnormal electrocardiogram, or unexplained LVH discovered by echocardiography. Symptomatic patients that will have an adverse clinical course will typically follow along one of the several pathways: (1) those at high risk for sudden cardiac death, (2) progressive symptoms of exertional dyspnea and chest pain associated with presyncope or syncope in the setting of preserved LV function, (3) development of progressive congestive heart failure due to severe LV remodeling resulting in systolic dysfunction, and (4) consequences of supraventricular or ventricular arrhythmias.[1,7,11–13]

Sudden cardiac death (SCD) is a common presentation and source of mortality in HCM.[1,7,12,14,15] Although obviously the most fearsome and dramatic complication of HCM, those at high risk for SCD actually constitute only a small fraction of the disease spectrum[1,6,7,16,17] and much effort has been devoted to the premorbid identification of this subset of patients. Currently identified risk factors for SCD include prior cardiac arrest, family history of SCD, unexplained syncope or near syncope, left ventricular thickness greater than 30 mm, a high-risk genetic mutation (e.g., β-myosin heavy-chain mutations Arg403Gln and Arg719Gln), hypotensive response during exercise stress testing, and nonsustained VT on Holter monitoring.[1,7,12,16,18–23] In addition, an LVOT gradient greater than 30 mm Hg has been associated with an increased risk of SCD, progression to heart failure, and morbidity related to arrhythmia including stroke.[24,25] However, incremental increase in the subaortic gradient above 30 mm Hg has not been demonstrated to impart any additional risk. It is uncommon that HCM patients suffer SCD without at least one of the aforementioned risk factors ($<3\%$).[16] It has been suggested that the etiology of SCD in this population is related to the development of complex ventricular tachyarrhythmia[7,26,27] often during mild-to-moderate physical exertion and with a circadian predilection for the early morning hours.[28]

Over the last 4 to 5 decades, the evolution of cardiovascular imaging techniques, both invasive and noninvasive, has helped us to understand its pathophysiology and selecting and guiding appropriate therapy. In this chapter, we discuss the existing imaging methodologies, with emphasis on current and emerging applications in HCM patients.

ECHOCARDIOGRAPHY

Cardiac morphology

Echocardiography is the most commonly utilized diagnostic imaging modality to gain insight into this complex disease. Along with LV dimensions and volumes, the pattern and extent of LVH can be determined. The most commonly observed pattern is that of asymmetric upper septal hypertrophy (Fig. 23.1).[29] However, mid-ventricular, apical (Fig. 23.2), or posterolateral hypertrophy can also occur. In addition, up to 5% of patients have concentric LVH. Maximal wall thickness is a simple and important measurement as it has been demonstrated to predict SCD in this population.[17] Because of its perceived importance in the literature, accurate measurement is imperative and care should be taken to avoid oblique transection of the septum by the ultrasound beam to exclude right ventricular myocardium on the right ventricular side. Also, the identification of the apical variant can be challenging. Quantification of LV mass should preferably be done using semiquantitative scores such as the Wigle[29] and the Maron and Spirito score.[30] More recently, real-time three-dimensional (3D) echocardiography and cardiac magnetic resonance (CMR) have been applied to determine LV mass (Figs.23.1 and 23.2).

Differential diagnosis

Because of clinical and familial implications, it is important to exclude other etiologies of LVH, such as hypertension and aortic stenosis. Although it is relatively easy to diagnose HCM in gene-positive patients or those with a positive family history, the diagnosis is difficult in patients with mild concentric LVH and hypertension or aortic stenosis. Recently, more severely reduced systolic compression (by strain Doppler echocardiography) along with asymmetric LVH readily identified biopsy-proven HCM patients from those with hypertension.[31]

Distinguishing HCM from athlete's heart is very important, given the high propensity to SCD in HCM patients engaging in competitive sports. The criteria for diagnosis of HCM in athletes include the presence of wall thickness >12 mm (11 mm in women) in the presence of a nondilated LV[32] in HCM, because HCM patients usually have normal or reduced LV dimensions and no cavity dilatation (>55 mm is common in athletes), except with disease progression and systolic dysfunction. Also, HCM patients have abnormal myocardial function as detected by tissue Doppler (TD) imaging.[33] In borderline cases, it is reasonable to recommend stopping exercise with repeat imaging, when one would expect regression of physiologic but not pathologic LVH.

Assessment of systolic function

Most HCM patients have hyperdynamic ejection fraction (EF), whereas a small subset might develop LV enlargement along with depressed EF. In HCM, a normal EF does not exclude contractile dysfunction, which can be detected by more sensitive techniques such as myocardial systolic velocities, strain rate, and strain.[31,33]

Assessment of diastolic function

In multiple cross-sectional studies, no close correlation was observed between Doppler filling patterns, extent of LVH, and invasive indexes of diastolic function,[34] with the exception of the atrial flow signal recorded from the pulmonary veins, which has a significant correlation with LV end-diastolic pressure.[35] However, TD imaging in combination with transmitral inflow can provide reasonably accurate predictions of filling pressures.[35] E/E_a ratio has been demonstrated to detect changes in filling pressures after alcohol-induced septal ablation[36,37] and cardiac surgery[37] and predicts exercise tolerance in adults[38] and children[39] with HCM. In addition, septal Ea is an independent predictor of death and ventricular dysrhythmia in children with HCM.[39] Left atrial volume reflects the LA hemodynamic burden from LV diastolic dysfunction, mitral regurgitation (MR), and atrial myopathy. A number of studies have now reported a significant association between LA dimensions and subsequent development of atrial fibrillation as well as adverse outcomes after myectomy.[40]

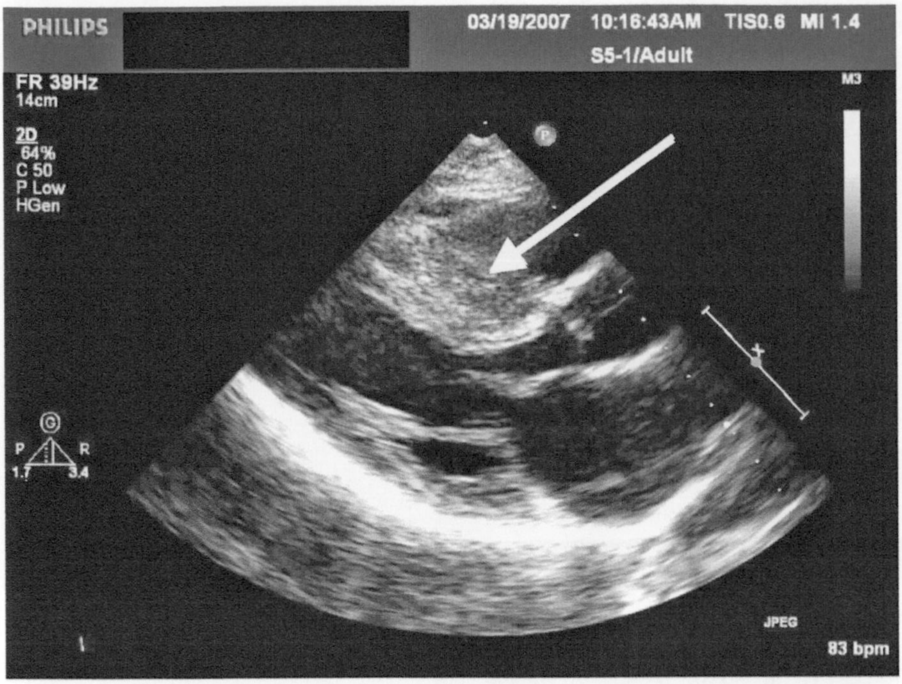

A

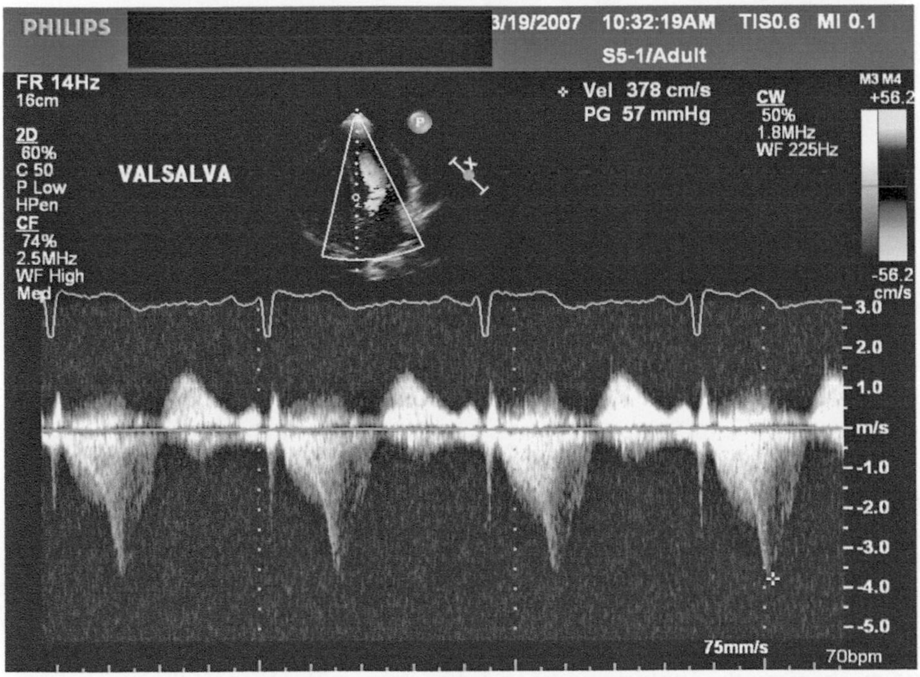

B

Figure 23.1 A 25-year-old male with palpitations and syncope. (**A**) Parasternal 2D echocardiographic view demonstrating severe upper septal hypertrophy (*arrow*). (**B**) Doppler envelope across the left ventricular outflow tract following Valsalva maneuver demonstrating a gradient of 4 m/sec. (**C**) Black-blood cardiac magnetic resonance image demonstrating severe septal hypertrophy (*arrow*). (**D**) short-axis delayed hyperenhancement magnetic resonance image demonstrating fibrosis (*arrows*) at right ventricular insertion points. Patient was diagnosed with classic form of hypertrophic obstructive cardiomyopathy. (*Continued*)

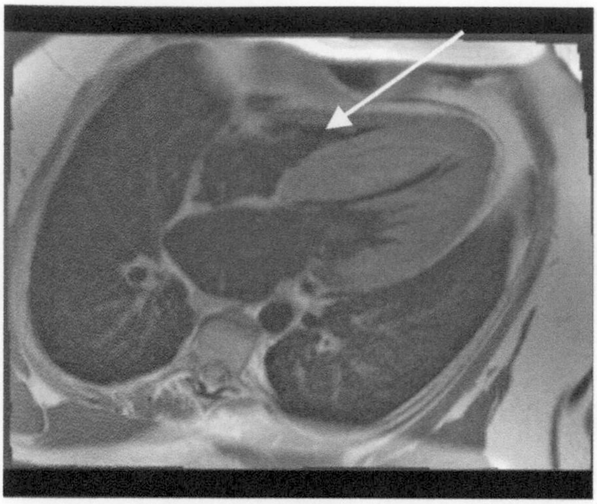

C

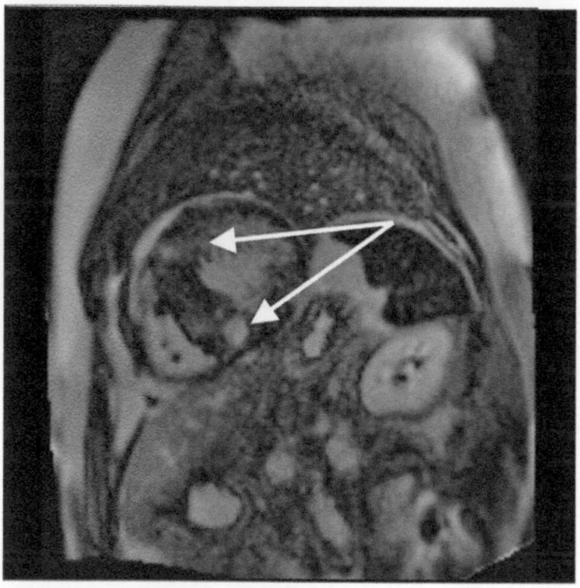

D

Figure 23.1 (*Continued*)

Dynamic LVOT obstruction

This is a unique feature of HCM, occurring at multiple levels in the same patient and can vary with time and physiologic states,[41] dependent on intravascular blood volume, afterload, and cardiac contractility. The exact location of the obstruction should be identified by careful mapping by pulse wave Doppler. Continuous wave Doppler is used o determine peak LVOT gradient with caution exercised to exclude the MR jet. Multiple theories have been attempted to explain this mechanism: the Venturi effect[29] and drag forces. The Venturi theory proposes that the earliest event is an increased ejection velocity, leading to an increase in kinetic energy. The increase in kinetic energy is accompanied by a decrease in potential energy and local pressure leading to the anterior motion of the mitral valve. This in turn leads to a gap between the anterior and posterior mitral leaflets through which MR occurs (i.e., "eject, obstruct, leak" sequence).[29] In contrast, the theory implicating drag forces[42] looks at anterior movement of the mitral valve because of drag forces, which act on the posterior surface of the valve and are proportional to the surface area of the leaflets exposed to these forces and systolic flow velocity.

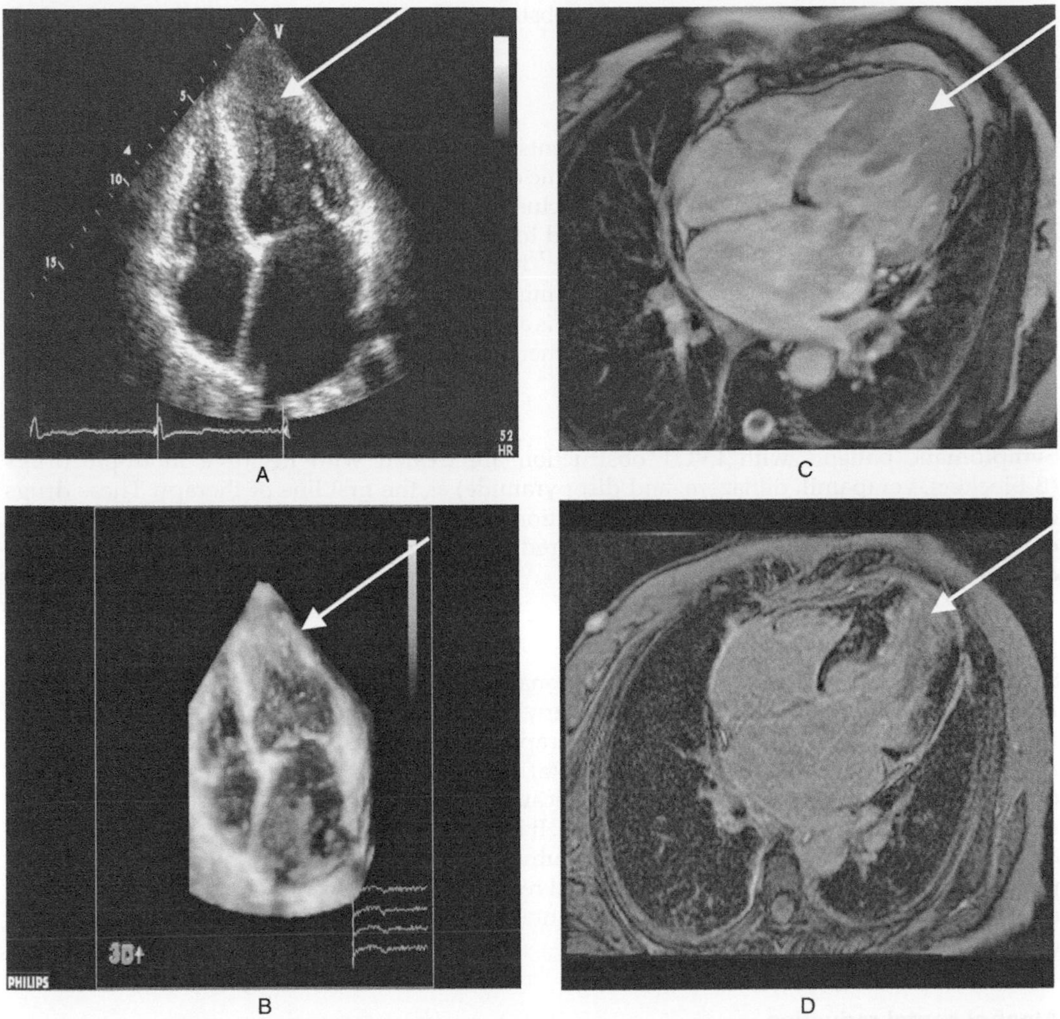

Figure 23.2 A 19-year-old college student with abnormal electrocardiogram identified on routine sports physical. (**A**) Four-chamber view on surface echocardiography demonstrating markedly thickened apex (*arrow*). (**B**) Three-dimensional echocardiogram demonstrating apical hypertrophy (*arrow*). (**C**) Cardiac magnetic resonance image (four-chamber cine image) confirming apical hypertrophy (*arrow*). (**D**) Four-chamber delayed hyperenhancement magnetic resonance image demonstrating significant fibrosis in the apex (*arrow*). Patient was diagnosed with apical (Yamaguchi) type-cardiomyopathy.

This mechanism is supported by the presence of SAM at a time when the LVOT velocity is not increased.[43] Irrespective of the underlying mechanism(s), LVOT obstruction is associated with worse clinical outcomes, including death and heart failure.[24]

Provocable LVOT obstruction

A number of methods can provoke obstruction in the echocardiography laboratory, including Valsalva maneuver, amyl nitrite, exercise, and dobutamine. It is relatively easy to acquire data during the strain phase of Valsalva in most patients, but when the gradient is <30 mm Hg, particularly in highly symptomatic patients, it is reasonable to proceed to other methods of provoking obstruction. For those able to exercise, exercise Doppler should be used,[44] because exercise is the modality that most closely simulates physiologic stress. For patients unable or unwilling to exercise, medical provocation is a viable alternative. Isoproterenol, because of its positive inotropic properties, has been used for decades in the catheterization laboratory, providing the rationale and precedent for dobutamine injection in the echocardiography laboratory. Importantly, treating provocable obstruction has resulted in significant clinical, exercise, and hemodynamic improvement.[45]

Mitral regurgitation

Mitral regurgitation can occur in HCM patients because of rheumatic heart disease or myxomatous degeneration. In patients with dynamic obstruction, MR jet is directed posterolaterally. The direction of the MR jet is an important clue for the underlying mechanism,[46] because an anteriorly/medially directed jet is not related to dynamic obstruction but is due to a primary leaflet pathology. Echocardiographic studies[47] have drawn attention to the reduced mobility and length of the posterior mitral leaflet leading to a shorter coaptation length and therefore a longer free segment of the anterior leaflet that is amenable to drag forces. MR related to dynamic obstruction is improved by septal reduction therapy.[48]

Guidance of treatment in HCM

Symptomatic patients with LVOT obstruction are treated with negative inotropic drugs (β-blockers, verapamil, diltiazem, and disopyramide) as the first line of therapy. These drugs decrease LVOT gradient by reducing acceleration rate of LV systolic flow and prolonging acceleration time relative to ejection time, thereby reducing the time available for the build up of the dynamic gradient.[49]

Evaluation for septal reduction therapy

Septal reduction is performed using intracoronary alcohol and surgical myectomy. For symptomatic patients, on maximally tolerated therapy, with dynamic obstruction at rest (>30 mm Hg) or provocation (>50 mm Hg), definitive therapy using surgical myectomy or alcohol septal ablation needs to be considered. Before septal reduction, it is important to identify the site of obstruction (mid or distal obstruction), because reduction of septal base thickness will not result in an improvement of distal obstruction. It is also important to identify coexisting valvular disease that warrants surgery, for example, subvalvular-fixed stenosis, anomalous insertion of papillary muscle, or a flail valve. When septal reduction therapy cannot be performed because of inadequate septal thickness, plication of anterior mitral leaflet or mitral valve replacement can be considered.

Alcohol septal reduction

During alcohol septal reduction therapy, procedural guidance with myocardial contrast echocardiography is important.[50] It is possible to identify the myocardial territory of septal perforator branches that arise from vessels other than the left anterior descending coronary artery. Contrast opacification of other LV/RV segments or papillary muscle precludes the injection of ethanol, which would result in infarction outside the culprit septal segments but not septal reduction. The reduction of LVOT gradient in the acute phase is related to the decrease in systolic thickening and excursion of septal base due to necrosis/ischemia-stunning as well as global decrease in LV systolic function.[48] Later on, LVOT widening, reduction in drag forces, and decrease in peak LV ejection acceleration rate account for the reduction in LVOT obstruction.[48]

Surgery

During surgery, transesophageal echocardiography is needed[51] to determine the adequacy of septal resection, because inadequate septal resection is an important cause of residual obstruction. Additional reasons for repeat surgery include mid-ventricular obstruction and anomalous papillary muscle insertion.[52] Both can be identified by echocardiography and surgical inspection of the LVOT. In contrast to alcohol septal reduction therapy, most of the reduction in LVOT gradient after surgery occurs acutely owing to widening of the LVOT, which is maintained at follow-up. Transesophageal echocardiography is also important in determining the adequacy of mitral valve repair in cases with MR due to primary leaflet pathology or with additional surgical procedures, such as valve plication/extension.

Preclinical diagnosis of HCM

Echocardiography is the most practical technique at the present time for HCM screening. It is considered in first-degree relatives and potentially in other family members of the index cases. Given the adolescent growth spurt, repeat imaging at yearly intervals is reasonable during this time period.[53] Repeat imaging is also considered for adults at longer time intervals of 5 years because of the possibility of later development of LVH.[53]

CARDIAC MAGNETIC RESONANCE

Because of persistent challenges in the noninvasive evaluation of HCM, better characterization of patients is likely to benefit from effective but expensive therapies (including implantable defibrillators). CMR has the incremental capacity to aid in a comprehensive assessment, over and above echocardiography. CMR has following advantages: ability to image in any plane, superb visualization of epicardial and endocardial borders, visualization of apex and inferior walls, no geometric assumptions in evaluating overall dimensions, mass, and function.

Assessment of cardiac morphology

CMR can measure LV dimensions, volumes, and EF with high reproducibility,[54] including patients with LVH. CMR, because of its 3D capabilities, can improve identification of atypical forms of HCM, including those involving the anterolateral free wall[55] and apical variant.[56] CMR might be a vital adjunct to echocardiography, when evaluating patients with anterolateral T-wave abnormalities and no obvious underlying etiology. In addition, given its accuracy, this technique might be useful for familial screening and genetic linkage studies. In summary, CMR is considered a Class I indication for patients with apical HCM (Fig. 23.2) and a Class II indication for other phenotypic variants of HCM (Fig. 23.1).[54] Also, recently, CMR has been utilized to further assess papillary muscle morphology in HCM patients.[57] A subset of patients with dynamic LVOT obstruction have normal LV thickness; and the only abnormality noted involves abnormal orientation of papillary muscles.[57] In such patients, an alteration in surgical technique, using a unique "papillary muscle realignment" procedure has been developed to relieve LVOT obstruction.[58]

Regional function

CMR studies have shown reduced circumferential shortening in hypertrophied segments with an inverse relation to local thickness and with most shortening occurring in early systole.[59,60] Longitudinal shortening is likewise reduced in the basal septum.[60] On a global basis, the number of hypokinetic segments is a strong independent predictor of LV mass, confirming the association of LVH with myocardial dysfunction.[61]

Flow mapping by CMR

In patients with LVOT obstruction, phase velocity flow mapping is useful to determine the peak velocity in a manner similar to TD by echocardiography.

Both in-plane and through-plane velocities can be assessed. The relation of the pressure gradient assessed by TTE and the CMR-derived planimetry of the LVOT has been recently studied in 37 patients with HCM and 14 healthy controls using standard sequences with 3D coverage of the LVOT. A cutoff value of 2.7 cm^2 appears to identify obstruction as defined by TTE with 100% accuracy. CMR planimetry at rest may therefore have an incremental role to flow mapping in HCM.[62] The amount of MR can be calculated either from the difference in LV and RV stroke volumes or by the difference in aortic output measured by phase velocity flow mapping and the LV stroke volume.

Detection of fibrosis

An important strength of CMR compared with other imaging modalities is the ability to determine myocardial tissue characteristics in vivo using the delayed hyperenhancement technique (Figs. 23.1D and 23.2D). In patients with HCM, the pattern of replacement fibrosis is distinct to that seen in coronary artery disease or patients with dilated cardiomyopathy. Typically, it is patchy, mid-wall, with multiple foci and most commonly found in regions of hypertrophy. Several patterns are seen with a diffuse transseptal or RV septal pattern at one end of the spectrum and a confluent pattern that may affect the interventricular junction or be multifocal at the other end. The mechanism for development of scarring may reflect microvascular ischemia. A study by Maron et al.[63] found areas of scarring correlated with areas of abnormal intramural coronary arteries, and suggested that it was ischemia that led to this scarring process. The pattern, distribution, and amount of fibrosis as determined in vivo seen in HCM patients correlates closely with histopathology in explanted hearts of patients undergoing cardiac transplantation.[64] Choudhury et al. demonstrated that myocardial replacement fibrosis was detectable in over 80% of asymptomatic HCM patients and correlated with wall thickness and inversely with regional function.[65] In a study of 68 HCM patients, with preserved LVEF, Kwon et al. demonstrated a strong association between LV thickness and degree of myocardial fibrosis.[66] In a prospective cohort of HCM patients with known troponin I mutations, 80% of patients with underlying LVH demonstrated late enhancement.[67] Teraoka et al. reported that myocardial fibrosis was observed in 75% of patients with HCM, typically small and patchy and mostly distributed in the interventricular septum.[68] The clinical significance of fibrosis is still uncertain. Current data indicate that particularly in younger patients (<40 years), its extent is associated with clinical markers of SCD (21% with >two risk factors). In patients over 40 years, it is associated with a greater likelihood for progressive disease. Kwon et al. demonstrated an association between degree of myocardial fibrosis and ventricular arrhythmia noted on Holter monitoring.[66] In the study by Teraoka et al., the extent and the presence of fibrosis correlated directly with the development of ventricular arrhythmias[68] and as such may help aid in risk stratification of HCM patients at higher risk of SCD and those that may need ICD implantation over and beyond current risk stratification algorithms.

Assessment of treatment

Following alcohol ablation, CMR is helpful to assess early and mid-term LV remodeling based on the size and location of the induced infarct. Work by van Dockum et al.[69] has shown that myocardial hypertrophy is, at least in part, afterload dependent and reversible and not caused exclusively by the genetic disorder. CMR has been used to study patients who underwent ethanol septal reduction therapy. With gradient echo sequences in 10 patients, a continuous and nonlinear improvement of the outflow tract area was noted during a 12-month period of follow-up, which correlated well with symptomatic improvement.[70]

Differential diagnosis

CMR has a similar utility as echocardiography in the differential diagnosis of HCM (e.g., hypertension, aortic stenosis, and athlete's heart). Indeed, CMR can be used if echocardiography is suboptimal or inconclusive. About 5% of patients with phenotypes of HCM will have Fabry's disease, which is an X-linked recessive glycolipid storage disease characterized by deficient α-galactosidase activity. Delayed hyperenhancement studies in these patients show a predilection for mid-wall fibrosis of the basal lateral wall unlike HCM. The pattern of hypertrophy is usually more concentric than in HCM.[64] Amyloidosis has a characteristic hyperenhancement pattern on delayed CMR images.[71]

CATHETERIZATION AND HEMODYNAMICS

Given the wealth of hemodynamic and anatomical data that can be derived noninvasively, cardiac catheterization is generally not required for the diagnosis of HCM. Catheterization is generally employed, however, if noninvasive imaging is of insufficient quality to quantify the degree or location of obstruction, to evaluate for coronary disease prior to a planned surgical therapy (i.e., myectomy or pacemaker), or if anginal symptoms are present in older patients that may be attributable to ischemia. The coronary arteries in patients with HCM are usually normal and typically of large caliber. Occasionally, compression of the left anterior descending artery may be observed during systole due to contraction of the hypertrophied ventricle resulting in a "sawfish" appearance.[72] Ventriculogram may demonstrate systolic cavity obliteration, varying degrees of MR, and occasionally the hypertrophied septum prolapsing into the LVOT.

Direct measurement and localization of the gradient is easily obtained by passing a multipurpose catheter into the apical portion of the left ventricle and slowly withdrawing while continuously monitoring the pressure waveform. Use of a wire via a guide-catheter often

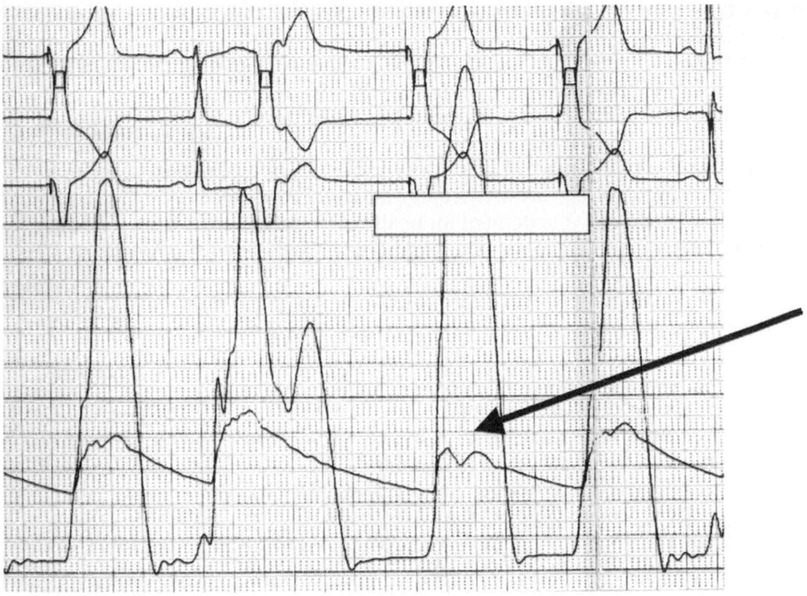

Figure 23.3 Brockenbrough–Braunwald–Morrow sign (postextrasystolic potentiation): simultaneous LV and aortic pressure tracing demonstrating the augmentation in LV pressure with concomitant decrement in the aortic systolic and pulse pressures as a result of increased LVOT obstruction following premature ventricular contraction (*arrow*).

results in increased control during the pullback and a more accurate determination of the level of obstruction. As opposed to what is observed in aortic stenosis, the gradient is reduced prior to crossing the aortic valve. This same technique can be performed using simultaneous aortic and LV pressure waveforms to allow side-by-side comparison. The gradient in HCM is characteristically labile and various pharmacologic and physiologic maneuvers similar to echocardiography may be employed to accentuate the obstruction while in the catheterization laboratory. Postextrasystolic potentiation refers to the augmentation of LV pressure with a concomitant decrement in the aortic systolic and pulse pressures as a result of increased LVOT obstruction in the cardiac cycle that follows a premature ventricular contraction (Fig. 23.3). Postextrasystolic increase in gradient between LV and aorta is seen even with aortic stenosis but unlike HCM, pulse pressure (stroke volume) does not decrease because in aortic stenosis, larger stroke volume of the postextrasystolic beat leads to higher gradient with no change in severity of obstruction.

CONCLUSIONS

In summary, imaging can provide important information that is needed for the appropriate evaluation of HCM patients. In addition to clinical risk factors, imaging studies can play a critical role in risk stratification for sudden cardiac death. However, their full potential remains to be realized.

REFERENCES

1. Maron BJ. Hypertrophic cardiomyopathy: A systematic review. JAMA 2002; 287:1308–1320.
2. Braunwald E, Lambrew CT, Rockoff SD, et al. Idiopathic hypertrophic subaortic stenosis. I. A description of the disease based upon an analysis of 64 patients. Circulation 1964; 30(Suppl. 4):3–119.
3. Maron BJ, Spirito P. Impact of patient selection biases on the perception of hypertrophic cardiomyopathy and its natural history. Am J Cardiol 1993; 72:970–972.
4. Maron BJ, Casey SA, Poliac LC, et al. Clinical course of hypertrophic cardiomyopathy in a regional United States cohort. JAMA 1999; 281:650–655.
5. Spirito P, Chiarella F, Carratino L, et al. Clinical course and prognosis of hypertrophic cardiomyopathy in an outpatient population. N Engl J Med 1989; 320:749–755.

6. Elliott P. Relation between the severity of left ventricular hypertrophy and prognosis in patients with hypertrophic cardiomyopathy. Lancet 2001; 357:420–424.
7. Maron BJ, McKenna WJ, Danielson GK, et al. ACC/ESC Expert Consensus Document on Hypertrophic Cardiomyopathy. J Am Coll Cardiol 2003; 42.
8. Ho CY, Seidman CE. A contemporary approach to hypertrophic cardiomyopathy. Circulation 2006; 113:e858–e862.
9. Maron BJ, Moller JH, Seidman CE, et al. Impact of laboratory molecular diagnosis on contemporary diagnostic criteria for genetically transmitted cardiovascular diseases: Hypertrophic cardiomyopathy, long-QT syndrome, and Marfan syndrome. A statement for healthcare professionals from the Councils on Clinical Cardiology, Cardiovascular Disease in the Young, and Basic Science, American Heart Association. Circulation 1998; 98:1460–1471.
10. Richard P, Charron P, Carrier L, et al. Hypertrophic cardiomyopathy: Distribution of disease genes, spectrum of mutations, and implications for a molecular diagnosis strategy. Circulation 2003; 107:2227–2232.
11. Maron BJ. Hypertrophic cardiomyopathy. Lancet 1997; 350:127–133.
12. Spirito P. The management of hypertrophic cardiomyopathy. N J Med 1997; 336:775–785.
13. Maron BJ. Clinical profile of stroke in 900 patients with hypertrophic cardiomyopathy. J Am Coll Cardiol 2002; 39:301–307.
14. Elliott P, McKenna WJ. Hypertrophic cardiomyopathy. Lancet 2004; 363:1881–1891.
15. Spirito P, Autore C. Management of hypertrophic cardiomyopathy. BMJ 2006; 332:1251–1255.
16. Elliott PM, Poloniecki J, Dickie S, et al. Sudden death in hypertrophic cardiomyopathy: Identification of high risk patients. J Am Coll Cardiol 2000; 36:2212–2218.
17. Spirito P, Bellone P, Harris KM, et al. Magnitude of left ventricular hypertrophy and risk of sudden death in hypertrophic cardiomyopathy. N Engl J Med 2000; 342:1778–1785.
18. Monserrat L, Elliott PM, Gimeno JR, et al. Non-sustained ventricular tachycardia in hypertrophic cardiomyopathy: An independent marker of sudden death risk in young patients. J Am Coll Cardiol 2003; 42:873–879.
19. Yoshida N, Ikeda H, Wada T, et al. Exercise-induced abnormal blood pressure responses are related to subendocardial ischemia in hypertrophic cardiomyopathy. J Am Coll Cardiol 1998; 32:1938–1942.
20. Olivotto I, Cecchi F, Casey SA, et al. Impact of atrial fibrillation on the clinical course of hypertrophic cardiomyopathy. Circulation 2001; 104:2517–2524.
21. Cecchi F, Olivotto I, Montereggi A, et al. Prognostic value of non-sustained ventricular tachycardia and the potential role of amiodarone treatment in hypertrophic cardiomyopathy: Assessment in an unselected non-referral based patient population. Heart 1998; 79:331–336.
22. Moolman JC, Corfield VA, Posen B, et al. Sudden death due to troponin T mutations. J Am Coll Cardiol 1997; 29:549–555.
23. Watkins H. Sudden death in hypertrophic cardiomyopathy. N Engl J Med 2000; 342:422–424.
24. Maron MS, Olivotto I, Betocchi S, et al. Effect of left ventricular outflow tract obstruction on clinical outcome in hypertrophic cardiomyopathy. N Engl J Med 2003; 348:295–303.
25. Kofflard MJ, Ten Cate FJ, van der Lee C, et al. Hypertrophic cardiomyopathy in a large community-based population: Clinical outcome and identification of risk factors for sudden cardiac death and clinical deterioration. J Am Coll Cardiol 2003; 41:987–993.
26. Elliott PM, Sharma S, Varnava A, et al. Survival after cardiac arrest or sustained ventricular tachycardia in patients with hypertrophic cardiomyopathy. J Am Coll Cardiol 1999; 33:1596–1601.
27. Maron BJ, Shen WK, Link MS, et al. Efficacy of implantable cardioverter-defibrillators for the prevention of sudden death in patients with hypertrophic cardiomyopathy. N Engl J Med 2000; 342:365–373.
28. Maron BJ, Kogan J, Proschan MA, et al. Circadian variability in the occurrence of sudden cardiac death in patients with hypertrophic cardiomyopathy. J Am Coll Cardiol 1994; 23:1405–1409.
29. Wigle ED, Sasson Z, Henderson MA, et al. Hypertrophic cardiomyopathy. The importance of the site and the extent of hypertrophy. A review. Prog Cardiovasc Dis 1985; 28:1–83.
30. Spirito P, Maron BJ. Relation between extent of left ventricular hypertrophy and occurrence of sudden cardiac death in hypertrophic cardiomyopathy. J Am Coll Cardiol 1990; 15:1521–1526.
31. Kato TS, Noda A, Izawa H, et al. Discrimination of nonobstructive hypertrophic cardiomyopathy from hypertensive left ventricular hypertrophy on the basis of strain rate imaging by tissue Doppler ultrasonography. Circulation 2004; 110:3808–3814.
32. Sharma S, Maron BJ, Whyte G, et al. Physiologic limits of left ventricular hypertrophy in elite junior athletes: Relevance to differential diagnosis of athlete's heart and hypertrophic cardiomyopathy. J Am Coll Cardiol 2002; 40:1431–1436.
33. Rajiv C, Vinereanu D, Fraser AG. Tissue Doppler imaging for the evaluation of patients with hypertrophic cardiomyopathy. Curr Opin Cardiol 2004; 19:430–436.

34. Nishimura RA, Appleton CP, Redfield MM, et al. Noninvasive Doppler echocardiographic evaluation of left ventricular filling pressures in patients with cardiomyopathies: A simultaneous Doppler echocardiographic and cardiac catheterization study. J Am Coll Cardiol 1996; 28:1226–1233.
35. Nagueh SF, Lakkis NM, Middleton KJ, et al. Doppler estimation of left ventricular filling pressures in patients with hypertrophic cardiomyopathy. Circulation 1999; 99:254–261.
36. Nagueh SF, Lakkis NM, Middleton KJ, et al. Changes in left ventricular filling and left atrial function six months after nonsurgical septal reduction therapy for hypertrophic obstructive cardiomyopathy. J Am Coll Cardiol 1999; 34:1123–1128.
37. Sitges M, Shiota T, Lever HM, et al. Comparison of left ventricular diastolic function in obstructive hypertrophic cardiomyopathy in patients undergoing percutaneous septal alcohol ablation versus surgical myotomy/myectomy. Am J Cardiol 2003; 91:817–821.
38. Matsumura Y, Elliott PM, Virdee MS, et al. Left ventricular diastolic function assessed using Doppler tissue imaging in patients with hypertrophic cardiomyopathy: Relation to symptoms and exercise capacity. Heart 2002; 87:247–251.
39. McMahon CJ, Nagueh SF, Pignatelli RH, et al, Characterization of left ventricular diastolic function by tissue Doppler imaging and clinical status in children with hypertrophic cardiomyopathy. Circulation 2004; 109:1756–1762.
40. Woo A, Williams WG, Choi R, et al. Clinical and echocardiographic determinants of long-term survival after surgical myectomy in obstructive hypertrophic cardiomyopathy. Circulation 2005; 111:2033–2041.
41. Maron BJ, McKenna WJ, Danielson GK, et al. American College of Cardiology/European Society of Cardiology Clinical Expert Consensus Document on Hypertrophic Cardiomyopathy. A report of the American College of Cardiology Foundation Task Force on Clinical Expert Consensus Documents and the European Society of Cardiology Committee for Practice Guidelines. Eur Heart J 2003; 24:1965–1991.
42. Sherrid MV, Chu CK, Delia E, et al. An echocardiographic study of the fluid mechanics of obstruction in hypertrophic cardiomyopathy. J Am Coll Cardiol 1993; 22:816–825.
43. Sherrid MV, Gunsburg DZ, Moldenhauer S, et al. Systolic anterior motion begins at low left ventricular outflow tract velocity in obstructive hypertrophic cardiomyopathy. J Am Coll Cardiol 2000; 36:1344–1354.
44. Maron BJ, McKenna WJ, Danielson GK, et al. American College of Cardiology/European Society of Cardiology clinical expert consensus document on hypertrophic cardiomyopathy. A report of the American College of Cardiology Foundation Task Force on Clinical Expert Consensus Documents and the European Society of Cardiology Committee for Practice Guidelines. J Am Coll Cardiol 2003; 42:1687–1713.
45. Lakkis N, Plana JC, Nagueh S, et al. Efficacy of nonsurgical septal reduction therapy in symptomatic patients with obstructive hypertrophic cardiomyopathy and provocable gradients. Am J Cardiol 2001; 88:583–586.
46. Yu EH, Omran AS, Wigle ED, et al. Mitral regurgitation in hypertrophic obstructive cardiomyopathy: Relationship to obstruction and relief with myectomy. J Am Coll Cardiol 2000; 36:2219–2225.
47. Schwammenthal E, Nakatani S, He S, et al. Mechanism of mitral regurgitation in hypertrophic cardiomyopathy: Mismatch of posterior to anterior leaflet length and mobility. Circulation 1998; 98:856–865.
48. Flores-Ramirez R, Lakkis NM, Middleton KJ, et al. Echocardiographic insights into the mechanisms of relief of left ventricular outflow tract obstruction after nonsurgical septal reduction therapy in patients with hypertrophic obstructive cardiomyopathy. J Am Coll Cardiol 2001; 37:208–214.
49. Sherrid MV, Pearle G, Gunsburg DZ. Mechanism of benefit of negative inotropes in obstructive hypertrophic cardiomyopathy. Circulation 1998; 97:41–47.
50. Nagueh SF, Lakkis NM, He ZX, et al. Role of myocardial contrast echocardiography during nonsurgical septal reduction therapy for hypertrophic obstructive cardiomyopathy. J Am Coll Cardiol 1998; 32:225–229.
51. Ommen SR, Park SH, Click RL, et al. Impact of intraoperative transesophageal echocardiography in the surgical management of hypertrophic cardiomyopathy. Am J Cardiol 2002; 90:1022–1024.
52. Minakata K, Dearani JA, Schaff HV, et al. Mechanisms for recurrent left ventricular outflow tract obstruction after septal myectomy for obstructive hypertrophic cardiomyopathy. Ann Thorac Surg 2005; 80:851–856.
53. Maron BJ, Seidman JG, Seidman CE. Proposal for contemporary screening strategies in families with hypertrophic cardiomyopathy. J Am Coll Cardiol 2004; 44:2125–2132.
54. Pennell DJ, Sechtem UP, Higgins CB, et al. Clinical indications for cardiovascular magnetic resonance (CMR): Consensus panel report. J Cardiovasc Magn Reson 2004; 6:727–765.
55. Rickers C, Wilke NM, Jerosch-Herold M, et al. Utility of cardiac magnetic resonance imaging in the diagnosis of hypertrophic cardiomyopathy. Circulation 2005; 112:855–861.

56. Moon JC, Fisher NG, McKenna WJ, et al. Detection of apical hypertrophic cardiomyopathy by cardiovascular magnetic resonance in patients with non-diagnostic echocardiography. Heart 2004; 90:645–649.
57. Kwon D, Setser R, Thamilarasan M, et al. Abnormal papillary muscle morphology is independently associated with increased left ventricular outflow tract obstruction in hypertrophic cardiomyopathy. Heart 2007.
58. Bryant R III, Smedira NG. Papillary muscle realignment for symptomatic left ventricular outflow tract obstruction. J Thorac Cardiovasc Surg 2008; 135:223–224.
59. Dong SJ, MacGregor JH, Crawley AP, et al. Left ventricular wall thickness and regional systolic function in patients with hypertrophic cardiomyopathy. A three-dimensional tagged magnetic resonance imaging study. Circulation 1994; 90:1200–1209.
60. Kramer CM, Reichek N, Ferrari VA, et al. Regional heterogeneity of function in hypertrophic cardiomyopathy. Circulation 1994; 90:186–194.
61. Sipola P, Lauerma K, Jaaskelainen P, et al. Cine MR imaging of myocardial contractile impairment in patients with hypertrophic cardiomyopathy attributable to Asp175Asn mutation in the alpha-tropomyosin gene. Radiology 2005; 236:815–824.
62. Schulz-Menger J, Abdel-Aty H, Busjahn A, et al. Left ventricular outflow tract planimetry by cardiovascular magnetic resonance differentiates obstructive from non-obstructive hypertrophic cardiomyopathy. J Cardiovasc Magn Reson 2006; 8:741–746.
63. Maron BJ, Wolfson JK, Epstein SE, et al. Intramural ("small vessel") coronary artery disease in hypertrophic cardiomyopathy. J Am Coll Cardiol 1986; 8:545–557.
64. Moon JC, Sheppard M, Reed E, et al. The histological basis of late gadolinium enhancement cardiovascular magnetic resonance in a patient with Anderson-Fabry disease. J Cardiovasc Magn Reson 2006; 8:479–482.
65. Choudhury L, Mahrholdt H, Wagner A, et al. Myocardial scarring in asymptomatic or mildly symptomatic patients with hypertrophic cardiomyopathy. J Am Coll Cardiol 2002; 40:2156–2164.
66. Kwon DH, Setser RM, Popovic ZB, et al. Association of myocardial fibrosis, electrocardiography and ventricular tachyarrhythmia in hypertrophic cardiomyopathy: A delayed contrast enhanced MRI study. Int J Cardiovasc Imaging 2008.
67. Moon JC, Mogensen J, Elliott PM, et al. Myocardial late gadolinium enhancement cardiovascular magnetic resonance in hypertrophic cardiomyopathy caused by mutations in troponin I. Heart 2005; 91:1036–1040.
68. Teraoka K, Hirano M, Ookubo H, et al. Delayed contrast enhancement of MRI in hypertrophic cardiomyopathy. Magn Reson Imaging 2004; 22:155–161.
69. van Dockum WG, Beek AM, ten Cate FJ, et al. Early onset and progression of left ventricular remodeling after alcohol septal ablation in hypertrophic obstructive cardiomyopathy. Circulation 2005; 111:2503–2508.
70. Schulz-Menger J, Strohm O, Waigand J, et al. The value of magnetic resonance imaging of the left ventricular outflow tract in patients with hypertrophic obstructive cardiomyopathy after septal artery embolization. Circulation 2000; 101:1764–1766.
71. Maceira AM, Joshi J, Prasad SK, et al. Cardiovascular magnetic resonance in cardiac amyloidosis. Circulation 2005; 111:186–193.
72. Brugada P. "Sawfish" systolic narrowing of the left anterior descending artery: An angiographic sign of hypertrophic cardiomyopathy. Circulation 1982; 66:800–803.

24 The role of the cath lab in patients with advanced heart failure and cardiac transplantation

Anuj Gupta and LeRoy E. Rabbani

Patients with advanced heart failure (HF) often require extensive evaluation in the cardiac catheterization laboratory. The rationale and method of the most common procedures performed on these complex patients is described below.

Patients presenting with new onset HF associated with left ventricular systolic dysfunction of unknown etiology require evaluation of the extent of coronary artery disease (CAD), as CAD is the most common cause of cardiomyopathy in the United States. The ACC/AHA guidelines give coronary angiography a Class 1 indication for patients in HF with either angina or regional wall motion abnormalities, with or without evidence of reversible ischemia, and a Class 2a indication in patients with systolic dysfunction of unexplained etiology despite noninvasive testing.[1] Right-heart catheterization is also routinely performed in these patients to evaluate volume status and determine whether elevated filling pressures explains dyspnea. In unusual circumstances, where amyloidosis, hemochromatosis, or giant cell myocarditis is suspected as the cause of HF, endomyocardial biopsy may be performed (more below).

In patients with HF in whom significant obstructive coronary disease is discovered, percutaneous coronary intervention (PCI) has been offered as a means of relieving ischemia, improving myocardial perfusion, and potentially improving myocardial function. High-risk PCI (especially those procedures involving left main or proximal left anterior descending artery lesions) may be performed with intra-aortic balloon pump (IABP) support, both to improve coronary perfusion pressures and decrease afterload.

In patients with HF in whom PCI is being considered on the last remaining vessel (e.g., proximal left anterior descending artery which feeds collaterals to occluded circumflex and right coronary arteries), percutaneous left ventricular assist devices, such as the TandemHeart® or Impella® devices, may be used. The TandemHeart works via a 21F cannula advanced through the venous system over a guidewire across the intra-atrial septum, and therefore requires an operator experienced in transeptal puncture. This cannula withdraws oxygenated blood and introduces it into the femoral artery via a 15F arterial sheath. The TandemHeart device provides approximately 4–5 L/min of cardiac output and may generally be left in for 2 to 3 days.[2] The Impella device is a 12F transaortic valve microaxial flow catheter that propels blood across the valve and provides a cardiac output of approximately 2.5 L/min, and is maintained for short periods of time, generally less than 24 hours. Protect 1 is a Phase 1 feasibility trial evaluating the device in high-risk PCI, while Protect 2 is a planned Phase 2 trial comparing the Impella device to IABP.

A special situation is that of the patients with low cardiac output HF and aortic stenosis present on echocardiography or cardiac catheterization. The low cardiac output may prevent adequate opening of the sclerotic valve and appear as aortic stenosis. Right-heart catheterization is performed with infusion of dobutamine, usually starting at 5 μg/kg/min, increasing to 10 μg/kg/min with subsequent stepwise increases of 10 μg/kg/min, with a maximum dose of 40 μg/kg/min.[3] If the heart rate does not respond, atropine 0.6 mg may be given. Generally, dobutamine infusion is completed when the heart rate reaches about 110 beats per minute. Patients are considered to have fixed aortic stenosis if they have a mean gradient at rest or at peak dobutamine infusion of 30 mm Hg or greater, or an aortic valve area that remains below 1.2 cm^2.

For patients with HF and systolic dysfunction being considered for heart transplantation, elevated irreversible pulmonary vascular resistance is a predictor of early mortality after heart transplantation, as the donor right ventricle rapidly fails against increased pulmonary vascular resistance (PVR) of the recipient.[4] Right-heart catheterization with vasodilators, particularly with nitroprusside, has been shown to predict which patients with elevated PVR will do well post–heart transplantation.[5] Typically, right-heart catheter placement and measurement of pulmonary artery pressure, pulmonary capillary wedge pressure, pulmonary artery oxygen saturations, and cardiac outputs are followed by infusion of nitroprusside at 10 μg/min, with a stepwise increase in the infusion dose by 10 μg/min every 3 minutes. The infusion continues until hypotension is reached (generally to systolic pressures in the low 80's are tolerated), or PVR is reduced to below 2 Woods units.

An alternative test for reversibility of PVR is a single bolus infusion of milrinone given at 50 μg/kg over 10 minutes, followed by evaluation of hemodynamics.[6] Milrinone causes fewer episodes of hypotension and reduces PVR in all patients. Although outcome data is directly lacking, patients whose PVR reduces to below 2 Woods units continue to candidates for heart transplantation. Patients whose CO increases or wedge pressure decreases by 20% may be considered for continuous home infusion of milrinone. Patients who meet these criteria are eligible for Medicare reimbursement.

Inhaled nitric oxide at a rate of 40–80 ppm provides another means of demonstrating reversible PVR without causing significant systemic hypotension and is able to lower PVR to a greater extent than the maximally tolerated dose of nitroprusside.[7] It is generally reserved for patients with elevated pulmonary pressures but normal left-sided filling pressures. Although some labs titrate the INO in a stepwise progression, initiating INO at 80 ppm works safely. Responsiveness to INO may predict whether patients would benefit from oral sildenafil.[8] A 20% reduction of pulmonary artery pressures with oxygen is generally considered a reasonable indication for 24-hour home oxygen.

After transplantation, rejection, along with infection, causes a majority of deaths in the first year. Subsequently, most centers have aggressive early biopsy schedules, often occurring weekly in the first month, twice monthly in the second and third months, monthly for months 4 through 6, and bimonthly for the remainder of the first year. The right internal jugular vein remains the preferred access site, followed by femoral vein access site. Subclavian vein access is infrequent.

For the right internal jugular vein, the bioptome is inserted through an 8.5F sheath with the right hand, while the left hand controls the finger controls. The bioptome is oriented so that the operator's left thumb is pointed up and is to the left of the finger controls. As the bioptome is advanced under fluoroscopy, the left hand rotates roughly 90° to 120° counterclockwise, so that the bioptome goes through the tricuspid apparatus smoothly (the jaws of the bioptome are kept closed). As the bioptome reaches the apex of the right ventricle, the bioptome is further rotated 20° to 30° counterclockwise, to point to the posterior septum. Ventricular premature contractions (VPCs) indicate that the bioptome is in contact with the myocardium. At this time, the bioptome is withdrawn approximately 2 to 3 mm, the jaws are opened, the bioptome is advanced 2 to 3 mm till VPCs are again seen, and the jaws are closed and the bioptome promptly withdrawn. Rate of advancement too large may increase the risk of perforation and should be avoided. Generally, four samples are taken for histology, with 1 to 2 further samples taken for immunohistochemistry, as necessary.

Pitfalls include a donor/recipient anastamosis that may be irregular or narrow, preventing insertion of the bioptome. The short 8.5F sheath should be carefully exchanged over a wire using fluoroscopy to a long 8.5F sheath, with the tip of the sheath located at the junction of the SVC and the right atrium. This will bypass the restriction caused by the anastamosis. Another frequent occurrence is difficulty in having the bioptome cross the tricuspid valve; often, reshaping the bioptome with a lesser or greater curve will allow for the proper angulation. Buckling of the bioptome jaws, generally in the right atrium, is an indicator of being against a wall or the tricuspid apparatus; unlike with a right-heart catheter, the bioptome should be withdrawn and advanced where there is no resistance.

Generally, femoral vein approaches are reserved for patients with thrombosis of the jugular veins, or who are undergoing "annual" transplant evaluations (see below). Femoral artery access requires somewhat greater maneuvering. One set of equipment includes the St. Jude Fastcath sheath and the Cordis bioptome. The St. Jude sheath with dilator is advanced over a wire and maneuvered with wire across the tricuspid valve. Alternatively, the dilator is replaced with a

7F monitoring right-heart catheter, so that the tricuspid valve is crossed with a balloon-tipped catheter. The sheath is situated in a quiet place in the distal RV apex and the posterior orientation of the sheath is confirmed in the left anterior oblique (LAO) angle. The dilator (or right-heart catheter) is removed with the wire, and the biopsy is performed as described above.

In a prospective review of complications of endomyocardial biopsy in 464 cardiomyopathy patients undergoing 546 procedures, the incidence of access site complications was 2.7% of the procedures, but were not associated with adverse outcomes, while biopsy-related complications (arrhythmia and perforation) occurred 3.3% of the procedures. Perforations occurred 1% of the time and was associated with one death. The newly transplanted heart often has the thinnest myocardium with the least amount of fibrosis at the RV distal septum, and is therefore considered to be the time of greatest risk for perforation. Newer, noninvasive means to detect cellular rejection are in development,[10] and hopefully will add to the arsenal of tools for the transplant cardiologist to manage heart transplant patients.

Recommendations to reduce the risk of perforation from either jugular or femoral venous approach include posterior rotation of the bioptome towards the ventricular septum, the use of the LAO projection to confirm the posterior direction of the bioptome catheter, and minimal advancement of the bioptome after VPCs are induced. After the biopsy specimens are obtained, fluoroscopic visualization of the heart border or right-heart catheterization may be performed to detect either pericardial fluid or equalization of diastolic pressures. Suspicion of perforation, regardless of tamponade, should lead to immediate infusion of fluids and placement of a pericardial drain.

Another major cause of morbidity and mortality related to transplant heart disease is transplant allograft vasculopathy (TAV). This diffuse disease of the intima of the coronary arteries is caused by immune-mediated mechanisms (Fig 24.1). In a study of 143 transplanted patients who underwent surveillance coronary angiography and intravascular ultrasound (IVUS), 6-year survival was significantly diminished in those patients who had rapidly progressive transplant vasculopathy detected on IVUS at 1 year.[11] As the donor heart is denervated, the recipient often will be asymptomatic. Because of its role as a leading cause of mortality in heart transplant patients who have survived their first year, screening with annual or biannual angiography (with concomitant right-heart catheterization and biopsy) in patients with normal renal function is common in transplant centers. On a biannual schedule, the alternate year is replaced with noninvasive imaging, particularly dobutamine stress echo. Patients with symptoms of HF, new evidence of graft dysfunction not explained by rejection, or other evidence of myocardial ischemia alter this schedule as necessary.

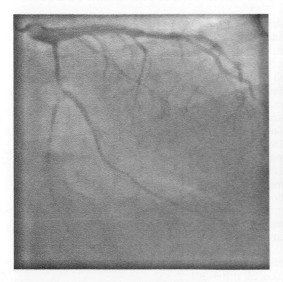

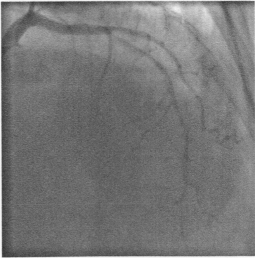

Figure 24.1 Coronary angiograms from a patient with severe transplant allograft vasculopathy marked by diffuse narrowing of the coronary arteries as well as pruning and beading of the tertiary branches.

During annual evaluation, screening right-heart catheterization, endomyocardial biopsy, and coronary angiography are performed. Left ventriculography can often be avoided with other noninvasive measurements of LV systolic function, such as multiple gated acquisition scan (MUGA) or echocardiography. Angiography should be performed after nitroglycerin 100 to 200 μg is administered intracoronary to reduce catheter-induced vasospasm of the coronary arteries, which transplant patients are particularly apt to experience. Angiographically, TAV generally manifests itself as diffuse narrowing of the coronary arteries, with pruning of the tertiary and quaternary branches of the arterial tree. Occasionally, it may manifest as a discrete stenosis. Importantly, discrete stenosis provides a visible indication of severe diffuse TAV in the rest of the coronary arterial tree and should be treated with aggressive medical therapy.

Discrete stenoses caused by TAV have been treated with balloon angioplasty,[12] bare metal stents,[13,14] and drug-eluting stents.[15,16] These data demonstrate reduction in restenosis with stents. Whether PCI in TAV improves long-term outcomes or provides only palliation remains unclear and awaits further study.

REFERENCES

1. Scanlon PJ, Faxon DP, Audet AM, et al. ACC/AHA guidelines for coronary angiography: A report of the American College of Cardiology/American Heart Association Task Force on Practice Guidelines (Committee on Coronary Angiography). J Am Coll Cardiol 1999; 33:1756–1824.
2. Burkhoff D, Cohen H, Brunckhorst C, et al. TandemHeart Investigators Group. A randomized multicenter clinical study to evaluate the safety and efficacy of the TandemHeart percutaneous ventricular assist device versus conventional therapy with intraaortic balloon pumping for treatment of cardiogenic shock. Am Heart J 2006; 152(3):469e1–469e8.
3. Nishimura RA, Grantham JA, Connolly HM, et al. Low-output, low-gradient aortic stenosis in patients with depressed left ventricular systolic function: The clinical utility of the dobutamine challenge in the catheterization laboratory. Circulation 2002; 106(7):809–813.
4. Costard-Jäckle A, Hill I, Schroeder JS, et al. The influence of preoperative patient characteristics on early and late survival following cardiac transplantation. Circulation 1991; 84(5 Suppl.):III329–III337.
5. Costard-Jäckle A, Fowler MB. Influence of preoperative pulmonary artery pressure on mortality after heart transplantation: Testing of potential reversibility of pulmonary hypertension with nitroprusside is useful in defining a high risk group. J Am Coll Cardiol 1992; 19(1):48–54.
6. Givertz MM, Hare JM, Loh E, et al. Effect of bolus milrinone on hemodynamic variables and pulmonary vascular resistance in patients with severe left ventricular dysfunction: A rapid test for reversibility of pulmonary hypertension. J Am Coll Cardiol 1996; 28(7):1775–1880.
7. Semigran MJ, Cockrill BA, Kacmarek R, et al. Hemodynamic effects of inhaled nitric oxide in heart failure. J Am Coll Cardiol 1994; 24(4):982–988.
8. Ghofrani HA, Wiedemann R, Rose F, et al. Sildenafil for treatment of lung fibrosis and pulmonary hypertension: A randomised controlled trial. Lancet 2002; 360(9337):895–900.
9. Deckers JW, Hare JM, Baughman KL. Complications of transvenous right ventricular endomyocardial biopsy in adult patients with cardiomyopathy: A seven-year survey of 546 consecutive diagnostic procedures in a tertiary referral center. J Am Coll Cardiol 1992; 19:43–47.
10. Deng MC, Eisen HJ, Mehra MR, et al. CARGO Investigators. Noninvasive discrimination of rejection in cardiac allograft recipients using gene expression profiling. Am J Transplant 2006; 6(1):150–160.
11. Tuzcu EM, Kapadia SR, Sachar R, et al. Intravascular ultrasound evidence of angiographically silent progression in coronary atherosclerosis predicts long-term morbidity and mortality after cardiac transplantation. J Am Coll Cardiol 2005; 45(9):1538–1542.
12. Halle AA, Disciascio G, Massin EK, et al. Coronary angioplasty, atherectomy and bypass surgery in cardiac transplant recipients. JACC 1995; 26(1):120–128.
13. McKay M, Pinney S, Gorwara S, et al. Anti-human leukocyte antigen antibodies are associated with restenosis after percutaneous coronary intervention for cardiac allograft vasculopathy. Transplantation 2005; 79(11):1581–1587.
14. Jonas M, Fang JC, Wang JC, et al. In-stent restenosis and remote coronary lesion progression are coupled in cardiac transplant vasculopathy but not in native coronary artery disease. J Am Coll Cardiol 2006; 48(3):453–461.
15. Bader FM, Kfoury AG, Gilbert EM, et al. Percutaneous coronary interventions with stents in cardiac transplant recipients. J Heart Lung Transplant 2006; 25(3):298–301.
16. Tanaka K, Li H, Curran PJ, et al. Usefulness and safety of percutaneous coronary interventions for cardiac transplant vasculopathy. Am J Cardiol 2006; 97(8):1192–1197.

25 Evaluation of common congenital heart defects in the adult

Christian Spies and Ziyad M. Hijazi

INTRODUCTION

The field of adult congenital heart disease

Congenital heart disease (CHD) occurs in approximately 5 to 10 per 1000 live births.[1] Over the past 50 years, improved medical and surgical therapies for children with congenital heart conditions have led to a growing population of adult patients with underlying CHD. The majority of patients, even those with complex cyanotic heart lesions, now survive into adulthood. It is estimated that there are about 800,000 to 1,200,000 adult patients in the United States with underlying CHD.[2,3] There are essentially three types of patients with adult CHD that the practicing cardiologist may have to face: (A) the patient with previously undiagnosed CHD. An example of this is a new patient that present with secundum atrial septal defect (ASD). (B) Patients may have prior recognized CHD in childhood, which did not require intervention, such as the patient with an uncomplicated, restrictive ventricular septal defect (VSD). (C) Commonly the most complex patients are those with prior surgical correction or palliation of underlying CHD.

Advances in noninvasive imaging including magnetic resonance imaging, echocardiography, and computed tomography have reduced the need for diagnostic cardiac catheterization procedures dramatically. Most infants and children with many forms of CHD commonly get operated based on these noninvasive imaging modalities. Invasive catheterization is nowadays usually performed to obtain data that is not readily available using noninvasive imaging or when a therapeutic intervention is planned in the same setting. The same holds partially true in the adult population with CHD. Hence, several maneuvers described later in this chapter are not necessarily needed in a purely diagnostic procedure to evaluate the defects appropriately, but rather commonly take place when a therapeutic intervention is performed. An example for this is a patent ductus arteriosus (PDA) or VSD, which can be sufficiently diagnosed with a shunt run, basic hemodynamic information, and an angiography; crossing the defect with a catheter or guidewire is only needed if one is planning to close those defects during the catheterization procedure or if one wants to evaluate the impact of possible closure of a shunt lesion on the pulmonary vasculature by temporary balloon occlusion of the defect.

In the real world, the vast majority of patients have a firm diagnosis following a noninvasive imaging study, most frequently transthoracic or transesophageal echocardiography. The patient is then taken to the catheterization laboratory with the intention to treat the underlying abnormality, with the diagnostic catheterization being part of the initial assessment in the catheterization site.

The basics of shunt calculation

Apart from the hemodynamic assessment with a right-heart catheterization and angiography, evaluation for the presence of a left-to-right shunt in a patient with suspected or known adult CHD is a basic component of every diagnostic catheterization procedure. Several basic principles should be observed when such a "shunt run" is performed. Obviously, the patient who is undergoing a diagnostic catheterization should be stable and off any supplemental oxygen. Ideally, blood samples should be obtained as quickly as possible to avoid any change in hemodynamics, because even the cardiac output itself impacts the ability to detect a left-to-right shunt. An end-hole catheter, such as a Swan-Ganz catheter is preferred to achieve the highest possible sampling accuracy. At least the blood samples should be obtained from the following sites: superior and inferior venae cavae, right atrium, right ventricle, left and/or right pulmonary arteries. If a patent foramen ovale (PFO) or ASD exists, the catheter should be directed into the left atrium and left ventricle to obtain hemodynamic measurements and blood samples for oximetry. If a left-sided cardiac chamber cannot be entered, femoral artery saturation can be used as the systemic arterial sample. If no arterial access is available, the reading of the pulse oximeter may be used as the systemic arterial value, provided a good waveform is present.

Although left-to-right shunts can be calculated using oxygen content in the obtained blood samples, if the patient is breathing room air, it is simpler to use oxygen saturation values provided the saturation ranges between 40% and 100%, since hemoglobin concentration is taken out of the equation. The three blood sources entering the right atrium, inferior and superior venae cavae (IVC and SVC), and coronary sinus have different oxygen saturations. The lowest oxygenation is originating in the coronary sinus blood, which is in the range of 40% to 50%. Usually, blood entering the right atrium from the superior vena cava is about 75% oxygenated, while blood from the inferior vena cava is normally more oxygenated due to the inherent shunt of the renal circulation. The oxygen saturation of the "receiving chamber" proximally to the right atrium is then calculated according to the formula by Flamm et al.: (3 × SVC O_2 saturation + 1 × IVC O_2 saturation)/4.[4] Given those three sources of blood, complete mixing with a true average of systemic venous return commonly does not occur until blood enters the pulmonary artery. Further, this leads to a rather large variation of oxygenation values among samples drawn from the same chamber. Hence, to avoid false-positive interpretation of a shunt run, a minimum step up in oxygen saturation needs to be achieved. There is no clear consensus as to what this minimum step up needs to be, but certain basic rules can help to quickly interpret shunt run findings: (A) a step up of 8% or greater between the superior vena cava and the pulmonary artery is highly suspicious for an underlying left-to-right shunt at either level (atrial, ventricular, pulmonary arterial). (B) A chamber-to-chamber increase in oxygen saturation of 3% should raise the suspicion that there may be an underlying left-to-right shunt, while (C) an increase of 5% or more from one chamber to the one following it, is a definite evidence for an underlying left-to-right shunt.

In order to quantify the cardiac shunt, a pulmonary (Q_p) to systemic (Q_s) blood flow ratio should be calculated (Table 25.1). In the presence of intracardiac shunt, the best-mixed venous oxygen saturation is in the superior vena cava.

Pure right-to-left shunts are encountered rather rarely in the adult patient with CHD. The majority of adult patients with CHD presenting with a right-to-left shunt will have Eisenmenger syndrome due to un-repaired ASD, VSD, or PDA. The site of right-to-left shunt can be localized if blood samples can be obtained from a pulmonary vein, left atrium, left ventricle, and aorta, in addition to the right-sided blood samples. Again, if the patient has an underlying PFO or ASD, these blood samples can be obtained fairly easy. However, if the atrial septum is intact,

Table 25.1 Formulas for shunt calculations and valve area

A. Quantifying shunt by oximetry:

$$\frac{Q_P}{Q_s} = \frac{(\%AO - \%MV)}{(\%PV - \%PA)}$$

where Q_P, pulmonary blood flow; Q_S, systemic blood flow; %, percent oxygen saturation in respective blood sample; AO, aortic or systemic saturation; MV, mixed venous saturation; PV, pulmonary venous saturation (in left-to-right shunt calculations assumed to be identical to AO saturation); PA, pulmonary arterial saturation.

B. Gorlin equation for calculation of aortic valve area:

$$AVA = \frac{[CO(mL/min)]/[HR(bpm) \times SEP(sec/beat)]}{44.3 \times \sqrt{MG(mm\,Hg)}}$$

where AVA, aortic valve area in cm^2; CO, cardiac output; HR, heart rate; SEP, systolic ejection period; MG, mean transvalvular gradient.

C. Hakki equation for calculation of valve:

$$AVA = \frac{CO\,(mL/min)}{\sqrt{PPG\,(mm\,Hg)}}$$

where AVA, aortic valve area in cm^2; CO, cardiac output; PPG, peak-to-peak transvalvular gradient.

detection of right-to-left shunts by oximetry is rather difficult and would involve transseptal puncture to gain access to the left atrium. Again, no clear cutoff has been defined for a drop in oxygenation for a right-to-left shunt to be considered significant, although a decrease of 3% may be reasonable.

Hemodynamic evaluation

Apart from the usual pressures gathered from a standard right-heart catheterization in the right atrium, right ventricle, left (or right) pulmonary artery, as well as the pulmonary capillary wedge pressure, the cardiologist evaluating an adult patient with CHD should measure the main pulmonary arterial pressure and, if a PFO or ASD is available, then he should measure the left atrial and left ventricular pressure. Most corrected congenital defects follow the basic underlying anatomy of the normal heart. However, in cases of repaired complex (cyanotic) lesions, such as transposition of the great arteries (TGA) with a Mustard or Senning procedure, or palliation of a single-ventricle physiology with a Fontan operation, require a firm knowledge of the underlying anatomy in order to direct the catheter in the appropriate direction. Generally, evaluation using an end-hole catheter is preferable, either as a balloon-tipped catheter such as the Swan-Ganz, or as a stiffer multipurpose catheter. For the evaluation of stenotic lesions, such as baffle or conduit stenosis, coarctation or valvular stenosis, simultaneous pressure recordings should be obtained when possible. This sometimes may be accomplished with dual-lumen catheters with a proximal and a distal port and two pressure transducers. Otherwise, a pullback across the lesion can be recorded, although it is imperative to strictly avoid using multiple side-hole catheters in that setting.

Angiography

Angiographic visualization of cardiovascular structures is the final component of the comprehensive evaluation of the adult patient with CHD in the catheterization laboratory. The operator should have a thorough understanding of the anticipated pathology and underlying anatomy prior to the procedure. Based on the results of the preceding noninvasive imaging tests, angiography commonly can be reduced to only few cine runs, allowing minimization of contrast exposure. Most frequently, angiography is only needed to allow measurements of the identified defect in order to guide the anticipated intervention. Biplane imaging is preferable and can be helpful, but is not a must to perform a diagnostic or even an interventional procedure in the adult patient with CHD. The projections used during angiography differ from the one the adult cardiologist may be used to. A standard view in the evaluation of patients with ASDs or muscular VSDs is the hepatoclavicular view at 30° to 45° LAO and 30° to 45° cranial. Each congenital lesion has its preferred specific projections, which will be further described in the individual section. Most angiograms are performed using either a Berman catheter or a pigtail catheter. The settings for the power injector depend on the location of the defect and the main purpose of the angiogram (evaluation of function or delineation of defect anatomy). The total contrast volume per angiogram is usually 30 to 40 mL at a rate of 10 to 25 mL/sec, again depending on the main purpose of the angiogram.

Catheter manipulation and equipment

Right-heart catheterization with a balloon-tipped catheter (Swan-Ganz or Berman) is most commonly accomplished via femoral vein access. In order to maneuver the catheter into the superior vena cava, once the catheter tip is at the right atrium-inferior vena cava junction, the operator has to apply and maintain counterclockwise torque on the catheter while advancing it cephalad to the superior vena cava. This usually straightens the tip of the catheter allowing passage into the superior vena cava. In order to maneuver the catheter into the right ventricle, the catheter is withdrawn to low right atrium with its tip oriented to the patients left side and then advanced with clockwise rotation all the way to the pulmonary artery. To direct a catheter into the left atrium via an ASD or PFO, the catheter tip has to be placed at the low right atrium with its tip oriented to the left side of the patient. Then, the operator has to maintain extreme clockwise torque while advancing cephalad near the fossa, above the mouth of the tricuspid valve into the left atrium. To enter the left upper pulmonary vein, one applies clockwise torque near the mid-spine area with forward advancement into the left upper pulmonary vein. If one is interested in the right upper pulmonary vein (for sampling or for angiography in ASD),

Table 25.2 Commonly used catheterization equipment

Catheters
5–7F Swan-Ganz
5–7F Berman angiographic catheter
5–6F pigtail (preferably with markers for calibration)
6F dual-lumen pigtail
5F JR3.0 to 4.0
5F multipurpose (MP-A)
5F Amplatz AL1
Guidewires
J-tipped, regular 0.035 in. wire (150–300 cm in length)
J-tipped 0.025 in. wire (150 cm)
Glidewire 0.035 in. (Terumo, 150–260 cm length; angled-tip and straight)
Amplatz super stiff 0.035 in. wire (Cook, 260 cm length)

the catheter is pulled back from mid–left atrium all the way until very close to the mid-spine, then with extreme clockwise rotation one can maneuver it to the right upper pulmonary vein. Finally, from the mid-left atrial level, a balloon-tipped catheter can be advanced with the balloon inflated with clockwise rotation to the mitral valve orifice to the left ventricle.

Diagnostic catheterization can be performed using an end-hole or side-hole balloon-tipped catheters or a multipurpose catheter. Other equipment that may be needed is listed in Table 25.2

SPECIFIC LESIONS

Right ventricular outflow tract obstruction

Isolated pulmonary valve stenosis is not uncommon in adults with CHD. It is typically caused by commissural fusion, although dysplastic, thickened valves can be encountered as well. Subvalvular stenosis is usually secondary to hypertrophy of the right ventricle's infundibulum as a consequence of an underlying valvular stenosis. Supravalvular stenosis is rare, while supravalvular dilatation of the pulmonary artery is the norm in stenotic pulmonary valves. The hemodynamic evaluation is notable for increased right ventricular pressures with a commonly peaked or triangular appearance of the waveform. Once the valve has been crossed, one will notice low-normal pulmonary artery pressures, although the pulse pressure is frequently greater in the left pulmonary artery compared to the right, this is because of the preferential jet of blood directed by the stenotic pulmonary valve. Stenosis severity is judged by the peak-to-peak gradient across the pulmonary valve. A gradient greater than 40 mm Hg is considered moderate and greater than 60 mm Hg is severe.

Right ventriculography should be performed in the lateral (90° LAO) projection and an AP with 30° cranial angulation, which opens the right ventricular outflow tract and allows evaluation of the main, right, and left pulmonary arteries as well. Measurements of the pulmonary valve annulus diameter should be taken in the lateral view where the hinge points of the leaflets are best visualized. When performing a right ventriculogram the operator should remember to stay on cine for a prolonged run to evaluate the left ventricular function on levophase, which not only allows evaluation of the left ventricular function, but with left atrial filling a concurrent ASD may be excluded.

A Swan-Ganz catheter for hemodynamic evaluation and a Berman catheter for the ventriculography are usually sufficient. Passage of an inflated balloon at the tip of a Swan-Ganz catheter is commonly prevented by the valvular stenosis. Partial or complete deflation of the balloon once its tip has been positioned in the right ventricular outflow tract may be enough to cross the stenotic valve. If passage is not possible with that method, attempts with wire support should be made using a floppy-tip 0.035-in. wire or an angled glide wire preloaded either through a Swan-Ganz catheter or for better steerability through a 5F to 6F JR3.5 or JR4 catheter.

Left ventricular outflow tract obstruction

This group of lesions includes valvular, subvalvular, and supravalvular stenosis. Most commonly encountered is valvular aortic stenosis due to a bicuspid valve. Although initially those valves are only stenotic due to commissural fusion, cases presenting in adulthood usually also have valvular calcifications. The hemodynamics of congenital aortic stenosis are similar to those of the acquired forms. The left ventricular pressure should be recorded well within the left ventricular cavity to avoid falsely low readings due to tapering high-velocity flow in the subvalvular region. Traditionally, severity of aortic stenosis in children has been judged based on the peak systolic pressure gradient across the valve. A gradient greater than 50 mm Hg is considered moderate, while a gradient greater than 75 mm Hg is classified as severe. A cardiac output should be determined and the valve area can be calculated using the Gorlin or the simpler Hakke equation (Table 25.1).[5,6]

If an echocardiogram is available, it remains debatable whether an aortogram of the aortic root is necessary to evaluate the presence and degree of aortic insufficiency. In the case of supra valvular stenosis, however, an aortogram in a 45° LAO projection is recommended. A 30° RAO projection provides the operator with a standard projection of the left ventricle and allows for evaluation and diameter measurements of the aortic valve prior to a planned valvuloplasty procedure. Otherwise, a 60° LAO with 20° to 30° cranial also outlines the aortic valve pathology as well as its subvalvular and supravalvular structures.

To measure an accurate transvalvular gradient, either a dual-lumen 6F pigtail catheter is placed in the left ventricle, or alternatively, the left ventricle is approached via a transseptal puncture and another catheter is positioned retrograde in the aortic root for simultaneous measurement of the gradient. If the valve is difficult to cross, variety of catheters can be used to direct a straight-tip 0.035-in. guidewire or straight glidewire into the left ventricle. Among these catheters is the Amplatz AL1, JR4, Feldman, or a multipurpose catheter. Once in the left ventricle, the catheter can be exchanged for a pigtail catheter over the wire.

Coarctation of the aorta

The discrete narrowing of a coarctation of the aorta is usually immediately distal to the takeoff of the left subclavian artery. Diagnostic catheterization of patients with coarctation is usually only performed when an interventional therapy is contemplated. Catheterization for this lesion is generally straightforward. It is usually sufficient to place a pigtail catheter into the aortic arch and following pullback a translesional gradient can be calculated. Usually, a peak-to-peak gradient greater than 20 mm Hg is considered significant, although the indication for coarctation repair is usually a clinical one, driven by upper extremity hypertension and a gradient of 10 mm Hg or greater between the upper and lower extremity based on noninvasive blood pressure measurements. Important to note is that the translesional gradient is dependent on the extent of collateral flow; the more collateral flow, the less the gradient is. On occasions, due to complete atresia (interruption) of the aortic segment, a catheter is placed from the left brachial or radial artery for angiography and possibly cross the coarctation from above (Fig. 25.1).

Aortography in a lateral projection (40–90° LAO) usually displays the coarctation nicely (Fig. 25.1). Occasionally, a little caudal angulation (10–15°) will help to reduce overlap with surrounding structures. An alterative projection is 30° LAO that also outlines the aortic arch.

Atrial septal defect

Of the three main types of ASDs, primum, secundum, and sinus venosus defect, the secundum ASD is the most prevalent. Not infrequently unrecognized in childhood, adult patients may present with an unrepaired ASD with symptoms of exertional dyspnea and palpitations. ASDs are usually large enough to allow free communication between the atria without any pressure gradient across the septum. Hence, the degree of shunting is largely affected by the compliances of the left- and right-sided cardiac chambers. With long standing left-to-right shunts pulmonary arterial hypertension may develop eventually leading to a reversal of shunt as seen in Eisenmenger physiology. Thus, apart from a regular hemodynamic evaluation and shunt run, pulmonary vascular resistance needs to be calculated and close attention needs to be paid to possible systemic hypoxia suggesting right-to-left shunting. A Q_p/Q_s greater than 1.5 is considered significant and usually indicates ASD closure. However, the most important

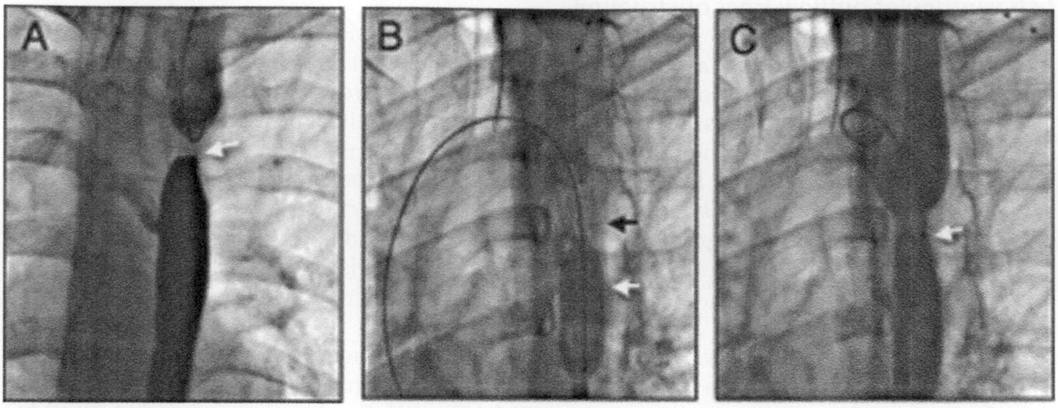

Figure 25.1 (**A**) Angiogram in 35° LAO projection in a 26-year-old patient with acquired aortic atresia (coarctation). The angiogram was done simultaneous contrast injection in the ascending aorta (using the left subclavian artery) and the descending aorta. This angiogram demonstrates the interruption (*arrow*). (**B**) Cine fluoroscopy after the lesion was crossed and a Genesis stent was deployed (*black arrow*). Note the distal part of the stent is being inflated by a balloon (*white arrow*), so that the distal part can appose the aortic wall. (**C**) Final angiogram demonstrating continuity (*arrow*) via the stent with good result.

indication to close an ASD is the presence of right ventricular volume overload as evidenced by the transthoracic echocardiogram. In the case of increased pulmonary vascular resistance, closure may be harmful if pulmonary-to-systemic vascular resistance ratio is 0.7 or greater (or an absolute pulmonary vascular resistance of greater than 10 Wood units) and the Q_p/Q_s ratio is less than 1.5:1.

Crossing a secundum ASD is usually a simple task if the catheter is advanced from the femoral vein, as mentioned above. Primum defects are located more inferiorly and a sinus venosus defect can be found more superiorly. When advancing a catheter into the superior vena cava close attention should be paid to the course of the catheter, as it may enter, if present, anomalous pulmonary veins. This is most apparent if the catheter tip takes a course outside of the cardiac silhouette, usually to the patient's right side.

During the shunt run of an uncomplicated ASD, a significant step up in oxygenation will be detected at the right atrial level. For the calculation of the Q_p/Q_s ratio, the mixed venous saturation obtained in the superior and inferior venae cavae should be used utilizing the prior-mentioned Flamm formula. Unfortunately, neither the presence nor the absence of a detected shunt guarantees or excludes the presence of an ASD. As in the case of a VSD with accompanying tricuspid regurgitation, the step up in oxygenation may be detected in the right atrium, leading to the false impression of an ASD. In contrast, an ASD with identical right and left heart compliance and equalization of atrial pressures may not allow a detectable step up in oxygenation in the right atrium.

With the advent of transcatheter closure, angiography in patients with an ASD has become important. When a Berman angiographic catheter is positioned in the right upper pulmonary vein, the frontal projection should be 30° to 35° LAO with 30° to 35° cranial. This allows not only visualization of the ASD, it also displays the superior portion of the septum and anomalous pulmonary vein drainage can be excluded. Device closure is an accepted approach for ASD closure (Fig. 25.2).

Ventricular septal defect

Isolated VSDs are common in childhood, but due to frequent spontaneous closure, VSDs are far less common in the adult patient population. VSDs are classified anatomically based on their location as muscular, perimembranous, or outlet VSDs. Further, they are classified physiologically based on their shunt volume as being restrictive or nonrestrictive. Restrictive VSDs produce a large pressure gradient across the ventricular septum and usually have a small shunt volume ($Q_p/Q_s < 1.5$). Common indications for VSD closure are a Q_p/Q_s greater than 1.5:1,

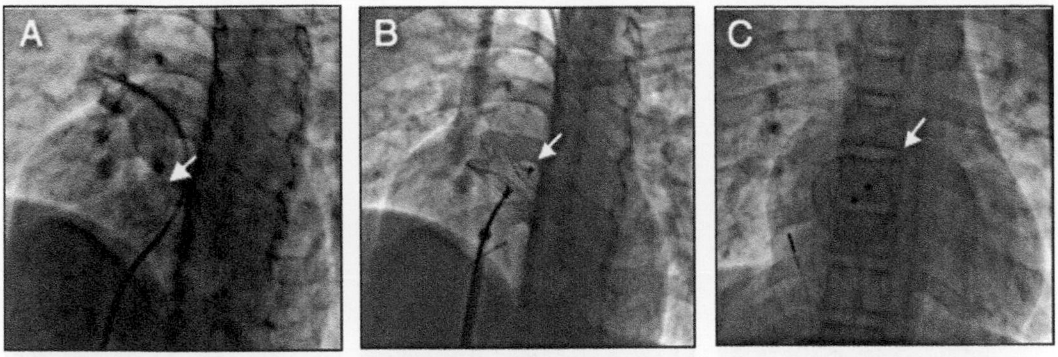

Figure 25.2 (**A**) Angiogram in the right upper pulmonary vein in a 13-year-old patient with a large secundum atrial septal defect demonstrating the left–right shunt (*arrow*). (**B**) Cine fluoroscopy in the four-chamber view after the right atrial desk of a 34-mm Amplatzer device (*arrow*) has been deployed. (**C**) Final cine fluoroscopy in the straight frontal projection after the device (*arrow*) has been released.

symptomatic patient in the absence of significantly increased pulmonary vascular resistance, left ventricle volume overload as evidenced by transthoracic echocardiography, or recurrent infective endocarditis.

Similar to the evaluation of a patient with ASD, patients with a VSD need a complete right-heart catheterization where close attention needs to be paid to the pulmonary vascular resistance. The step up in oximetry will be in the right ventricle; we prefer to use the superior vena cava as the mixed venous sample for the calculation of the Q_P/Q_S. Crossing of a VSD is usually unnecessary for a purely diagnostic procedure. However, with the advent of transcatheter closure options for patients with muscular and perimembranous VSDs, crossing of the defect becomes an important part of the interventionalist's skill set. There are multiple ways of crossing a VSD, however, given its left-to-right pressure gradient and the presence of right ventricular trabecultions with the possibility of entangling of equipment, we prefer entering the VSD from the left ventricular side. Using a 5F JR3–4 catheter placed in the left ventricle, the defect is crossed with a glidewire and advanced into the pulmonary artery. The catheter is advanced over the wire and the wire is then exchanged for a noodle wire that ultimately is snared and externalized from either the jugular vein or the femoral vein, depending on the VSD location. In patients with post-infarct VSD and due to the necrosis and friability of the septum, one should be very careful in using wires and/or stiff catheters. In such cases, we have found it very helpful to use balloon-tipped catheters, once in the left ventricle the balloon is inflated. Almost always, the balloon will be directed by the flow across the VSD to the pulmonary artery. Then as mentioned above, the wire can be snared from either jugular vein (mid, apical, and posterior VSDs) or femoral vein (anterior or perimembranous VSDs). Over this arteriovenous loop, the appropriate size delivery sheath can be advanced to the VSD from the venous side.

Using a pigtail catheter placed in the left ventricle a perimembranous and an anterior muscular VSD defect are best visualized angiographically in a 50° to 60° LAO with 15° to 30° cranial projection (Fig. 25.3). To better profile posteriorly located muscular VSDs, a shallower projection is preferred, while a steeper angulation helps to better visualize outlet VSDs and muscular defects located more anteriorly or apical. Additional helpful projections include a regular RAO view or even AP for high outlet VSDs.

Patent ductus arteriosus

A PDA represents the most common type of extracardiac shunt. This fetal connection between the pulmonary artery and the aorta usually closes within a few days following birth. The PDA takes off the superior aspect of the origin of the left pulmonary artery and inserts in the aorta, just distally to the left subclavian artery. Depending on the size and length of the PDA it allows various degrees of shunt volume. Large PDAs represent essentially a free communication between the systemic and pulmonary circulation, while small PDAs are restrictive enough to only enable

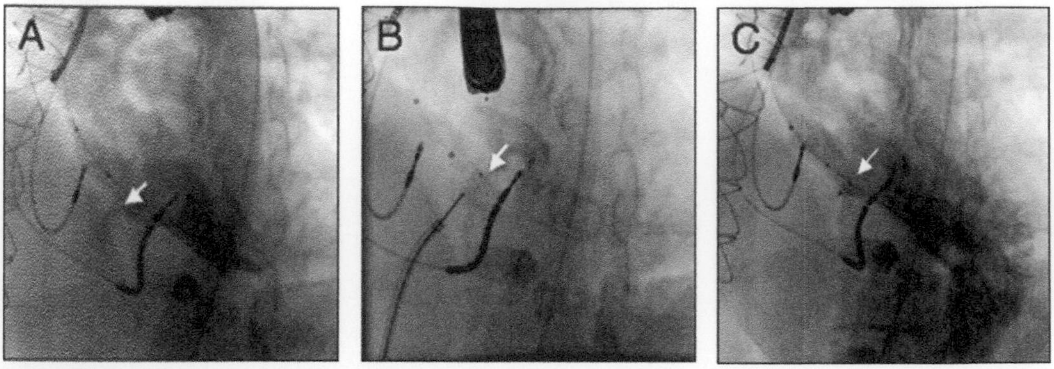

Figure 25.3 (**A**) Angiogram in the left ventricle in 50° LAO/15° cranial in a 32-year-old female patient who was status postseptal myomyctomy for hypertrophic cardiomyopathy that was complicated by small-to-moderate size high muscular perimembranous ventricular septal defect (*arrow*). Note the patient also had ICD leads placed. (**B**) Cine fluoroscopy prior to release of a 6-mm Amplatzer Muscular VSD device (*arrow*). (**C**) Final LV angiogram showing good device position and no residual shunt.

small amounts of left-to-right shunting. The shunting of blood leads to increased pulmonary arterial pressures, and left atrial and ventricular volume load. As a consequence, pulmonary arterial hypertension and right ventricular pressure load with secondary hypertrophy and/or failure may occur. Apart from the hemodynamic consequences, infective endarteritis poses a life-long risk; hence, all nonsilent PDAs should be closed as long as the ratio between pulmonary vascular resistance and systemic vascular resistance is not greater than 0.7 and the Q_p/Q_s is greater than 1.5.

During catheterization one may encounter various degrees of increased right ventricular and pulmonary arterial pressures. A significant step up in oximetry will be found in the main or left pulmonary artery. Crossing the PDA from the pulmonary side is usually not very difficult. Once in the proximal main pulmonary artery, a Swan-Ganz catheter with a deflated balloon or 5F multipurpose catheter can be used to cross the PDA by advancing the catheter with clockwise torque. The catheter may also be lead by a glidewire. Once the PDA is crossed, the wire's tip should be placed in the descending aorta. The catheter then can be exchanged for a delivery sheath in case transcatheter closure is planned.

Angiographically, the PDA is best visualized in a lateral projection. The pigtail catheter is placed in the descending aorta, just in the proximal descending aorta, to allow filling of the PDA prior to retrograde opacification of the aortic arch (Fig. 25.4). If biplane is used, another very useful projection is 25° to 30° RAO. To estimate the success of various PDA device closure

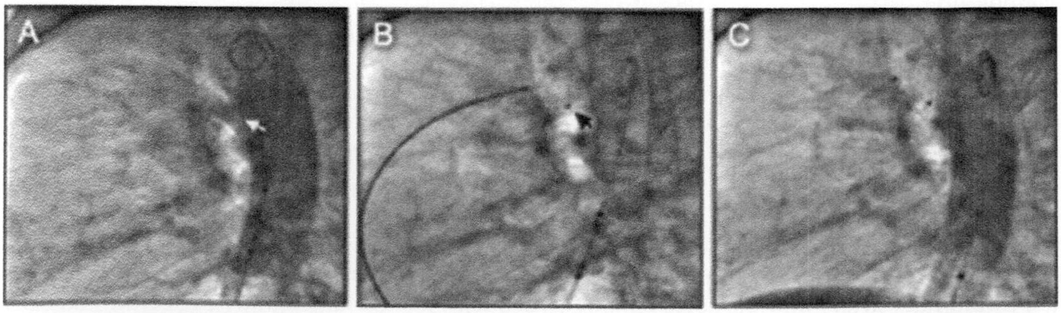

Figure 25.4 (**A**) Angiogram in the proximal descending aorta in the straight lateral projection in a 28-year-old female patient with 5-mm patent ductus arteriosus (*arrow*). (**B**) Cine fluoroscopy during deployment of a 10–8-mm Amplatzer Duct Occlud (*arrow*). (**C**) Final angiogram in the descending aorta after the device has been released demonstrating good device position and complete closure.

techniques, the lesion can be classified angiographically according to Krichenko's classification which considers the PDAs length and shape.[7]

Repaired transposition of the great arteries

Patients with complete transposition of the great arteries (TGA) have a very high mortality and do not survive until adulthood. With the introduction of the Senning and Mustard operations in the 1960s the group of adult patients with repaired TGA has been growing.[8,9] Using autologous tissue or synthetic material systemic venous blood is redirected via a baffle to the left ventricle which ejects into the pulmonary artery, while the blood from the pulmonary veins is drained into the right ventricle, which functions as the systemic ventricle, as it is connected to the aorta. Long-term follow-up has shown that baffle obstruction, arrhythmias, and systemic ventricular dysfunction are common problems. Hence, the arterial switch procedure was developed to essentially restore "normal" anatomy by transecting and re-anastomoses of the great arteries, as well as coronary arteries.[10] This operation was popularized in the 1980s and 1990s, therefore, the practicing adult cardiologist will start encountering young adult patients who underwent this arterial switch operation. However, the practicing cardiologist may still and will continue to encounter adult patients who underwent the Senning or Mustard atrial switch procedure in the past.

As it is true for most other CHD, diagnostic catheterization is rarely needed given the excellent noninvasive modalities available. Nevertheless, occasionally a patient following Mustard or Senning procedure is in need for a catheterization procedure. Right-heart catheterization, mainly done for hemodynamic evaluation of a possible baffle obstruction, is somewhat complex. Utilizing femoral vein access, the catheter course to the superior vena cava is anterior to the pulmonary venous atrium. Approaching from the inferior vena cava, the left ventricle can be entered using a regular balloon-tipped catheter. Care must be taken to measure any gradients upon pullback.

To evaluate the function of the systemic ventricle, ventriculography of the morphologically right ventricle needs to be performed. A pigtail catheter should be advanced retrograde via the aorta into the right ventricle. Helpful projections for ventriculography include AP and 90° LAO/lateral.

Repaired single ventricle lesions

"Single ventricle lesions" are part of a complex family of congenital heart lesions, which have a wide variety of underlying anatomy. The common denominator of those defects, however, is the presence of only one functional ventricular chamber. Among the single ventricle lesions are tricuspid atresia, pulmonary atresia with intact ventricular septum, double-inlet ventricle, and hypoplastic left heart syndrome. A full description of the underlying pathology and possible surgical approaches is beyond the scope of this chapter and the reader is referred to the standard pediatric cardiology textbooks. The best known and most likely encountered procedure is the Fontan operation, first described in the early 1970s.[11] All Fontan modifications have in common the basic principle that all systemic venous return is connected to the pulmonary arteries without interposition of a ventricle. Although early Fontan circuits created right atrial to pulmonary artery connections, the total cavopulmonary connection has emerged as the superior strategy. The superior vena cava is connected directly to the right pulmonary artery and the inferior vena cava is tunneled through the right atrium using a baffle to the pulmonary artery. This effectively excludes every right-sided cardiac chamber from the circulation, except for those cases that have received a fenestration in the tunnel. This fenestration was performed to allow "pop-off" and to unload the right-sided circulation. Given these complexities, it is obvious that the clinician needs to know exactly what kind of Fontan procedure the patient has received prior to proceeding with any invasive evaluation. Common indications for a diagnostic catheterization of a patient status post-Fontan procedure is congestive heart failure, venous hypertension or cyanosis caused by ventricular dysfunction, baffle obstruction or baffle leaks, and protein loosing enteropathy. It is recommended that patients should only undergo diagnostic catheterization at institutions with explicit expertise in the area of CHD. These procedures can be lengthy and sometimes difficult to interpret. Generally, using femoral vein access, an end-hole balloon-tipped flotation catheter can be used for hemodynamic evaluation of the Fontan circuit. Meticulous technique is important, as gradients as small as 2 mm Hg are considered significant in the conduit/baffle. Angiography of the baffle can be performed with a Berman or pigtail catheter placed in the inferior vena cava/conduit junction. The presence of veno-venous collaterals is important in patients who are cyanotic. These collaterals may lead to right–left shunt causing cyanosis. Newer modification of the Fontan is the extracardiac conduit where instead of performing surgery inside the right atrium, the surgeon reroutes the inferior vena cava blood to the pulmonary artery using an extracardiac tube. A retrograde catheter into the single ventricle should be advanced to measure the ventricular end-diastolic pressure and of course for angiographic assessment should the need arise.

Patients posttetralogy of Fallot repair

This by far comprises perhaps the largest group of patients the practicing adult cardiologist may encounter. Complete repair of tetralogy of Fallot was popularized in the 1950s and 1960s; therefore, many patients who are in their 40s and 50s are alive and doing well. Patients postrepair may have the following: residual defects, including ASDs and VSDs and branch pulmonary artery stenoses; right ventricular dysfunction; tricuspid regurgitation; and chronic pulmonary insufficiency. Most patients who underwent repair had transannular patch, thus by default have significant pulmonary insufficiency. Therefore, when catheterizing these patients, it is extremely important to evaluate the branch pulmonary arteries by catheter pullback technique in both pulmonary arteries and angiography. In unilateral pulmonary artery stenosis, it is not uncommon to have normal right ventricle pressure, therefore, the presence of normal right ventricle pressure does not necessarily rule out significant obstruction in one of the pulmonary arteries. Other noninvasive imaging (MRI/CT) should be incorporated in these patients' evaluations. Further, many patients had homografts placed between the right ventricle and pulmonary arteries. Such homografts may and do deteriorate with time. Therefore, evaluation using angiography and MRI/CT is essential. Currently, percutaneous pulmonary valve placement is gaining acceptance and may become readily available. Therefore, knowledge of the operative procedure that these patients had is important to help direct these patients to the appropriate therapy.

Other lesions

Obviously, the practicing cardiologist may encounter other congenital heart lesions in an adult patient. However, these usually may have been corrected in childhood or adolescence and present with at least near normal anatomy in adulthood, thus allowing a standard evaluation with a normal right- and left-heart catheterization. Among these lesions is the corrected atrioventricular canal. Others may present with other unrepaired CHD including coronary arteriovenous fistulae and pulmonary arteriovenous malformations. These are not rare and we encounter few patients each year that require a therapeutic intervention. Patients following complex, extra-anatomic repairs for congenital heart lesions should be referred to a center specialized in the care of those patients.

REFERENCES

1. Hoffman JI, Kaplan S, Liberthson RR. Prevalence of congenital heart disease. Am Heart J 2004; 147:425–439.
2. Warnes CA, Liberthson R, Danielson GK, et al. Task force 1: The changing profile of congenital heart disease in adult life. J Am Coll Cardiol 2001; 37:1170–1175.
3. Monro J. The changing state of surgery for adult congenital heart disease. Heart 2005; 91:139–140.
4. Flamm MD, Cohn KE, Hancock EW. Measurement of systemic cardiac output at rest and exercise in patients with atrial septal defect. Am J Cardiol 1969; 23:258–265.
5. Gorlin R, Gorlin SG. Hydraulic formula for calculation of the area of the stenotic mitral valve, other cardiac valves, and central circulatory shunts. Am Heart J 1951; 41:1–29.
6. Hakki AH, Iskandrian AS, Bemis CE, et al. A simplified valve formula for the calculation of stenotic cardiac valve areas. Circulation 1981; 63:1050–1055.
7. Krichenko A, Benson LN, Burrows P, et al. Angiographic classification of the isolated, persistently patent ductus arteriosus and implications for percutaneous catheter occlusion. Am J Cardiol 1989; 63:877–880.

8. Senning A. Surgical correction of transposition of the great vessels. Surgery 1959; 45:966–980.
9. Mustard WT. Successful two-stage correction of transposition of the great vessels. Surgery 1964; 55:469–472.
10. Jatene AD, Fontes VF, Paulista PP, et al. Anatomic correction of transposition of the great vessels. J Thorac Cardiovasc Surg 1976; 72:364–370.
11. Fontan F, Baudet E. Surgical repair of tricuspid atresia. Thorax 1971; 26:240–248.

26 Tips and tricks of the angiographic anatomy of the carotid arteries and vertebrobasilar system

Marco Roffi and Zsolt Kulcsár

INTRODUCTION

Selecting an appropriate imaging modality is an essential component of the management of patients with carotid or vertebral disease. The most frequently applied techniques include duplex ultrasound (DUS), computed tomography angiography (CTA), and magnetic resonance angiography (MRA). DUS remains the cornerstone of diagnostics of cervical vascular disease.[1] In experienced hands it has excellent sensitivity and specificity for the assessment of stenoses at the level of the proximal internal carotid artery (ICA) and of the distal common carotid artery (CCA). However, for proximal lesions of the CCA and for ostial lesions of the vertebral arteries (VA), the sensitivity and specificity of the DUS decreases.[2] In the presence of equivocal DUS findings, CTA and MRA may be performed.[3] CTA is fast, easily available, and has excellent sensitivity and specificity for the detection of both cervical and intracranial stenoses. Major limitations of this imaging modality are the use of iodinated contrast media, the radiation exposure, and the artifacts created by dense calcification or bone. MRA can also image accurately the entire cerebrovascular tree at once but has limited specificity for intracranial disease, particularly in severely tortuous vessels.

The imaging gold standard of the carotid and vertebral arteries remains the digital subtraction angiography (DSA). However, based on the mentioned excellent accuracy of noninvasive imaging, DSA is rarely required for diagnostic purposes. Catheter-based angiography remains an essential step in the planning and execution of endovascular procedures. Frequently, DSA is performed at the time of the intervention. In patients with symptomatic cerebral atherosclerosis undergoing diagnostic cerebral angiography, the reported risk of stroke ranged between 0.5% and 5.7%, and the risk of TIA was between 0.6% and 6.8%.[4] Recently, neurological complication rates of <1% associated with angiography were observed, suggesting that the risk may be lower than previously reported.[5] Possible explanations for these differences include improvements in equipment, technique, and operator experience; monitoring of catheter-tip pressure; and the use of procedural heparin and antiplatelet agents. The present chapter will cover anatomic features, angiographic views, and catheterization techniques of the cervical carotid and vertebral arteries, while a dedicated chapter will address the intracranial circulation.

GENERAL MEASURES

Carotid and vertebral angiographies are usually performed under local anesthesia using a femoral approach and 4F or 5F diagnostic catheters. Sedation should be avoided to adequately assess the neurologic status of the patients throughout the procedure.[6] In selected cases—for example, in the presence of advanced aortoiliac disease—the supraaortic vessel may be engaged using a brachial or radial approach. Accessing the supraaortic vessel using an upper extremity approach requires complex catheter manipulations at the level of the aortic arch and is therefore associated with higher embolic risk. It remains source of debate whether unfractionated heparin, usually at a dose ranging from 2000 to 5000 units, should be administered at the time of diagnostic angiography. Routine monitoring of the level of anticoagulation using the activated clotting time is not necessary. Neurologic complications of diagnostic angiography may be minimized by flushing the catheters, cleaning the wires, and gentle catheter manipulation. In addition, monitoring of catheter-tip pressure may be helpful in ensuring optimal catheter positioning in the vessel lumen.

AORTIC ARCH ANGIOGRAPHY

The performance of an aortic arch angiogram is an essential step in the evaluation of the supraaortic vessels and in the planning of an endovascular intervention. The suggested view

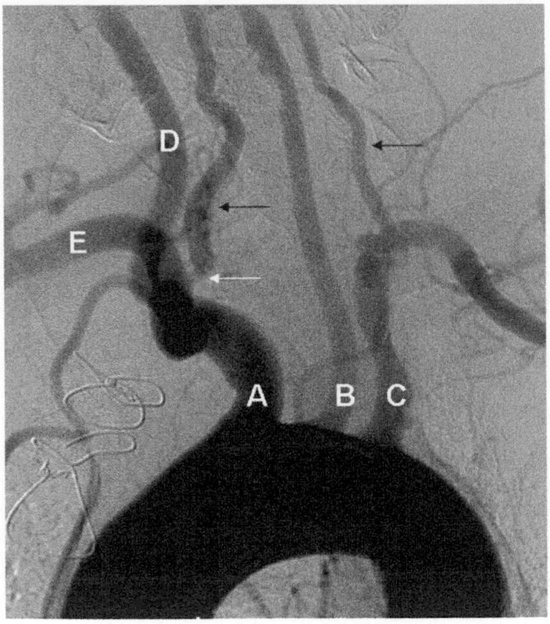

Figure 26.1 Left anterior oblique aortic arch digital subtraction angiogram revealing a normal configuration of the arch and great vessels. Note that this is a Type I arch as the origins of the brachiocephalic trunk (A), left common carotid artery (B), and left subclavian artery (C) all arise approximately at the same level (*horizontal line drawn through the arch apex*) from the aortic arch. The right vertebral artery (dominant) has a larger diameter than the left one (*black arrows*). There is mild disease at the ostium of the right vertebral artery (*white arrow*); D, right common carotid artery; E, right subclavian artery.

is 30° to 40° left anterior oblique (LAO). The most common aortic arch configuration is a "left aortic arch" with the innominate artery (also called brachiocephalic trunk), left CCA, and the left subclavian artery originating from the aortic arch in succession from proximal to distal (Fig. 26.1). In the most common variant of the aortic arch (~25%), the innominate artery and the left CCA share a common origin. The left CCA still arises from the arch but its proximal wall is fused with the distal wall of the innominate artery. Less common (~7%), but of greater impact on left CCA cannulation, is the "bovine arch" (Fig. 26.2). In this configuration there are

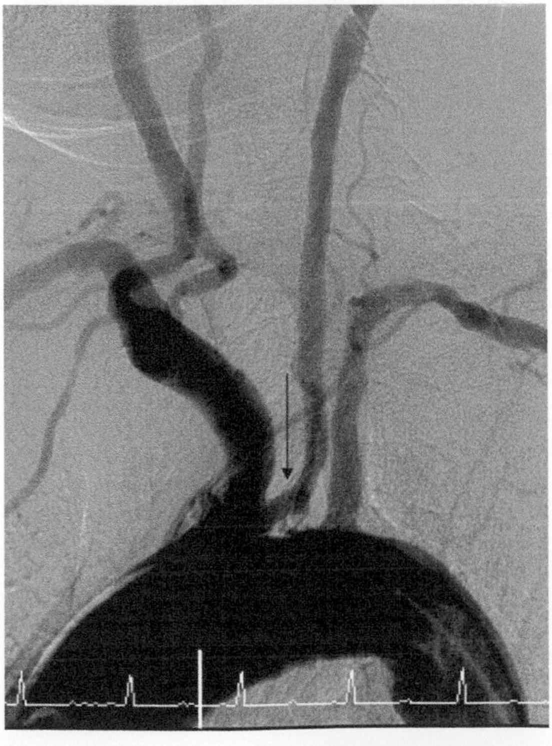

Figure 26.2 Aortic arch angiography showing that the left common carotid artery (*arrow*) originates from the innominate artery or brachiocephalic trunk (bovine arch). Note that the left vertebral artery is absent. This is also a Type I arch.

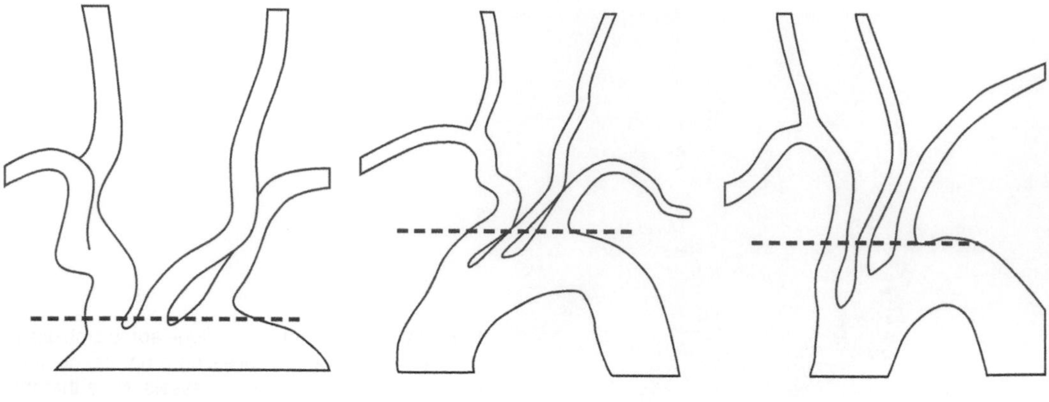

Figure 26.3 Classification of elongation and tortuousity of the aortic arch. Type I: all three great vessels arise from the apex of the aortic arch, so that a horizontal line drawn perpendicular to the long axis of the human body at the apex of the arch will intersect the origin of all three vessels. Type II and III arches: increasing elongation and rostral migration of the distal aortic arch with the innominate artery arising "lower." In the Type III arch the position of the innominate artery is lower than that of the origin of the subclavian artery by more than two "diameters" of the left common carotid artery. *Source*: Adapted from Ref. 8.

only two great vessels arising from the arch, the innominate and the left subclavian, and the left CCA originates from the innominate artery.[7] Rare variants include a left VA arising from the aortic arch (~5%), typically in between the left CCA and left subclavian artery and a left arch with an aberrant right subclavian artery that arises from the arch distal to the left subclavian artery (~0.5–2%).[7]

More frequently than congenital variants, challenging-acquired abnormalities of the aortic arch result in challenging cannulation of the supraaortic vessels. In the young nonhypertensive adult, all three great vessels usually arise from the apex of the aortic arch so that a horizontal line drawn perpendicular to the long axis of the human body at the apex of the arch will intersect the origin of all three vessels. However, elongation and rostral migration of the distal aortic arch with increasing age, atherosclerosis, and hypertension lead to a change in the relative positions of the great vessels. In these cases, left CCA and the left subclavian artery migrate rostrally along with the distal arch, which takes on a narrowed and peaked appearance rather than a smooth convex shape. This leads to a configuration change in which the origin innominate artery appears to migrate inferiorly, followed by the left CCA and the left subclavian artery (Fig. 26.3).[8] In the presence of excessive elongation/tortuousity, engagement of the supraaortic vessels may be difficult, if not impossible (Fig. 26.4). Minimal requirements to perform angiography of the cervico-cranial vessels include the use of DSA and of roadmap. As a general rule, a diagnostic catheter should not be advanced in the supraaortic vessels without prior advancement of a wire and the wire should preferably be advanced under roadmap.

CAROTID ANGIOGRAPHY

Anatomy

Blood supply to the brain is delivered by two carotid and two vertebral arteries. The paired ICA deliver about 80% of the cerebral blood flow. The right CCA is a branch of the innominate artery, while the left CCA arises directly from the aortic arch. The CCA measures approximately 7 to 8 mm in diameter and is generally a straight vessel, but in older and in hypertensive patients this may become tortuous. The CCA bifurcates into the ICA and the external carotid artery (ECA) (Fig. 26.5). The two vessels may be differentiated based on the diameter (ICA > ECA) and on the side branches. While the ECA has multiple side branches, the ICA has none in its extracranial portion. Due to superposition, sometimes multiple views are necessary to identify the vessels. The carotid bifurcation occurs most commonly near the angle of the jaw at the third to fourth cervical vertebral level, but it can be as low as the first thoracic and as high as the first

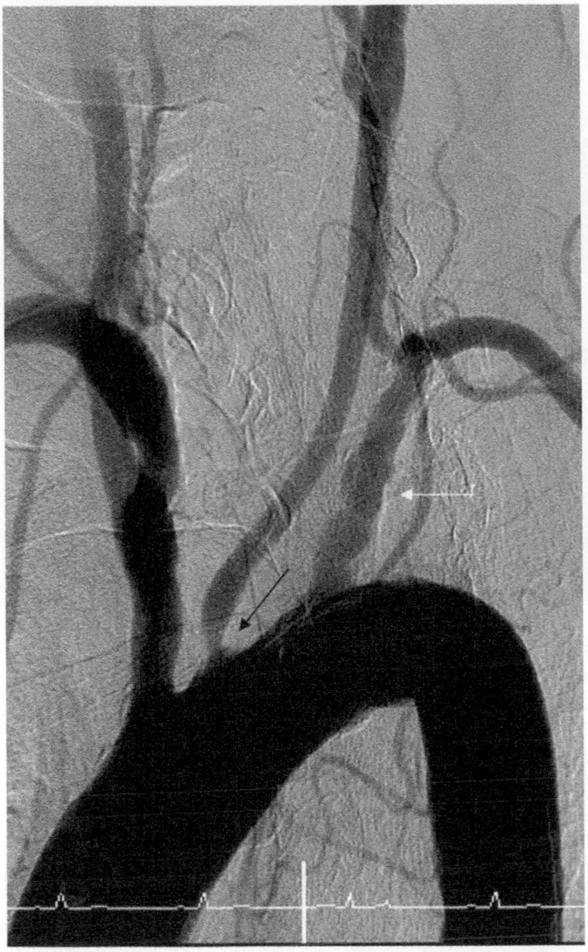

Figure 26.4 Type III aortic arch. The engagement of the supraaortic vessel from a femoral access is challenging, if not impossible. Note the moderate disease at the level of the origin of the left common carotid artery (*black arrow*) and the left subclavian artery (*white arrow*).

cervical vertebral levels. Multiple measurement modalities have been developed to quantify the severity of a carotid stenosis. Since each relies on a different reference segment, the absolute value in percentage also differs. Among them, the NASCET method—relying on the diameter of the proximal ICA above the carotid bulb as the reference diameter—has been widely embraced (Fig. 26.6).

The multiple branches of the ECA supply the soft tissues of the face, mouth, pharynx, larynx, and the neck. In the presence of severe cerebrovascular disease, the ECA may serve as a source of collateral blood flow to the intracranial ICA circulation and the vertebrobasilar system. The most important branches in relation to the cerebral circulation are the ascending pharyngeal, the occipital, and the middle meningeal arteries, and several small branches of the internal maxillary artery, all of which anastomose with the intracranial circulation. The ophthalmic artery is the major collateral source between the ECA and ICA and can, in the presence of cervical ICA occlusion, lead to reconstitution of the intracranial ICA. ECA collaterals to the VA occur most commonly through the occipital artery and muscular and spinal collaterals at the first and second cervical vertebral levels.

The carotid bulb defines a dilated vascular segment at the origin of the ICA. The diameters of the carotid bulb and of the cervical ICA range between 7 and 9 mm and between 4.5 and 6 mm, respectively. The bulb contains baroreceptors involved in regulation of arterial blood pressure and maintaining cerebral perfusion. During a hypertensive episode, the increased wall tension at the level of the carotid bulb activates baroreceptors producing reflex-mediated bradycardia and vasodilation. In addition, bulb chemoreceptors, capable of detecting arterial oxygen tension, can mediate an increase in ventilation in response to hypoxemia.

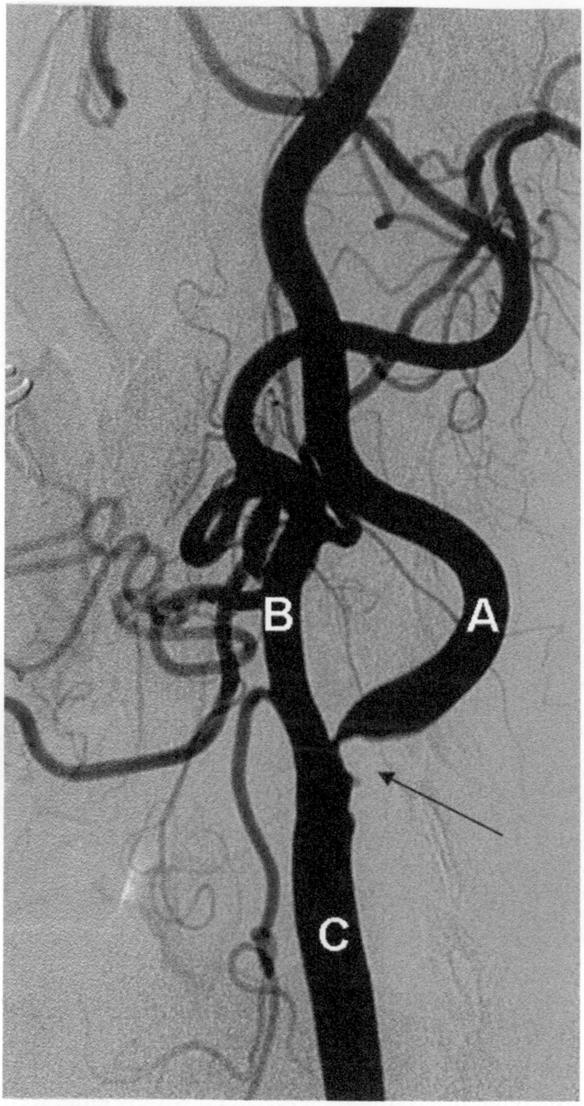

Figure 26.5 Forty-five degree left anterior oblique view of the carotid bifurcation showing a subtotal lesion at the origin of the internal carotid artery (A). The cervical internal carotid artery is mildly tortuous and has no branches. The external carotid artery (B) has multiple branches; C, common carotid artery.

Views

Intubation of the supraaortic vessels is performed under fluoroscopic guidance and usually in LAO projection. An aortic arch angiogram should be used to guide supraaortic cannulation in order to minimize catheter manipulations and the amount of contrast. While the left CCA is intubated directly, the innominate artery needs to be intubated first to selectively engage the CCA. Subsequently, a roadmap should be performed to guide advancement of the wire and subsequently of the catheter into the CCA. Although the best view to open the bifurcation between the right CCA and the right subclavian may be an anterior–posterior (AP) or right anterior oblique (RAO) view, the projection that allows optimal catheter control while cannulating the right CCA is the LAO. At the level of the carotid bifurcation, angiography may be performed in AP and in lateral views, as well as in ~30° RAO and ~30° LAO. Multiple views may be necessary to separate the ICA from the ECA and to adequately assess the severity of the ICA stenosis.

Catheterization technique

Intubation of the CCA may be achieved with a variety of diagnostic catheters. In the presence of a "friendly" aortic arch, CCA engagement can be achieved with catheter shapes such as

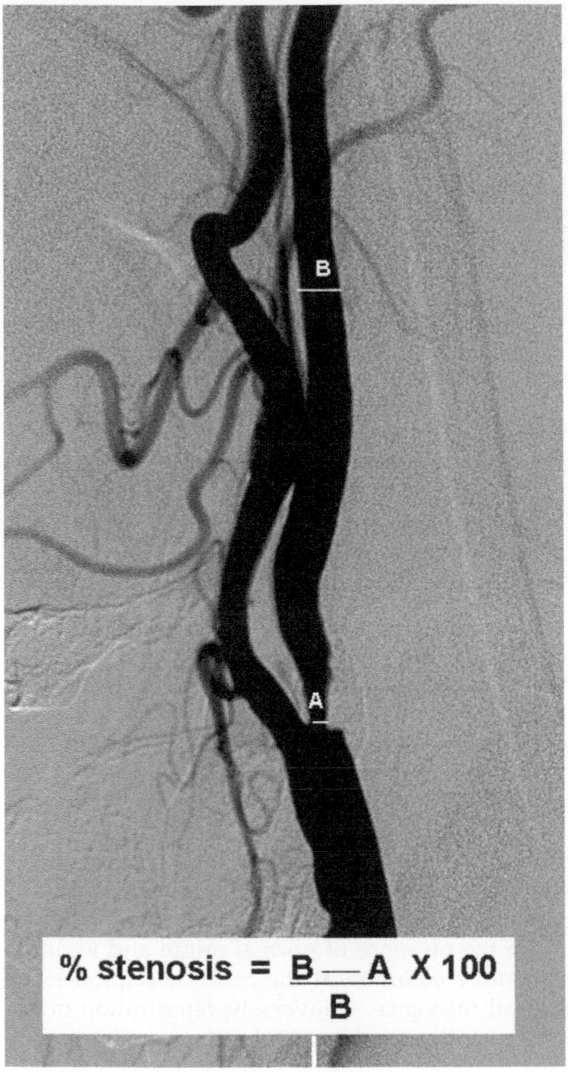

Figure 26.6 Angiographic method for determining the severity of internal carotid artery stenosis according to the NASCET study.

the Judkins right coronary or the vertebral/Bernstein catheters. Alternatively, the headhunter or the Benson diagnostic catheters can be used as routine. For more steep/tortuous aortic arches (i.e., Type III), shapes such as the Vitek or the Simmons/Sidewinder or the Benson may be used. The handling of these catheters is more challenging and may be associated with an increased risk of embolization. In order to engage selectively the right CCA, it is recommended to advance the diagnostic catheter over a steerable 0.035 in. wire after having performed a roadmap. In the presence of a "bovine arch" direct intubation of the left CCA may be achieved with a coronary Amplatz left catheter or a Simmons/Sidewinder or Benson shape. Alternatively, intubation of the left CCA in this particular anatomy may be achieved using a right radial or brachial approach. Selective cannulation of supraaortic vessels requires gentle manipulation and training. The intubation techniques with different catheters can be successfully trained at simulators.[9]

VERTEBRAL ARTERIES

Anatomy

The VA provides the main arterial supply to the posterior fossa structures and in 80% to 85% of cases to the territory of the posterior cerebral arteries. The VA is the first branch of the subclavian artery and arises from the superior aspect of the parent vessel in almost half of the cases, whereas in the other half the origin may be on the ventral, caudal, or dorsal aspect. The left VA may also arise directly form the aortic arch between the left CCA and the left subclavian artery in ~5% of cases.[10] The diameter of the VA is 3 to 5 mm and may vary to a great extent between the left and the right side. The left and the right VA are dominant in over half and 25% of cases, respectively. In the remaining the two vessels have similar caliber. In about 15% of the population one VA is atretic, that is, has a diameter <2 mm and supplies only the posterior inferior cerebellar artery (PICA) or gives only minimal contribution to the basilar system. In the absences of associated pathologies such as stenosis or aneurysms, these mentioned anatomical variations have no clinical relevance.

The anatomic course of the VA can be divided into the following four segments (Figs. 26.7 and 26.8):

1. The V1 (extraosseous) segment: extends from the origin to the transverse foramen of the 6th cervical (C6) vertebra.
2. The V2 (foraminal) segment: from the transverse foramen of C6 to C1.
3. The V3 (extraspinal) segment: from the transverse foramen of C1 to the foramen magnum, where it penetrates the dura.
4. The V4 (intradural segment): extends from entrance through the dura to the level of medulopontine junction, where it joins the VA from the other side.

During the ascent through the transverse foramina, the VA gives off multiple unnamed muscular branches that supply the deep cervical musculature, and also spinal segmental branches. The latter supply the vertebral bodies, the nerve roots, and the dura, and may give rise to branches to the spinal cord. Small rami of the segmental arteries may communicate with the other side at each vertebral level. The muscular branches of the V3 segment may have significant anastomotic connections with similar branches of the occipital artery. From the distal extracranial portion of the VA originate the anterior and posterior meningeal arteries for the dura of the foramen magnum and the posterior fossa.

The posterior spinal artery is usually originating from this segment, although it is rarely visible on vertebral angiograms (Fig. 26.7). Branches from the intracranial V4 segment include the anterior spinal artery and the PICA (Fig. 26.8). The PICA is the largest branch of the VA and may also be absent or originate extracranially from the V3 segment. Fenestration of the VA, defined as double lumen for part of its course in the presence of normal origin and location, is found in up to 2% of individuals, and it is more common at the atlanto-occipital level. Extracranial fenestrations usually have no clinical relevance. Conversely, fenestration of the basilar artery at the vertebrobasilar junction is frequently associated with aneurysm formation. Duplicate origin of the VA is rare.

Views

The evaluation of the origin and the proximal portion of the VA might be difficult because in more than half of the cases the vessel is not branching off from the superior aspect of the subclavian artery. As a consequence, the proximal part of the V1 segment and the aorta is often overlapped on the arch angiography. As atherosclerosis of the VA typically affects the ostium and/or the proximal segment (Fig. 26.9), it is mandatory to demonstrate these portions in the absence of vessel superimposition. Following intubation of the subclavian artery, the first contrast injection performed is in AP view. This will adequately demonstrate the ostium and proximal VA in the presence of a takeoff at the superior aspect of the subclavian artery. If the visualization is insufficient, an ~30° RAO and ~30° LAO projections may be used for both the right and left VA. Sometimes multiple views with craniocaudal angulation are necessary to exclude an ostial stenosis. The more distal segments of the VA are usually well visualized on AP and lateral views.

Catheterization technique

The left subclavian artery is usually easily accessible to catheterization with a variety of diagnostic catheters. Selective intubation of the right subclavian artery may pose difficulties in tortuous/steep aortic arches or in cases where the innominate artery has an elongated,

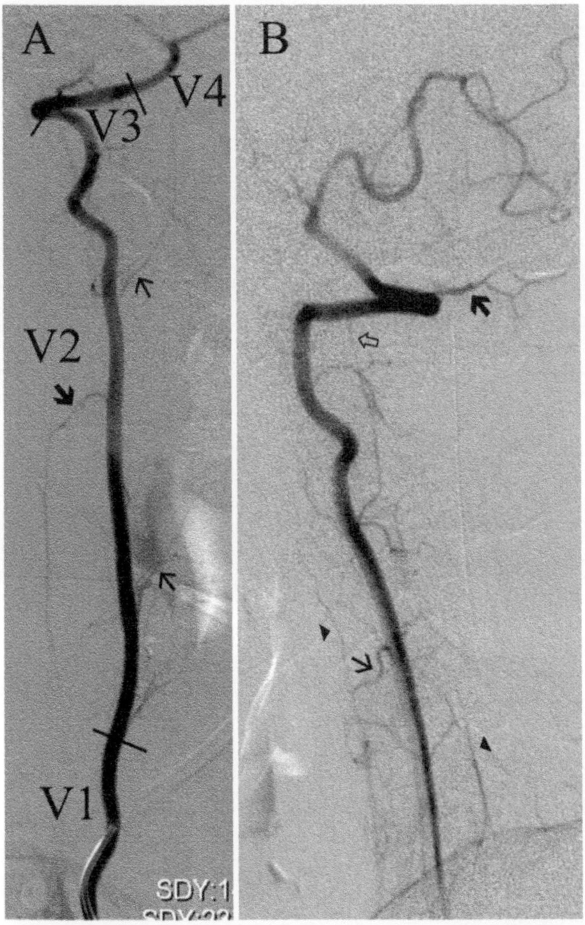

Figure 26.7 Selective right vertebral artery angiograms in anteroposterior (A) and lateral (B) views showing the cervical segments. Note the numerous segmental spinal (*thin arrows*) and muscular (*thick arrows*) branches that arise from the V2 and V3 segments. On the lateral view (B), note the segmental spinal rami supplying the spinal cord (*arrowheads*) and the posterior spinal artery arising from the V3 segment (*open arrow*).

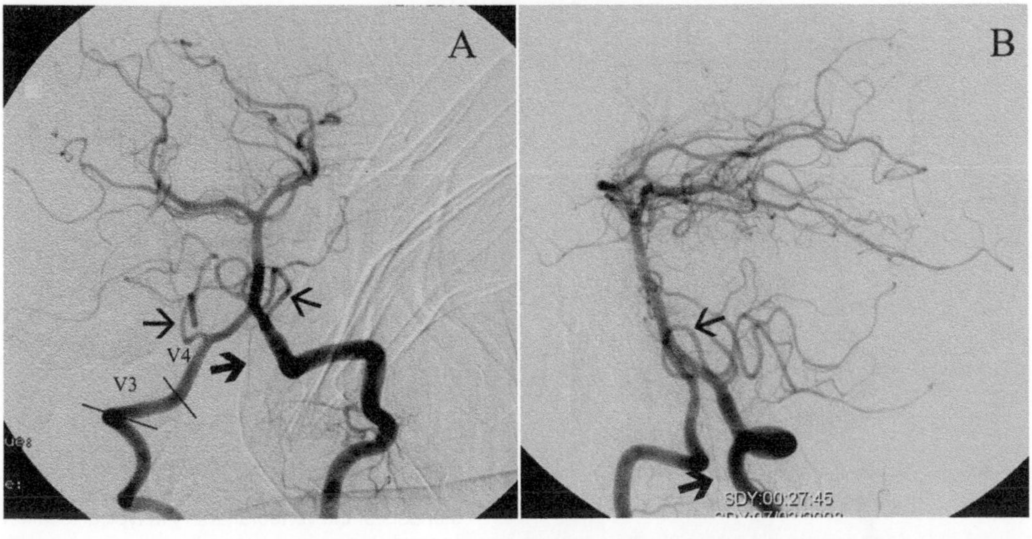

Figure 26.8 Simultaneous contrast injection in both vertebral arteries in slight anteroposterior (**A**) and lateral oblique views (**B**) showing the distal cervical and intracranial portions of the vertebral artery (V3 and V4 segments) and the vertebrobasilar system. Note the origin and the characteristic course of the posterior inferior cerebellar artery (PICA; *thin arrows*) and the very thin anterior spinal artery (*thick arrows*).

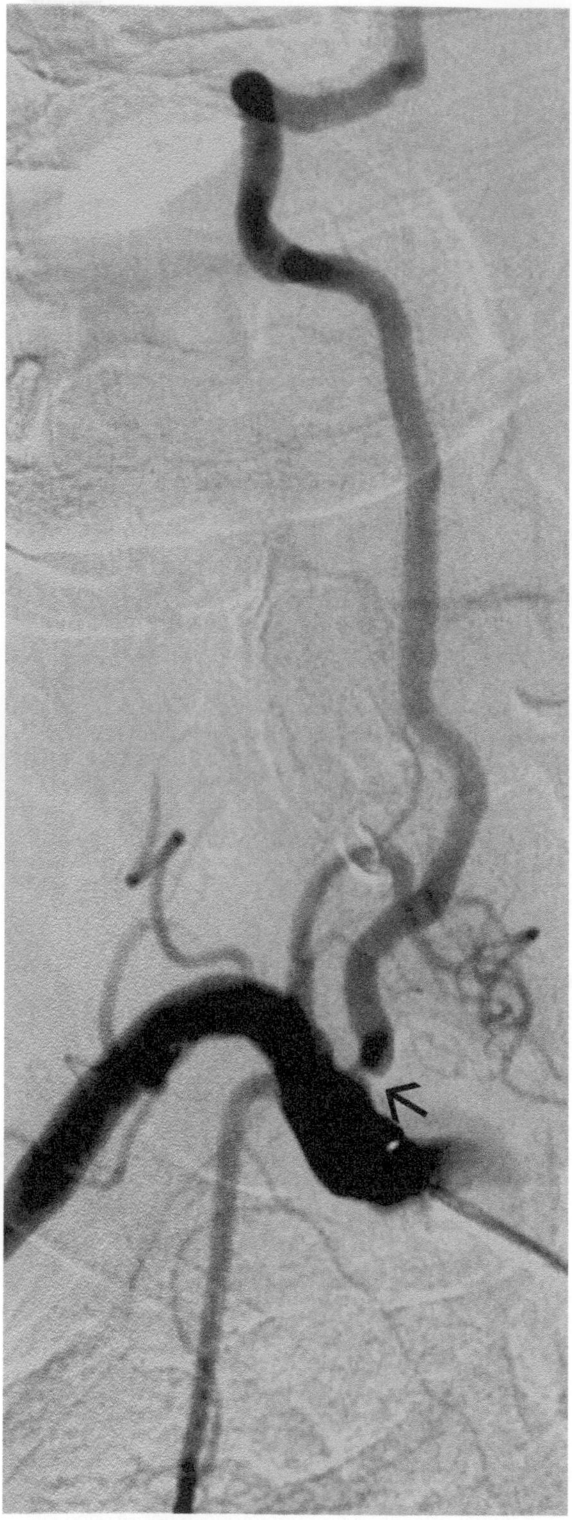

Figure 26.9 Left anterior oblique view of a right subclavian artery injection shows severe orifice stenosis of the vertebral artery in typical location (*arrow*).

tortuous course. For most cases, a vertebral, Judkins right, or headhunter diagnostic catheter will easily allow cannulation of the innominate artery. In more demanding aortic arches, this may be achieved with catheter shapes like Benson or Simmons/Sidewinder. A roadmap is than performed, and the catheter is advanced over a steerable 0.035 in. wire in the subclavian artery. Selective catheterization of the VA should be attempted only if clinically indicated and if an intact origin was well demonstrated. Frequently, selective intubation of the VA may not be necessary because good opacification of the cervical segments and of the intracranial vertebrobasilar circulation may be achieved by positioning the catheter in the subclavian artery and by inflating the blood pressure cuff on the ipsilateral arm over the systolic blood pressure at the time of injection. In addition, in the presence of challenging anatomy the intracranial vertebrobasilar system may be visualized by injection of the contralateral side.

Selective VA angiography requires gentle manipulation and for that purpose simple-shaped diagnostic catheters—like the vertebral, Judkins right, or headhunter—are preferred. The guidewire is positioned at the mid-distal third of the V2 segment avoiding hooking in small branches, and then the catheter is advanced in the VA over the wire. For diagnostic purposes the catheter should be kept in the V1 segment. In difficult anatomical situations the selective catheterization of the VA should be discouraged because of the associated dissection risk. Vessel wall injury may be the result of catheter manipulations or forced contrast injection.

REFERENCES

1. Qureshi AI, Alexandrov AV, Tegeler CH, et al. Guidelines for screening of extracranial carotid artery disease: A statement for healthcare professionals from the multidisciplinary practice guidelines committee of the American Society of Neuroimaging; cosponsored by the Society of Vascular and Interventional Neurology. J Neuroimaging 2007; 17(1):19–47.
2. Tay KY, U-King-Im JM, Trivedi RA, et al. Imaging the vertebral artery. Eur Rad 2005; 15(7):1329–1343.
3. Nonent M, Serfaty JM, Nighoghossian N, et al. Concordance rate differences of 3 noninvasive imaging techniques to measure carotid stenosis in clinical routine practice: Results of the CARMEDAS multicenter study. Stroke J Cereb Circ 2004; 35(3):682–686.
4. Connors JJ III, Sacks D, Furlan AJ, et al. Training, competency, and credentialing standards for diagnostic cervicocerebral angiography, carotid stenting, and cerebrovascular intervention: A joint statement from the American Academy of Neurology, American Association of Neurological Surgeons, American Society of Interventional and Therapeutic Radiology, American Society of Neuroradiology, Congress of Neurological Surgeons, AANS/CNS Cerebrovascular Section, and Society of Interventional Radiology. Radiology 2005; 234(1):26–34.
5. Fayed AM, White CJ, Ramee SR, et al. Carotid and cerebral angiography performed by cardiologists: Cerebrovascular complications. Catheter Cardiovasc Interv 2002; 55(3):277–280.
6. Roffi M, Abou-Chebl A, Mukherjee D. Principles of Carotid Artery Stenting. 1st ed. Bremen, Germany: Uni-Med; 2008; 1–80.
7. Osborn AG. Diagnostic Cerebral Angiography. 2nd ed. Phyladelphia, PA, USA: Williams & Wilkins, 1999.
8. Casserly IP, Yadav JS. Carotid interventions. In: Casserly IP, Sachar R, Yadav JS, eds. Manual of Peripheral Vascular Intervention. Philadelphia, PA, USA: Lippincott Williams & Wilkins, 2005:83–109.
9. Patel AD, Gallagher AG, Nicholson WJ, et al. Learning curves and reliability measures for virtual reality simulation in the performance assessment of carotid angiography. J Am Coll Cardiol 2006; 47(9):1796–1802.
10. Okahara M, Kiyosue H, Mori H, et al. Anatomic variations of the cerebral arteries and their embryology: A pictorial review. Eur Rad 2002; 12(10):2548–2561.

27 Invasive evaluation of renal artery stenosis

Stanley N. Thornton and Christopher J. White

INTRODUCTION

Atherosclerotic renal artery stenosis (RAS) is an increasingly recognized clinical entity, and is especially common among patients with atherosclerotic disease in other vascular beds. Ultrasound screening of an unselected Medicare population demonstrated a prevalence rate of 6.8% in RAS >60%.[1] In patients suspected of coronary artery disease (CAD) undergoing cardiac catheterization, RAS has been found in 15% to 30%.[2–7] Among patients with atherosclerotic disease of the lower extremities, the prevalence of RAS is estimated at greater than 30%.[8–10]

NATURAL HISTORY

The natural history of RAS is one of progressive diseases, resulting in functional loss and total occlusion. In a trial randomizing patients with significant RAS (>50%) to medical therapy or balloon angioplasty, progression to total occlusion over a 1-year period occurred in 16% of those treated with medical therapy as compared with none among those treated with angioplasty.[11] A second study demonstrated that progression to total occlusion occurred more commonly as the severity of stenosis increased.[12]

Atherosclerotic RAS is an independent predictor of mortality, even when comorbidities such as systolic heart failure, CAD, and renal insufficiency are taken into account. A study of nearly 4000 patients who underwent screening aortography at the time of cardiac catheterization for suspected CAD demonstrated that significant RAS (≥50%) had a 4-year mortality rate of 52%, as compared to 30% in those without RAS.[13]

CLINICAL MANIFESTATIONS

Clinical manifestations of RAS include ischemic nephropathy, renovascular hypertension, and cardiac destabilization syndromes such as "flash" pulmonary edema. RAS causing ischemic nephropathy leads to progressive loss of kidney function and is responsible for up to 15% of patients over the age of 50 who begin dialysis each year.[14–16] Renovascular hypertension, a renin–angiotensin driven cause of hypertension, causes approximately 5% of all hypertension cases and is the most common secondary (correctable) cause of hypertension. Cardiac destabilization syndromes are often a result of the peripheral vasoconstriction and volume retention, which are associated with increased renin–angiotensin production.

INVASIVE EVALUATION

Screening is indicated in patients who are at increased risk of having RAS as outlined in Table 27.1, and should be carried out through noninvasive means whenever possible. There are a number of imaging modalities available for screening, each with its own inherent strengths and weaknesses. Doppler ultrasound, computed tomographic angiography, and magnetic resonance angiography all have sufficient sensitivity and specificity for detecting significant RAS and have been given a Class I indication by the American College of Cardiology/American Heart Association's (ACC/AHA) *2005 Guidelines for the Management of Patients with Peripheral Arterial Disease*.[17] In most cases, the test of choice will be determined by availability, patient demographics, and local expertise. Any noninvasive screening test that proves inconclusive should be clarified with invasive angiography, which is still considered to be the "gold standard."

The issue of screening for RAS at the time of angiographic evaluation of other vascular beds, so called "drive by renal angiography," has been a source of contention among experts and payers alike. To help clarify this issue, the ACC/AHA has made recommendations outlining appropriate uses of this technique.[17] For patients with risk factors as outlined in Table 27.1 or clinical syndromes suggestive of RAS, aortography is given a Class I indication for screening at

Table 27.1 Causes of increased prevalence of RAS

Onset of hypertension ≤30 yr ≥55 yr
Malignant, accelerated, or resistant hypertension
Unexplained renal dysfunction
Development of azotemia with an ACE inhibitor or ARB medication
Unexplained size discrepancy of ≥1.5 cm between kidneys
Cardiac disturbance syndrome (flash pulmonary edema)
Peripheral arterial disease (abdominal aortic aneurysm or ABI <0.9)
Multivessel (≥2) coronary artery disease

Abbreviations: ACE, angiotensin-converting enzyme; ARB, angiotensin-receptor blocker; ABI, ankle brachial index.

the time of angiography performed for other reasons. There is a good evidence that nonselective renal angiography at the time of cardiac catheterization may be performed without incremental or additional risk.

CATHETER-BASED ANGIOGRAPHY

Angiography, although the gold standard for the evaluation and assessment of RAS, can be imprecise. Angiography is a luminogram, imaging radiopaque contrast material within the vessel lumen and not of the vessel wall. Proper angulation of the image intensifier is a key in demonstrating the true degree of stenosis and often proves difficult for aorto-ostial lesions. The angiographic appearance of a stenosis is an imprecise marker for clinically significant RAS. The overall incidence of blood pressure improvement following successful reperfusion of "angiographically significant" RAS is approximately 70%, despite an angiographic success rate of 95% or greater.[18,19] This suggests that the hypertension was independent of the RAS. Several methods have been proposed to investigate the physiologic significance of a lesion prior to intervention in hopes identifying patients who will benefit from revascularization.

We performed quantitative angiography in 121 peripheral arterial segments, including renal arteries, using three techniques: automated edge detection (Medis, Leiden, the Netherlands), manual electronic calipers (Toshiba, Irvine, CA), and visual estimation. While excellent overall correlation was noted between both quantitative systems [automated edge detection and manual electronic calipers ($r = 0.827$, $p < 0.0001$)], visual estimation correlated poorly with either of the quantitative methods (automated edge detection: $r = 0.51$, $p < 0.0001$; electronic calipers: $r = 0.56$, $p < 0.0001$) as shown in Figure 27.1. Clinicians should be aware that visual estimation of vessel diameters is an inconsistent and variable method of vessel sizing in the peripheral vasculature.

A visually estimated stenosis ≥70% is considered hemodynamically significant and is a generally accepted indication for revascularization, while a moderate stenosis of 50% to 69% generally requires hemodynamic confirmation.[20] Visual estimation of the severity of RAS has a high of degree interobserver variability and compares poorly with quantitative methods of lesion assessment.

Quantitative angiographic measurements of renal flow is approximated with the renal frame count (RFC), which is analogous to TIMI frame count in coronary angiography.[21] RFCs measured in a group of patients with fibromuscular dysplasia (FMD) of the renal arteries were compared to a group of patients with normal renal arteries. The RFC was defined as the number of cine frames required for contrast to reach the smallest visible distal branch of the renal parenchyma (Figs. 27.2 and 27.3). Compared to the group of normal patients, mean RFC for the FMD arteries was significantly prolonged (26.9 ± 9 vs. 20.4 ± 3; $p = 0.0001$, 95% CI = 21.4–32.4). RFC takes into account macrovascular blood flow in the main renal artery and its segmental branches as well as microvascular resistance in the cortex and medulla, and may prove to be a valuable angiographic tool for assessing renal blood flow.

INVASIVE FUNCTIONAL EVALUATION

Because the renin–angiotensin system is the pathophysiological mediator of hypertension from a hypoperfused kidney, efforts have been made to quantify the degree of anatomic stenosis

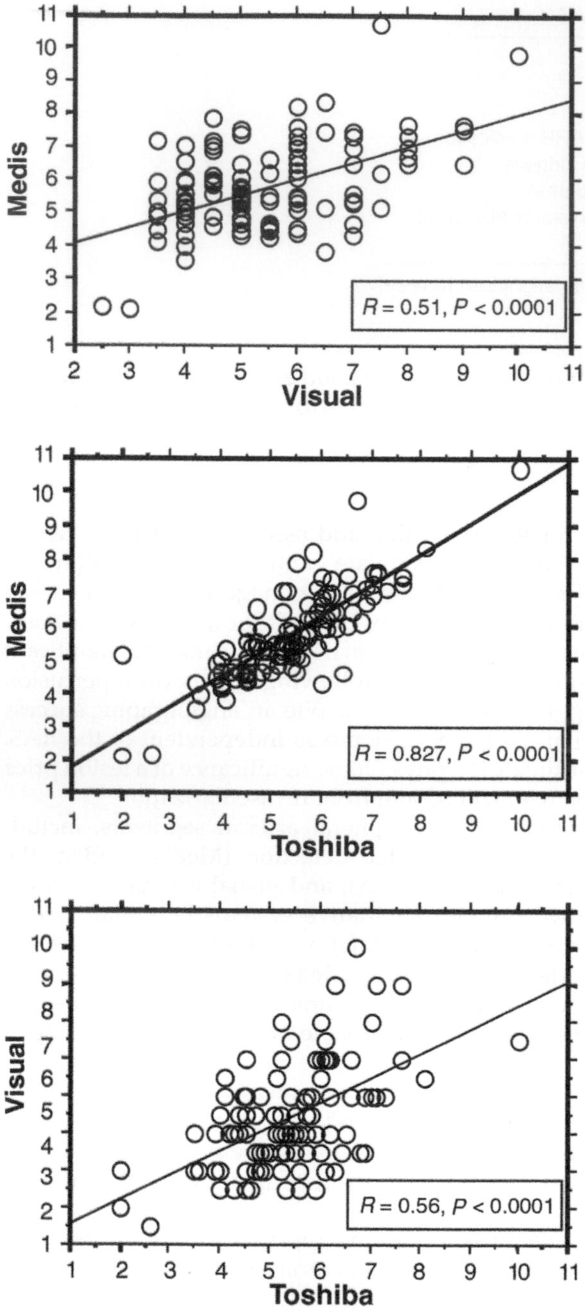

Figure 27.1 Comparison of three methods of vascular (noncoronary) angiography.

required to stimulate renin production. In 15 patients with bilateral renal vein sampling, a unilateral RAS was produced with a controlled balloon inflation while monitoring aortic and renal artery pressure distal to the partially occlusive balloon.[22] To compensate for varying levels of systemic aortic pressure, gradients were expressed as a ratio of distal renal pressure to the aortic pressure (P_d/P_a). Balloon inflations were performed to simulate progressive degrees of stenosis, from a P_d/P_a of 1.0 (no stenosis) to a P_d/P_a of 0.5. Renal vein renin samples were obtained with each balloon inflation. The results of this study established two important points relating to the functional significance of a stenotic renal artery. The first is that while there was good correlation between P_d/P_a and absolute pressure gradients, there is a much larger

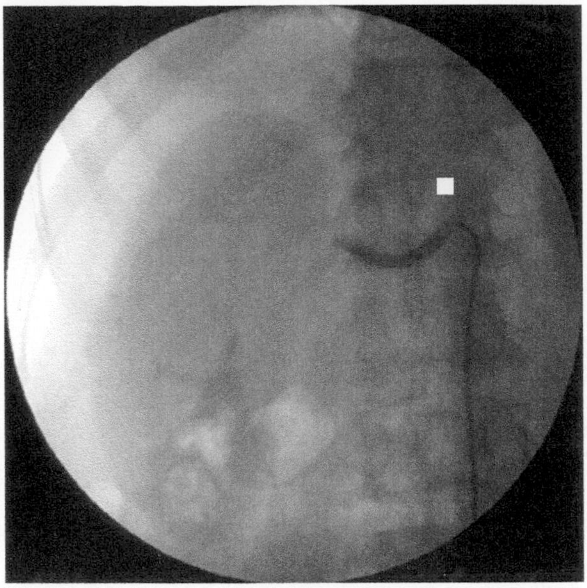

Figure 27.2 Renal frame count (RFC); first frame. A column of contrast extending the entire width of the main renal artery with antegrade flow.

variation in the absolute gradient for any given ratio of P_d/P_a (Fig. 27.4). Second, there was no significant increase in renal vein renin levels for degrees of $P_d/P_a > 0.9$, identifying a group of patients that are unlikely to benefit from renal artery revascularization (Fig. 27.5).

Renal fractional flow reserve (FFR) is another physiologic assessment method that has been validated in clinical trials.[22–24] This technique utilizes measurements taken under conditions of maximum hyperemia, using a nonendothelial-dependent vasodilator, measuring perfusion distal to a stenosis and is useful in predicting a positive clinical response to intervention[25] (Fig. 27.6). An FFR <0.8 indicates a significant impairment in flow and is associated with a therapeutic response after treatment of the RAS. In a study involving 17 patients with uncontrolled hypertension, those with a baseline FFR $\leq$0.8 had a significantly higher rate of blood pressure improvement following intervention than those with a normal FFR (86% vs. 30%; $p = 0.04$).[23] The poor correlation between angiographic percent diameter stenosis and FFR is shown in

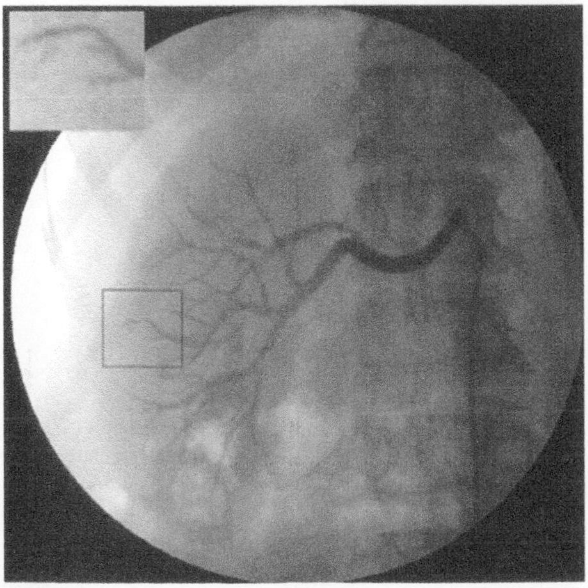

Figure 27.3 Renal frame count (RFC); final frame. Contrast filling the smallest visible branch in the distal renal parenchyma.

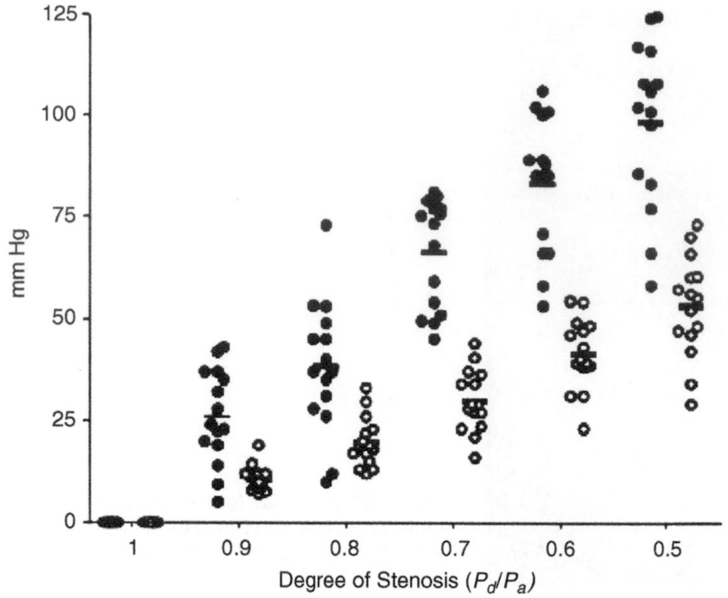

Figure 27.4 Relationship between the individual values of mean aortic pressure (P_d) and mean pressure distal to the renal artery stenosis (P_a) ratios and the corresponding systolic pressure gradients (*closed circles*) and mean pressure gradients across the stenosis (*open circles*). *Source*: Adapted from Ref. 22.

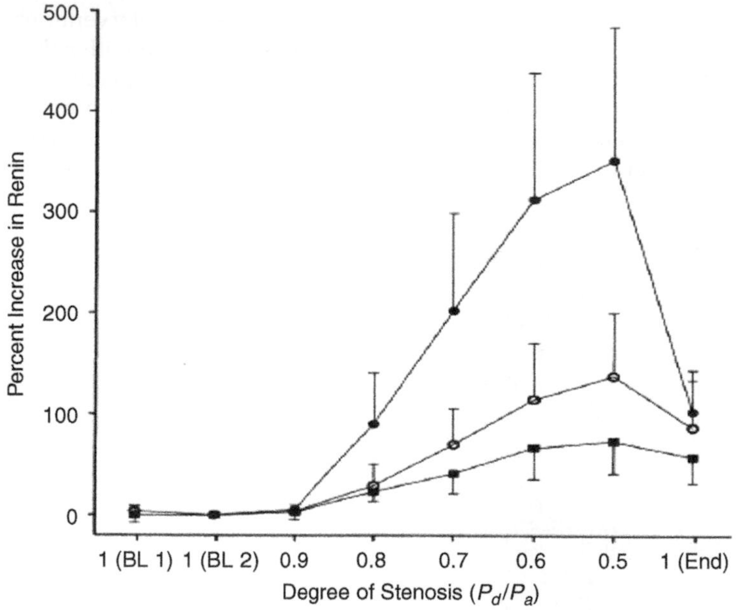

Figure 27.5 Effects of a balloon-induced, unilateral, controlled, graded stenosis (expressed as P_d/P_a ratio) on plasma renin concentration in the aorta (*squares*), in the vein of the stenotic kidney (*closed circles*), and in the vein of the nonstenotic kidney (*open circles*). BL 1, baseline before stenting; BL 2, baseline after stenting; other abbreviations as in Figure 27.4. *Source*: Adapted from Ref. 22.

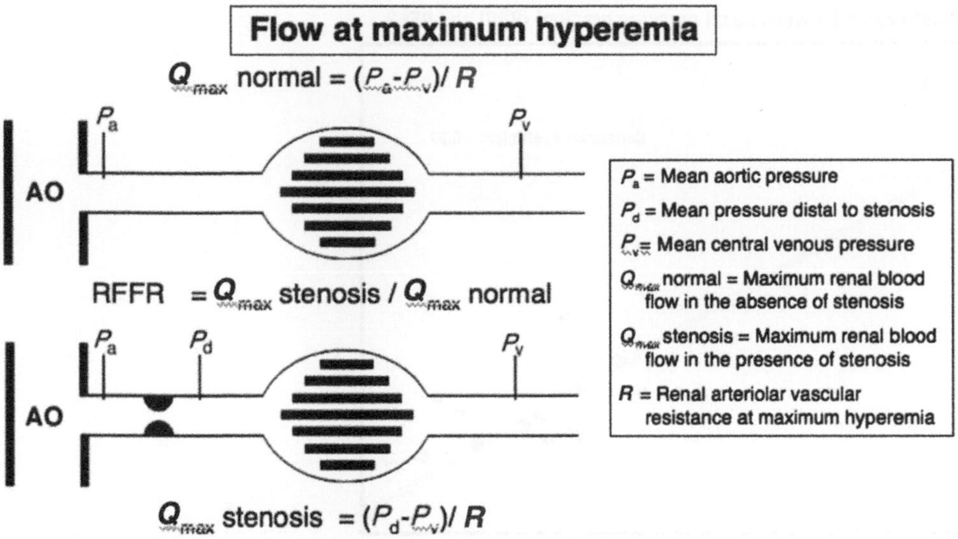

Figure 27.6 Pressure-derived renal FFR. *Source*: Adapted from Ref. 25.

Figure 27.7, while an excellent relationship between FFR and a resting translesional pressure gradient is shown in Figure 27.8. Despite this correlation, a borderline resting pressure gradient in RAS was not adequate to predict responders to revascularization as did in the FFR (Fig. 27.9).

SUMMARY

As awareness of the prevalence and potential consequences of RAS continues to increase, it is important to properly screen those who are at increased risk and to identify those who are most likely to benefit from revascularization. Renal angiography is the gold standard for identifying renovascular disease, but other parameters of the renal circulation are being investigated to determine the optimal management of these patients.

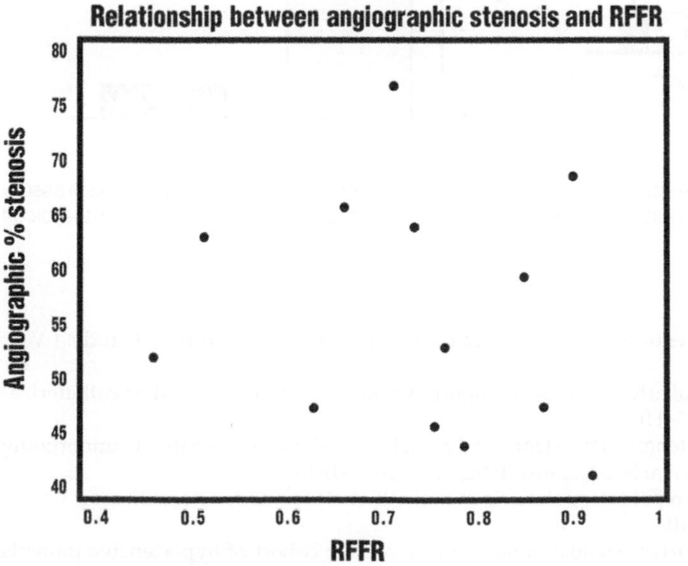

Figure 27.7 The correlation between renal artery angiographic percent diameter stenosis and the renal FFR was poor. *Source*: Adapted from Ref. 24.

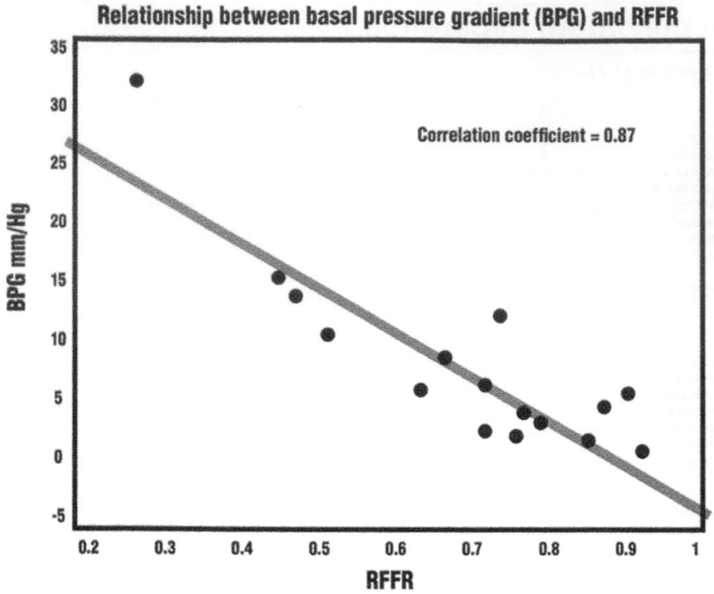

Figure 27.8 There was an excellent correlation between renal FFR and the baseline pressure gradient. *Source*: Adapted from Ref. 24.

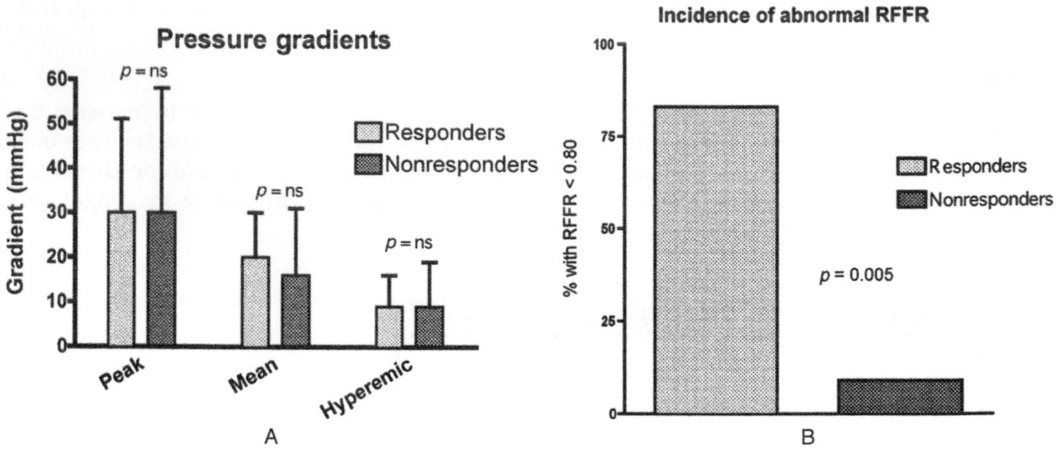

Figure 27.9 (**A**) Peak, mean, and hyperemic translesional pressure gradients did not differentiate blood pressure responders from nonresponders. (**B**) An abnormal renal FFR was present in approximately 80% of the blood pressure responders.

REFERENCES

1. Hansen KJ, et al. Prevalence of renovascular disease in the elderly: A population-based study. J Vasc Surg 2002; 36(3):443–451.
2. Aqel RA, et al. Prevalence of renal artery stenosis in high-risk veterans referred to cardiac catheterization. J Hypertens 2003; 21(6):1157–1162.
3. Harding MB, et al. Renal artery stenosis: Prevalence and associated risk factors in patients undergoing routine cardiac catheterization. J Am Soc Nephrol 1992; 2(11):1608–1616.
4. Jean WJ, et al. High incidence of renal artery stenosis in patients with coronary artery disease. Cathet Cardiovasc Diagn 1994; 32(1):8–10.
5. Rihal CS, et al. Incidental renal artery stenosis among a prospective cohort of hypertensive patients undergoing coronary angiography. Mayo Clin Proc 2002; 77(4):309–316.
6. Vetrovec GW, Landwehr DM, Edwards VI. Incidence of renal artery stenosis in hypertensive patients undergoing coronary angiography. J Interv Cardiol 1989; 2:69–76.

7. Weber-Mzell D, et al. Coronary anatomy predicts presence or absence of renal artery stenosis. A prospective study in patients undergoing cardiac catheterization for suspected coronary artery disease. Eur Heart J 2002; 23(21):1684–1691.
8. Olin JW, et al. Prevalence of atherosclerotic renal artery stenosis in patients with atherosclerosis elsewhere. Am J Med 1990; 88(1N):46N–51N.
9. Schwartz CJ, White TA. Stenosis of renal artery: An unselected necropsy study. Br Med J 1964; 2(5422):1415–1421.
10. Valentine RJ, et al. Detection of unsuspected renal artery stenoses in patients with abdominal aortic aneurysms: Refined indications for preoperative aortography. Ann Vasc Surg 1993; 7(3):220–224.
11. van Jaarsveld B, Krijnen P, Pieterman H, et al. The effect of balloon angioplasty on hypertension in atherosclerotic renal artery stenosis. N Engl J Med 2000; 342:1007–1014.
12. Caps MT, et al. Prospective study of atherosclerotic disease progression in the renal artery. Circulation 1998; 98(25):2866–2872.
13. Conlon PJ, et al. Severity of renal vascular disease predicts mortality in patients undergoing coronary angiography. Kidney Int 2001; 60(4):1490–1497.
14. Mailloux LU, et al. Renal vascular disease causing end-stage renal disease, incidence, clinical correlates, and outcomes: A 20-year clinical experience. Am J Kidney Dis 1994; 24(4):622–629.
15. Rimmer JM, Gennari FJ. Atherosclerotic renovascular disease and progressive renal failure. Ann Intern Med 1993; 118(9):712–719.
16. Scoble JE, et al. Atherosclerotic renovascular disease causing renal impairment—A case for treatment. Clin Nephrol 1989; 31(3):119–122.
17. Hirsch AT, et al. ACC/AHA 2005 guidelines for the management of patients with peripheral arterial disease (lower extremity, renal, mesenteric, and abdominal aortic): Executive summary a collaborative report from the American Association for Vascular Surgery/Society for Vascular Surgery, Society for Cardiovascular Angiography and Interventions, Society for Vascular Medicine and Biology, Society of Interventional Radiology, and the ACC/AHA Task Force on Practice Guidelines (Writing Committee to Develop Guidelines for the Management of Patients With Peripheral Arterial Disease) endorsed by the American Association of Cardiovascular and Pulmonary Rehabilitation; National Heart, Lung, and Blood Institute; Society for Vascular Nursing; TransAtlantic Inter-Society Consensus; and Vascular Disease Foundation. J Am Coll Cardiol 2006; 47(6):1239–1312.
18. Leertouwer TC, et al. Stent placement for renal arterial stenosis: Where do we stand? A meta-analysis. Radiology 2000; 216(1):78–85.
19. Safian RD, Textor SC. Renal-artery stenosis. N Engl J Med 2001; 344(6):431–442.
20. Rundback JH, et al. Guidelines for the reporting of renal artery revascularization in clinical trials. American Heart Association. Circulation 2002; 106(12):1572–1585.
21. Mulumudi MS, White CJ. Renal frame count: A quantitative angiographic assessment of renal perfusion. Catheter Cardiovasc Interv 2005; 65(2):183–186.
22. De Bruyne B, et al. Assessment of renal artery stenosis severity by pressure gradient measurements. J Am Coll Cardiol 2006; 48(9):1851–1855.
23. Mitchell JSR, Stewart R, White C. Pressure-derived renal fractional flow reserve with clinical outcomes following intervention. Catheter Cardiovasc Interv 2005; 65:135.
24. Subramanian R, et al. Renal fractional flow reserve: A hemodynamic evaluation of moderate renal artery stenoses. Catheter Cardiovasc Interv 2005; 64(4):480–486.
25. Pijls NH, De Bruyne B. Coronary pressure measurement and fractional flow reserve. Heart 1998; 80(6):539–542.

28 Angiographic assessment of lower extremity arterial insufficiency

Guillermo E. Pineda and Debabrata Mukherjee

INTRODUCTION

Catheter-based angiography allows direct visualization of blood vessels by the injection of iodinated contrast agents directly into an artery or a vein. Although noninvasive imaging techniques, including CT and MR angiograms, have made significant strides in recent years, catheter-based angiography has similarly undergone a new level of complexity and sophistication and to date, remains the "gold standard" for definitive evaluation of peripheral vascular beds and is a necessary initial step prior to percutaneous revascularization. The selective intubation and cannulation of lower extremity arteries has been facilitated by the development of multiple catheter shapes now available in catheterization laboratories.

The purpose of this chapter is to provide an overview of the angiographic techniques and equipments most commonly used during lower extremity diagnostic angiography, and a description of some of the fundamental principles involved in these procedures. The goals of preangiographic assessment should be to determine (a) the suitability for angiography and therapy, (b) the most likely level of disease, and (c) the preprocedure status as a baseline against which the results of therapy will be gauged.

Before performance of contrast angiography, a full history and complete vascular examination should be performed. This is usually followed by the use of noninvasive vascular tests which will optimize decisions regarding the access site, as well as to minimize contrast dose and catheter manipulation.

Lower extremity peripheral pulses at the access sites and distal to these sites must be thoroughly evaluated and documented prior to the angiographic study; this includes the calculation of the ankle-brachial index (ABI), which is a simple, accurate, inexpensive, and painless noninvasive test. It may also serve as a reference if complications should occur during the angiographic study. The ABI is calculated by dividing the systolic blood pressure obtained with a handheld Doppler in the ankle by the higher of the systolic blood pressures in the arms. A normal resting ABI is 1.0 to 1.29. An ABI <0.9 has a sensitivity of 95% and a specificity of 99% for angiographically demonstrated peripheral arterial disease.[1,2]

The primary objective of peripheral arteriography is to identify and characterize the lesions responsible for the patient's symptoms. Full characterization should include a description of lesion morphology, location within the vessel, extent of disease, and the presence of similar disease in adjacent vascular beds. Such characterization will help in determining the best treatment option and revascularization strategy, if needed.

RADIOGRAPHIC IMAGING

For the adequate angiographic assessment of lower extremity vasculature, it is particularly important to have a large image intensifier that will provide a larger field of view, ideally 15 to 16 in. The angiographic table should be sufficiently long to provide working space caudal to the feet. During angiography, the settings of the examination console are adjusted for lower extremity angiography using preset vascular packages. The frame rates for peripheral angiography are generally set at 3/sec. For these static vascular structures, digital subtraction angiography (DSA) is the ideal imaging modality. The DSA imaging modality requires that the patient does not move during image acquisition to avoid registration artifacts.

When performing a runoff of the arterial system in the legs, the interactive mode permits complete imaging of one or both the lower extremities with a single bolus given in the external iliac artery (EIA) or distal abdominal aorta. The first step is to establish the beginning and end positions of the moving table. A dry cineangiographic run is then performed; this dry run is stored and will be then subtracted from the contrast angiogram using the same starting and finishing points. The bolus of contrast is chased by moving the table proximally, relative to the image intensifier. The resultant subtracted angiograms sharply delineate the vascular anatomy and lesions of interest. An alternative mode is to obtain sequential, stepped, static angiographic images from each vascular territory from multiple small contrast injections. Complete opacification of the runoff vessels is important not only for planning therapy but also for predicting its success. The status of the distal runoff has been shown to correlate with the success of angioplasty in the superficial femoral and popliteal arteries.[3]

For added safety while advancing wires and catheters, trace-subtract fluoroscopy or road mapping is used. Like DSA, following the subtraction of the initial fluoroscopic image, contrast is injected to completely opacify the vessel. The pedal is then released and the subtracted image with contrast-filled vessel remains on the screen; this map of the vessel is then used for the safe advancement of equipment and to help minimize contrast use.

RADIOGRAPHIC CONTRAST AGENTS

The practice of endovascular diagnostic angiography has been made possible by advances not only in diagnostic equipments and techniques but also in the contrast media that permits visualization of the anatomic details of vascular structures. The remarkably high tolerance of modern contrast media has been achieved through successive developments in chemical pharmacological technology that allows them to be cleared from the system rapidly and naturally, usually with minimal or no adverse effects.

There are several types of contrast agents available today for angiography. Before the late 1960s, all iodinated contrast agents used for radiologic imaging were ionic monomers with an ionizing carboxyl group attached to the first carbon of the iodine-containing benzene ring. Significant adverse effects were related to hyperosmolar ionic contrast agents.

As a result of this, nonionic monomers were developed (iohexol, iopamidol, and ioversol), whose osmolality was substantially lower than previous agents, but they were still hyperosmolar relative to plasma—in the range of 600 to 850 mOsm/kg. Third-generation nonionic contrast agents reduce osmolality even further by creating a dimer. Iodixanol is a dimeric contrast agent in this class and is iso-osmolal with plasma. Nonionic, low-osmolal contrast agents are now routinely used for angiography. Besides being safer, newer contrast agents are much better tolerated.[4]

Low-osmolal or preferably iso-osmolal agents are preferred in patients with severe congestive heart failure, hypotension, history of contrast allergy, severe bradycardia, renal insufficiency (serum creatinine >2 mg/dL), and peripheral vascular contrast studies. A history of contrast reaction should be documented prior to the performance of contrast angiography and appropriate pretreatment should be administered before contrast is given.

TECHNIQUES AND CATHETERS

Clinical anatomy

Lower extremity vasculature can be broadly classified into three functional segments: the inflow vessels, which include the common iliac and the external iliac arteries; the outflow vessels, which include the common femoral, superficial femoral, and the profunda femoris arteries; and the runoff, which includes the anterior tibial, posterior tibial, and the peroneal (PER) arteries. Based on the territory affected, patients are said to have inflow, outflow, distal, or multilevel disease if more than one territory is affected.

The iliac vessels

These vessels are the continuation of the distal abdominal aorta with a diameter that ranges from 7 to 10 mm. The common iliac artery (CIA) subsequently divides into two terminal branches at the lumbosacral junction, the internal and external iliac arteries. The internal iliac artery (IIA) takes off medially and posteriorly to supply the pelvic organs, and the external iliac artery (EIA), which is the in-line continuation of the CIA, travels anteriorly and laterally to the groin to exit the pelvis just posterior to the inguinal ligament to become the common femoral artery (CFA) (Fig. 28.1).

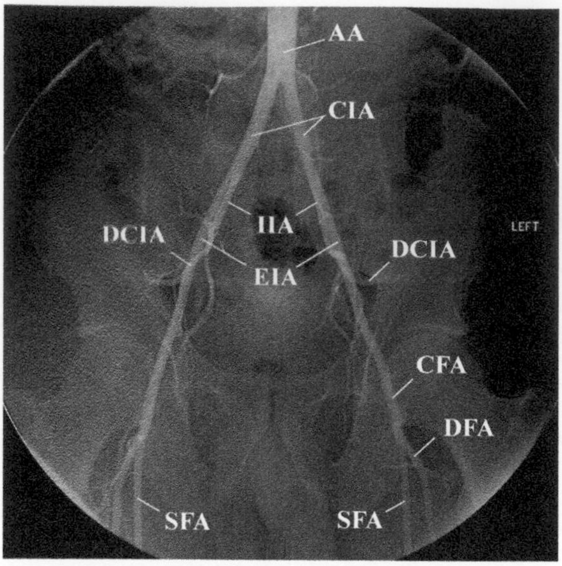

Figure 28.1 Pelvic aortogram showing common iliac arteries and their bifurcation. Common femoral artery and its bifurcation is also displayed. *Abbreviations*: AA, abdominal aorta; CIA, common iliac artery; EIA, external iliac artery; IIA, internal iliac artery; DCIA, deep circumflex iliac artery; CFA, common femoral artery; SFA, superficial femoral artery; DFA, deep femoral artery.

The femoral vessels

The CFA is the in-line continuation of the EIA below the inguinal ligament. On average, it is 2.5 to 4-cm long and 6 to 8 mm in diameter. The CFA bifurcates into the profunda femoris or deep femoral artery (DFA) posterolaterally and superficial femoral artery (SFA) anteromedially, commonly at the level of the mid-femoral head; this bifurcation is best visualized with an ipsilateral anterior oblique angulation of 30° to 40° (Fig. 28.2).

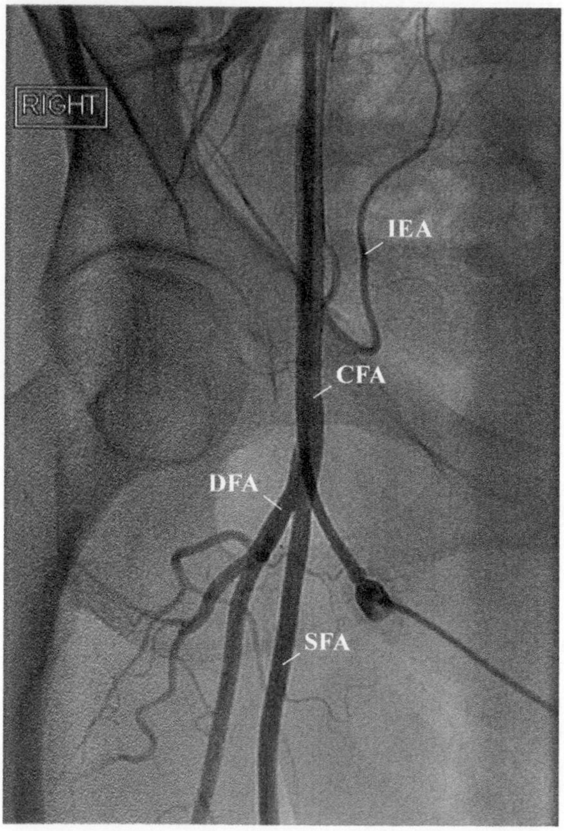

Figure 28.2 Right common femoral artery angiogram. Sheath positioned proximal to bifurcation at the level of the middle of the femoral head. *Abbreviations*: CFA, common femoral artery; IEA, inferior epigastric artery; SFA, superficial femoral artery; DFA, deep femoral artery.

The DFA runs along posteriorly and laterally along internal aspect of the femur. It provides several branches along its course, which are an important source of collateral flow to the leg and the foot, in patients with significant SFA stenosis or occlusion.

The SFA represents the direct continuation of the CFA and extends from the CFA bifurcation to the adductor (Hunter's) canal. It exits the adductor canal through the tendinous opening in the adductor magnus muscle to reach the popliteal fossa, located in the distal portion of the posterior surface of the femur where it becomes the popliteal artery. No major branches originate from the SFA throughout its course; this explains the constant diameter of this vessel, typically 6 to 7 mm. It provides multiple small muscular branches and gives off the descending genicular branch, just above the adductor canal, which contributes to collateral circulation at the knee.

The popliteal artery

This vessel is the continuation of the SFA below the adductor canal. It has a gradual medial to lateral course as it travels through the popliteal fossa and is usually 5 to 7 mm in diameter (Fig 28.3). Along its course, it gives origin to small muscular branches, two sural branches, and three geniculate arteries (the superior, middle, and inferior) which have the potential to provide collateral flow to reconstitute the popliteal or tibial vessels. The popliteal artery usually bifurcates into the anterior tibialis (AT) and the tibioperoneal trunk (TPT) approximately 5 cm below the tibial plateau at the level of the popliteous muscle.

The tibial arteries

These vessels are the terminal branches of the popliteal artery which commonly divides below the knee into the AT and the TPT (Fig. 28.3). The TPT courses for 3 to 4 cm before it bifurcate into the posterior tibialis (PT) and peroneal (PER) arteries. This branching pattern is seen in over 90% of patients; in the remaining cases a variant branching is observed. The most commonly

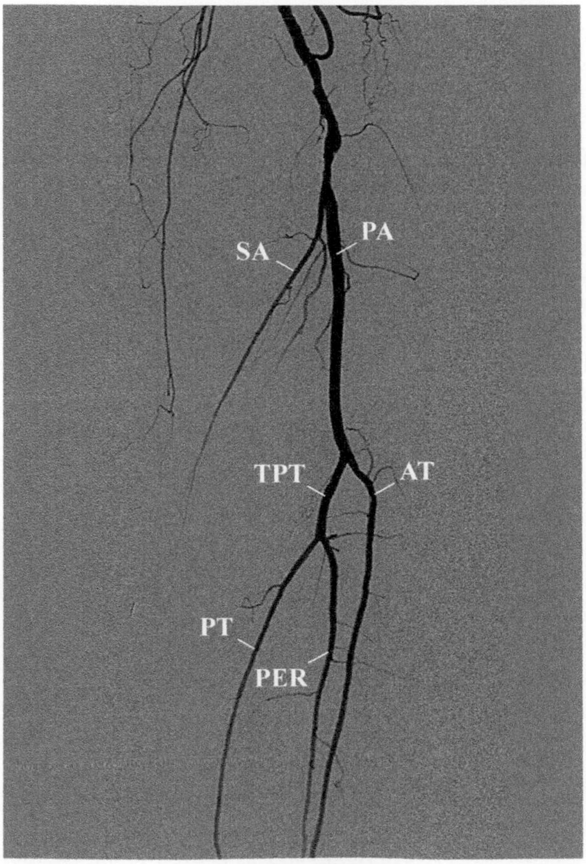

Figure 28.3 Digital subtraction angiogram of left popliteal artery (PA) bifurcating into the anterior tibial (AT), and the tibioperoneal trunk (TPT), which then divides into the posterior tibial (PT) and peroneal arteries (PER); Sural artery (SA).

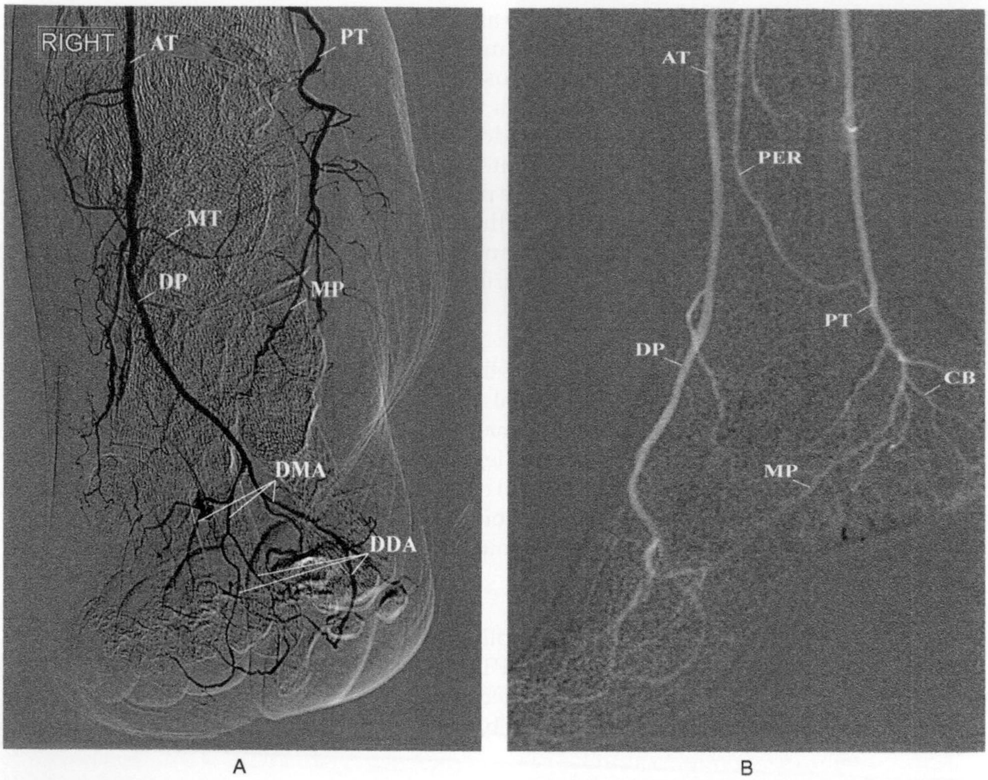

Figure 28.4 Arterial circulation of the right ankle and foot. Digital subtraction angiogram in anteroposterior (**A**) and lateral (**B**) projections. *Abbreviations*: AT, anterior tibial; PT, Posterior tibial; PER, peroneal; MT, medial tarsal; DMA, dorsal metatarsal arteries; DDA, dorsal digital arteries; MP, medial plantar; CB, calcaneal branches.

encountered variants are the trifurcation of the popliteal artery into its terminal branches which include the AT, PT and PER arteries, and origin of the PER artery from the AT.

The pedal arteries

The AT and PT continue into the foot as the DP and the PT arteries. The PER artery runs near the fibula between the AT and PT arteries and terminates at the ankle providing terminal branches to the DP and PT arteries. The DP provides the medial and lateral tarsal arteries before terminating as the arcuate artery from which the dorsal, metatarsal, and subsequent dorsal digital arteries originate. The terminal branches of the PT are the lateral and medial plantar arteries which provide the plantar cutaneous arch from which the plantar metatarsal and subsequent plantar digital arteries originate. In addition, there are multiple perforating branches which are pathways that link the ventral and dorsal circulation in the foot (Fig. 28.4).

Access for vascular angiography

One of the first and crucial steps of any endovascular procedure is to determine the most appropriate site for arterial access. Optimal access reduces the likelihood of complications and shortens the duration of the procedure. As a general rule, and for the purposes of angiographic assessment, the location of the lesion determines the access site in most cases. A couple of principles are worth highlighting.

Vascular anatomy

If available, one must be aware of the vascular anatomy of the patient at hand. Previous angiographic studies and noninvasive studies (e.g., CT or MR angiography, ultrasound) must be reviewed. Known occlusions, significant stenosis, and severe tortuosity proximal to a potential access site are helpful points to know in advance. If not available, a lower abdominal aortogram should be performed and evaluated before selective lower extremity angiography is carried out. Acute angulation of the aortic bifurcation increases the difficulty in performing crossover techniques, and severe atherosclerotic disease of aortic arch and great vessels increase the risk of cerebral embolization if upper extremities are utilized for arterial access. In addition, it is imperative to carefully document the peripheral pulses as described above.

Previous revascularization

The timing and nature of previous surgical revascularization must be available, as percutaneous puncture of grafts is generally avoided in the first 6 to 12 months. It is also crucial to know the direction of flow if a femoral–femoral bypass is present, as this will determine the site to be accessed. With the above information in mind, the access site that will provide the safest approach for an adequate diagnostic or interventional procedure is determined.

Common femoral artery (CFA)

The retrograde CFA is the most common access site used for diagnostic angiography and intervention. It is centrally located and provides greater distance from the X-ray source and more spacious workplace compared to the arm. The puncture of the CFA should be performed proximal to its bifurcation using the front wall technique (Fig. 28.2). The site should be checked under fluoroscopy to identify bony landmarks prior to arterial puncture, as its bifurcation usually occurs at the level of the mid-femoral head.

Although many operators use crossover techniques from the contralateral CFA, antegrade puncture via the ipsilateral CFA is an effective approach to SFA, popliteal, or infrapopliteal disease. It is technically more challenging and limits angiography to ipsilateral leg but offers stable platform for interventions. As in retrograde access, the desired site of entry is the CFA below the inguinal ligament.

Upper extremity access: Brachial and radial arteries

This site offers the advantage of early ambulation and reduced risk of bleeding complications. It is generally considered in individuals with bilateral CIA or distal aortic occlusions, severe downward angulation of aortic visceral branches, and acutely angulated CIA bifurcation, which makes the crossover technique unfavorable. The left brachial approach is preferable since instrumentation and passage of equipment across the origin of the vertebral and right common carotid artery exposes the patient to a risk of cerebral embolization when the right-sided vessels are used.

Diagnostic catheters

Knowledge of appropriate catheters, angulations, and injection rates is of vital importance in performing safe and optimal vascular angiography.

Several catheter shapes have been designed, which ultimately determines a specific function. They fall into the following general families:

(a) Side-hole catheters: These allow for large volumes of contrast to be infused safely in large vessels at a rapid rate via power injection. By having multiple side holes along the distal shaft of the catheter, the likelihood of catheter whipping or subintimal dissection is decreased.
(b) End-hole, simple-curve, and complex reverse-curve catheters permit selective angiography by manual injection of contrast material into a specific vessel.

The use of DSA permits the use of 5F catheters with excellent angiographic results. A general recommendation for catheter selection, injection rates, and angiographic projections for optimal separation of arterial branches in different vascular territories is displayed in Table 28.1.[5] Some of the most commonly used catheters for abdominal aorta and lower extremity angiography are shown (Fig. 28.5A–I).

Table 28.1 Catheters for peripheral angiography and recommended radiographic filming projections

Artery	Catheter	Angulation	Injection
Pelvic/abdominal aortogram	5F straight pigtail between L1 and L2	Anteroposterior	20 mL/sec for 1 sec
Distal aorta for bolus chase and runoff[a]	5F straight pigtail between L2 and L3	Anteroposterior	8 mL/sec for 10 sec using DSA
Common iliac artery	5F MP, straight pigtail	Anteroposterior	10 mL/sec for 1 sec
External–internal iliac artery bifurcation	5F MP, straight pigtail	Contralateral anterior oblique at 30–35°	10 mL/sec for 1 sec
Common femoral artery and SFA/DFA bifurcation	Access sheath	Ipsilateral anterior oblique at 30–35°	Hand injection or 10 mL/sec for 1 sec
Infrainguinal segments (SFA, popliteal, trifurcation, and tibial arteries)	Access sheath or antegrade: MP, JR4 or crossover: IMA, MP	Anteroposterior	10 mL/sec for 1 sec
Pedal arteries	Antegrade: MP, JR4 or crossover: IMA, MP	Anteroposterior and lateral	10 mL/sec for 1 sec

[a]The volume should be reduced by 50% if each leg is injected separately.
Abbreviations: SFA, superficial femoral artery; DFA, deep femoral artery; JR4, Judkins right; IMA, internal mammary artery; MP, multipurpose catheter.

Pelvic and lower extremity angiography

The diagnostic lower extremity arteriogram should image the iliac, femoral, and popliteal trifurcation in profile without vessel overlap. The indications for pelvic and lower extremity angiography include ischemia (either resting or exertional) owing to atherosclerosis, embolism, thrombosis, and vasculitis.[6] Other potential indications include peripheral aneurysms, vascular tumors, trauma, and extrinsic compression. The preliminary digital subtraction pelvic aortogram is obtained by placing a multiholed catheter (straight pigtail or Omni Flush) at the level of L3 slightly above the aortoiliac bifurcation (usually the aorta bifurcates at L4–L5 level).

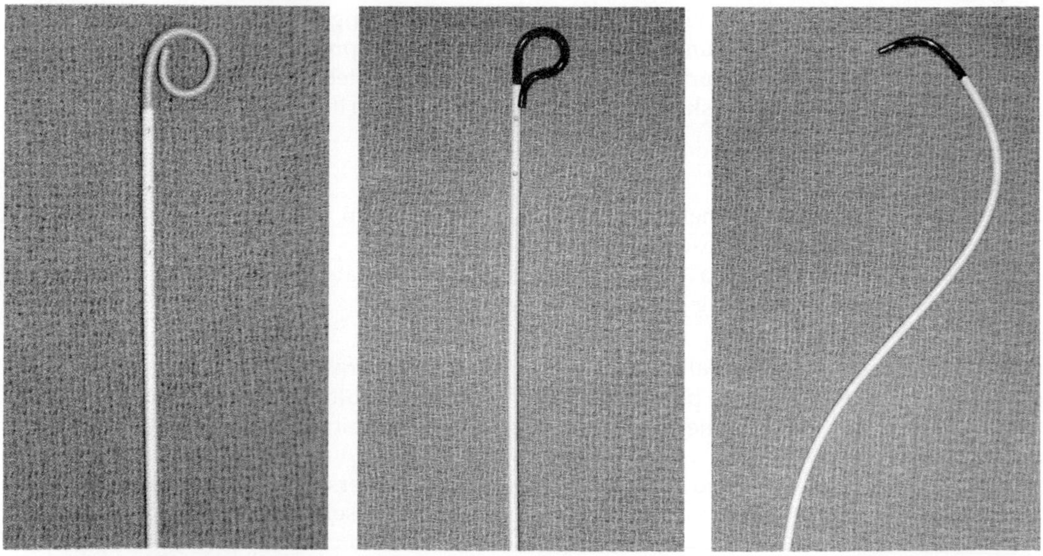

A B C

Figure 28.5 Commonly used catheters for pelvic aorta, its branches, and lower extremity angiography. Side-hole catheters: (**A**) pigtail and (**B**) Omni Flush. End-hole catheters: (**C**) cobra, (**D**) Judkins right (JR), (**E**) internal mammary (IMA), (**F**) renal double curve (RDC), (**G**) SOS-OMNI, (**H**) Simmons-1, and (**I**) multipurpose (MP). (*Continued*)

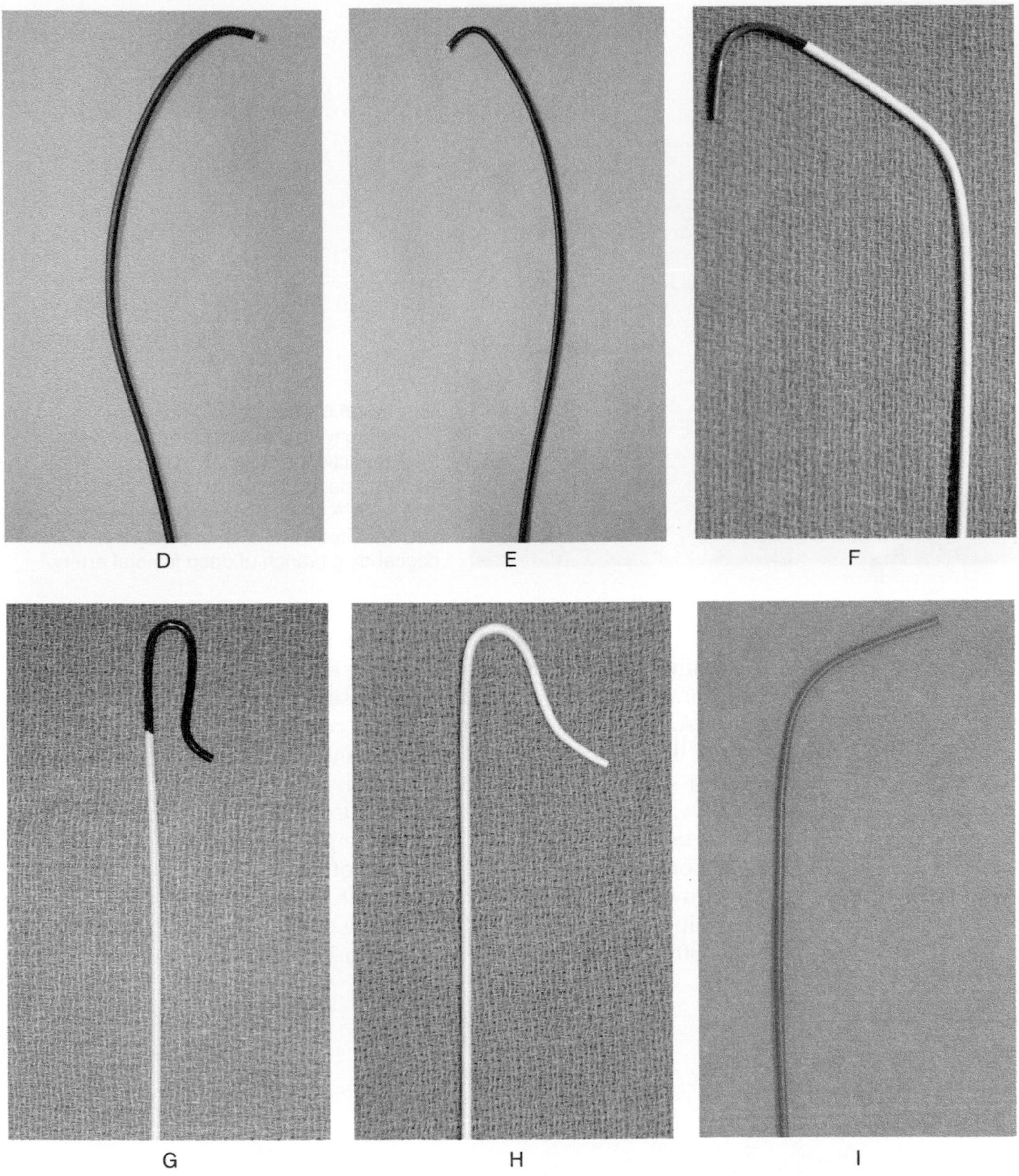

Figure 28.5 *(Continued)*

The digital run is obtained at 6 frames/sec using a contrast injection rate of 15 cc/sec for a total of 20 to 25 cc at a maximum of 800 to 1200 psi. This allows excellent visualization of the distal aorta, common iliacs, external iliacs, and the common femoral arteries (Fig. 28.1).

Following the adequate visualization of the inflow vessels with the pelvic aortogram, runoff angiography with DSA with a moving table and bolus chase technology is performed. Contrast material is injected at a rate of 7 to 10 cc/sec for a total of 10 to 12 seconds (i.e., 70–120 cc). Filming is begun after a 2-second delay and the bolus of contrast is then chased from the pelvis to the feet (Fig. 28.6). The transit of contrast material is dependent on the patient's cardiac output and severity of underlying vascular disease.

Selective angiography of the iliac arteries can also be achieved via the brachial or femoral approach. If the ipsilateral femoral artery is used (retrograde approach), contrast is injected directly through the arterial sheath or via a short catheter (multipurpose catheter (MP), pigtail)

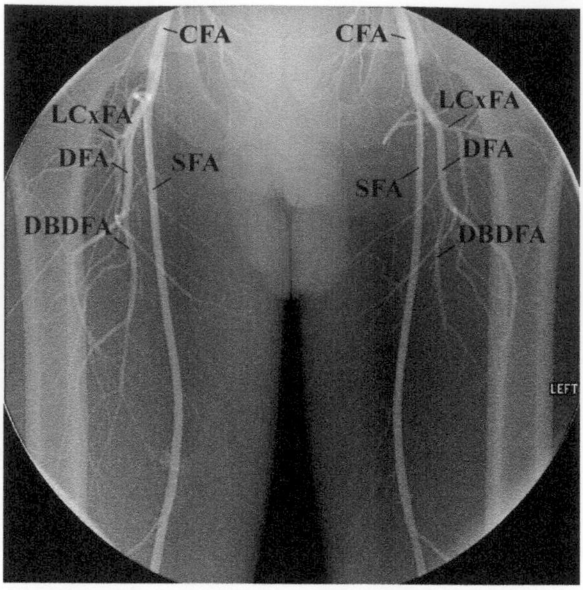

Figure 28.6 Bilateral lower extremity runoff angiography; anteroposterior view with digital subtraction technique. *Abbreviations*: CFA, common femoral artery; DFA, deep femoral artery; SFA, superficial femoral artery; LCxFA, lateral circumflex femoral artery; DBDFA, descending branch of deep femoral artery.

placed in external iliac or CIA. With a brachial artery access, a multipurpose catheter is used to selectively engage each common iliac vessel. An alternative and commonly used approach is from the contralateral femoral artery, which requires crossing the aortic bifurcation and engagement of the opposite CIA. To accomplish this, catheters commonly used are an internal mammary or Cobra. When the iliac bifurcation is at an acute angle, a shepherd crook–shaped catheter like the Simmons-1 or -2 or the SOS-OMNI (Angiodynamics, Inc.) may be used to cannulate the contralateral CIA. Alternatively, the CIA can also be engaged by unfolding a pigtail or Omni Flush catheter using an angled 0.035 in. stiff-angled glide wire (Terumo, BSC, Watertown, MA). Once the tip of the catheter is at the ostium of the contralateral CIA, a glide wire is then advanced gently down the CFA and the catheter exchanged for an angiographic one (pigtail, tennis racquet, or multipurpose), which is placed in the distal CIA. An angulated view (contralateral anterior oblique 30° to 40° with caudal angulation 20°) allows visualization of the

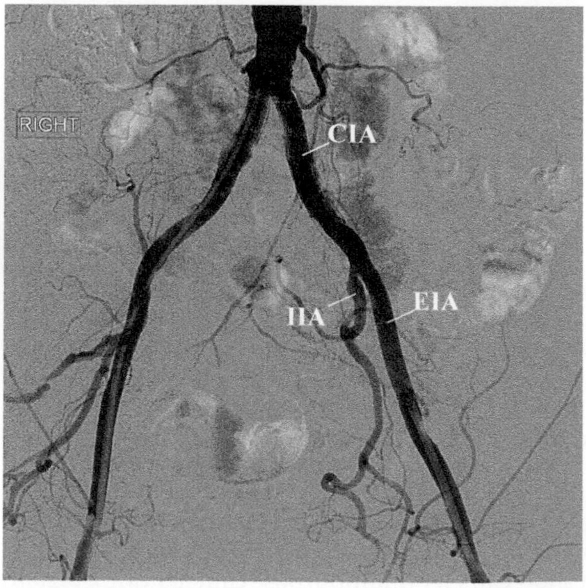

Figure 28.7 Left common iliac artery angiogram. Contralateral anterior oblique with caudal angulation (10°) displays left CIA bifurcation. *Abbreviations*: CIA, common iliac artery; EIA, external iliac artery; IIA, internal iliac artery.

common iliac bifurcation without overlap (Fig. 28.7). Hand or power injection at 10 mL/sec for a total of 10 mL is sufficient for adequate visualization. Pressure gradients across iliac artery stenosis aid in determining the hemodynamic significance of common iliac stenosis. A pressure gradient >15 mm Hg is typically considered significant.

For a more detailed image of a particular arterial segment, the use of sequential stations allows for better resolution and angulated views if stenosis is suspected. The catheters used should be as small as possible, usually 5F to 6F in size, and always advanced over a guidewire to avoid trauma to the vessel. If DSA is used, an image rate of 4 frames/sec is used for above the knee and 2 frames/sec for below the knee.

COMPLICATIONS

Angiography is an established, safe, and effective method to visualize the lower extremity circulation. Nonetheless, complications still occur and vary widely by disease state and vascular bed being treated. The most common complications are related to the access site and the adverse effects of iodinated contrast.

Contrast-induced nephropathy (CIN)

Nephropathy induced by contrast medium remains one of the most clinically important complications of the use of iodinated contrast medium. CIN is the third most common cause of hospital-acquired renal failure. CIN is usually defined as an acute decline in renal function, expressed as a relative increase in serum creatinine concentration of at least 25%, or an absolute increase in serum creatinine of 0.5 mg/dL (44.2 μmol/L) in the absence of other etiologies.[7] Although the risk of renal function impairment in the general population is low (<1%), it is very high in selected patient subsets, estimated at 5.5% of patients with underlying renal insufficiency and up to 50% of patients with both renal insufficiency and diabetes.[8] Recent studies have shown high in-hospital mortality (34%) and poor long-term survival (19% at 2 years) for those patients started on emergency dialysis.[9]

A recently proposed CIN risk stratification score based on eight readily available variables, showed that an increasing score number conferred an exponentially increased CIN risk to the patient.[10,11] The use of intravenous fluids for hydration remains crucial in the prevention of CIN; this approach is simple and carries minimal risks of adverse effects if appropriate care is taken.[12] Most recently, the periprocedural use of sodium bicarbonate infusion has decreased even further the incidence of nephropathy following radiographic contrast administration.[13,14]

Access site

One of the most common complications of both diagnostic and interventional endovascular procedures involves the vascular access site and is an important cause of procedure-related morbidity and mortality.[15] The femoral approach is the most commonly used site of vascular access and is associated with the lowest incidence of complications with rates ranging from 0.1% to 2% for diagnostic and from 0.5% to 5% for interventional procedures. Following transbrachial and transradial catheterization, local vascular complications amount to 1% to 3% after diagnostic and 1% to 5% after interventional procedures.

The most frequently encountered complication following transfemoral catheterization is bleeding and local hematoma followed by pseudoaneurysm formation, which may not be evident for days to even weeks after the procedure. Small-sized pseudoaneurysms (≤2 cm) may be observed and are likely to close spontaneously. Larger aneurysms may be closed with thrombin injection (not FDA approved), ultrasound-guided compression, and surgical repair. Retroperitoneal hemorrhage, although infrequent (0.2% with diagnostic procedures), can be life-threatening with rates increasing with high levels of anticoagulation, such as those used during interventions (~3%).[16] Such bleeding is not evident from the surface, but should be considered whenever a patient develops unexplained hypotension (particularly if it responds only briefly to volume loading), fall in hematocrit, or ipsilateral flank following a femoral catheterization procedure. The best prevention for retroperitoneal bleeding is careful identification of the puncture site to avoid entry of the femoral artery above the inguinal ligament where the arteriotomy site is poorly compressible.[17]

Other less-frequently encountered complications include arterial thrombosis, femoral nerve injury, peripheral embolization, dissection, AV fistula, infection, and venous thrombosis, all of which occur in less than 1% of procedures. Instances of femoral or lateral cutaneous nerve compression from groin hematomas, however, may lead to sensory and motor deficits that may take weeks or even months to resolve.[11]

Risk factors for femoral access complications include female gender, older age, uncontrolled hypertension, high or low body mass index, high level of anticoagulation, prolonged sheath duration, larger arterial sheaths, presence of peripheral vascular disease, and location of the arteriotomy site.[17,18]

As described above, the radial and brachial arteries are also feasible access sites for lower extremity angiography. Because of the smaller size of the brachial artery, arterial thrombosis (~5%) is the most common complication, followed by pseudoaneurysm formation (3–5%). Median nerve injury is infrequently encountered (<1%), mostly due to external compression by a brachial fossa hematoma or direct injury during arterial access. Due to the superficial course of the radial artery, it offers the lowest risk of bleeding complication and has the least classic major complications of any access site. However, it is imperative to have a normal Allen's test, which verifies patency of the ulnar artery and palmar arch before any attempt is made to cannulate this vessel. The traumatic or thrombotic occlusion of this vessel will not endanger the viability of the hand if adequate collateral blood supply from the ulnar artery is present.

By using smaller sized catheters and an adequate anticoagulation regimen, the rate of arterial access site complications may be reduced.

Access site closure devices have been developed for the use in the femoral artery, and although they have been demonstrated to shorten the time to ambulation and improvement of patient comfort, they have not been convincingly demonstrated to reduce major complications.[19] Given the common and troublesome nature of postprocedure vascular complications, all catheterization operators must understand vascular access and closure techniques completely to recognize and treat each type of complication.

KEY POINTS

- The history, clinical examination, and noninvasive imaging allow a targeted approach to peripheral angiography.
- Review noninvasive tests beforehand. It provides critical information of the vasculature to be imaged. This forward planning will help to ensure that the right access site is used and the necessary equipment is at hand for the successful completion of study.
- Adequate intravenous hydration and contrast dosage limitation can reduce the morbidity and mortality associated with contrast-induced nephropathy.
- Use of nonionic, iso-osmolal radiocontrast agents in patients with underlying impaired renal function is indicated.
- Always advance catheters and sheath over a wire.
- For diagnostic angiography, obtain orthogonal views of suspected lesions and identify the view that produces the least foreshortening of the lesion.
- Complete opacification of the runoff vessel is important for planning therapy and predicting success.

REFERENCES

1. Leng GC, Fowkes FG, Lee AJ, et al. Use of ankle brachial pressure index to predict cardiovascular events and death: A cohort study. BMJ 1996; 313(7070):1440–1444.
2. Newman AB, Shemanski L, Manolio TA, et al. Ankle–arm index as a predictor of cardiovascular disease and mortality in the cardiovascular health study. The Cardiovascular Health Study Group. Arterioscler Thromb Vasc Biol 1999; 19(3):538–545.
3. Morin JF, Johnston KW, Wasserman L, et al. Factors that determine the long-term results of percutaneous transluminal dilatation for peripheral arterial occlusive disease. J Vasc Surg 1986; 4(1):68–72.
4. Aspelin P, Aubry P, Fransson SG, et al. Nephrotoxic effects in high-risk patients undergoing angiography. N Engl J Med 2003; 348(6):491–499.
5. Mukherjee D. Diagnostic catheter-based vascular angiography. First ed. Philadelphia: Lippincott Williams & Wilkins, 2005.

6. Hirsch AT, Haskal ZJ, Hertzer NR, et al. ACC/AHA 2005 Practice Guidelines for the management of patients with peripheral arterial disease. Circulation 2006; 113(11):e463–e654.
7. Murphy SW, Barrett BJ, Parfrey PS. Contrast nephropathy. J Am Soc Nephrol 2000; 11(1):177–182.
8. Parfrey PS, Griffiths SM, Barrett BJ, et al. Contrast material-induced renal failure in patients with diabetes mellitus, renal insufficiency, or both. A prospective controlled study. N Engl J Med 1989; 320(3):143–149.
9. Levy EM, Viscoli CM, Horwitz RI. The effect of acute renal failure on mortality. A cohort analysis. JAMA 1996; 275(19):1489–1494.
10. Mehran R, Aymong ED, Nikolsky E, et al. A simple risk score for prediction of contrast-induced nephropathy after percutaneous coronary intervention: Development and initial validation. J Am Coll Cardiol 2004; 44(7):1393–1399.
11. Butler R, Webster MW. Meralgia paresthetica: An unusual complication of cardiac catheterization via the femoral artery. Catheter Cardiovasc Interv 2002; 56(1):69–71.
12. Stacul F, Adam A, Becker CR, et al. Strategies to reduce the risk of contrast-induced nephropathy. Am J Cardiol 2006; 98(6A):59K–77K.
13. Merten GJ, Burgess WP, Gray LV, et al. Prevention of contrast-induced nephropathy with sodium bicarbonate: A randomized controlled trial. JAMA 2004; 291(19):2328–2334.
14. Masuda M, Yamada T, Mine T, et al. Comparison of usefulness of sodium bicarbonate versus sodium chloride to prevent contrast-induced nephropathy in patients undergoing an emergent coronary procedure. Am J Cardiol 2007; 100(5):781–786.
15. Chandrasekar B, Doucet S, Bilodeau L, et al. Complications of cardiac catheterization in the current era: A single-center experience. Catheter Cardiovasc Interv 2001; 52(3):289–295.
16. Kent KC, Moscucci M, Mansour KA, et al. Retroperitoneal hematoma after cardiac catheterization: Prevalence, risk factors, and optimal management. J Vasc Surg 1994; 20(6):905–910; discussion 10–13.
17. Sherev DA, Shaw RE, Brent BN. Angiographic predictors of femoral access site complications: Implication for planned percutaneous coronary intervention. Catheter Cardiovasc Interv 2005; 65(2):196–202.
18. Waksman R, King SB III, Douglas JS, et al. Predictors of groin complications after balloon and new-device coronary intervention. Am J Cardiol 1995; 75(14):886–889.
19. Nikolsky E, Mehran R, Halkin A, et al. Vascular complications associated with arteriotomy closure devices in patients undergoing percutaneous coronary procedures: A meta-analysis. J Am Coll Cardiol 2004; 44(6):1200–1209.

Index

Printed and bound by CPI Group (UK) Ltd, Croydon, CR0 4YY
18/10/2024
01776249-0008